OBSTETRICS AND GYNECOLOGY FOR MEDICAL STUDENTS

CHARLES R. B. BECKMANN, M.D., M.H.P.E.
Professor of Obstetrics and Gynecology and Associate Residency Director
Department of Obstetrics and Gynecology
University of Wisconsin at Milwaukee
Director of Ambulatory Care
Sinai Samaritan Medical Center West
Milwaukee, Wisconsin

FRANK W. LING, M.D.
Associate Professor, Division of Gynecology
Director, Residency Training Program
Department of Obstetrics and Gynecology
University of Tennessee
Memphis, Tennessee

BARBARA M. BARZANSKY, Ph.D., M.H.P.E.
Associate Director, Division of Undergraduate Medical Education
The American Medical Association
Chicago, Illinois

G. WILLIAM BATES, M.D.
Professor of Obstetrics and Gynecology
University of South Carolina
Vice President, Medical Education
Greenville Hospital System
Greenville, South Carolina

WILLIAM N. P. HERBERT, M.D.
Professor and Director
Division of Maternal and Fetal Medicine
Department of Obstetrics and Gynecology
Duke University School of Medicine
Durham, North Carolina

DOUGLAS W. LAUBE, M.D, M.Ed.
Professor and Chairman
Department of Obstetrics and Gynecology
University of Wisconsin Medical School
Madison, Wisconsin

ROGER P. SMITH, M.D.
Professor and Director, General Obstetrics and Gynecology
Department of Obstetrics and Gynecology
Medical College of Georgia
Augusta, Georgia

OBSTETRICS AND GYNECOLOGY
FOR MEDICAL STUDENTS

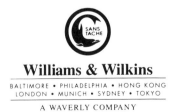

Williams & Wilkins

BALTIMORE • PHILADELPHIA • HONG KONG
LONDON • MUNICH • SYDNEY • TOKYO

A WAVERLY COMPANY

Editor: Timothy S. Satterfield
Managing Editor: Linda Napora
Copy Editor: Klemie Bryte
Designer: Dan Pfisterer
Illustration Planner: Ray Lowman
Production Coordinator: Charles E. Zeller

Accurate indications, adverse reactions, and dosage schedules for drugs are provided in this book, but it is possible that they may change. The reader is urged to review the package information data of the manufacturers of the medications mentioned.

Printed in the United States of America

Library of Congress Cataloging-in-Publication Data

Obstetrics and gynecology for medical students / editors, Charles R.B. Beckmann, Frank
    W. Ling; education editor, Barbara M. Barzansky; associate editors, G. William Bates
    . . . [et al.]. — 1st ed.
       p.   cm.
    Includes index.
    ISBN 0-683-0500-6
    1. Gynecology.   2. Obstetrics.   I. Beckmann, Charles R. B.
II. Ling, Frank W.
    [DNLM: 1. Genital Diseases, Female.   2. Labor.   3. Pregnancy.
WP 140 014]
RG101.024   1992
618—dc20
DNLM/DLC
for Library of Congress   92-5111
                                                CIP

94 95 96
3 4 5 6 7 8 9 10

FOREWORD

Most of us who teach obstetrics and gynecology are aware that the comprehensive standard textbooks in our field often fail to meet the unique needs of medical students engaged in their clerkships. *Obstetrics and Gynecology for Medical Students* offers a new approach to the subject and fulfills the critical need for a text for *all* medical students, not just those interested in our specialty.

The authors all teach in our specialty, and each has enjoyed a long career and taken an active interest in medical education. Their book, unlike others in the field, includes objectives and self-evaluation materials that make it a most useful learning tool. It is complete and well organized, striking a balance between detailed books for the specialist and outline books used for review. Although directed to medical students, the book's special approach will also make it suitable as a resource for residents and practitioners.

The authors are to be congratulated on their concept for this new approach to learning and on their success in achieving their objectives. I recommend it without reservation and predict it will become the standard text for all obstetric-gynecologic clerkships.

MARTIN L. STONE, M.D.
PROFESSOR EMERITUS
SUNY STONY BROOK, NEW YORK

PREFACE

Obstetrics and Gynecology for Medical Students is written *specifically for medical students taking their clerkship in obstetrics and gynecology.* The goal of the book is to provide the basic information about obstetrics and gynecology that all medical school graduates should possess, that is, *the information needed to successfully complete an obstetrics and gynecology clerkship and pass national standardized examinations in this content area.*

Obstetrics and Gynecology for Medical Students is *unique* in two important ways:

1. This textbook was *written by seven professional medical educators. Six are experienced obstetrician-gynecologists who have expertise and interest in education*, including additional degrees in education, experience as clerkship directors, and involvement in the preparation of national standardized examinations. *The seventh author is a professional educator and anatomist* with extensive experience in curriculum development and evaluation. With the exception of special sections and one chapter that were written by four contributors, the entire book was written, reviewed, and revised by these seven individuals.

2. This textbook was *designed to facilitate student learning and self-evaluation.* To do this, the book is based on the Instructional Objectives for a Clinical Curriculum in Obstetrics and Gynecology of the Association of Professors of Gynecology and Obstetrics, sixth edition. These national standards are used to organize most OB-GYN clerkships in the United States and Canada, and they are used as a guideline in the development of national standardized examinations. *A summary of these objectives is provided* in the book as well as a comprehensive *Objectives Index* that will facilitate access to the objectives. This *APGO Objectives Index* will provide students with a fast method of studying a particular topic across all the chapters of the book. In addition, at the end of each chapter there is a *Self-Evaluation* section so that students may gauge their progress and focus their efforts with maximum efficiency. The use of these special facets of the book is discussed in the introductory section, "How to Use This Book."

Medical school textbooks often contain large amounts of information more useful to residents and practicing physicians than to medical students. In contrast, *Obstetrics and Gynecology for Medical Students* focuses specifically on the needs of medical students during the six- to eight-week OB-GYN clerkship and has been written by professional educators according to sound educational principles to accomplish this goal. The concise and easy-to-read chapters, correlated with national learning objectives, and the self-evaluation sections for measuring progress fulfill our intention: to provide the basic information about obstetrics and gynecology required by all medical school graduates.

ACKNOWLEDGMENTS

We extend our appreciation to Tim Satterfield, Linda Napora, Chuck Zeller, Dan Pfisterer, Ray Lowman, and Klemie Bryte and all the staff at Williams & Wilkins for their seemingly tireless help and encouragement during the arduous preparation of *Obstetrics and Gynecology for Medical Students*. Likewise, we appreciate the innovative educational art provided by Joyce Lavery, which adds so much to the usefulness of the book. We also extend thanks to Ruthe Bady for her coordination of the manuscript chapters and figures and to our secretaries for their good-spirited efforts as we produced revision after revision of each chapter. Finally, we extend a special thanks to Carol-Lynn Brown, our first editor at Williams & Wilkins, for her foresight and support in the early development of this book.

CONTRIBUTORS

BARBARA F. SHARF, Ph.D.
Head, Medical Humanities Program
Associate Professor of Health Communication and Medical Education
Department of Medical Education
University of Illinois College of Medicine
Chicago, Illinois
   Contributor, Chapter 1, "Patient Evaluation and Management"

DANIEL L. CLARKE-PEARSON, M.D.
Professor and Director, Division of Gynecologic Oncology
Department of Obstetrics and Gynecology
Duke Medical Center
Durham, North Carolina
   Contributor, Chapter 1, "Patient Evaluation and Management"

LEE P. SHULMAN, M.D.
Assistant Professor of Obstetrics and Gynecology
Division of Reproductive Genetics
Department of Obstetrics and Gynecology
University of Tennessee
Memphis, Tennessee
   Contributor, Reproductive Genetics in Chapter 3, "Embryology and
   Anatomy of the Female Reproductive System"

JOANNA M. CAIN, M.D.
Associate Professor of Obstetrics and Gynecology
Division of Gynecologic Oncology
University of Washington
Seattle, Washington
   Author, Chapter 47, "Ethics in Obstetrics and Gynecology"

HOW TO USE THIS BOOK

Obstetrics and Gynecology for Medical Students is specifically written to help the medical student learn the basics of obstetrics-gynecology. It is useful in studying during the clerkship and in reviewing for standardized national examinations. The following suggestions will make the use of the book most efficient.

Indexes

There are *two indexes* in this book. The first is a traditional *Subject Index* giving the page references for specific topics. The second is an *APGO Objectives Index* based on the sixth edition of the objectives of the Association of Professors of Gynecology and Obstetrics (APGO). Each APGO objective has been condensed, and the pages where content relating to that objective can be found are listed. It would be useful for you to review these objectives at the start of the clerkship to get an idea of the basic content that you will be expected to master during the clerkship.

To Study a Topic for the First Time

Each chapter covers a general topic and most of the chapters are directly related to one of the APGO objectives. Locate the appropriate objective summary and read it carefully. Then read the chapter and attempt to answer the study questions at the end. The multiple choice questions are to help you assess whether you have learned the chapter's main points. If you answer one or more questions incorrectly, go back and reread the relevant portion of the chapter. The "questions for further consideration" are to help you summarize and synthesize the information. They also can be used during review.

Many chapters contain references to content contained in other parts of the book. Sometimes this information is required in order for you to understand the topic that you are studying. In this case, you should read these additional pages. For example, terms in the book are defined only once in any detail. You will need to find the definition of important terms related to the topic and learn these. To ensure that you have read all the information about a topic, consult both the Subject Index and the *APGO Objectives Index* and read the cited pages.

After you have studied a chapter and completed the study questions, go back and reread the APGO objective. Make sure that you know the information asked for in the objective.

To Review for Examinations after the Clerkship

Begin by attempting to answer the study questions again. If you answer the questions correctly, you should briefly reread the chapter to stimulate your memory. If you cannot answer the study questions, read the chapter carefully, along with related content that is contained elsewhere in the book.

APGO OBJECTIVES (condensed)

The following is a condensation of the "Instructional Objectives for a Clinical Curriculum in Obstetrics and Gynecology" (Sixth Edition) of the Association of Professors of Gynecology and Obstetrics (APGO). The numbers correspond to the numbers of the APGO objectives.

The student should be able to:

Unit 1 : Approach to the Patient

1. HISTORY
   Take a thorough obstetric-gynecologic history, utilizing appropriate communication skills, and transmit the results in written and oral form.
2. PHYSICAL EXAMINATION
   a. Perform a thorough obstetric-gynecologic examination (breasts, abdomen, pelvis), utilizing appropriate communication skills, and transmit the results in written and oral form.
   b. Explain breast self-examination to the patient.
3. PAP SMEAR AND CULTURES
   Obtain and properly handle specimens for a Pap smear and microbiologic cultures to detect sexually transmitted diseases and explain the purpose of these tests to the patient.
4. DIAGNOSIS AND MANAGEMENT PLAN
   Based on the results of the patient history and physical examination, generate a problem list, identify likely diagnoses, and develop a management plan (laboratory and diagnostic studies, patient education, plans for continuing care and treatment).

Unit 2 : Obstetrics

SECTION A : NORMAL OBSTETRICS

5. MATERNAL-FETAL PHYSIOLOGY
   Explain the maternal physiologic changes associated with pregnancy and the physiology of the placenta and fetus.
6. ANTEPARTUM CARE
   a. Explain the initial and ongoing elements of antepartum care, including methods to diagnose pregnancy and establish gestational age; determination of obstetric risk status; techniques to assess fetal growth, maturity, and well-being; and appropriate diagnostic studies.

b. Perform a physical examination on an obstetric patient, and develop a problem list and management plan based on the initial assessment and ongoing evaluation.

c. Answer commonly asked questions concerning pregnancy, labor, and delivery.

7. INTRAPARTUM CARE

Describe the stages and mechanisms of labor, including the differences between false and true labor; the initial and ongoing assessment of the fetus and the laboring patient; the management of normal labor and delivery, including the indications for operative delivery; and the immediate postpartum care of the mother.

8. IMMEDIATE CARE OF THE NEWBORN

Explain the assessment and immediate postpartum care of the newborn, including situations requiring immediate intervention.

9. POSTPARTUM CARE

Explain normal postpartum care and the appropriate counseling of the postpartum patient. Explain the normal physiologic changes in the postpartum period.

SECTION B : ABNORMAL OBSTETRICS

10. ECTOPIC PREGNANCY

Describe the diagnosis and management of ectopic pregnancy, including risk factors, symptoms/physical findings, diagnostic procedures and treatment options.

11. SPONTANEOUS ABORTION

Explain the diagnosis and management of the causes of first trimester bleeding, including incomplete, threatened, and missed abortion, as well as the potential complications of spontaneous abortion.

12. MEDICAL AND SURGICAL CONDITIONS IN PREGNANCY

Describe the diagnosis and management of the common medical and surgical complications in the pregnant patient, including their effects on the pregnancy and the effects of pregnancy on the condition, including: anemia, diabetes, urinary tract disease, infectious disease (herpes, rubella, streptococcus, hepatitis B, HIV), cardiac disease, asthma, substance abuse, and acute abdominal symptoms.

13. PREGNANCY-INDUCED HYPERTENSION

Define pregnancy-induced hypertension and describe the pathophysiology, diagnosis, management, and potential maternal and fetal complications of this condition.

14. RH ISOIMMUNIZATION

Describe the circumstances leading to Rh isoimmunization and the techniques utilized to determine its presence in the mother, the methods used to assess the severity of disease in the fetus and newborn, and the appropriate use of immunoglobulin prophylaxis.

15. MULTIPLE GESTATION

Describe the mechanism of twinning and the altered physiology associated with multiple gestation. Describe the diagnosis and the antepartum, intrapartum, and postpartum management of multiple gestation.

16. FETAL DEATH

Describe the diagnosis and management of fetal death, including methods to determine the cause, the potential maternal complications (including disseminated intravascular coagulation), and the emotional consequences.

17. ABNORMAL LABOR

a. Describe the causes, labor patterns, evaluation, and management of abnormal labor, fetopelvic disproportion, and abnormal fetal presentations.

b. Describe the indications and contraindications for oxytocin administration and vaginal birth after cesarean section.

c. Describe the maternal and fetal complications resulting from abnormal labor.

18. THIRD TRIMESTER BLEEDING

Describe the approach to the patient with third trimester bleeding, including the methods to differentiate among the causes (such as placenta previa and abruptio placentae), the maternal and fetal complications, and the management of shock secondary to bleeding.

19. PRETERM LABOR

Describe the predisposing factors and causes of preterm labor and the approach to the patient with premature contractions, including the principles of tocolysis.

20. PREMATURE RUPTURE OF MEMBRANES

Describe the diagnosis and management of premature rupture of the membranes, including the indications for expectant management versus immediate delivery and the methods used to monitor maternal and fetal status during expectant management.

21. INTRAPARTUM FETAL DISTRESS

Explain the techniques for intrapartum electronic and biochemical fetal monitoring. Describe normal and abnormal fetal heart rate patterns and the approach to management when there is an abnormal fetal heart rate.

22. POSTPARTUM HEMORRHAGE

Describe the likely causes and predisposing factors of postpartum hemorrhage and the approach to its diagnosis and management.

23. POSTPARTUM INFECTION

Describe the risk factors associated with postpartum infection, the possible causes and the means to distinguish among them, and the approach to the management of a patient with fever and presumed postpartum infection.

24. ANXIETY AND DEPRESSION

Describe the factors commonly associated with anxiety and depression in normal and high risk pregnancy and the symptoms commonly exhibited by patients.

25. MORTALITY

Define, supply the common causes of, and describe the formula for calculating the rate of maternal death, fetal death, neonatal death, and perinatal death.

26. POSTDATES PREGNANCY

Define and describe postdates pregnancy and its associated risks and complications, and explain the methods used in antepartum monitoring of the fetus.

27. FETAL GROWTH ABNORMALITIES

Define macrosomia and intrauterine growth retardation, and for each describe the associated risk factors, recognized causes, methods used in diagnosis and management, and associated maternal and fetal morbidities.

SECTION C : PROCEDURES

28. OBSTETRICAL PROCEDURES

a. Define, supply the indications and contraindications for, and list the risks of the following procedures: ultrasonography, episiotomy, cesarean delivery, forceps delivery, induction of labor, vacuum-assisted delivery, antepartum fetal assessment, amniocentesis, chorionic villus sampling, and newborn circumcision.

b. Explain each of the above procedures in language understandable to the patient.

Unit 3 : Gynecology

SECTION A : GYNECOLOGY

29. CONTRACEPTION

Describe the mechanism of action, degree of effectiveness, advantages and disadvantages, contraindications, and potential complications for each commonly utilized method of contraception.

30. STERILIZATION

Describe the advantages and disadvantages, contraindications, and potential complications for each commonly used method of male and female sterilization.

31. VULVITIS AND VAGINITIS

Describe the physiologic or infectious causes, history/physical findings, methods of diagnosis and management of vaginitis, vulvitis, and Bartholin's gland disease.

32. SEXUALLY TRANSMITTED DISEASES

Describe the causative agent, method of transmission, symptoms/physical findings, and methods of diagnosis/screening and management for gonorrhea, chlamydia, herpes, syphilis, condyloma acuminatum (HPV) and HIV infection.

33. SALPINGITIS

Describe the anatomical location, causes, symptoms/physical findings, methods of diagnosis, and possible sequelae of acute and chronic salpingitis.

34. PELVIC RELAXATION

Explain the types of pelvic relaxation and describe their signs/symptoms and managment.

35. ENDOMETRIOSIS

Describe the theories of pathogenesis and anatomic sites affected by endometriosis, as well as its signs and symptoms, method of diagnosis and treatment, and chronic sequelae including pelvic pain, infertility, and menstrual dysfunction.

36. ADENOMYOSIS

Explain the differences between endometriosis and adenomyosis. Describe the history/physical findings characteristic of adenomyosis and the methods used in diagnosis.

SECTION B : BREASTS

37. DISORDERS OF THE BREAST

a. Describe the indications for and timing of breast self-examination, physical examination of the breast, and mammography.

b. Describe the diagnostic approach to a woman with a breast mass, nipple discharge, or breast pain.

c. Explain the history/physical findings associated with intraductal papilloma, fibrocystic changes in the breast, fibroadenoma, and breast carcinoma.

SECTION C : PROCEDURES

38. GYNECOLOGIC PROCEDURES

a. Define and describe the indications and contraindications for and the risks of the following gynecologic procedures: dilation and curettage, colposcopy and cervical biopsy, endometrial biopsy, cone biopsy, culdocentesis, hysterosalpingography, laparoscopy, hysterectomy, pregnancy termination, hysteroscopy, laser vaporization, vulvar biopsy, cryotherapy, mammography, and needle aspiration of the breast.

b. Explain each of the above procedures in language understandable to the patient.

Unit 4 : Reproductive Endocrinology, Infertility, and Related Topics

39. PUBERTY

a. Describe the physiologic and psychologic events associated with normal puberty and the approximate ages at which these occur.

b. Explain the causes, characteristics, diagnostic approach to, and counseling issues about abnormal puberty.

c. Define true precocious puberty, pseudoprecocious puberty, and delayed puberty.

40. AMENORRHEA
    a. Define primary amenorrhea, secondary amenorrhea, and oligomenorrhea.
    b. Describe the physical, endocrinologic, and psychologic causes of amenorrhea and the diagnostic approach to the patient with this problem.

41. HIRSUTISM AND VIRILIZATION
    a. Define hirsutism, defeminization, and virilization.
    b. Describe the causes of hirsutism and virilization and the diagnostic approach to the patient with this problem.

42. ABNORMAL UTERINE BLEEDING
    a. Define abnormal uterine bleeding and dysfunctional uterine bleeding.
    b. Describe the causes of abnormal uterine bleeding and the diagnostic approach to the patient with this problem.

43. DYSMENORRHEA
    Define primary and secondary dysmenorrhea and describe the causes and approach to the evaluation and management of each.

44. MENOPAUSE
    a. Describe the physiologic changes in the hypothalamic-pituitary-ovarian axis related to menopause and the associated physical, emotional, and sexual symptoms/physical findings.
    b. Describe the indications, contraindications, and method of hormone replacement therapy.

45. INFERTILITY
    a. Define infertility.
    b. Describe the causes of infertility and the diagnostic methods used to evaluate the presence of each.

46. PREMENSTRUAL SYNDROME
    a. Describe the premenstrual syndrome and its possible causes.
    b. Describe the diagnostic and therapeutic options for symptomatic patients with premenstrual syndrome.

Unit 5 : Neoplasia

47. GESTATIONAL TROPHOBLASTIC DISEASE
    a. List symptoms/physical findings commonly found in patients with gestational trophoblastic disease.
    b. Describe the diagnostic methods used to confirm this condition, and the management and follow-up of patients.

48. VULVAR NEOPLASMS
    a. Define the risk factors for vulvar neoplasia.
    b. Describe the diagnostic approach to the patient with vulvar symptoms.

49. CERVICAL DISEASE AND NEOPLASIA
    a. Describe the risk factors, symptoms, and physical findings characteristic of cervicitis and cervical neoplasia.
    b. Describe the management of a patient with an abnormal Pap smear.
    c. Explain the common course of cervical neoplastic disease, including the histologic categories of cervical neoplasia.

50. UTERINE MYOMA
    Describe the symptoms/physical findings characteristic of uterine myoma; the diagnostic methods employed to confirm the condition; and the management options, including indications for surgical intervention.

51. ENDOMETRIAL CARCINOMA
    a. Describe the approach to the patient with postmenopausal bleeding.
    b. Describe the risk factors and the symptoms/physical findings characteristic of endometrial carcinoma, the methods used in diagnosis and staging of the disease, and the typical disease course.

52. OVARIAN NEOPLASMS
    a. Describe how specific factors (such as patient age, characteristics of the mass) affect the approach to the patient with an adnexal mass.
    b. Describe the symptoms/physical findings, methods used in diagnosis and staging, and histologic systems used for classification of functional and benign ovarian neoplasia and ovarian carcinoma.

Unit 6 : Human Sexuality

53. SEXUALITY
    a. Explain the phases of the female sexual response and the physiologic basis of each.
    b. Describe the influences on sexuality at various stages in the female life cycle.
    c. List and answer commonly asked questions about sexual function.
    d. Describe common examples of sexual dysfunction and their preliminary assessment and identify those problems that require referral.

54. ALTERNATIVE MODES OF SEXUAL EXPRESSION
    Define heterosexual, homosexual, bisexual, transsexual, and transvestite.

55. PHYSICIAN SEXUALITY
    a. Demonstrate empathetic and nonjudgmental behaviors in interactions with patients.
    b. Demonstrate awareness of the influence of the physician's own sexuality on his/her interactions with patients.
    c. Describe the behavioral patterns of seductive patients.

56. SEXUAL ASSAULT
    a. Define the rape trauma syndrome.
    b. Describe the management of suspected cases of sexual assault in children and adults.

Unit 7 : Professional Behavior / Ethics / Law

57. PERSONAL INTERACTION AND COMMUNICATION SKILLS
    a. Establish rapport and work dependably with patients.
    b. Work cooperatively and dependably with other members of the health care team.
    c. Recognize personal limitations.
58. LAW IN OBSTETRICS AND GYNECOLOGY
    a. Demonstrate a knowledge of the elements of informed consent: right to refuse care, outcomes, options, capacity to choose, surrogate decision makers.
    b. Describe the following legal obligations to protect patient interests: advance directives for health care, confidentiality, abandonment, contractual nature of medical benefits, fraud.
59. ETHICS IN OBSTETRICS AND GYNECOLOGY
    a. Describe approaches to the definition of ethical problems and the bases of ethical conflict in maternal/fetal medicine.
    b. Describe how the concept of justice applies to access to care in obstetrics and gynecology.
    c. Describe the ethical issues raised by termination of pregnancy and reproductive technology.

Unit 8 : Preventive Care and Health Maintenance

60. PREVENTIVE CARE
    a. Describe the indications for and appropriate intervals between the following screening procedures that are part of routine health surveillance: Papanicolaou smear, mammograms, blood pressure monitoring, blood lipid profiles.
    b. Describe the appropriate patient education associated with the following: contraception, STD prevention, diet, exercise, stress management, smoking, immunization.
    c. Describe the cost/benefit of routine health surveillance.

CONTENTS

chapter 1

PATIENT EVALUATION AND MANAGEMENT

During the initial evaluation, the physician and patient should establish a *professional relationship of mutual trust and respect.* The physician gathers the historical and physical information needed for the patient's care, makes differential and presumptive diagnoses, and formulates a management plan. At the same time, the patient usually decides if the physician is knowledgeable and trustworthy and whether she will accept and follow the regimens recommended. The process begins with an appropriate *greeting*, which deserves special attention because of the importance of initial impressions. A handshake is commonly used. Surnames should generally be used. First names are more appropriate for friendship relationships, whereas the patient-physician relationship, while friendly, is professional. "What brought you to the office today?" or "How may I help you today?" are neutral opening statements that allow the patient to frame a response that includes her problems, concerns, and/or reasons for the visit.

Attentive, thoughtful listening is essential for accurate patient evaluation. Many issues are quite personal, potentially eliciting negative reactions. In selected cases, such responses can be minimized by an explanatory preamble such as: "I must ask some questions that are quite personal. I am not doing so to pry into your private life, nor do the questions imply anything about you. I am trying to get all the information I can to provide you with the best health care. So, . . ." followed by the question. Such a preamble is not needed in all cases, but should be considered when the

clinician suspects that a negative response may ensue. When faced with a negative, perhaps hostile, response, such a comment may help the physician resolve the conflict and reestablish a positive interaction. Ignoring such a negative response usually dooms the professional relationship. Further, such a response may be the first indication of an unstated problem that requires evaluation and management.

HISTORY
Chief Complaint

The chief complaint is the reason for the patient's visit. This may be expressed and recorded as a quote or as a paraphrased statement, although care must be taken in the latter case to avoid obscuring the patient's true meaning with medical jargon. Establishing the *chronology* of a problem carefully is important because chronological organization of symptoms may suggest a specific disorder.

Menstrual History

Menstrual history begins with *menarche*, the age at which menses began. The *basic menstrual history* should then include the duration of bleeding, the interval between menstrual periods, the frequency of menses, and the *last menstrual period (LMP)*, dated from the first day of the last normal period. Episodes of bleeding that are "light but on time" should be noted as such, as they may have diagnostic significance. Estimation of the *amount of menstrual flow* can be made by asking whether the patient uses pads or tampons, how many are used during the heavy days of her flow, and whether they are soaked or just soiled when they are changed. It is normal for women to pass *clots* during menstruation, but not larger than dime size. Asking the size of clots relative to coins is useful because it provides patient and clinician with a standard reference. Specific inquiry should be made about *irregular* or *intermenstrual bleeding or spotting* and *contact bleeding (postcoital or postdouching bleeding or spotting)*. Such abnormal bleeding must be correlated with information about contraceptive method, infections, concurrent gynecologic problems, and sexual practices. The menstrual history also includes *perimenstrual symptoms* (molimina) such as anxiety, fluid retention, nervousness, mood fluctuations, food craving, variations in sexual feelings, and difficulty sleeping. Any medications used during this time should be noted. *Crampy pain* during the menses is common. It is abnormal when it interferes with daily activities or when it requires more analgesia than provided by plain aspirin or acetaminophen. Inquiry about duration, quality, radiation of the pain to areas outside the pelvis, and association with body position or daily activities completes the pain history.

For older women, the menstrual history will end, as do the menses themselves, with the *climacteric*. The climacteric history begins for most women with increasing menstrual irregularity and varying or decreased flow, associated with hot flashes, nervousness, mood changes, and decreased vaginal lubrication. The physician should ask the patient whether she has had or is undergoing hormonal therapy (estrogen replacement with or without progestin and/or other hormonal treatment) as well as other medical treatment such as psychoactive medications. A history of medical (radiation or chemotherapy) or surgical oophorectomy should be taken. *Postmenopausal bleeding* is abnormal and usually defined as bleeding 6 months after cessation of menses. It is an important historical fact that should be documented or stated as a pertinent negative because of its association with genital malignancy, especially endometrial carcinoma.

Obstetric-Gynecologic History

Obstetric history includes the number of pregnancies (gravidity) and outcomes of each (parity). The following abbreviation may be used:

Gravida (G) *a* Para (P) *b c d e*
where:
a Number of pregnancies
b Number of term pregnancies ($\geq$37 weeks)
c Number of preterm pregnancies (viability through 36 weeks)
d Number of abortions (spontaneous or induced) and ectopic pregnancies
e Number of living children

Specific information about each item should be included. For term and preterm deliveries, determine the outcome, any complications, and mode of delivery. For abortions and ectopic pregnancies, determine any known causes, medical therapy and/or surgical procedure(s) done, complications, and feelings about events.

The *gynecologic history* includes information about any *gynecologic disease and/or treatment* the patient has had, including the diagnosis or as much as the patient can remember about her illness, the medical and/or surgical treatment, and the results. Questions about *previous gynecologic surgery* should include what surgery, reason for the surgery, when and where and by whom the surgery was performed, the results as the patient understands them and whether they agree with her expectations for the surgery, and the emotional and physical effects of the surgery.

Information about *sexually transmitted and infectious disease* should be obtained. Information about *vaginitis* should include frequency, duration, treatment, and effect of treatment. *Vaginal discharge* should be characterized by color, odor, consistency, quantity, association with rectal or urethral discharge, associated symptoms such as pain or pruritus, relationship to medication such as antibiotics and exogenous steroids, and to exacerbations of diseases such as diabetes. *Localized lesions or ulcerations* should be characterized by date of recognition, location, growth, associated symptoms (pain, pruritus, bleeding, discharge), similar nonperineal lesions, treatment, and results of treatment. *Pelvic inflammatory disease* (PID) is a frequently encountered history. PID is classically characterized by fever, chills, abdominopelvic pain, and an appropriate response to oral or parenteral antibiotic therapy. PID is often confused with vaginitis, which may be differentiated by the different history of vaginal discharge, characterized by local symptoms such as pruritus or irritation and treatment with topical medications. The patient should be asked specifically about a history of sexually transmitted disease such as gonorrhea, herpes, chlamydia, warts (condyloma), and syphilis, as well as the use of intrauterine devices (IUDs) since these have been associated with PID. Finally, patients should be asked about behaviors that are "high risk" for the acquisition of the *HIV virus*, including parenteral drug use, sexual relationships with drug users or bisexuals, transfusion before approximately 1980, or prostitution or promiscuity.

A history about *breast disease and breast cancer* should include previous known breast disease or cancer, previous breast biopsy, previous mammography or other imaging study, family history of breast cancer, or appreciation by the patient of a mass, discharge, or painful area. Correlation with the patient's age, menstrual status, and hormonal therapy should be made.

Some couples will have a history of *infertility*, which involves questions concerning partners, including previous diseases or surgery that may affect fertility, previous fertility (previous children with the same or other partners), duration of time that pregnancy has been attempted, and a history of sexual practices.

Finally, *diethylstilbestrol (DES)* use by the patient's mother during her pregnancy should be noted, since it may be associated with infertility problems and/or vaginal carcinoma in the daughter. A *personal hygiene*

history should address the use of douching and vaginal "feminine sprays," deodorants, or self-medications. A history of gastrointestinal and urinary disorders completes the gynecologic history.

Sexual and Contraceptive History

Taking a *sexual history* will be facilitated by behaviors, attitudes, and direct statements by the physician that project a nonjudgmental manner of acceptance and respect for the patient's life style. The initial questions are often the most difficult. A good opening question is: "Please tell me about your sexual partner or partners." This question is gender neutral, leaves the issue of number of partners open, and also gives the patient considerable latitude for response. In the final analysis, however, these questions must be individualized to each patient. If faced with an untoward emotional response, the physician should address the situation directly, assuring the patient that no disrespect or judgment was meant or implied and that the goal is solely to provide good care. Data to be elicited should include age at first intercourse, the patient's present sexual partner(s) and their sex, types of sexual practices, and the patient's level of satisfaction with her sex life. A chronological history is also useful, especially focusing on changes in the patient's life style. Finally, comment needs to be made about the possibility of child and adult *sexual abuse and assault* in the patient's past or present.

A patient's *contraceptive history* should include the contraceptive method currently used, when begun, any problems or complications, and the patient's and her partner's satisfaction with the method. Previous contraceptive methods should also be noted, with the reasons they were discontinued. The history concludes with inquiry about the patient's future conceptive or contraceptive plans.

PHYSICAL EXAMINATION

Preparation for the pelvic examination begins with the patient emptying her bladder and donning an examination gown. An *assistant*

Table 1.1
The OB-GYN History and Physical
Examination: Generalized Report Format

History
  Chief complaint
  Menstrual history
    Menarche
    Menstrual history
      Normal menses
      Menstrual flow
      Abnormal menses
      Pain
    Climacteric
      Peri- and postmenopausal history
      Postmenopausal bleeding
  Obstetric history: gravidity and parity
  Gynecologic history
    Gynecologic diseases and treatment, including
      surgery and medical treatment
    Sexually transmitted diseases and pelvic
      inflammatory disease
      Vaginitis, vulvitis
      Local lesions
      Pelvic inflammatory disease
    Breast disease
    Infertility
    DES
    Personal hygiene
    Gastrointestinal (GI) and genitourinary (GU)
      review of systems
  Sexual and contraceptive history
    Sexual history
      Present and past sexual history
      Sexual assault and abuse
    Contraceptive history
      Present contraception
      Past contraception
      Conception plans
Physical Examination
  Height, weight, and blood pressure
  Breast examination
  Examination of the abdomen, back, and
    lymphatics
  Pelvic examination
    Vulva
    Clitoris
    BUS (Bartholin's, urethra, Skene's glands)
    Vagina
    Cervix
    Uterus
    Adnexa
    Rectovaginal examination (guaiac
      determination, if needed)

should usually be present for the pelvic examination to assist in the preparation of spec-

imens and act as a chaperone. It is important to *thoroughly explain everything that is going to happen to a patient before it happens.* The cardinal rule is *"TALK BEFORE YOU TOUCH,"* as an unexpected touch is disconcerting. Gentle, deliberate movements will allow the patient to remain relaxed. If any maneuvers require deep palpation or may cause discomfort, the patient should be told what to expect before they are done.

Abdominal and especially pelvic examination require *relaxation of the muscles.* An abrupt or stern command, such as "Relax now; I'm not going to hurt you," may raise the patient's fears, whereas the phrase "Try to relax as much as you can, although I know that that is a lot easier for me to say than for you to do" sends two messages: (1) that the patient needs to relax and (2) that you recognize that it is difficult, both of which demonstrate patience and understanding. The phrase "Let me know if anything is uncomfortable, and I will stop and then we will try to do it differently" tells the patient that there might be discomfort but that she has control and can stop the examination if discomfort occurs. Few positions leave a woman with such a feeling of helplessness as the lithotomy position; returning a degree of control to her is most helpful. The term "we" also demonstrates that the examination is a cooperative effort. Techniques that help the patient to relax include encouraging the patient to breathe in and out gently and regularly rather than holding her breath and helping the patient to identify specific muscle groups (such as the abdominal muscle groups or the perineal muscle groups) that need to be relaxed.

Table 1.1 presents a useful *format for the oral and written report.*

Breast Examination

The breast examination by a physician remains the most cost-effective and reliable means of early detection of breast cancer when combined with appropriately scheduled mammography. It should be combined with patient education, includ-

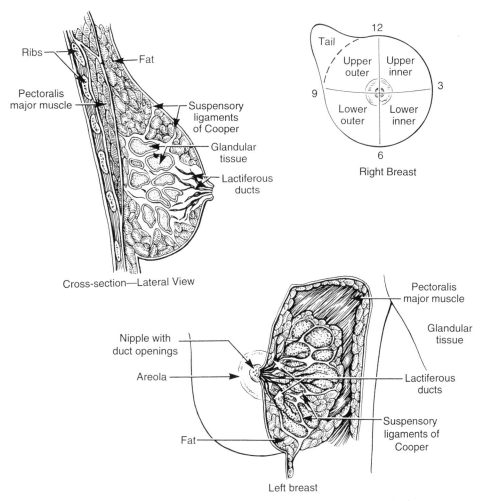

Figure 1.1. Clinical anatomy and associated examination schema of the breast.

ing teaching the technique of the breast self-examination.

The *results of the breast examination* may be expressed by description or diagram or both, usually with reference to four quadrants and the tail region of the breast or by allusion to the breast as a clock face with the nipple at the center (Fig. 1.1) Development of the female breast as described in Tanner's sex maturity ratings is used in description of the breast examination (Fig. 1.2).

The breasts are first examined by *inspection*. Inspection is first done with the pa-

tient's arms at her side and then with her hands pressed against her hips and/or her arms raised over her head. If the patient's breasts are especially large and pendulous, leaning forward so that the breasts hang free of the chest may facilitate inspection. The patient's breasts are observed before and after these maneuvers, which alter the relations of the supportive fascia of the breast tissue as the arms move. Tumors often distort the relationships of these tissues, causing disruption of the shape, contour, or symmetry of the breast or position

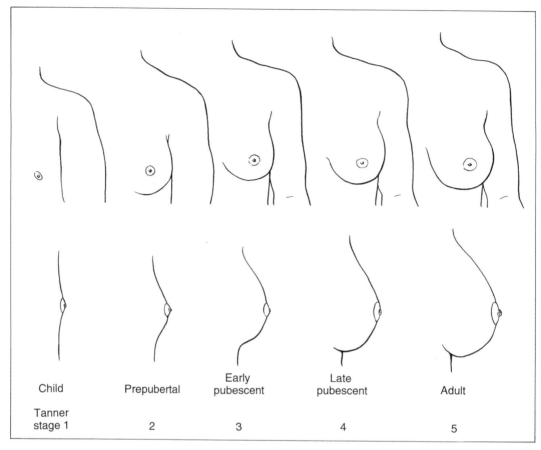

Child	Prepubertal	Early pubescent	Late pubescent	Adult
Tanner stage 1	2	3	4	5

Figure 1.2. Tanner classification: Breasts.

of the nipple. Some asymmetry of the breasts is common, but marked differences or recent changes deserve further evaluation. Discolorations or ulcerations of the skin of the breast or areola/nipple, or edema of the lymphatics (causing a leathery puckered appearance of the skin, like an orange skin, hence called peau d'orange) are not normal except in the lactating patient and require evaluation. A clear or milky breast discharge (galactorrhea) requires a specific evaluation. Bloody discharge from the breast is abnormal, but usually does not represent carcinoma but rather inflammation of a breast structure. Pus usually indicates infection of the breast, although an underlying tumor may be encountered.

Palpation follows inspection, first with the patient's arms at her side and then raised over her head. This is usually done in the supine position, although sometimes use of the sitting position with the patient's arm resting on the examiner's shoulder or over her head for examination of the most lateral aspects of the axilla is helpful. Palpation should be done with slow, careful maneuvers using the flat of the fingers and not the tips. The fingers are moved up and down in a wavelike motion, moving the tissues under them back and forth. By so doing breast masses are moved so that they may be more easily felt. A spiral or radial pattern is described over each breast to uniformly cover all of the breast tissue, including that of the axillary tail. If masses are found, their size, shape, consistency (soft,

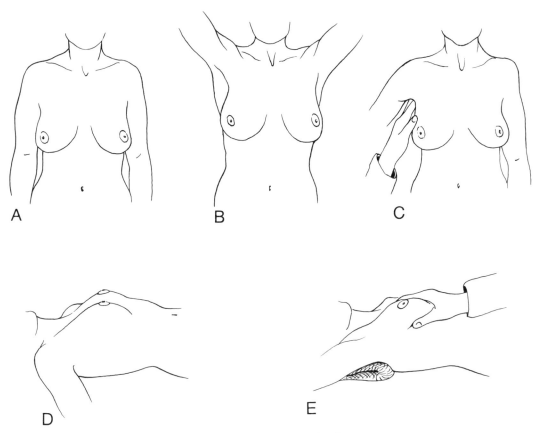

Figure 1.3. Breast examination.

hard, firm, cystic), and mobility, as well as their position, should be determined. Women with large breasts may demonstrate a firm ridge of tissue found transversely along the lower edge of the breast. This is the inframammary ridge and is a normal finding. The examination is concluded with gentle pressure inward and then upward at the sides of the areola, a gentle "squeezing" action to express fluid. If fluid is expressed, it should be sent for culture and sensitivity and cytopathology if indicated by its character and the clinical situation (Fig. 1.3).

Pelvic Examination

The patient is asked to sit at the edge of the examination table and an opened *draping sheet* is placed over the patient's knees. Draping respects the patient's sense of modesty and protects the patient from exposure to un-

comfortable drafts. If a patient requests that a drape not be used, the request should be honored.

Positioning the patient for examinations begins with *elevation of the head of the examining table* about 30° from the horizontal, which serves three purposes: (*a*) it allows eye contact and facilitates communication between physician and patient during the entire examination; (*b*) it relaxes the abdominal wall muscle groups, making the examination much easier; and (*c*) it allows the clinician to observe the patient for responses to the examination, which may provide valuable information, e.g., wincing as evidence of pain on examination. The physician and/or an assistant should *help the patient assume the lithotomy position*. The patient should be asked to lie back, place her heels in the stirrups, and then slide down to the end of the table until her buttocks are flush with the edge of the table.

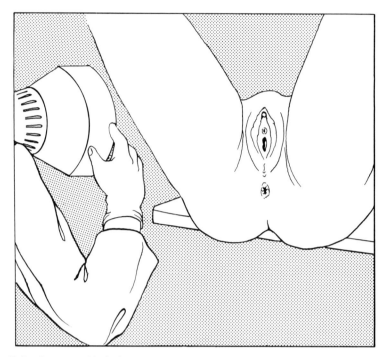

Figure 1.4. Position of light for inspection of the vulva/perineum and speculum examination.

After the patient is in the lithotomy position, the drape is adjusted so that it does not obscure the clinician's view of the perineum nor obscure eye contact between patient and physician.

The physician should sit at the foot of the examining table with the *examination lamp* adjusted to shine on the perineum. The lamp should be positioned in front of the physician's chest a few inches or so below the level of the chin, just at the level of the perineum but at about an arm's length distance from it, allowing the examination maneuvers (see Fig. 1.4). The assistant should have prepared the *materials for specimen collection* (slides, culture materials, etc.) prior to the examination. The physician should *glove both hands*. This protects the patient's modesty and sense of privacy and also protects the clinician from sexually transmitted disease. After contact with the patient, there should be minimal contact with equipment such as the lamp (Fig. 1.4).

The pelvic examination begins with the *inspection and examination of the external genitalia*. The physician begins by firmly placing the back of his hand on the patient's lower inner thigh, progressing to both hands touching the external genitalia, and thereafter to a sequential inspection and palpation of the external genitalia. Initial touching of the inner thigh begins the examination in a "personal and sensitive" area, yet not so sensitive as the perineum. Throughout the pelvic examination, the examiner should *make use of the bilateral symmetry of the body*. Dissymmetry shows that one side is different from the other, perhaps because of disease, which then requires explanation. All maneuvers should be performed gently yet with a firmness that is comfortable. Deliberate speed is important but not abruptness; neither linger beyond the time needed to do the task nor move too quickly, failing to gain the needed information.

Inspection should include the *mons pubis, labia majora and labia minora, perineum*, and *perianal area*. Inspection continues as palpation is performed in an orderly sequence, starting with the clitoral hood which may be pulled back to inspect the glans proper. The

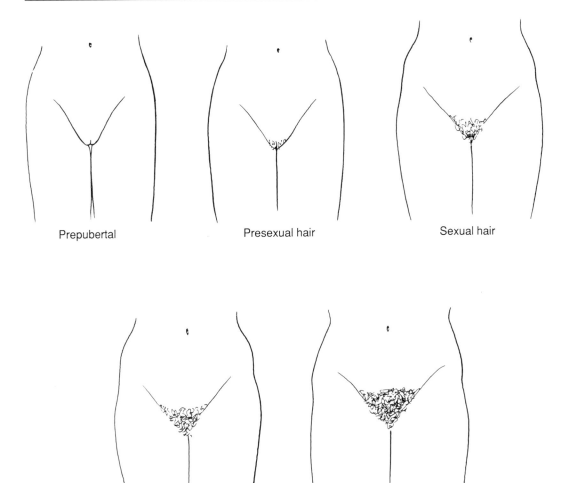

Prepubertal   Presexual hair   Sexual hair

Mid-escutcheon   Female escutcheon
Figure 1.5. Tanner classification: Pubic hair.

labia are spread laterally to allow inspection of the introitus and outer vagina. The *urethral meatus* and the areas of the *urethra and Skene's glands* should be inspected. After forewarning the patient about the possible sensation of having to urinate, the forefinger is placed an inch or so into the vagina to gently milk the urethra. A culture should be taken of any discharge from the urethral opening. The forefinger is then rotated posteriorly to palpate the area of the *Bartholin's glands* between that finger and the thumb. The patient is then asked to bear down slightly as if she were going to have a bowel movement while the *vaginal walls* are inspected for cystocele

or rectocele. Just as with the breast examination, women at different ages will demonstrate different stages of development of the genitals and associated hair, as seen in Tanner's classification (Fig. 1.5).

The next step is the *speculum examination*. The parts of the speculum are seen in Figure 1.6. There are two types of specula in common use for the examination of adults. The *Pederson speculum* has flat and narrow blades that barely curve on the sides. The *Pederson* works well for most nulliparous women and postmenopausal women with atrophic, narrowed vaginas. The *Graves speculum* has blades that are wider, higher, and curved on

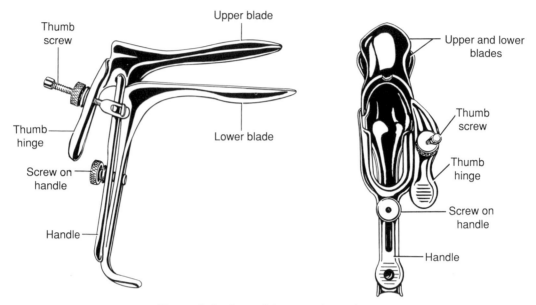

Figure 1.6. Parts of the vaginal speculum.

the sides and is more appropriate for most parous women. Its wider, curved blades keep the looser vaginal walls on the multiparous women separated for visualization (Fig. 1.7). A Pederson with extra narrow blades may be used for visualizing the cervix in pubertal girls.

First, *the speculum is examined* to be sure it is clean and in proper working order. Then, *the speculum is warmed.* If the speculum has not been kept warm, it can be warmed by running warm water over it or by holding the blades in the examiner's hand.

Speculum insertion and visualization of the vagina and cervix is performed in a stepwise manner (Fig. 1.8). Moistening the speculum with warm water may help with insertion. Lubricants should not be used routinely as they interfere with cytologic and microbiologic specimens. Situations that require their use are encountered infrequently; examples include some prepubertal girls, some postmenopausal women, and patients with irritation or lesions of the vagina making manipulative examination uncomfortable.

Most physicians find the *control of pressure and movement of the speculum* facilitated by holding the speculum with the dominant hand. The speculum is held by the handle with the blades completely closed. The first two fingers of the opposite hand are placed upon the perineum laterally and just below the introitus and pressure is applied downward and slightly inward until the introitus is opened slightly. If the patient is sufficiently relaxed, this downward pressure upon the perineum results in an open introitus into which the speculum may be easily inserted. The speculum is initially inserted in a horizontal plane with the width of the blades perpendicular to the vertical axis of the introitus. The speculum is then inclined at approximately a 45° angle from the horizontal, with adjustment of the angle as the speculum is inserted so that the speculum slides into the vagina with minimal resistance (Fig. 1.8). Inserting the speculum in a more vertical plane and then rotating the speculum is another method of insertion that is widely used. If the patient is not relaxed, posterior pressure from a finger inserted in the vagina will sometimes relax the perineal musculature.

As the speculum is inserted, a slight continuous *downward pressure* is exerted so that distention of the perineum is used to create space into which the speculum may advance.

Adult Speculae

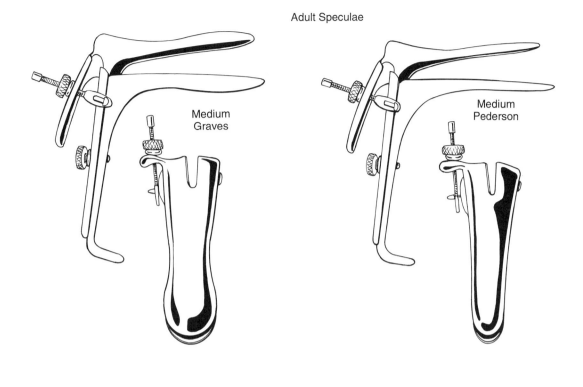

Medium
Graves

Medium
Pederson

Pediatric Speculae

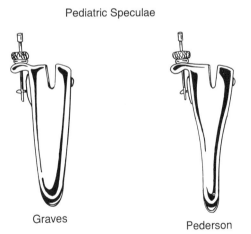

Graves

Pederson

Figure 1.7. Types of speculae.

Taking advantage of the distensibility of the perineum and vagina posterior to the introitus is a crucial concept for the efficient and comfortable manipulation of the speculum (and later for the bimanual and rectovaginal) examinations. Pressure superiorly causes pain in the sensitive area of the urethra and clitoris. The speculum is inserted as far as it will go, which in most women means insertion of the entire speculum length. The speculum is then opened in a smooth deliberate fashion. With slight tilting of the specu-

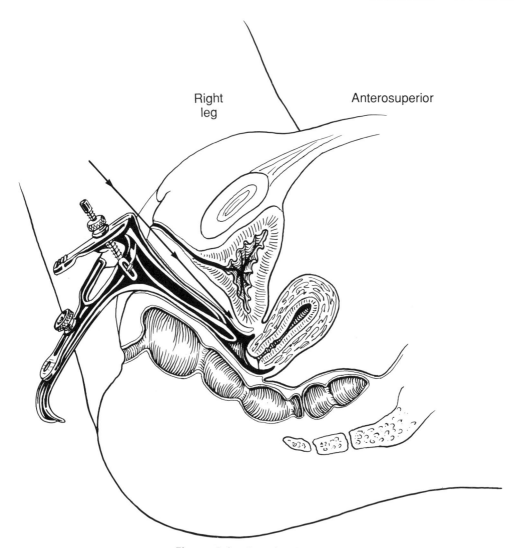

Right
leg

Anterosuperior

Figure 1.8. Speculum insertion.

lum, the cervix will slide into view between the blades of the speculum. The speculum is then locked into the open position using the thumb screw for the speculum blades. The patient is told that she may feel a sensation of pressure or of having to urinate while the speculum is in place, and that the sensation will pass when the speculum is removed.

Failure to find the cervix most commonly results from not having the speculum inserted far enough. Keeping the speculum fully inserted while opening the speculum does not result in discomfort. The lower blade of the speculum is slightly longer than the upper blade, a design that takes advantage of the deeper posterior fornix and the fact that the uterus and cervix are quite mobile. Thus, when the speculum is fully inserted and then opened, the cervix and uterus move upward slightly into the pelvis and then fall back into the space created, with the cervix coming into view. If the cervix cannot be found, one first determines if the speculum is in far enough. If only the vaginal wall is seen bulging into the space created by the opened speculum, the speculum is probably not in far enough and it should be removed and reinserted. If it appears that the cervix is "close" but trapped above or below the speculum, the speculum may be withdrawn slightly; if the cervix slides into view, the speculum may be gently reinserted and locked in the open position. Upward and downward searching movements of the speculum with full insertion is another way to find a "lost cervix," again with great care to use gentle movements of the speculum. A forefinger may be inserted to "find" a "lost cervix," an especially useful maneuver in a patient with a sharply flexed uterus.

When the speculum is locked into position, it will usually stay in place without being held. For most patients, the speculum is opened sufficiently by use of the upper thumb screw. In some cases, however, more space is required. This may be obtained by gently expanding the vertical distance between the speculum blades by use of the lower thumb screw on the handle of the speculum.

With the speculum in place, the cervix and the deep lateral vaginal vault may be inspected. The *Pap smear*, "wet prep," and/or cultures may be taken at this time. Materials needed for the Pap smear include: instrument(s) for exocervical and endocervical sample collection, glass slides with frosted ends, and a specimen bottle filled with 95% ethanol or spray fixative. Each individual slide should be labeled appropriately including the anatomic source of the specimen.

Before obtaining the Pap smear, the patient should be told that she may feel a slight "scraping" sensation, but no pain. Specimens are collected in order to fully evaluate the transformation zone where cervical intraepithelial neoplasia is more likely to be encountered. Both an *endocervical sample* as well as an *exocervical sample* are obtained using appropriate sampling devices. The material is thinly smeared on a slide, avoiding large accumulations of mucus and other material. Thick accumulations of material cannot be accurately evaluated. If indicated, a direct scrape from any vaginal lesion or from the

vaginal walls of an in utero exposed DES daughter using a second spatula can be obtained. *Immediate fixation* is important to avoid air drying artifacts, which compromise cytopathologic evaluation. Slides left in air longer than 10 seconds demonstrate a very high incidence of such artifacts (Fig. 1.9). Cultures are usually obtained for sexually transmitted diseases (STDs), including gonorrhea and chlamydia.

When specimen collection is completed, it is time for *speculum withdrawal and inspection of the vaginal walls*. After telling the patient that the speculum is to be removed and that she should not tighten her vaginal muscles upon movement of the speculum, the blades of the speculum are opened very slightly by pressure upon the thumb hinge and the thumbscrew is completely loosened. Opening the speculum blades slightly farther before starting to withdraw the speculum avoids pinching the cervix between the blades. The speculum is withdrawn about 1 inch before pressure on the thumb hinge is slowly released. The speculum is withdrawn slowly enough to allow inspection of the vaginal walls. As the end of the speculum blades approaches the introitus, there should be no pressure on the thumb hinge, otherwise the anterior blade can "flip up" hitting the sensitive vaginal, urethral, and clitoral tissues.

The *bimanual examination* uses both hands (the "vaginal hand" and the "abdominal hand") to entrap and palpate the pelvic organs. The bimanual examination begins by exerting gentle pressure on the abdomen about halfway between the umbilicus and the pubic hair line with the abdominal hand, while at the same time inserting one finger of the vaginal hand into the vagina to about 2 inches and gently pushing downward, distending the vaginal canal. The patient is asked to feel the muscles being pushed upon and to relax them as much as possible. This helps the patient relax and simultaneously creates space into which both vaginal examining fingers will usually fit. Then, both fingers are inserted into the vagina until they rest at the limit of the vaginal vault in the

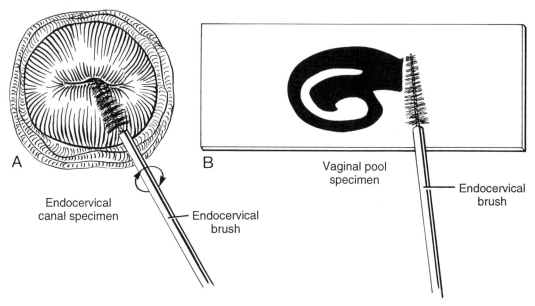

Figure 1.9. Pap smear.

posterior fornix behind and below the cervix. A great deal of space may be "created" by posterior distention of the perineum. During the examination care must be taken not to "forget" to continue downward pressure. Many clinicians find it useful to rest the elbow of the vaginal hand on their leg or knee (or against their side). The angle of the hands and the anatomy of the pelvis allow the examiner's right hand to examine the patient's right side slightly more easily and vice versa.

During the bimanual examination, the pelvic structures are "caught" and palpated between the abdominal and vaginal hands. Whether to use the dominant hand as the abdominal or vaginal hand is a question of personal preference. The most common error in this part of the pelvic examination is failure to make *effective use of the abdominal hand*. Pressure should be applied with the flat of the fingers, not the tips, starting midway between the umbilicus and the hairline, moving downward in conjunction with upward movements of the vaginal hand. The bimanual examination continues with the circumferential examination of the *cervix* for its *size, shape, position, mobility*, and the *presence or ab-*

sence of tenderness or mass lesions. Cervical position is often related to uterine position. A posterior cervix is often associated with an anteverted or midposition uterus, whereas an anterior cervix is often associated with a retroverted uterus. Sharp flexion of the uterus, however, may alter these relationships. Bimanual examination of the *uterus* is accomplished by lifting the uterus up toward the abdominal fingers so that it may be palpated between the vaginal and abdominal hands. The uterus is evaluated for its *size, shape, consistency, configuration*, and *mobility*, as well as *masses* or *tenderness* and for *position* (anteversion, midposition, retroversion, anteflexion, retroflexion). The technique varies somewhat with the position of the uterus. Examination of the anterior and midposition uterus is facilitated with the vaginal fingers lateral and deep to the cervix in the posterior fornix. The uterus is gently lifted upward to the abdominal fingers and a gentle side-to-side "searching" motion of the vaginal fingers is combined with steady pressure and palpation by the abdominal hand to determine the characteristics of the uterus (Fig. 1.10). Examination of the retroverted uterus is more

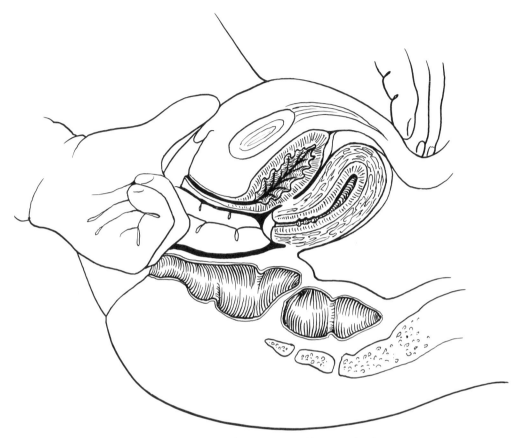

Figure 1.10. Bimanual examination: Uterus and adnexae.

difficult. In some cases the vaginal fingers may be slowly pushed below or at the level of the uterine fundus, after which gentle pressure exerted inward and upward will cause the uterus to antevert or at least move "upward," somewhat facilitating palpation. Then palpation is accomplished as in the normally anteverted uterus. If this cannot be done, a waving motion in the vaginal fingers in the posterior fornix must be combined with an extensive rectovaginal examination to assess the retroverted uterus.

Bimanual examination of the *adnexa* to assess the ovaries, fallopian tubes, and support structures begins by placing the vaginal fingers to the side of the cervix deep in the lateral fornix. The abdominal hand is moved to the same side just inside the flare of the sacral arch and above the pubic hairline. Pressure is then applied downward and toward the symphysis with the abdominal hand while at the same time lifting upward with the vaginal fingers. The same movements of the fingers of both hands used to assess the uterus are used to assess the adnexal structures, which are brought between the fingers by these maneuvers to evaluate their *size, shape, consistency, configuration, mobility,* and *tenderness,* as well as to palpate for *masses*. Special care must be taken when examining the ovaries, which are sensitive such that excessive pressure or sudden movements causes a deep visceral pain. It is important to note that the ovaries are palpable in normal menstrual women about one-half of the time, whereas palpation of ovaries in postmenopausal women implies ovarian pathology requiring further evaluation.

The *rectovaginal examination* is an integral part of the complete pelvic examination on ini-

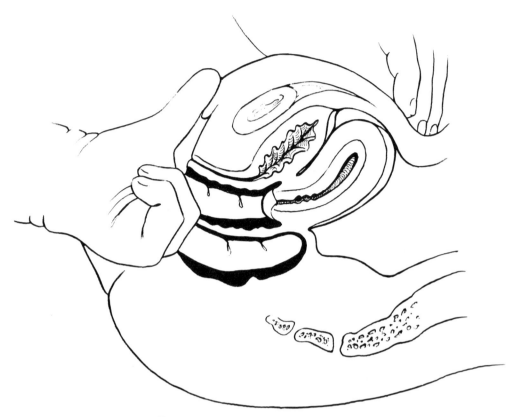

Figure 1.11. Rectovaginal examination.

tial and annual examination, as well as at interval examinations whenever clinically indicated. Full evaluation of the posterior aspect of the pelvic structures and of the support structures is possible only by this method in many patients. As patients may have had bad experiences with this part of the pelvic examination, a careful explanation of the value of the examination and reassurance that the examination will be gently done is helpful.

The rectovaginal examination is begun by *changing the glove on the vaginal hand* and using a *liberal supply of lubricant*. The examination may be comfortably performed if the natural inclination of the rectal canal is followed: upward at a 45° angle for about 1–2 cm, then downward (Fig. 1.11). This is accomplished by positioning the fingers of the vaginal hand as for the bimanual examination except that the index finger is also flexed. The second finger is then gently inserted through the rectal

opening and inserted to the "bend" where the angle turns downward. The index (vaginal) finger is inserted into the vagina, and both fingers are inserted until the vaginal finger rests in the posterior fornix below the cervix and the rectal finger rests as far as it can go into the rectal canal. Asking the patient to bear down as the rectal finger is inserted is not necessary and may add to the tension for the patient. Palpation of the pelvic structures is then accomplished as in their vaginal palpation. The *uterosacral ligaments* are also palpated to determine if they are symmetrical, smooth, and nontender (as normally) or if they are nodular, slack, or thickened. The *rectal canal* is evaluated as is the integrity and function of the *rectal sphincter*. After palpation is complete, the fingers are rapidly but steadily removed in a reversal of the sequence of movements used on insertion. Care should be taken to avoid contamination of the vagina with fecal matter. A *guaiac determination* is made from fecal material collected on the rectal finger.

At the *conclusion of the pelvic examination*, the patient is asked to move back up on the table and thereafter to sit up. It is both good manners and helpful to offer a hand to the patient when she sits up. *Discussion of the findings and recommendations for further care* should be done after the patient has had a chance to clean herself, go to the washroom if needed, and dress.

PATIENT MANAGEMENT

Based on the information gained, the physician then has five "management" tasks:

1. Formulation of Differential Diagnosis

The differential diagnosis is a list of conditions whose characteristics may correspond to one or more of the historical, physical examination, and/or laboratory findings. This list should be inclusive of all entities that reasonably may fit the information at hand, not exhaustive of all that in theory could fit the situation. The purpose of a differential diagnosis is to avoid failure to consider unusual or rare conditions and to provide a list for reconsideration should the presumptive diagnosis prove to be in error.

2. Selection of Laboratory Testing

Only those laboratory tests that are sufficient and necessary to select among the elements of the differential diagnosis and confirm the presumptive diagnosis should be obtained. Each test should be valid (validity is the closeness with which the measurements reflect the true value) and reliable (reliability is the property of a test to reproducibly identify the testable goal when present) and should not impose risks for the patient disproportionate to the severity of the malady under evaluation nor be more costly than justifiable for the same reason. As a general policy, the minimum number of tests needed to confirm

the presumptive diagnosis and allow management to begin should be obtained.

3. Formulation of a Presumptive Diagnosis

That diagnosis that best fits the information at hand is chosen as the presumptive diagnosis. At times this will clearly be the correct diagnosis; other times the correctness of the selection may be very much in doubt. In addition, a patient may often have more than one problem.

4. Development of a Management Plan

The management selected should be an effective treatment for the presumptive diagnosis and the benefits and risks of the proposed therapy should outweigh the risk of no treatment. In some cases, there will be only one management that fits these requirements; in other cases several management alternatives may exist.

Whether there are one or more possible managements, an informed consent for treatment must be made by the patient prior to treatment. Informed consent is an educational process wherein the physician explains the diagnosis, the natural course of the process if untreated (i.e., risk of no treatment), and the management(s) available including the risks, benefits, and anticipated results of each. The patient and physician should discuss this information until both are satisfied with their understandings of the situation. The patient then consents to treatment, which is begun. In the case of a surgical procedure, participation in a research protocol, or at times in other situations, a written "consent form" is completed to document that this process has occurred.

5. Follow-Up Management

During/after treatment, the patient's clinical course should be followed to ascertain if the desired outcome is achieved. If not, the presumptive diagnosis may be in error, the management plan or its execution may be faulty, or both. Reconsideration of the diagnosis and management is made and a new or revised diagnosis/management plan instituted. This process is iterated until the desired outcome is achieved.

PREVENTIVE HEALTH CARE (HEALTH MAINTENANCE)

While much of medical education is focused on the treatment of disease, it is clear that a major focus of medical care must be preventive health care, also called health maintenance. There are two basic components of this aspect of comprehensive health care. The first involves routine history and physical examination and the use of screening laboratory testing to identify problems early in their natural course. Examples include the yearly breast and pelvic examination with PAP smear, instruction in breast self-examination, instruction or referral for dietary counseling, etc. The second involves patient education about aspects of their health that may be improved by specific interventions. Perhaps the most obvious example is the cessation of tobacco abuse with its associated detrimental effects. The importance of these "routine" aspects of health care cannot be overemphasized, for if done well on a routine basis, a significant reduction in avoidable morbidity and mortality for all patients can be expected.

PRIMARY CARE AND OBSTETRICS AND GYNECOLOGY

The only physician seen regularly by many women is their obstetrician-gynecologist. In the rapidly changing health care system, this may alter the role of the obstetrician-gynecologist to include not only "speciality related activities" such as the care of pregnancy but also care not part of the traditional purview of the speciality. For example, the obstetrician-gynecologist may be more involved in the evaluation of hypercholesteremia or hypertension, and either its treatment or appropriate referral. This has been called "primary care," a specific and expanded relationship between patient and physician rather than an identified medical discipline. The result will be a primary health care role coupled with the traditional obstetrician-gynecologist's role as a consultant. There will also be a broad spectrum of practice patterns within obstetrics and gynecology that will allow the potential obstetrician-gynecologist expanded practice opportunities and an expanded, rewarding diversity of patient care experiences.

chapter 2

OBSTETRIC AND GYNECOLOGIC PROCEDURES

Any physician who cares for women must be familiar with some of the procedures common in obstetric and gynecologic practice. Whether the physician performs the procedure or not, he or she should understand the indications, contraindications, risks, benefits, and the appropriate language needed to inform the patient about her therapeutic options.

OBSTETRIC PROCEDURES
Amniocentesis

Amniocentesis is the withdrawal of fluid from the amniotic sac to obtain fluid and cells for a variety of tests. Biochemical studies can identify the presence of fetal physiologic markers (deficiency of hexosaminidase A, or Tay-Sachs disease) or the presence of substances indicating fetal abnormalities (e.g., α-feto-protein in neural tube defects, or bilirubin in Rh incompatibility). Tissue culture of fetal cells allows genetic evaluation of the fetus.

In more advanced gestations, amniocentesis is used to obtain fluid to assess the degree of fetal lung maturity. This indication of fetal lung readiness is extremely valuable in the management of premature labor or the timing of delivery for patients with medical complications.

Amniocentesis is associated with a 0.5% risk of fetal loss because of bleeding, infection, preterm labor, or fetal injury (Fig. 2.1). To reduce this risk, the procedure is usually performed under ultrasound.

Chorionic Villus Sampling

In chorionic villus sampling, a small cannula is passed through the cervix to aspirate villus cells for genetic analysis of an early gestation. Cells may also be acquired via transabdominal aspiration. The cells that are obtained are cultured for genetic studies.

Since chorionic villus sampling carries about a 0.5% risk of fetal loss, it is usually reserved for patients with a greater than 0.5% chance of abnormality (those over the age of 35 or with a history of genetic abnormalities). Bleeding or infections are infrequent complications. Compared with amniocentesis, chorionic villus sampling can be performed earlier in pregnancy with a more rapid availability of results. This allows for an earlier decision regarding possible pregnancy termination in the case of significant fetal abnormality.

Forceps Delivery and Vacuum Extraction

Vaginal delivery may be assisted with obstetrical forceps or a vacuum extractor. These methods augment the expulsive forces during the second stage of labor, as well as direct these forces in an optimal manner.

Obstetric forceps are designed either to provide traction or to facilitate the rotation of the fetal head (Fig. 2.2). Each type is applied to the fetal head and is classified as low (or outlet), mid, or high, based on the level of descent of the fetal head (station) at the time the forceps are applied. In general, low or outlet forceps describe application when the fetal scalp is visible at the introitus; midfor-

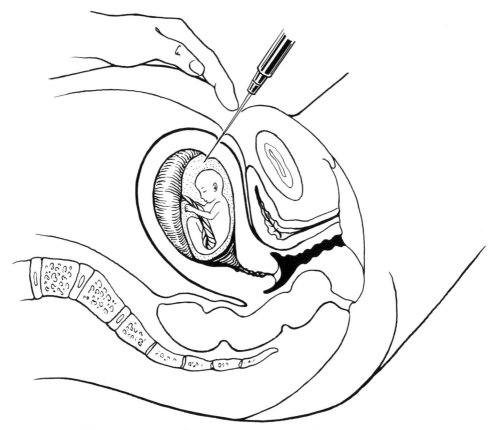

Figure 2.1. Cross-section of uterus and fetus with needle in pocket of amniotic fluid.

ceps, when the head is engaged but above the pelvic outlet, or in those cases in which a forceps rotation of the head is performed; and high forceps, when the presenting part is above zero station. High forceps should not be utilized because the risk of fetal or maternal injury is too high. Piper forceps are specially designed to facilitate the delivery of the "after-coming head" in vaginal breech deliveries (Fig. 2.3).

Forceps may cause injury to either the fetus or mother unless applied carefully and used judiciously. Transient bruising over the zygomatic arch is common and is generally of little consequence. More dangerous are lacerations of the birth canal or cervix that may result from excessive force or improper manipulation of the forceps during delivery.

The vacuum extractor is a suction cup-like device that is applied to the fetal scalp (Fig.

2.4). Traction is then used to aid expulsive efforts and expedite delivery. Although damage to maternal structures is less likely with the use of the vacuum extractor than with forceps, hematomas or abrasions of the fetal scalp can occur.

Cesarean Delivery

Cesarean delivery (or cesarean section) is the delivery of the fetus through an abdominal incision. This route may be chosen when rapid delivery is required and vaginal delivery is not imminent (e.g., fetal distress, abruptio placentae), when vaginal delivery is not advisable (e.g., placenta previa, fetal anomalies, malpresentation), or when vaginal delivery cannot be accomplished by the normal forces of labor (e.g., cephalopelvic disproportion, macrosomia). Cesarean deliveries are classified as "lower uterine segment" (transverse

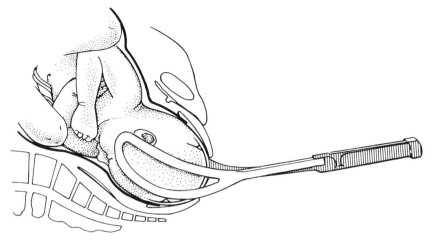

Figure 2.2. Correct biparietal, bimalar, cephalic forceps application.

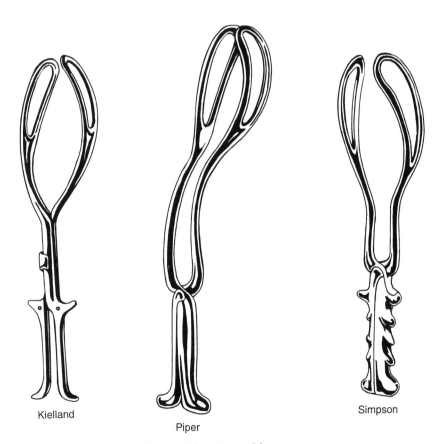

Kielland

Piper

Simpson

Figure 2.3. Types of forceps.

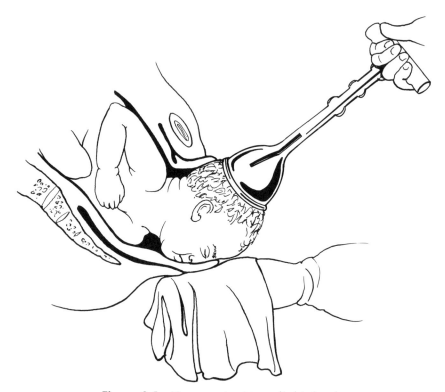

Figure 2.4. Vacuum extractor applied to head.

or vertical), when the incision is in the lower uterine segment, or "classical," when the incision is in the upper, contractile portion of the uterus (Fig. 2.5). Patients with lower uterine segment cesarean deliveries may be candidates for future vaginal delivery (**vaginal birth after cesarean (VBAC)**) if careful maternal and fetal monitoring is available as well as staff and facilities for emergency cesarean section. Patients with classical incisions are at greater risk of rupture of the uterine scar before or during labor and are generally not allowed to labor in subsequent pregnancies.

Although cesarean delivery offers some advantages in the management of problem pregnancies, its operative nature significantly increases the maternal morbidity from infection, bleeding, hematoma, or anesthetic complications.

Circumcision

Circumcision of the newborn (the removal of the foreskin from the penis) has been prac-

ticed for centuries for both religious and health reasons. Controversy continues over the health value of this surgical procedure. It has been argued that circumcision represents mutilation, reduces penile sensitivity, and carries a greater risk of operative complications (surgical damage, bleeding, infection) than is warranted by its benefits. Opposing arguments point to improved hygiene and a dramatically reduced prevalence of penile cancer.

GYNECOLOGIC PROCEDURES
Imaging

The ability to image various parts and organs of the body has dramatically enhanced our diagnostic capabilities. These methods do not replace a careful and thoughtful history and physical evaluation. The effective use of these modalities requires that the physician be familiar with the benefits and limitations of each.

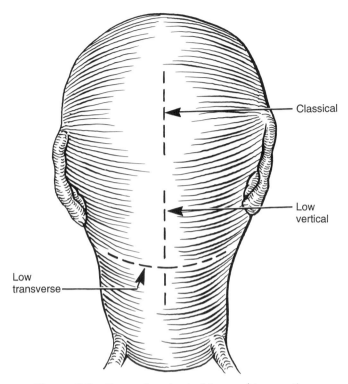

Figure 2.5. Types of uterine incision used in c. sections.

Ultrasonography

Ultrasonography is based on the use of high frequency sound reflections to identify different body tissues and structures. The term sonography literally means "sound writing" and is often described as using sound waves to make a picture. Very short bursts of low energy sound waves are sent into the body. When these waves encounter the interface between two tissues that transmit sound differently, some of the sound energy is reflected back toward the sound source (Fig. 2.6). The returning sound waves are detected and the distance from the sensor is deduced using the elapsed time from transmission to reception. This information is displayed graphically as a cross-sectional view of the structure encountered by the beam.

Since ultrasonography uses low energy sound waves, it is considered safe for use in pregnancy. Its reliance on subtle tissue differences limits the ability to distinguish some tissues. It is also affected by interference from substances such as bowel gas. Despite these limitations, ultrasonography is very good at distinguishing solid from cystic structures and for fetal assessments (Fig. 2.6). In obstetrics, measurement of fetal anatomy to infer age and weight is often carried out. Detailed evaluations of fetal structures such as heart, brain, spinal column, or kidneys are often possible. Fetal gender may frequently be determined as well.

In gynecology, ultrasonography may be used to distinguish the character of pelvic masses (solid versus cystic) or to provide accurate measurement of tumors such as fibroids. These applications often have little impact on clinical management or decision making and provide only a false sense of precision. Because of cost and limited return, ultrasonography should be used only to evaluate pelvic masses when an adequate examination is not possible (e.g., extreme obesity) or when the information gathered will alter patient management. Routine ultrasonography to confirm findings on pelvic examination is not warranted.

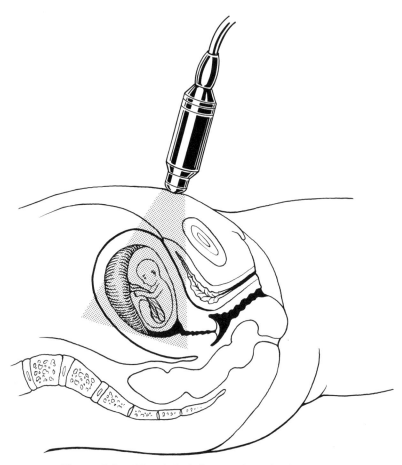

Figure 2.6. "Curtain" of ultrasound passing into uterus.

Improved resolution for imaging intrauterine and adnexal structures may be obtained by placing the ultrasound transducer inside the vagina. The higher frequencies of sound used for transvaginal imaging allow enhanced details to be seen but limit the depth of penetration of the sound. Therefore, transvaginal ultrasound is used only for structures located near the apex of the vagina. Transvaginal ultrasonography has proven especially useful for evaluating very early gestations, possible ectopic pregnancies, and for follicle monitoring during assisted reproduction.

"Doppler ultrasound" is a form of ultrasonography that uses changes in the frequency of the reflected sound to infer motion of the reflecting surface. This can be useful in detecting cardiac motion or assessing blood flow. A growing application of Doppler ultrasound has been the evaluation of blood flow patterns in the umbilical vessels, as changes in these patterns may be an indication of fetal stress.

Computed Axial Tomography

Computed axial tomography (CAT scanning) uses computer algorithms to construct cross-sectional images based on x-ray information. This technique involves slightly greater radiation exposure than a conventional single-exposure x-ray, but provides significantly more information. With the use of contrast agents, this modality can be very helpful in evaluating pelvic masses, looking for signs of adenopathy, or planning radiation therapy.

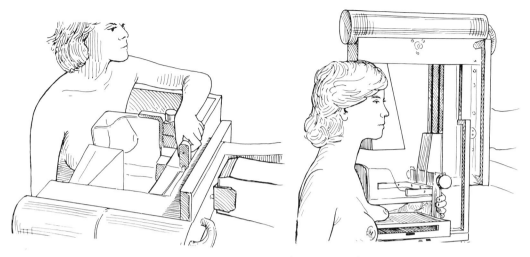

Figure 2.7. Technique of mammography.

Magnetic Resonance Imaging

Magnetic resonance imaging (MRI) is based on the magnetic characteristics of various atoms and molecules in the body. Because of the variations in chemical composition of body tissues (especially the content of hydrogen, sodium, fluoride, or phosphorus), MRI offers exceptional images of many soft tissues. The relatively longer time needed to form images and MRI's somewhat experimental nature make this modality exciting in its possibilities, but limited in direct clinical application in obstetrics and gynecology.

Mammography

The need to develop an effective screening method for breast cancer has prompted the evaluation of many imaging technologies such as thermography (based on skin temperature patterns), ultrasonography, transillumination by light, and x-ray. It has been the latter (mammography) that has proven to be the most effective for screening and in the evaluation of recognized abnormalities. In mammography, breast tissue is compressed against an imaging plate and a small amount of radiation used to form the image (Fig. 2.7). Improved films, imaging screens, and xerographic technologies have all led to improved images with the lower radiation exposures.

Hysterosalpingography

In hysterosalpingography, contrast material is introduced through the cervix into the uterine cavity and fallopian tubes and then an x-ray is taken (Fig. 2.8). This technique is useful for evaluation of the size, shape, and configuration of the uterine cavity as part of the evaluations for infertility or genital anomalies. The passage of contrast material through the fallopian tubes will spill into the peritoneal cavity and can be a good indicator of tubal patency. The absence of spill from the tube, however, may be an indication of tubal obstruction.

This procedure is associated with the risk of infection of the uterus or pelvis, as well as bleeding or pain. With the increasing availability and reliance on hysteroscopy and laparoscopy, the role of hysterosalpingography in clinical practice continues to evolve.

Genital Tract Biopsy

The removal of tissue from genital tract lesions for histologic study may be safely obtained from the vulva, vagina, cervix, and endometrial cavity. Usually performed in the office, most of these procedures require little

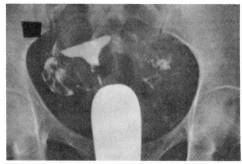

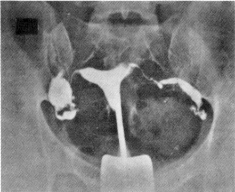

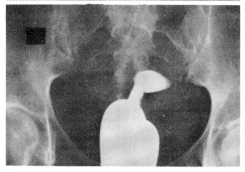

Figure 2.8. Hysterosalpingography.

or no anesthetics and are associated with minimal risk.

Vulvar biopsies are generally accomplished with the use of a local anesthetic. Tissue may be removed by elevating a portion of the tissue and cutting at the base a hollow punch ("Keyes" biopsy) or with a "pinch" biopsy (Fig. 2.9). Local pressure or the use of styptics such as Monsel's solution (ferric subsulfate) are usually adequate for hemostasis; sutures are seldom required.

Biopsy of vaginal lesions is generally carried out using either the pinch technique for lesions low in the canal or a biopsy forceps. This instrument is also used for biopsy of the cervix. Local anesthesia is often not required for vaginal lesions and is not used for cervical biopsy.

An *endometrial biopsy* may be obtained in several ways. A small hollow tube may be passed through the cervix and tissue fragments aspirated (Fig. 2.10). Larger, more rigid cannula may be used to aspirate or even curet the endometrium. Sharp curettage may be used to sample the endometrium, but this often requires greater cervical dilation and produces more discomfort so that a paracervical block is indicated.

Colposcopy

Colposcopy employs a horizontally mounted type of dissecting microscope and specialized light source to facilitate evaluation of the surface structure of the cervix, vagina, and vulva. Through the use of green filters (to make blood vessels more easily visible) and a 1% acetic acid wash (to bring out epithelial changes), colposcopy is the most sensitive technique for the identification of early dysplastic or neoplastic changes. Based on the colposcopic findings, biopsies are taken of the area(s) with the most significant abnormalities.

Cryotherapy

Cryotherapy is the term used to describe tissue destruction by freezing. Cryotherapy is most frequently used to treat dysplastic changes (Fig. 2.11). It may also be used for the treatment of vulvar lesions such as condyloma of the cervix although other modalities such as chemical therapy and laser are more successful and more frequently used. The formation of ice crystals within the cells of the treated tissue leads to tissue destruction and slough. As a result, patients who have had cryotherapy of the cervix can be expected to have a watery discharge for several weeks as the tissue sloughs and healing occurs. Cryotherapy is inexpensive and generally effective but is less precise than laser therapy.

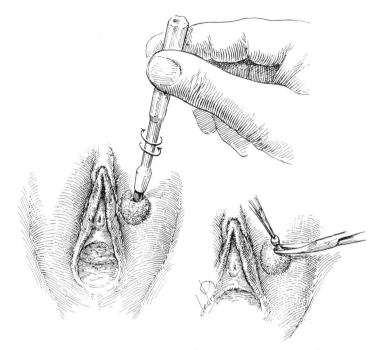

Figure 2.9. Biopsy of vulvar skin with Keyes punch.

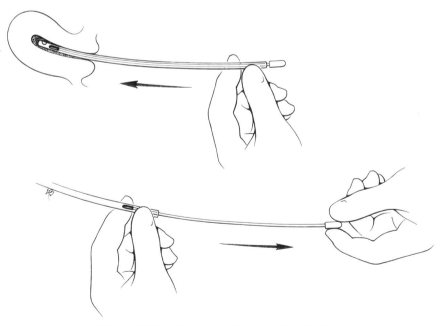

Figure 2.10. Endometrial biopsy using Pipelle.

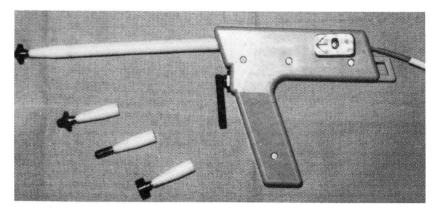

Figure 2.11. Cryosurgical equipment.

Laser Vaporization

Energy from intense beams of light may be transferred to tissue to produce a therapeutic effect. This effect may vary from "sunburn" to explosive vaporization of the tissue. Light from laser (**l**ight **a**mplification by **s**timulated **e**mission of **r**adiation) sources is used because of its coherence (allowing the beam to be manipulated) and the purity of wavelength (decreasing extraneous effects and interactions). The interaction of the light and tissue is dependent on the wavelength of light and the "power density," or intensity, of the beam.

One of the most common lasers used in gynecology is the infrared laser. The infrared energy emitted by this device is readily absorbed by the water molecules in tissue. This results in efficient energy transfer and relatively shallow depth of penetration. These two characteristics allow for precise control and selective tissue destruction. Laser therapy may be used to remove tissue by vaporization or to act as a "light knife" to excise tissues. The precise control possible with this technique makes its use for cervical and vulvar lesions attractive. Laser light may also be used for operative procedures during laparoscopy. Other laser light sources are used for purposes such as endometrial ablation, although these applications are still being evaluated.

Dilation and Curettage

Dilation and curettage, or D&C, was once one of the most common surgical procedures. Supplanted in part by today's more easily accomplished endometrial biopsy techniques, D&C allows the lining of the uterus to be explored and tissues removed for diagnosis or therapy. The "dilation" of D&C refers to opening the cervix to allow access to the endometrial cavity. This is usually done by gently using a series of graduated dilators to stretch the cervical opening. Because stretching of the cervix is painful, D&C is usually performed under a local (paracervical) or general anesthetic in an operating room. The "curettage" is a scraping of the uterine lining.

Pregnancy Termination

This term refers to the planned interruption of a pregnancy prior to viability and is often referred to as induced abortion. It is generally accomplished surgically through dilation of the cervix and evacuation of the uterine contents (sometimes called D&E). Removal of the products of conception in the first and early second trimester uses either a suction or sharp curette. Suction curettes are often preferred because they are less likely to cause uterine damage such as endometrial scarring or perforation. Later in the second trimester, grasping forceps or medication induction of labor are utilized.

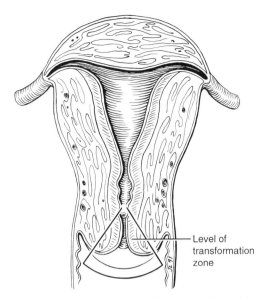

Level of transformation zone

Figure 2.12. Cone biopsy showing wedge of tissue.

Cervical Conization

Conization is a surgical procedure performed for either diagnostic or therapeutic purposes in which a cone-shaped sample of tissue, which encompasses the entire cervical transformation zone and extends up the endocervical canal, is removed from the cervix (Fig. 2.12). Conization is required for the definitive evaluation of patients with abnormal Pap smears where adequate colposcopic examinations are impossible or are inconsistent with Pap smear data.

Conization may be performed using a variety of techniques including sharp dissection (cold knife cone), laser excision, or electrocautery (loop electrosurgical excisional of the transformation zone (LEETZ)). An early complication of conization is excessive bleeding, which can occur 5–10 days after surgery. Cervical stenosis or incompetence are infrequent complications.

Laparoscopy

Laparoscopy (or pelviscopy) involves inspection and manipulation of tissue within the abdominal cavity using endoscopic instruments. The laparoscope is inserted into the abdominal cavity through a periumbilical incision. To facilitate viewing and to decrease the chance of bowel injury, the abdominal cavity is distended with either carbon dioxide or nitrous oxide gas. Additional incisions in the lower abdomen may be made to allow supplementary instruments to be placed into the abdominal cavity for surgical or other manipulations (Fig. 2.13). A probe or other device is often inserted into the uterine cavity to facilitate uterine manipulations.

Laparoscopy is used for diagnostic or therapeutic purposes. Laparoscopic inspection of the pelvis can be invaluable in the diagnosis of pelvic pain, infertility, congenital abnormalities, or small pelvic masses. Operative laparoscopy may be used to lyse adhesions, treat endometriosis, or carry out surgical sterilizations and other gynecology procedures.

Because laparoscopy involves the penetration of the abdominal cavity, it is considered major surgery. Even though it is usually done on an outpatient basis under local or general anesthesia, the surgical nature of the procedure must be recognized. Serious complications from injury to the bowel or great vessels can occur. Intraperitoneal bleeding or injuries from intraperitoneal manipulations (e.g., unappreciated damage to bowel during fulguration or laser) also pose a risk. Anesthetic complications are possible, as are infections and bleeding at the incision site.

Hysteroscopy

Improved optics have led to the availability of small endoscopes that allow a direct view of the endocervix and endometrial cavity. These endoscopes may be used for diagnosis (such as the evaluation of bleeding or congenital malformations, the staging of cancer, or the location of missing intrauterine devices) or for therapy (such as polypectomy, myomectomy, endometrial ablation, or removal of a uterine septum). Usually done as an outpatient procedure under local or general anesthesia, hysteroscopy shares most of the same

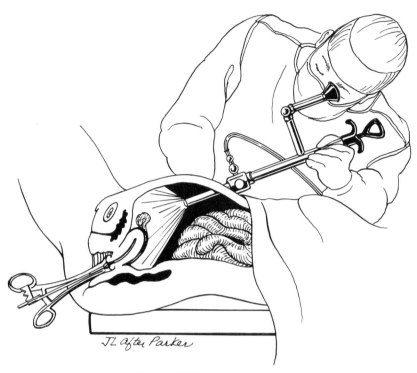

Figure 2.13. Laparoscopy.

problems and complications found in dilation and curettage.

Hysterectomy

Hysterectomy, the removal of the uterus, is still one of the most common surgical procedures performed. In the United States, approximately 500,000 hysterectomies are performed each year. Removing the uterus may be indicated for patients with benign or malignant changes in the uterine wall or cavity, abnormalities of the cervix, or menstrual disturbances that do not respond to more conservative therapy. Hysterectomy provides protection from further pregnancy, cessation of menses, and prevention of cervical disease. Despite this, hysterectomy is sufficiently expensive, time consuming, and risky that it cannot be recommended for the sole purpose of sterilization.

In discussing hysterectomy with patients, it is important to realize the correct use, and common misuse, of terms associated with the procedure. When physicians use the term "total hysterectomy," it refers to the removal of all of the uterus. It does not indicate removal of the ovary (oophorectomy) or fallopian tube (salpingectomy). These distinctions are important and should be emphasized during history taking or preoperative counseling. A "sub-total" or "supracervical" hysterectomy is one in which the body of the uterus is removed near the level of the inner cervical os, leaving the cervix in place. A "radical" hysterectomy is a cancer surgery procedure in which the uterus is removed with very wide margins of surrounding tissues.

Removal of the uterus may be accomplished by entering the abdominal cavity from above (abdominal hysterectomy) or by extracting the uterus through the vagina (vaginal hysterectomy). Each has advantages and disadvantages that must be evaluated for each patient. With either approach, certain steps must be accomplished to allow safe removal of the uterus. The blood supply to the uterus is interrupted by ligation of the uterine arteries and the anastomotic connections to the vaginal and ovarian blood supplies. The latter is ligated at the level of the utero-ovarian ligament, if the ovaries are to be preserved, or at the level of the infundibulopelvic ligament, if oophorectomy is planned. The supporting structures of the uterus (round ligaments, cardinal ligaments, uterosacral ligaments, and the leaves of the broad ligament) are severed. The sequence of these steps is dictated by the route of surgery chosen (fundus to cervix for the abdominal route, cervix to fundus for the vaginal route) and local exigencies mandated by the pathology encountered (e.g., distortion of anatomy by fibroids).

Abdominal Hysterectomy

Removal of the uterus through an abdominal incision allows the surgeon maximal exposure and latitude in performing the procedure. This approach is used when substantial pathology is anticipated (as with large fibroids or pelvic scarring), wide margins or further exploration is required (as in cancer surgery), or additional abdominal procedures are contemplated (such as bladder suspension), or at the time of cesarean section. Abdominal hysterectomies generally involve longer operating times. This is due to the time spent making and repairing the abdominal wall incision and to the more involved procedures often performed via this route. As might be expected, this route is also associated with a greater rate of morbidity and longer hospital stay.

Vaginal Hysterectomy

Vaginal hysterectomy is generally associated with a faster recovery period and less patient discomfort. Offsetting this is the higher incidence of fever and infection although the use of prophylactic antibiotics has reduced this to a minimum. Vaginal hysterectomy is often chosen when the uterus is not enlarged and other adnexal or pelvic pathology is not anticipated. Vaginal hysterectomy is especially appropriate for patients who require repair of a cystocele, rectocele, or enterocele. Vaginal hysterectomy is typically avoided with the uterus is larger than 10–12 weeks size, movement of the pelvic organs is restricted by scarring or endometriosis, or further abdominal exploration is required.

FURTHER READING

Jones HW III, Wentz AC, Burnett LS, eds. Novak's textbook of gynecology, 11th ed. Baltimore: Williams & Wilkins, 1988.

chapter 3

EMBRYOLOGY AND ANATOMY OF THE FEMALE REPRODUCTIVE SYSTEM

A knowledge of the embryology of the female reproductive system is helpful in understanding both normal anatomy and the structural anomalies that can sometimes occur. Although this chapter concentrates on development in the female, comparisons to the development of the male reproductive system are made for illustration.

The genital system develops from embryonic intermediate mesoderm. With the folding of the embryo, the intermediate mesoderm comes to lie as two longitudinal rods on either side of the primitive aorta. In the trunk region, the rods are called nephrogenic cords (Fig. 3.1*A*). There is a dorsal outgrowth of each nephrogenic cord, which bulges into the celomic cavity. These bulges, called the *urogenital ridges*, are covered with celomic epithelium. The urogenital ridges give rise to elements of both the urinary and reproductive systems (Fig. 3.1*B*).

In general, the elements of the reproductive system pass through an undifferentiated stage in the early embryo. That is, development in the male and female is identical. Later, sex-specific differentiation occurs.

Development of the Ovary

Genetic sex, determined at fertilization, depends on whether the X-bearing oocyte is fertilized by an X- or Y-bearing sperm. However, early in development, the gonads are undifferentiated, that is, the sex of the embryo cannot be determined from the appearance of the gonad.

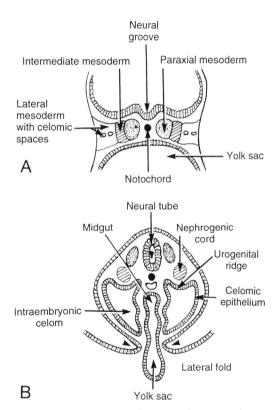

Figure 3.1. Early development of urogenital system.

The gonads begin to develop during the 5th week when a portion of the urogenital ridge on the medial side of the mesonephric kidney thickens to form the *gonadal ridge*. The celomic epithelium divides to form finger-like bands of cells (the *primary sex cords*), which project into the underlying mesodermal mesenchyme of the gonadal ridge. In the female, it is the cortical area that predomi-

33

nates in the mature gonad and it is this corti-cal tissue that contains the follicles. This growth results in the creation of a cortex and a medulla in the indifferent (undifferentiated) gonad.

During the 4th week, the *primordial germ cells* (which will eventually give rise to the ga-metes) can be identified in the yolk sac. As the embryo folds, some of the yolk sac is in-corporated into the embryo. During the 6th week, the primordial germ cells migrate into the mesenchyme of the gonadal ridge, where they become associated with the primary sex cords. In the female, the primordial germ cells become oogonia, which divide by mito-sis during fetal life. No oogonia form after birth.

If a Y chromosome is present, the tunica albuginea of the testis will begin to form in the mesenchymal tissue of the medulla dur-ing the 8th week. This is the first indication of the sex of the embryo. In the absence of a Y chromosome, the undifferentiated gonad will develop into an ovary, which will be identifiable by about the 10th week of devel-opment. In the ovary, the primary sex cords degenerate, and secondary sex cords (cortical cords) appear and extend from the surface epithelium into the underlying mesenchyme. The *oogonia* are incorporated into them, and, at about 16 weeks of development, the corti-cal cords organize into *primordial follicles*. Each follicle eventually consists of an oogo-nium, derived from a primary germ cell, sur-rounded by a single layer of squamous follic-ular cells, derived from the cortical cords. *Follicular maturation* begins when the oogonia enter the first stage of meiotic division (at which point they are called oocytes). Oocyte development is then arrested until puberty, when one or more follicles are stimulated to continue development each month (see Chapter 34, "Reproductive Cycle," and Chapter 35, "Puberty").

Development of the Genital Ducts

In both the male and female, two pairs of ducts initially develop, the mesonephric or wolffian and the paramesonephric or müller-ian. As with the gonad, there is an indiffer-ent, or undifferentiated, stage in ductal de-velopment. During this stage, both sets of ducts are present in both the male and the female.

In the male, the *mesonephric ducts*, which drain the embryonic mesonephric kidneys, eventually form the *epididymis, ductus deferens*, and *ejaculatory ducts*. In the female, the meso-nephric ducts almost completely disappear.

In the female, it is the *paramesonephric* (or müllerian) *ducts* that persist to form major parts of the reproductive tract (the *fallopian tubes, uterus*, and *parts of the vagina*). The par-amesonephric ducts start to develop early in the 6th week, beginning as invaginations of the celomic epithelium in the vicinity of the mesonephric kidneys (Fig. 3.2*A*). For each duct, the invagination fuses to form a tube. The cranial end of each duct opens into the celomic (future peritoneal) cavity. The ducts grow caudally, and the caudal segments fuse at about the 8th week of development into the Y-shaped *uterovaginal primordium or canal* (Fig. 3.2*B*). The cranial (unfused) portion of each duct becomes a fallopian tube and the fused portions become the uterus and parts of the vagina. This differentiation is not de-pendent upon the presence of ovaries.

When the two paramesonephric ducts fuse, two peritoneal folds are brought to-gether. This creates the broad ligaments of the uterus (Fig. 3.2*C*).

Development of the Vagina

Between weeks 5 and 7, the *primitive cloaca*, a pouch-like enlargement of the caudal end of the hindgut, is divided into the *urogenital si-nus* (ventral) and the *anorectal canal* (dorsal). The contact of the caudally growing utero-vaginal primordium with the urogenital sinus results in the formation of a solid mass of cells called the vaginal plate. The vaginal plate extends from the urogenital sinus into the caudal end of the uterovaginal primor-dium. The central cells of the vaginal plate disappear, forming the lumen of the vagina.

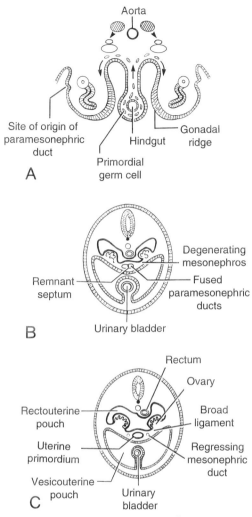

Figure 3.2. Formation of uterus.

The peripheral cells of the plate persist as the vaginal epithelium. In addition to contributing to the *vagina*, the urogenital sinus also gives rise to the *epithelium of the urinary bladder*, the *urethra*, the *greater vestibular glands*, and the *hymen*.

Development of the External Genitalia

The external genitalia also pass through an indifferent stage. Early in the 4th week, the *genital tubercle* or phallus develops at the cranial end of the cloacal membrane. Soon after, labioscrotal swellings and urogenital folds appear at either side of the cloacal membrane

(Fig. 3.3*A*). The genital tubercle (phallus) enlarges in both the male and the female (Fig. 3.3*B*).

The division of the cloaca by the urorectal septum divides the cloacal membrane into the dorsal anal membrane and the ventral urogenital membrane. At about week 7, these membranes rupture.

At about 9 weeks, distinguishing sexual characteristics begin to appear, but the external genital organs are not fully formed until week 12. In the absence of androgens, the external genitalia are feminized (Fig. 3.3*C*). The phallus develops into the relatively small *clitoris*. The unfused urogenital folds form the *labia minora* and the labioscrotal swellings become the *labia majora* (Fig. 3.3*D*).

ANATOMY OF THE FEMALE REPRODUCTIVE SYSTEM

This section first describes the normal anatomy of the female reproductive system. Anomalies, arising from defects in development, will then be discussed.

Bony Pelvis

The bony pelvis is composed of the paired *innominate bones* and the sacrum. The innominate bones are joined anteriorly to form the symphysis pubis, and each is articulated posteriorly with the sacrum through the sacroiliac joint (Fig. 3.4).

The innominate bones are composed of three portions—the *ilium*, the *ischium*, and the *pubis*—which become fused during adolescence. The three parts come together to contribute to the acetabulum. The sacrum is composed of five or six sacral vertebrae, which are fused in adulthood. The sacrum articulates with the coccyx inferiorly and with the fifth lumbar vertebra superiorly.

The pelvis is divided into the pelvis major (*false pelvis*) and the pelvis minor (*true pelvis*), which are separated by the linea terminalis. The false pelvis, whose main function is to support the pregnant uterus, is bounded by the lumbar vertebrae posteriorly, an iliac

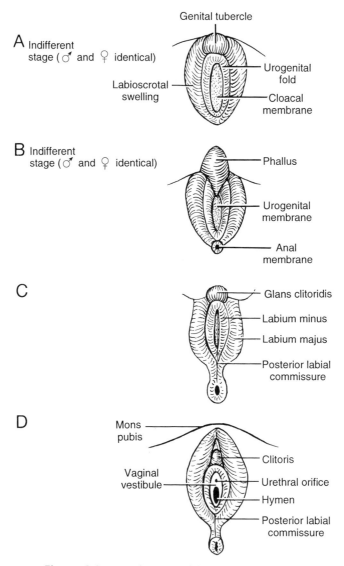

Figure 3.3. Development of the external genitalia.

fossa bilaterally, and the abdominal wall anteriorly.

The *true pelvis* is formed by the sacrum and coccyx posteriorly and by the ischium and pubis laterally and anteriorly. Concern arises when its dimensions are inadequate to permit passage of the fetus.

There are *four pelvic planes*: the *pelvic inlet*, the *plane of the greatest diameter*, the *plane of least diameter* (midplane), and the *pelvic outlet*. The pelvic inlet is bounded posteriorly by the promontory and alae of the sacrum, later-ally by the linea terminalis, and anteriorly by the superior surface of the pubic bones. Thus, the plane of the inlet separates the false pelvis and the true pelvis. The plane of the greatest diameter is bounded by the junction of the second and third sacral vertebrae posteriorly, the upper part of the obturator foramina laterally, and the midpoint of the pubis anteriorly. The plane of least diameter (the midplane) extends from the lower border of the pubis anteriorly to the lower sacrum at the level of the ischial spines. This

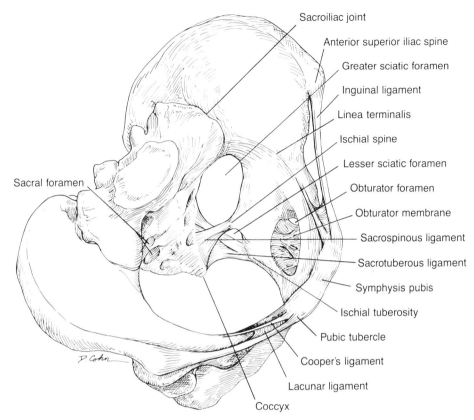

Sacroiliac joint

Anterior superior iliac spine

Greater sciatic foramen

Inguinal ligament

Linea terminalis

Ischial spine

Lesser sciatic foramen

Obturator foramen

Obturator membrane

Sacrospinous ligament

Sacrotuberous ligament

Symphysis pubis

Ischial tuberosity

Pubic tubercle

Cooper's ligament

Lacunar ligament

Coccyx

Sacral foramen

D Cohn

Figure 3.4. View of the pelvis from above, showing bones, joints, ligaments, and foramina.

Table 3.1
Length of Pelvic Plane Diameters

Pelvic plane	Diameter	Average length
		cm
Inlet	True conjugate	10.5–11.5
	Obstetric conjugate	10.0–11.0
	Diagonal conjugate	12.5
	Transverse diameter	13.5
	Oblique diameter	12.5
Greatest	Anterior-posterior	12.75
diameter	Transverse	12.5
Midplane	Anterior-posterior	11.5–12
	Bispinous	10.5
Outlet	Anterior-posterior	11.5
	Bituberous	8.0–11.0

plane is most important clinically, since arrest of fetal descent occurs most frequently at this point. The plane of the outlet is irregular, consisting of two intersecting triangles. It is bounded posteriorly by the tip of the sacrum, laterally by the ischial tuberosities and the sacrotuberous ligaments, and anteriorly by the lower border of the symphysis. There are certain key diameters of the pelvis, which are important in assessing the space available during fetal descent (Table 3.1).

The female pelvis is classified into four basic types, according to the scheme of Caldwell and Moloy (Fig. 3.5). The most common type is the *gynecoid*, occurring in about 40–50% of women. In this type, the inlet is rounded, the side walls are straight, the sacrum is well curved, and the sacrosciatic notch is adequate. In general, this gives the pelvis a cylindrical shape, which has adequate space along its length. The *android* pelvis occurs in about 30% of all women, but in only 10–15% of black women. There is a wedge-shaped inlet, the side walls converge, the sacrum in inclined forward, and the sacrosciatic notch is narrow. This pelvic type has limited space at

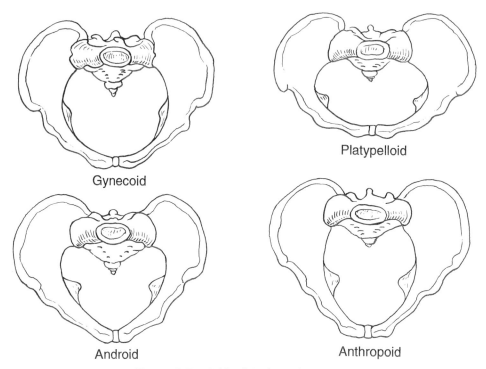

Figure 3.5. Caldwell-Moloy pelvic types.

the inlet, and the funnel shape results in even less space below. Fetal descent may be arrested at the midpelvis. The *anthropoid* type occurs in about 20% of all women (and in about 40% of black women). The inlet is oval, long, and narrow; the side walls are straight (do not converge); the sacrum is long and narrow; and the sacrosciatic notch is wide. Both the interspinous and intertuberous diameters are somewhat smaller than in the gynecoid pelvis. The *platypelloid* pelvis occurs in only about 2–5% of women. There is an oval inlet, the sacrum is normal, the side walls are straight, the sacrosciatic notch is narrowed, and the interspinous and intertuberous diameters are increased. Any individual may be of a pure or mixed pelvic type.

Vulva and Perineum

The vulva contains the labia majora, the *labia minora*, the mons pubis, the clitoris, the vestibule, and the ducts of glands that open into the vestibule (Fig. 3.6). The labia majora are

folds of skin with underlying adipose tissue, which are fused anteriorly with the mons pubis and posteriorly with the perineum. The skin of the labia majora contains hair follicles and sebaceous and sweat glands. The *labia minora* are narrow skin folds, which lie inside the labia majora. The labia minora merge anteriorly with the prepuce and frenulum of the clitoris and posteriorly with the labia majora and the perineum. The labia minora contain sebaceous and sweat glands but no hair follicles, and there is no underlying adipose tissue. The *clitoris*, which is located anterior to the labia minora, is the embryologic homologue of the penis. It consists of two crura (corresponding to the corpora cavernosa in the male) and the glans, which is found superior to the point of fusion of the crura. On the ventral surface of the glans is the *frenulum*, the fused junction of the labia minora. The *vestibule* lies between the labia minora and is bounded anteriorly by the clitoris and posteriorly by the perineum. The urethra and the vagina open into the vestibule in the midline. The ducts of *Skene's*

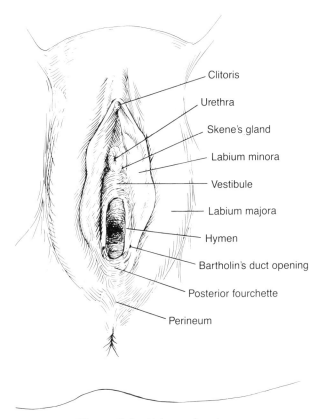

- Clitoris
- Urethra
- Skene's gland
- Labium minora
- Vestibule
- Labium majora
- Hymen
- Bartholin's duct opening
- Posterior fourchette
- Perineum

Figure 3.6. Vulva and perineum.

(*paraurethral*) *glands* and *Bartholin's glands* also empty into the vestibule.

The *muscles of the vulva* (the superior transverse perineal, the bulbocavernosus, and the ischiocavernosus) lie superficial to the fascia of the urogenital diaphragm. The vulva rests on the triangular-shaped urogenital diaphragm, which lies in the anterior part of the pelvis between the ischiopubic rami. The urogenital diaphragm surrounds and supports the urethra and the vagina.

Vagina

The vagina is a muscular tube that extends from the vestibule to the uterus (Fig. 3.7). The long axis of the vagina is approximately parallel to the lower portion of the sacrum. The uterine cervix projects into the upper portion of the vagina. Therefore, the anterior vaginal wall is about 2 cm shorter than the posterior wall. The area around the cervix, the fornix, is divided into four regions: the *anterior fornix*, two *lateral fornices*, and the *posterior fornix*. The posterior fornix is in close proximity to the peritoneum that forms the floor of the posterior pelvic cul-de-sac (pouch of Douglas). This allows access to the peritoneal cavity from the vagina, for example during culdocentesis.

At its lower end, the vagina traverses the urogenital diaphragm and is then surrounded by the two bulbocavernosus muscles. These act as a sphincter. The *hymen*, a fold of mucosal-covered connective tissue, somewhat obscures the external vaginal orifice in the child. The hymen is fragmented into irregular remnants with sexual activity and childbearing.

The major *blood supply* to the vagina is from the vaginal artery, a branch of the hypogastric artery. The veins follow the path of the arteries.

The *vaginal wall* consists of a mucous membrane and an external muscular layer.

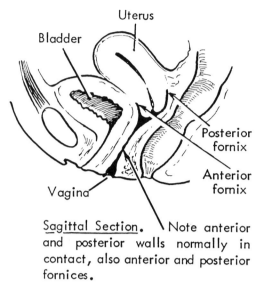

Uterus

Bladder

Posterior fornix

Anterior fornix

Vagina

Sagittal Section. Note anterior and posterior walls normally in contact, also anterior and posterior fornices.

Figure 3.7. Relationship of vagina to uterus and bladder.

The lumen is lined by a stratified squamous epithelium. Beneath this is a submucosal layer of connective tissue, which contains a rich supply of veins and lymphatics. Submucosal rugae throw the lumen of the vagina into a characteristic H shape in the young; these folds become less prominent with age. The muscular wall has three layers of smooth muscle. The vaginal wall is extremely distensible, especially during childbirth.

Uterus

The uterus is covered on each side by the two layers of the broad ligament, and it lies between the rectum and the bladder (Fig. 3.8). The two major portions of the uterus are the *cervix* and the body (*corpus*), which are separated by a narrower isthmus. Before puberty, the length of the cervix and the body are approximately equal; after puberty the ratio of the body to the cervix is between 2:1 and 3:1. The part of the body where the two uterine (fallopian) tubes enter is called the *cornu*. The part of the corpus above the cornu is termed the *fundus*. In the nonparous adult, the uterus is about 7–8 cm long and 4–5 cm wide at the widest part. The cervix is relatively cylindrical in shape and is 2–3 cm long. The corpus is generally pear shaped, with the anterior surface being flat and the posterior surface convex. In cross-section, the lumen of the corpus is triangular.

The normal position of the uterus is variable. The angle between the long axis of the corpus and the cervix varies from *anteflexion* to *retroflexion* and the angle between the cervix and the vagina varies from *anteversion* to *retroversion*. Unless caused by underlying pathology, these variations are normal. The uterus is supported by the uterosacral ligaments, the *cardinal ligaments*, the *round ligaments*, and the *broad ligaments*. The *blood supply* to the uterus comes primarily from the uterine and also from the ovarian arteries, whereas the venous plexus drains through the uterine vein (Fig. 3.9).

The *cervix* joins the vagina at an angle between 45 and 90°. The opening to the vagina, the external os, is round to oval in nonparous women, but is a transverse slit after childbirth. The portion of the cervix that projects into the vagina is covered with stratified squamous epithelium that resembles the vaginal epithelium. The squamous epithelium changes to a simple columnar epithelium in the *transition zone* (*transformation zone*). This zone is found at about the level of the external cervical os, although it is found higher in the endocervical canal in postmenopausal women. The importance of this zone in the process of neoplastic transformation is discussed in Chapter 42, "Cervical Neoplasia and Carcinoma."

There are *three basic layers in the wall of the uterine body*. The inner mucosa (the endometrium) consists of the simple columnar epithelium with underlying connective tissue. The changes in the structure of this layer that occur during the normal menstrual cycle are described in Chapter 44, "Endometrial Hyperplasia and Cancer." Beneath the musosa is a thick muscular layer (the myometrium), covered by a peritoneal serosa.

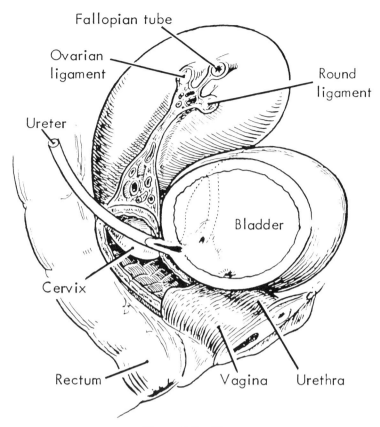

Figure 3.8. Uterus.

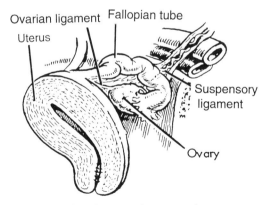

Figure 3.9. Ovary and associated structures.

Fallopian Tubes

The fallopian tubes (the oviducts) average about 7–14 cm in length. Each tube can be divided into *three portions*: a narrow and straight isthmus that adjoins the opening into the peritoneal cavity, the ampulla or central portion, and the finger-shaped fimbriae at the end, which surround the ovary and help to collect the oocyte at the time of ovulation. The epithelial lining of the fallopian tube is ciliated columnar. The cilia beat toward the uterus, assisting in oocyte transport.

Ovaries

Each ovary is about 3–5 cm long, 2–3 cm wide, and 1–3 cm during the menstrual years. The size decreases by about two thirds after the menopause, when follicular development ceases. The ovary is attached to the broad ligament by the mesovarium, to the uterus by the ovarian ligament, and to the side of the pelvis by the suspensory ligament of the ovary (infundibulopelvic ligament), which is

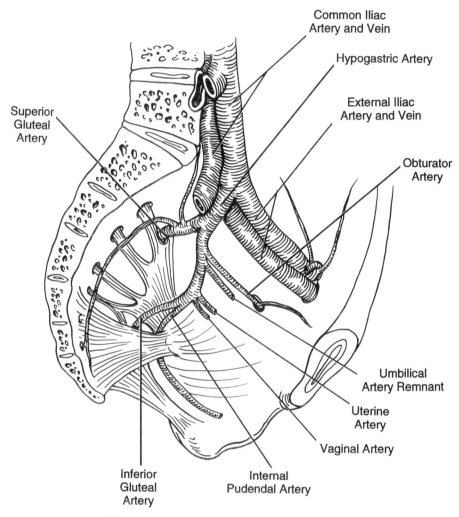

Figure 3.10. Arterial system of the female pelvis.

the lateral margin of the broad ligament (Fig. 3.9).

The outer ovarian cortex consists of follicles embedded in a connective tissue stroma. The connective tissue medulla contains smooth muscle fibers, blood vessels, nerves, and lymphatics.

The ovaries are mainly supplied by the ovarian arteries, which are direct branches of the abdominal aorta, but there also is a blood supply from the uterine artery, a branch of the hypogastric artery (internal iliac artery). Venous return via the right ovarian vein is directly into the inferior vena cava, and from the left ovary into the left renal vein (Fig. 3.10).

ANOMALIES OF THE FEMALE REPRODUCTIVE SYSTEM

Anatomic anomalies arise from defects during embryologic development and all occur very infrequently. Absence of the ovary is rare and usually associated with other genital tract anomalies. Ectopic ovarian tissue may occur, as supernumerary ovaries or as accessory ovarian tissue. In general, various kinds of uterine and vaginal malformations can arise from incomplete fusion of the paramesonephric ducts, incomplete development of one or both paramesonephric ducts, or incomplete canalization of the vaginal plate.

Absence of the uterus occurs when the paramesonephric ducts degenerate. This condition is associated with vaginal anomalies (such as absence of the vagina), because vaginal development is stimulated by the developing uterovaginal primordium. A double uterus (uterus didelphys) occurs when the inferior parts of the paramesonephric ducts do not fuse; this condition may be associated with a double or a single vagina. A bicornuate uterus results when lack of fusion is limited to the superior portion of the uterine body. If one of the paramesonephric ducts is poorly developed and fusion with the other duct does not occur, the result is a bicornuate uterus with a rudimentary horn. This horn may or may not communicate with the uterine cavity.

Absence of the vagina occurs when the vaginal plate does not develop. It is usually coupled with the absence of the uterus. If the vaginal plate does not canalize, the result is vaginal atresia. Imperforate hymen is a minor example of this.

REPRODUCTIVE GENETICS

Genetics is an integral part of obstetric care. Obstetricians must identify women at increased risk for fetal abnormalities and offer appropriate genetic screening and testing to appropriate patients. This section reviews current indications and techniques of genetic screening and testing applicable to the pregnant patient.

Genetic Counseling

Genetic counseling serves two important functions: (*a*) to obtain information from the patient in order to properly assess her risk for developing disease and for being delivered of an infant with congenital abnormalities; and (*b*) to provide information to the patient regarding appropriate screening or diagnostic tests. Data forms, questionnaires, pedigree construction, and patient interviews are all effective methods for obtaining information concerning personal and family medical history, parental exposure to potentially harmful

substances, or other issues that may impact on risk assessment. No single method or combination thereof is universally effective in obtaining all appropriate patient information. The specific methods used to gather information depend on the type of information required and the availability of trained personnel.

Genetic counseling should never be used to coerce a patient to undergo or forego certain tests or pregnancy management decisions: Information should be obtained and provided in a "nondirective" fashion so that the counselor acts in a completely objective manner, never interjecting his or her own personal opinions into the counseling session. Patients may then arrive at reproductive decisions based on their own values, ethics, and desires and not on those of the counselor. In addition to decisions concerning genetic screening or testing, counselors must be able to review alternative reproductive options (e.g., pregnancy termination, permanent sterilization, selective pregnancy reduction, donor insemination) with their patients in an empathetic yet nondirective manner.

Chromosome Abnormalities

In the United States, the most common indication for invasive prenatal diagnostic testing is increased risk for fetal chromosome abnormalities. Chromosome abnormalities (Table 3.2) also play an important role in spontaneous abortion and infertility; at least 50–60% of first trimester spontaneous abortions, 5% of stillbirths, and 2–3% of couples experiencing multiple miscarriage or infertility will be found to have an abnormal chromosome complement. Overall, 0.6% of all liveborn infants have a chromosome abnormality.

Couples who desire chromosome analysis because of a history of multiple miscarriage or infertility are evaluated by cytogenetic analysis of cultured lymphocytes obtained from their peripheral blood (Fig. 3.11). However, determination of fetal chromosome complement is not as simple or safe because obtaining fetal cells involves invasive

Table 3.2
Common Cytogenetic Abnormalities

Chromosome abnormality	Livebirth incidence	Characteristics
Trisomy 21 (Down syndrome)	1/800	Moderate to severe mental retardation; characteristic facies; cardiac abnormalities; increased incidence of respiratory infections and leukemia; only 2% live beyond 50 years
Trisomy 18 (Edwards syndrome)	1/8,000	Severe mental retardation; multiple organic abnormalities; less than 10% survive 1 year
Trisomy 13 (Patau syndrome)	1/20,000	Severe mental retardation; neurologic, ophthalmologic, and organic abnormalities; less than 5% survive 3 years
Trisomy 16	0	Lethal anomaly occurs frequently in first trimester spontaneous abortions; no infants are known to have trisomy 16
45,X (Turner syndrome)	1/10,000	Occurs frequently in first trimester spontaneous abortions; associated primarily with unique somatic features; patients are not mentally retarded, although IQ of affected individuals is lower than sibs
47,XXX 47,XYY 47,XYY 47,XXY (Klinefelter syndrome)	each approximately 1/900	Minimal somatic abnormalities; individuals with Klinefelter syndrome are characterized by a tall, eunuchoid habitus and small testes. 47,XXX and 47,XYY individuals do not usually exhibit somatic abnormalities, but 47,XYY individuals may be tall and may exhibit social pathology
del(5p) (cri-du-chat syndrome)	1/20,000	Severe mental retardation; microcephaly; distinctive facial features; characteristic "cat's cry" sound

procedures that increase fetal morbidity and mortality. Fetal chromosome analysis, either of continuing pregnancies or of spontaneous or induced abortions, is currently performed on cells obtained from amniotic fluid, placenta (chorionic villi), or fetal tissue. The procedures used to obtain these specimens are described later in this section.

INDICATIONS FOR PRENATAL CYTOGENETIC ANALYSIS
Advanced Maternal Age

The most common indication for invasive prenatal diagnosis is advanced maternal age. The incidence of Down syndrome among newborns is approximately 1:800; however, the incidence of Down syndrome among newborns delivered to 35-year-old women is 1:385, and the incidence among 45-year-old women is 1:33. Down syndrome is not the only chromosome abnormality that increases in frequency with advanced maternal age; other autosomal trisomies and some sex chromosome polysomies (Table 3.2) increase in incidence as parturients get older. In the

United States, it is now standard obstetric practice to offer all women who are 35 years old or older at their estimated day of delivery invasive prenatal diagnostic testing to detect fetal chromosome abnormalities.

The incidence of fetal chromosome abnormalities is higher at midtrimester (e.g., 16th week gestation) than at term because many chromosomally abnormal fetuses will be aborted spontaneously after the 16th gestational week. It is therefore important to use consistently either midtrimester or liveborn data when counseling patients concerning risks for fetal chromosome abnormalities.

Previous Child with Chromosome Abnormality

Women who have been delivered of a trisomic child may be at increased risk for subsequent trisomy. If a woman is younger than 30 years old at the time of delivery, the recurrence risk for a subsequent trisomic newborn is estimated to be 1–2%. However, if a woman is 30 years old or older and is delivered of a trisomic infant, the risk for subse-

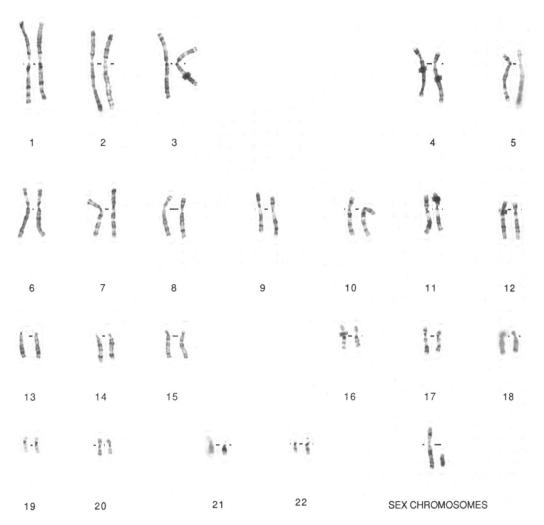

1   2   3   4   5

6   7   8   9   10   11   12

13   14   15   16   17   18

19   20   21   22   SEX CHROMOSOMES

Figure 3.11. Normal (46,XY) metaphase spread of a cultured lymphocyte obtained from peripheral blood. Metaphases from other cell types have the same appearance.

quent trisomy is maintained at the estimated maternal age risk. It remains unclear whether delivery of a trisomic abortus or stillbirth also confers a similar increase in risk.

Parental Chromosome Abnormality

Although an unbalanced parental chromosome complement is a rare occurrence, a balanced parental chromosome rearrangement is not uncommon. Approximately 4% of Down syndrome children are the result of an unbalanced robertsonian translocation (see below) between chromosome 21 and either chromosome 13, 14, 15, 21, or 22. Although 60% of these unbalanced translocations are the result of a de novo, i.e., new rearrangement, the other 40% are the result of an *unbalanced* gamete inherited from a parent with a *balanced* chromosome rearrangement (Fig. 3.12).

Three types of parental chromosome rearrangements that can result in chromosomally abnormal offspring are robertsonian translocations, reciprocal translocations, and inversions. Robertsonian translocations involve

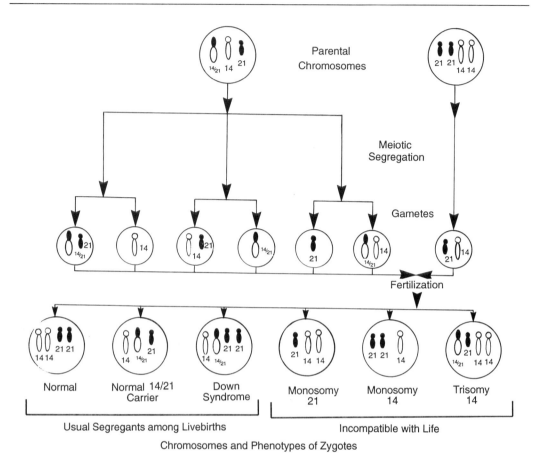

Chromosomes and Phenotypes of Zygotes

Figure 3.12. Possible gametic products of a parental balanced translocation. Although theoretical risk for abnormal liveborns is 33%, the empiric risk is frequently lower.

the two groups of acrocentric chromosomes, namely the D group (chromosomes 13, 14, and 15) and the G group (chromosomes 21 and 22); it is this type of balanced parental translocation that most frequently results in Down syndrome in offspring. The theoretical risk for a parent who has a balanced robertsonian translocation involving chromosome 21 to have a child with Down syndrome is 33%. However, the actual risk for Down syndrome in offspring is dependent on which parent has the translocation and the chromosomes involved. For example, if the mother carries a balanced robertsonian translocation involving chromosomes 14 and 21 $(45,XX, -14, -21, +t(14q;21q))$, the risk is approximately 10%, whereas if the father carries the same translocation, the risk is 1%

or less. In addition, if the balanced translocation involves two number 21 chromosomes, the risk for Down syndrome in liveborns is 100%, irrespective of which parent carries the translocation.

Balanced reciprocal translocations may involve any chromosome and are the result of a reciprocal "trade" of chromosome material between two or more chromosomes. This results in a rearranged complement characterized by the same amount of genetic material found in a "normal" complement. Similar to robertsonian translocations, empiric risk for newborn chromosome abnormality is less than the theoretical risk (33%). However, unlike robertsonian translocations, empiric risk of newborn chromosome abnormalities is approximately 11%, irrespective of which

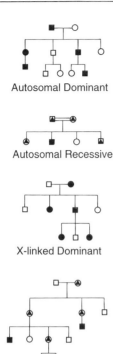

Autosomal Dominant

Autosomal Recessive

X-linked Dominant

X-linked Recessive

□   Males
○   Females
■● Affected
□○ Unaffected but heterozygous
═   Consanguineous

Figure 3.13. Patterns of familial transmission expected for autosomal dominant, autosomal recessive, X-linked recessive, and X-linked dominant inheritance.

parent carries the translocation or the chromosomes involved.

Detection of a parental inversion resulting in fetal or newborn chromosome abnormalities is rare, despite the relatively common occurrence of certain specific inversions (e.g., inv9(p11q13)) in the population. Such commonly occurring inversions do not apparently place couples at increased risk for chromosome abnormalities in offspring. Empiric data for unique inversions that result in chromosomally unbalanced progeny are unavailable; theoretical risks are dependent on whether the centromere is involved and the size of the inverted portion.

Screening Tests

In addition to the aforementioned indications, results from noninvasive screening techniques such as ultrasonography and maternal serum screening for Down syndrome (including measurement of maternal serum levels of α-fetoprotein (AFP), human chorionic gonadotropin (hCG), and/or unconjugated estriol (uE3)) may prompt a woman to consider invasive prenatal diagnostic testing. A thorough discussion of the particular protocol used to detect women at increased risk for Down syndrome or other chromosome abnormalities should be undertaken, as results may significantly alter pregnancy management.

Mendelian Disorders

Mendelian disorders result from mutations of specific genes. Expression of a disease or trait may result from expression of a single gene at a specific genetic locus on an autosomal chromosome (autosomal dominant) (Fig. 3.13) or may require expression of two genes at an autosomal locus (autosomal recessive) (Fig. 3.13). In addition, those genes located on the X chromosome that result in specific disorders or traits are known as "X-linked"; X-linked conditions may also be dominant or recessive. As males have only one X chromosome, those males possessing a single X-linked gene that is associated with a recessive condition will express that condition despite having only a single copy of the gene (hemizygosity) (Fig. 3.13). Expression of the same condition in females would require two copies of the same gene.

A plethora of mendelian disorders and traits have been described, and a description of them is beyond the scope of this section. Many mendelian disorders occur more frequently in certain groups (e.g., sickle cell diseases in blacks, cystic fibrosis in whites, Tay-Sachs disease in Ashkenazic Jews, β-thalassemia in southern Europeans and α-thalassemia in Asians) and usually have frequencies of less than 1:1000 in the at-risk group. Although screening for certain mendelian disorders is now available (e.g., sickle cell disease, Tay-Sachs disease, thalassemia) or is being developed (e.g., cystic fibrosis), couples found to be at risk for having children affected with most mendelian disorders are usually discovered as a result of a history of affected offspring or relatives. In addition, increased paternal age (usually 50 years old or older) has been shown to place couples at increased risk for new mutations, e.g., autosomal dominant disorders like achondroplasia or Marfan syndrome. Counseling thus plays a critical role in determining risk for a couple having a child with a specific mendelian disorder; information that better defines a couple's risk for affected offspring includes other family members with mendelian conditions or conditions similar to mendelian disorders and the race, religion, or national origin of relatives. This information helps reassess risk and permit couples undergoing screening tests to further delineate their risk or, in appropriate situations, to undergo invasive prenatal testing.

Prenatal detection of many mendelian disorders is now possible as result of recent advances in molecular biology. The association of certain DNA sequences (adenine, guanine, cytosine, and guanine) arranged in specific sequences and lengths is called a restriction fragment length polymorphism (RFLP). RFLPs are not genes that cause disorders, but rather are sequences physically close to the actual genes; the number and constitution of RFLPs differ among individuals. The association of certain RFLPs with specific mendelian disorders has permitted us to prenatally diagnose mendelian disorders, albeit using a nonabsolute mathematical algorithm determining the "linkage" or proximity of a specific RFLP to a specific gene. The sensitivity of RFLP analysis depends on the proximity of the RFLP to the gene; that is, the closer the RFLP to the gene in question, the more sensitive the analysis. It is therefore important to recognize the presence of a RFLP does not always indicate presence of a mutant gene, and conversely, absence of the same does not always indicate a disease-free state. More recently, direct detection of specific gene mutations, detection of abnormal proteins associated with specific diseases, and gene sequencing have permitted us to directly diagnose certain mendelian disorders (e.g., sickle cell disease) without the inherent inaccuracies of RFLP analysis.

Irrespective of the specific DNA analytic method used, all DNA tests require recovery of DNA; this is accomplished by obtaining nucleated cells. For DNA analysis of newborns, children, or adults, nucleated cells are easily recoverable from peripheral blood samples. However, prenatal DNA analyses require fetal nucleated cells, and obtaining fetal cells is currently performed by chorionic villus sampling (CVS), amniocentesis, or percutaneous umbilical blood sampling (PUBS). As sequences of more genes are delineated, diagnosis of mendelian disorders heretofore undetectable will be possible.

Polygenic/Multifactorial Disorders

Certain relatively common disorders result in a 2–5% recurrence risk if first-degree relatives (parents, siblings, children) are affected. Such recurrence risks suggest a polygenic/multifactorial etiology in which undetermined genes and environmental stimuli are involved in disease expression. Many of these disorders are manifest by anatomical abnormalities. Some examples include: cardiac anomalies such as ventricular and atrial septal defects and hypoplastic left heart syndrome; gastrointestinal anomalies including omphalocele, small bowel atresia, and diaphragmatic hernia; and urologic anomalies including renal agenesis and ureteropelvic junction obstruction.

An example of polygenic/multifactorial disorder is neural tube defects, a group of disorders that occurs relatively frequently in populations in both the United Kingdom and United States. The spectrum of neural tube defects ranges from anencephaly (absence of a portion or all of the forebrain) to spina bifida (spinal column closure defects). Neural tube defects occur in approximately 1 in 1500 births in the United States; however, in certain regions of the United States, neural tube defects occur more frequently (1 in 750 livebirths), whereas in some parts of the United Kingdom, the rate is 1 in 200 livebirths. Fetal neural tube defects are prenatally diagnosed by ultrasonography and α-fetoprotein and acetylcholinesterase assays of amniotic fluid obtained by amniocentesis. However, approximately 85% of newborns with neural tube defects are born to women with no family or medication history that would have indicated their being at increased risk and resulted in their being offered amniocentesis.

Fortunately, we are now able to offer all low risk women, between 15 and 20 weeks gestation, a screening blood test that measures maternal serum levels of α-fetoprotein (MSAFP), the fetal protein that is elevated in the amniotic fluid in cases of open fetal neural tube defect and which has been found to be elevated in the serum of most women carrying fetuses with open neural tube defects. However, as with most screening tests, many women found to have elevated MSAFP levels are not carrying an affected fetus. Accordingly, physicians and health care professionals who provide MSAFP screening must inform their patients of possible false-positive and false-negative results, as well as availability of further diagnostic testing if screening results are abnormal.

Invasive Prenatal Diagnostic Procedures

Amniocentesis has been used for prenatal diagnosis for almost 20 years. The procedure involves removing, usually under concurrent ultrasound guidance, 20–40 ml of amniotic fluid. Traditionally, amniocentesis is performed between 15 and 20 weeks gestation. Cytogenetic and DNA analysis of amniotic fluid specimens requires culture of amniotic fluid cells, as most cells obtained from amniocentesis are not in metaphase and the number of viable cells is relatively small. Direct analysis of the amniotic fluid supernatant (amniotic fluid liquor) is possible for α-fetoprotein and acetylcholinesterase assays; such analyses permit detection of fetal neural tube defects and other fetal structural defects (e.g., omphalocele, gastroschisis). In addition, some centers have begun to perform amniocentesis before 15 weeks gestation; however, the safety and accuracy of "early amniocentesis" are still undetermined.

Chorionic villus sampling was developed to provide early prenatal diagnosis. CVS is performed by transcervical or transabdominal aspiration of chorionic villi (immature placenta) under concurrent ultrasound guidance, usually between 9 and 12 weeks gestation. Recent multicenter trials have demonstrated CVS to have similar safety and accuracy to that of "traditional" (i.e., performed at or after 15 weeks gestation) amniocentesis. Another benefit of CVS is direct, and therefore rapid, cytogenetic and DNA analysis; this is possible because cytotrophoblasts obtained from first trimester placentas are more likely to be viable and in metaphase than amniotic fluid cells. However, disorders that require analysis of amniotic fluid liquor, such as neural tube defects, are not amenable to prenatal diagnosis by CVS.

Percutaneous umbilical blood sampling is usually performed after 20 weeks gestation and is used to obtain fetal blood for blood component analyses (e.g., hematocrit, Rh status, platelet count), as well as cytogenetic and DNA analyses. One major benefit of PUBS is the ability to obtain rapid (18–24 hours) fetal karyotypes. However, the safety of PUBS remains undetermined; accordingly, PUBS should not be utilized when amniocentesis or CVS can obtain similar diagnostic results in a timely fashion.

Other prenatal diagnostic procedures include fetal skin sampling, fetal tissue (muscle, liver) biopsy, and fetoscopy. These procedures are used only for the diagnosis of rare disorders not amenable to diagnosis by less invasive methods.

Teratogenesis

Teratogenesis is the development of fetal defects as a result of maternal exposure to specific compounds (agents) in the environment. Potential teratogenetic agents range from viruses and bacteria to heavy metals and organic compounds. Some agents are obviously teratogenetic (e.g., isotretinoin); other agents are not. Determination of teratogenicity of a specific agent is frequently difficult, and counseling women exposed to a particular agent is invariably incomplete. Many agents will be teratogenetic in some species, but not in others; for example, cortisol causes cleft palate in mice but not in humans. In addition, some agents may be teratogenetic only at certain doses, at certain stages of embryonic or fetal development, in combination with other specific agents, or in specific groups or populations more susceptible to the agent's embryotoxic effects than other groups or populations. Despite the inherent difficulty in arriving at an accurate risk assessment, a thorough review of maternal drug ingestion and environmental exposure is essential to estimate a woman's risk for fetal malformation and should be a part of the initial antenatal assessment, along with family and medical-surgical history.

Future Trends

The ultimate prenatal diagnostic test would have high sensitivity and specificity, but would not increase maternal or fetal morbidity and mortality. To this end, several centers are currently attempting to identify and isolate fetal cells in maternal circulation. If fetal cells can be isolated from maternal blood, and if these cells can be analyzed for cytogenetic and mendelian disorders, a noninvasive method for prenatal screening, and possibly diagnosis, would be possible. Even if fetal cells can be consistently isolated from maternal blood, the clinical application of this technology is years away; however, initial results are promising.

Ethics

Our increasing ability to detect fetal abnormalities by ultrasound and invasive prenatal diagnostic techniques has permitted couples to make pregnancy management decisions in cases in which fetal abnormalities are detected. However, our ability to detect fetal sex and other nonlethal characteristics creates a great ethical dilemma; that is, to what extent should prenatal diagnostic techniques be used to prenatally identify fetal characteristics, and which characteristics, traits, or disorders are appropriate for prenatal diagnosis. Accordingly, new applications of current prenatal diagnostic techniques and development of new prenatal diagnostic modalities should be undertaken only with due consideration of the ethical, moral, and social ramifications of such new applications or technologies.

FURTHER READINGS

Elias S, Annas GJ. Reproductive genetics and the law. Chicago: Year Book, 1987.

Gelehrter TD, Collins FS. Principles of medical genetics. Baltimore: Williams & Wilkins, 1990.

Simpson JL, Golbus MS. Genetics in obstetrics and gynecology, 2nd ed. Philadelphia: WB Saunders, 1992.

chapter 4

MATERNAL-FETAL PHYSIOLOGY

MATERNAL PHYSIOLOGY

There are many normal physiologic changes in pregnancy. Some mimic the signs, symptoms, or laboratory findings of disease in the nonpregnant patient, yet are normal in pregnancy. Therefore, knowledge of normal maternal physiology will help avoid unnecessary diagnostic or therapeutic interventions.

Gastrointestinal Changes

One of the earliest symptoms of pregnancy is *nausea and vomiting* or *"morning sickness."* Morning sickness typically begins between 4 and 8 weeks of gestational age and abates by the middle of the second trimester, usually by 14–16 weeks. Although the exact etiology of this nausea is unknown, it appears related to elevated levels of progesterone, human chorionic gonadotropin (hCG), and also to relaxation of the smooth muscle of the stomach. There are usually no significant nutritional deficits or weight loss associated with this distressing but transient symptom complex (Table 4.1).

Treatment consists primarily of reassurance, frequent small meals, and inclusion of bland foods as well as avoidance of those foods found to exacerbate the nausea and vomiting. If the symptoms persist beyond the middle of the second trimester or if there is an associated weight loss, ketonemia, and electrolyte imbalance at any time, the diagnosis of *hyperemesis gravidarum* should be considered. Patients with this severe nausea and vomiting must be hospitalized to receive parenteral fluid replacement and electrolytes. Environmental stressors and/or other psychological underpinning are common in

these patients, and evaluation should attempt to assess these and reduce them, if possible.

Despite the gastrointestinal upset seen in early pregnancy, many patients report *dietary cravings* during pregnancy. Some may be due to the patient's perception that a particular food may help with nausea and heartburn. *Pica* is an especially intense craving for such things as ice, laundry starch, or clay. Other patients develop dietary aversions during pregnancy. *Ptyalism* is perceived to be the excessive production of saliva but probably represents the inability of a nauseated patient to swallow the normal amounts of saliva that are produced.

In general, there is *decreased gastrointestinal motility* during pregnancy due to increasing levels of progesterone. As a result, gastric emptying time is prolonged and there is decreased esophageal tone and incompetence of the esophageal-stomach sphincter. The result is gastric reflux and heartburn, a common complaint in pregnancy. Gallbladder function is also delayed in pregnancy with the subsequent cholestasis resulting in an increased ten-

Table 4.1
Key Gastrointestinal Changes in Pregnancy

Appetite	Usually *increased*, sometimes with unusual *cravings* (pica)
Gastric reflux	Caused by cardiac *sphincter* relaxation and *anatomic displacement*
Gastric motility	*Decreases*
Intestinal transit time	*Slower*
Liver	Functionally *unchanged*
Gallbladder	*Dilated*
Bile composition	*Unchanged*

Table 4.2
Key Pulmonary Changes in Pregnancy

Oxygen requirement	Increased		
Carbon dioxide pressure		Decreased	
Oxygen pressure	Increased		
Arterial pH			Unchanged
Tidal volume	Increased		
Expiratory reserve volume		Decreased	
Residual volume		Decreased	
Inspiratory capacity	Increased		
Vital capacity	Increased		
Minute volume	Increased		

dency to form gallstones. Elevated liver enzymes and lowered serum protein levels are seen with resultant signs of spider angioma and palmar erythema, which are commonly found in association with liver disease. Mild elevations of alkaline phosphatase are seen as is a fall in serum albumin. Serum cholesterol levels are increased during pregnancy.

Pulmonary Changes

Pregnancy-related changes of the respiratory systems are the result of both anatomic and functional changes (Table 4.2). Mucosal hyperemia results in marked nasal stuffiness and an increased amount of nasal secretions. Patients often complain of allergy-like symptoms or chronic colds. Anatomically, there are also pregnancy-induced accommodations for the enlarging uterus. The subcostal angle increases from 68 to 103°, the chest circumference increases up to 7 cm and the chest diameter increases 1–2 cm. There is increased diaphragmatic excursion and the diaphragm is elevated approximately 4 cm.

Pulmonary functions are altered in pregnancy. There is a 30–40% increase in tidal volume. Inspiratory capacity increases approximately 5%, with respiratory rate, vital capacity, and inspiratory reserve remaining the same as in the nonpregnant state. The functional residual capacity, expiratory volume, and residual volume are all decreased by approximately 20%. The total lung capacity is also decreased by 5% with a resulting increase and minute ventilation of 30–40%. Arterial blood gases reflect this change in pulmonary function in the following ways: oxygen is increased, carbon dioxide is decreased, and serum bicarbonate is reduced. In summary, there is a mild respiratory alkalosis with the patient being aware of dyspnea, hyperventilation, and a relative decrease in exercise tolerance.

Cardiovascular Changes

The dramatic changes in the maternal cardiovascular system during pregnancy improve oxygenation and flow of nutrition to the fetus. (Table 4.3). Cardiac output increases up to 50% as a result of an increase in both heart rate and stroke volume. Particularly late in pregnancy, however, cardiac output may be decreased because of maternal position. In the supine position, the inferior vena cava is compressed by the enlarged uterus, resulting in decreased venous return to the heart with decreased cardiac output. Although most women do not become overtly hypotensive when lying supine, some may have symptoms including dizziness, lightheadedness, and syncopy. This is often termed the *"inferior vena cava syndrome."*

Due to the smooth muscle relaxing effect of increased levels of progesterone during pregnancy, *peripheral vascular resistance* is decreased. There is a decrease in arterial *blood pressure* during the first 24 weeks of pregnancy with a gradual rise returning to nonpregnant levels by term. Blood pressures higher than the nonpregnant values for a par-

Table 4.3
Key Cardiovascular Changes in Pregnancy

	Increased	Decreased	Unchanged
Blood flow			
Uterus	Increased		
Kidneys	Increased		
Breasts	Increased		
Skin	Increased		
Brain			Unchanged
Circulating tissue			Unchanged
Blood pressure			
Peripheral resistance		Decreased	
Arterial blood pressure[a]			
Systolic			Unchanged
Diastolic			
Venous pressure			
Arms			Unchanged
Legs	Increased		
Pulmonary blood pressure			Unchanged
Heart			
Size	Increased		
Cardiac output	Increased		
Stroke volume	Increased		
Rhythm: extrasystoles common			
Murmurs: systolic and diastolic common			
Electrocardiogram (ECG): changes due to positional changes			

[a]Decreased midpregnancy; increases third trimester to nonpregnant levels at term.

ticular patient should be considered abnormal.

Because the cardiovascular system is in a hyperdynamic state, normal physical findings on *cardiovascular examination* during pregnancy include an increased second heart sound split with inspiration, distended neck veins, and low grade systolic ejection murmurs. Most normal pregnant women will have an S_3 gallop or third heart sound after midpregnancy. Systolic ejection murmurs are felt to be caused by a normal increased blood flow across the aortic and pulmonic valves. Diastolic murmurs should not be considered normal findings in pregnancy.

Anatomically, the heart is displaced upward and to the left. Because the diaphragms are elevated and because the heart is in a more horizontal position, chest x-rays might appear to demonstrate cardiomegaly when no such abnormality exists.

During the course of *labor*, cardiac output increases approximately 40% above that in late pregnancy. Much of this is a result of pain and apprehension, as these findings are significantly reduced when a patient has an epidural anesthetic administered. Mean arterial blood pressure rises approximately 10 mm Hg during each contraction unless adequate analgesia is provided. Immediately *postpartum*, because the obstruction to venous return is released and because extracellular fluid is quickly mobilized, cardiac output increases 10–20%.

Hematologic Changes

Maternal *plasma volume* begins to increase as early as the sixth week of pregnancy and reaches maximum at approximately 30–34 weeks, after which it is stable. The mean increase in plasma volume is approximately 50% with a greater increase in patients with multiple gestation. Similarly, larger babies are associated with a greater increase of maternal plasma volume, whereas a pregnancy complicated by intrauterine growth retardation is often associated with a less than normal increase in blood volume.

Table 4.4
Key Hematologic and Biochemical Changes in Pregnancy

Hematologic			
Plasma volume	Increased		
Hemoglobin concentration		Decreased	
Hematocrit		Decreased	
Total erythrocyte volume	Increased		
Mean cell volume	Increased		
Erythrocyte sedimentation rate	Increased		
Serum iron		Decreased	
Total iron binding capacity	Increased		
Serum transferrin	Increased		
Serum ferritin		Decreased	
Clotting			
Fibrinogen (factor I)	Increased		
Factor VII, VIII, X	Increased		
Factor IV, VII	Increased		
Factor IX, XII		Decreased	
Fibrin	Increased		
Fibrinogen degradation products	Increased		
Biochemical			
Blood glucose			
Fasting		Decreased	
Postprandial	Increased		
Sodium		Decreased	
Potassium		Decreased	
Bicarbonate		Decreased	
Blood urea nitrogen (first trimester) increases toward term		Decreased	
Creatinine (first trimester) increases toward term		Decreased	
Uric acid (first trimester) increases toward term		Decreased	
Total lipids	Increased		
Cholesterol	Increased		
Total protein		Decreased	
Albumin		Decreased	
Osmolality		Decreased	
Lactic acid dehydrogenase (LDH)			Unchanged
Glutamic oxaloacetic transaminase (GOT)			Unchanged
Glutamic pyruvic transaminase (GPT)			Unchanged
Alkaline phosphatase	Increased		
Amylase			Unchanged

Red cell mass begins to increase later in pregnancy and increases to a lesser degree than does plasma volume. As a result, there is a "physiologic" anemia due to dilution of approximately 15% compared to nonpregnancy levels. Whereas erythrocyte volume increases by approximately 18% without iron supplementation, it can increase up to 30% when iron supplements are utilized. After 30–34 weeks, the hematocrit may increase somewhat as erythrocyte volume continues to increase while plasma volume is stable (Table 4.4).

White blood cell (WBC) counts also rise as pregnancy advances. This progressive increase may reach 20,000/ml during the late third trimester. During labor, the WBC count may further rise to 30,000/ml with a return to nonpregnant levels during the puerperium. The increase in the WBC count is due primarily to an increased number of granulocytes. Platelet counts during pregnancy may decline slightly but remain within the normal range of those of nonpregnant patients.

Pregnancy is considered a hypercoaguable state with an increased risk of *venous thromboembolism* both during pregnancy and the puerperium. The risk of thromboembolism is approximately two times normal during pregnancy and rises to 5.5 times normal during the puerperium. Fibrinogen (factor I) increases to a level of 400–500 mg/dl. There is an increase in fibrin split products and in factors VII, VIII, IX, and X. Prothrombin (factor II) and factors V and XII remain unchanged during pregnancy. *Bleeding time and clotting time* do not change during a normal pregnancy.

The normal pregnant patient requires a total of 1000 mg of additional iron: 500 mg are used to increase maternal red cell mass, 300 mg are transported to the fetus, and the additional 200 mg are utilized to compensate for normal iron loss. Iron use in pregnancy is intended to prevent iron deficiency in the mother. It is not intended to either prevent iron deficiency in the fetus or maintain maternal hemoglobin concentration. Since iron is actively transported to the fetus, fetal hemoglobin levels will be maintained despite maternal anemia. To supply their needs, 60 mg of elemental iron is recommended daily for the nonanemic patient. This is provided in 300 mg of ferrous sulfate. Patients who are anemic should receive twice this dose.

Renal Changes

Kidneys enlarge about 1 cm during pregnancy as measured on intravenous pyelography or ultrasonography. This is due to an increase in interstitial volume as well as distended renal vasculature. Both the renal pelves as well as the ureters are dilated during pregnancy due to the relaxing effect of progesterone. Typically, the right ureter is more dilated than the left. Mechanical compression of the ureters, both by the ovarian venous plexus as well as the enlarging uterus, contributes to uretal dilation. Because progesterone also decreases *bladder* tone, there is increased residual volume and, with the dilated collecting system, urinary stasis results, predisposing to an increased incidence of pyelonephritis in patients with asympto-

Table 4.5
Key Renal Changes in Pregnancy

Renal plasma flow	Increased	
Glomerular filtration rate	Increased	
Urinary output		Unchanged
Renin	Increased	
Angiotensin I and II	Increased	
Renin substrate	Increased	
24-h protein excretion		Unchanged

matic bacteriuria. There is also loss of urinary control as pregnancy advances due to the enlarging uterus. Bladder capacity decreases resulting in urinary frequency (Table 4.5).

Renal plasma flow (RPF) begins to increase early in the first trimester and increases to as much as 75% over nonpregnant levels at term. Similarly, *glomerular filtration rate (GFR)* increases to 50% over the nonpregnant state. The *creatinine clearance* is markedly increased in pregnancy with 150–200 ml/min being considered normal. Serum levels of creatinine, uric acid, and blood urea nitrogen decrease in normal pregnancy. *Plasma osmolality* is decreased primarily due to reduction in the serum *sodium concentration.* The tendency to lose sodium due to the increased GFR and the elevated levels of progesterone are compensated for by an increase in renal tubule reabsorption of sodium as well as by the increased levels of aldosterone, estrogen, and desoxycorticosterone. The plasma renin activity is up to 10 times that of the nonpregnant state. Similarly, renin substrate (angiotensinogen) is increased approximately fivefold. Angiotensin levels are also increased approximately fivefold. During pregnancy, the body retains approximately 1000 mEq of sodium in the fetus, placenta, and maternal intravascular and extracellular fluid spaces. Normal pregnant patients are relatively resistant to the hypertensive effects of the increased levels of renin-angiotensin-aldosterone whereas patients with hypertensive disease of pregnancy are not.

Because of the increase in GFR, there is a greatly increased load of glucose presented to the renal tubules. As a result, *glucose excretion* increases in virtually all pregnant patients.

Therefore, quantitative urine glucose measurements are not clinically useful in managing patients with diabetes, as they do not reflect blood glucose levels.

There is no significant increase in *protein loss* in the urine during pregnancy. There are increases in urinary excretion of *vitamin B_{12}* and folate.

Skin Changes

During pregnancy, *vascular spiders* (spider angiomata) are most common on the upper torso, face, and arms. *Palmar erythema* occurs in over half of patients. Both are due to increased levels of circulating estrogen and regress after delivery. *Striae gravidarum* can be either purple or pink initially and appear on the lower abdomen, breasts, and thighs. They are not related to weight gain but solely due to the stretching of normal skin. There is no effective therapy to prevent these "stretch marks" nor can they be eliminated once they appear. They do eventually become white or silvery in color.

Hyperpigmentation is felt to be due to elevated levels of estrogen and melanocyte-stimulating hormone. It commonly affects the umbilicus and perineum, although it may affect any skin surface. The lower abdomen linea alba darkens to become the linea nigra. The "mask of pregnancy," or *chloasma* (melasma), is also common. *Skin nevi* can increase in size and in pigmentation but resolve after pregnancy. Removal of rapidly changing nevi is recommended during pregnancy. *Eccrine sweating* and *sebum production* are increased during normal pregnancy, with many patients complaining of *acne*. Melasma may never disappear completely.

Hair growth during pregnancy is maintained. The anagen (growth) phase normally lasts up to 6 years. Fewer follicles are in the telogen (resting) phase. Late in pregnancy, the number of hairs in telogen is approximately one half of the normal 20% so that postpartum, the number of hairs entering telogen increases with a result in significant hair loss 2–4 months after pregnancy. Hair growth typically returns to normal 6–12 months after delivery.

Breast Changes

Blood flow increases to the breast as the breasts develop to support lactation. Some patients may complain of breast tenderness and a tingling sensation. Estrogen stimulation also results in ductal growth with alveolar hypertrophy a result of progesterone stimulation. Montgomery's follicles, the small elevations surrounding the areolae, enlarge and become more prominent during pregnancy. During the latter portion of pregnancy, a thick yellow fluid can be expressed from the nipples. This *colostrum* is more common in parous women. Ultimately, lactation will be dependent upon synergistic actions of estrogen, progesterone, prolactin, human placental lactogen, cortisol, and insulin.

Musculoskeletal Changes

As pregnancy progresses, a compensatory lumbar lordosis is apparent. As a result, virtually all women complain of low back pain. Beginning early in pregnancy, the effects of relaxin and progesterone result in a relative laxity of the ligaments. The pubic symphysis separates at approximately 28–30 weeks. Patients often complain of an unsteady gait and may fall more commonly during pregnancy than during the nonpregnant state as a result of both these changes and an altered center of gravity.

To provide for adequate calcium supplies to the fetal skeleton, mobilization of calcium stores occurs. Maternal serum ionized calcium is unchanged from the nonpregnant state, but maternal total serum calcium decreases. There is a significant increase in maternal parathyroid hormone, which acts to maintain serum calcium levels by increasing absorption from the intestine and decreasing the loss of calcium through the kidney. The skeleton is well maintained despite these elevated levels of parathyroid hormones. This may be due to the effect of calcitonin. Although the rate of bone turnover increases, there is no loss of bone density during a normal pregnancy.

Ophthalmic Changes

The most common visual complaint of pregnant women is blurred vision. This is due primarily to swelling of the lens and resolves after pregnancy. Changes in corrective lens prescriptions should therefore not be encouraged during pregnancy.

Reproductive Tract and Abdominal Wall Changes

The effects of pregnancy on the *vulva* are similar to the effects on other skin. Because of an increase in vascularity, *vulvar varicosities* are very common. These usually regress after delivery. An increase in vaginal transudation as well as stimulation of the vaginal mucosa result in a thick profuse *vaginal discharge*. The epithelium of the endocervix everts onto the ectocervix with an associated mucous plug being produced. The *uterus* undergoes an enormous increase in weight from a 70 g nonpregnant size to approximately 1100 g at term. Similarly, the uterine cavity, which in the nongravid state has a volume of less than 10 ml, increases anywhere from 500 to 1000 times. Cardiac output to the uterus is less than 2% in the nongravid state but increases to approximately 10% at term, that is, 500–700 ml/min. There is also increasing pressure caused by intraabdominal growth of the uterus, resulting in an exacerbation of *hernia* defects, most commonly seen at the umbilicus and in the abdominal wall (diastasis recti).

Endocrinologic Changes

Carbohydrate Metabolism

Several hormones secreted by the placenta are responsible for the *diabetogenic effect of pregnancy*. Human placental lactogen (hPL) increases the resistance of peripheral tissues and liver to the effects of insulin. Because hPL is secreted in proportion to placental mass, resistance to insulin increases as pregnancy progresses. Progesterone and estrogen also contribute to insulin resistance during pregnancy, and insulin is broken down by the placental production of insulinase. *Pregnancy is characterized by hyperglycemia, hyperinsulinemia, hypertriglyceridemia, and reduced tissue response to insulin.* The typical fasting glucose level is lower than that in the nonpregnant state, as the fetoplacental unit serves as a constant drain on maternal glucose levels. As a result, in response to maternal starvation, the patient demonstrates exaggerated hypoglycemia and hypoinsulinemia. Delivery of glucose from the mother to the fetus occurs by facilitated diffusion and, as a result, fetal glucose levels are dependent on maternal levels. The fetus is not, however, dependent on the mother for insulin, as fetal insulin is apparent at 9–11 weeks gestation (Table 4.6).

The major change in blood glucose levels in the pregnant woman is a lower fasting level with a prolonged elevation of glucose values after a glucose load is administered. The lower fasting levels result from the constant diffusion to the fetus where glucose is utilized as the primary energy source. In addition, there is hypertrophy of the beta cells of the maternal pancreas, which secrete two to three times the nonpregnant level of insulin late in pregnancy.

Thyroid Function

Several changes in the pregnant patient relate to thyroid function, with the net effect being that *the normal pregnant woman is euthyroid*. Estrogen induces an increased level of thyroxine-binding globulin (TBG), resulting in an increase in total thyroxine (T_4) and total triiodothyronine (T_3) beginning early in pregnancy. Free (T_4) and free (T_3), the active hormones, are unchanged from the normal range for nonpregnant patients (Table 4.6).

Adrenal Function

During pregnancy, there is an estrogen-induced increase in the plasma concentration of corticosteroid-binding globulin (CBG), resulting in elevated levels of plasma cortisol. Like thyroid hormone, only the portion of cortisol that is unbound is metabolically active. Unlike thyroid hormone, however, the concentration of free plasma cortisol is ele-

Table 4.6
Key Endocrine Changes in Pregnancy

Thyroid			
Thyroxine (T$_4$)		Total increased	
			Free unchanged
Triiodothyronine (T$_3$)		Total increased	
			Free unchanged
Thyroid-binding globulin (TBG)	Increased		
Adrenal			
Corticosteroid-binding globulin (CBG)	Increased		
Cortisol	Increased		
Androstenedione	Increased		
Deoxycorticosterone (DOC)	Increased		
Aldosterone	Increased		
Pituitary			
Prolactin	Increased		
Follicle-stimulating-hormone (FSH)		Decreased	
Luteinizing hormone (LH)		Decreased	
Adrenocorticotropic hormone (ACTH)	Increased		
Thyroid-stimulating hormone (TSH)			Unchanged
Oxytocin			Unchanged
Ovaries and placenta			
Progesterone	Increased		
17-Hydroxyprogesterone	Increased		
Estradiol	Increased		
Estriol	Increased		
Human placental lactogen (hPL)	Increased		
Human chorionic gonadotropin (hCG)	Increased (peak between 8 and 10 weeks)		

vated, progressively increasing from the first trimester until term. There is also increased plasma concentration of deoxycorticosterone (DOC) while dehydroepiandrosterone sulfate (DHEAS) is decreased (Table 4.6).

FETAL PHYSIOLOGY
Placental Physiology

Fetal Circulation

The umbilical vein, which carries oxygenated blood, enters the fetus and gives off branches to the left lobe of the liver. It then becomes the origin of the ductus venosus. Another branch joins blood flow from the portal vein that is flowing to the right lobe of the liver. Fifty percent of the umbilical blood supply goes through the ductus venosus. The blood flow from the left hepatic vein is mixed with the blood in the inferior vena cava and is directed toward the foramen ovale. As a result, the well oxygenated umbilical vein blood enters the left ventricle and supplies the carotid arteries. The relatively less oxygenated blood in the right hepatic vein, having entered the inferior vena cava, flows through the tricuspid valve into the right ventricle. Blood from the superior vena cava also preferentially flows through the tricuspid valve to the right ventricle. Blood from the pulmonary artery primarily flows through the ductus arteriosus into the aorta. Less than 10% of cardiac output goes to the lung with blood flow through the foramen ovale accounting for approximately one third of the cardiac output.

PLACENTAL PHYSIOLOGY

Glucose is the primary substrate for placental metabolism. It is estimated that as much as 70% of the glucose transferred from the mother is used by the placenta. Also, solutes that are transferred from the mother to the fetus are dependent on the concentration gradient, as well as on their size and lipid solubility. With regard to respiratory gases, fetal uptake of O_2 and excretion of CO_2 depend on the maternal and fetal blood carrying capacities for these gases as well as on uterine and umbilical blood flows. There is active transport of amino acids, whereas free fatty acids have very limited placental transfer.

Fetal Hemoglobin and Oxygenation

Although the partial pressure of oxygen in fetal arterial blood is only 20–25 mm Hg, the fetus is adequately oxygenated because of its higher cardiac output in organ blood flow. In addition, the higher hemoglobin concentration in the fetus than in the adult as well as higher oxygen saturation are also responsible for the oxygenation of the fetus. At any given oxygen tension, the fetal blood has a higher oxygen saturation than does adult blood.

Fetal Kidney

The fetal kidney forms urine and, as a result, amniotic fluid. Fetal urine is hypotonic compared with that of a newborn.

Fetal Liver

The fetal liver is not fully functional even at term. Bilirubin is primarily eliminated through the placenta.

Fetal Thyroid Gland

The fetal thyroid gland develops without direct influence from the mother. The placenta does not transport thyroid-stimulating hormone (TSH) and only minimal amounts of T_4 and T_3 cross the placenta.

Fetal Gonads

The primordial germ cells migrate during the eighth week of life from the endoderm of the yolk sac to the genital ridge. At this point, the gonads are undifferentiated. Differentiation into the testes occurs 6 weeks after conception if the embryo is 46,XY. This testicular differentiation appears dependent upon the presence of the H-Y antigen. The Y chromosome is also necessary for testicular differentiation. If the Y chromosome is ab-

sent, however, an ovary develops from the undifferentiated gonad. Development of the fetal ovary begins at about 7 weeks. The development of other genital organs depends on the presence or absence of specific hormones and is independent of gonadal differentiation. If the fetal testes are present, testosterone and müllerian inhibitory factor (MIF) inhibit the development of female external genitalia. If these two hormones are not present, the female genitalia develop with regression of the wolffian ducts.

IMMUNOLOGY OF PREGNANCY

Although the maternal immune system is not altered in pregnancy, the antigenically dissimilar fetus is able to survive in the uterus without being rejected. This fetal allograft appears to be somehow protected in this "privileged immunologic" site.

The placenta serves as an effective interference between the maternal and fetal vascular compartments by keeping the fetus from direct contact with the maternal immune system. The placenta also produces estrogen, progesterone, hCG, and human placental lactogen (HPL), all of which may contribute to suppression of maternal immune responses on a local level. The placenta is, in addition, the site of origin for blocking antibodies and masking antibodies, which alter the immune response.

The mother's systemic immune system remains intact as evidenced by leukocyte count, B and T cell count and function, and immunoglobin levels. As IgG is the only immunoglobin that can cross the placenta, maternal IgG comprises a major proportion of fetal immunoglobin both in utero and in the early neonatal period. It is in this fashion that passive immunity can be passed to the fetus.

Fetal lymphocyte production begins as early as 6 weeks gestation. By 12 weeks gestation, IgG, IgM, IgD, and IgE are present and are produced in progressively increasing amounts throughout pregnancy.

FURTHER READINGS

Cunningham FG, MacDonald PC, Gant NF, eds. Williams obstetrics. 18th ed. East Norwalk, CT: Appleton-Century-Crofts, 1989:129.

Gabbe SG, Niebyl JR, Simpson JL, eds. Obstetrics: normal and problem pregnancies. 2nd ed. New York: Churchill-Livingstone, 1991:93.

chapter 5

ANTEPARTUM CARE

The purpose of antepartum care is to help achieve as good a maternal and infant outcome as possible. Complete obstetric care includes the correct diagnosis of pregnancy followed by an initial thorough assessment early in pregnancy, periodic examinations and screening tests as appropriate through the course of gestation, patient education addressing pregnancy care, labor and delivery, nutrition and exercise, and early infant care; management of the patient during labor, delivery, and the postpartum period. Antepartum care ends with a final visit, generally 6 weeks following delivery. Most pregnant women will deliver healthy infants without any prenatal care. Therefore, obstetric care is designed to promote good health throughout the course of normal pregnancy, while screening for and managing any complications that may develop. The American College of Obstetricians and Gynecologists (ACOG) has prepared a standardized antepartum care form, which is presented in Figures 5.1 and 5.2. It is suggested that the reader refer to these forms as the details of antepartum care are discussed.

Ideally, obstetric care should commence prior to pregnancy as a *preconception visit* where a thorough family and medical history for both parents and a physical examination of the prospective mother is done. Preexisting conditions that may affect conception and/or pregnancy are identified and appropriate management plans formulated with the goal of a "healthy" subsequent pregnancy. Unfortunately, the idea of prepregnancy evaluation is uncommon; instead, most women seek care after pregnancy has begun.

Unfortunately, too many pregnant women have only episodic care, which contributes to increased perinatal and maternal morbidity and mortality. Educating patients on the benefits of regular, early care and motivating them to seek it is one of the most important public health goals of our time. For these reasons, obstetric care should be designed (*a*) to provide easy access to care, (*b*) to promote patient involvement, (*c*) to provide a team approach to ongoing surveillance and education for the patient and her fetus, and (*d*) to establish protocols for screening for high risk conditions, along with an organized plan to address any complications that may arise.

DIAGNOSIS OF PREGNANCY

The *diagnosis of pregnancy* should not be made based solely on symptoms and physical findings, which may be misleading in early pregnancy. *A pregnancy test is used to make an accurate diagnosis.* Even when the pregnancy test is positive, complications such as spontaneous abortion, ectopic pregnancy, and trophoblastic disease may make the diagnosis of a normal intrauterine pregnancy difficult.

In a woman with regular menstrual cycles, a history of one or more missed periods, especially if associated with fatigue, nausea/vomiting, and breast tenderness, strongly suggests pregnancy. Urinary frequency caused by the enlarging uterus pressing on the bladder is another common finding.

On *physical examination*, softening and enlargement of the pregnant uterus become apparent 6 or more weeks after the last normal menstrual period. A *pelvic examination* in early pregnancy is one of the better ways to establish a due date (estimated date of confinement [EDC]). Beginning at about 12–14 weeks gestation, the uterus is enlarged sufficiently to be palpable in the lower abdomen. Other genital tract findings early in pregnancy include congestion and a bluish discoloration of the vagina (Chadwick's sign) and softening of the cervix (Hegar's sign). Increased pigmentation of the skin and the appearance of striae on the abdominal wall occur later in pregnancy. *Palpation of fetal parts and the appreciation of fetal movement and fetal heart tones* are diagnostic of pregnancy, but at a more advanced gestational age. Perception of fetal movement (called "quickening") is not usually reported before 16–18 weeks of gestation.

Detection of *fetal heart tones* is also evidence of a viable ongoing pregnancy. With a traditional, nonelectronic fetoscope, auscultation of fetal heart tones is possible at or beyond 18–20 weeks gestational age. The commonly used electronic Doppler devices can detect fetal heart tones approximately 12 weeks from the onset of the last menses. With this device, the patient and her family can also hear the fetal heart beat, a strong bonding experience that also can provide reassurance.

Several types of *urine pregnancy tests* are available, all of which measure *human chorionic gonadotropin (hCG)* produced in the syncytiotrophoblast of the growing placenta. Because hCG shares an α subunit with luteinizing hormone (LH), interpretation of any test that does not differentiate LH from hCG must take into account this overlap in structure. The concentration of hCG necessary to evoke a positive test result must therefore be high enough to avoid a false-positive diagnosis of pregnancy, i.e., a positive test result when the patient is not pregnant. *Standard laboratory urine pregnancy tests become positive 4–6 weeks following the 1st day of the last menstrual period.* Home urine pregnancy tests are now available, which are said to have a low false-positive rate but a high false-negative rate (the test result is negative when the patient is pregnant). These tests may actually be more expensive than a more reliable test available through a health care facility. All urine pregnancy tests are best performed on early morning urine specimens, which contain the highest concentration of hCG.

Serum pregnancy tests are more specific and sensitive because they test for the unique β subunit of hCG. This allows detection of pregnancy very early in gestation, even before the patient has missed a period. Further information about a pregnancy may be obtained by the quantification of hCG. Curves of the normal quantitative values of β-hCG and the expected rate of production can help differentiate normal from abnormal pregnancies (Fig. 5.3). These more reliable and sensitive tests are both more expensive and difficult to perform.

Ultrasound examination can detect pregnancy early in gestation. With abdominal ultrasound, a gestational sac is initially seen 5–6 weeks after the beginning of the last normal menstrual period (corresponding to β-hCG concentrations of 5000–6000 mIU/ml). The newer transvaginal techniques can detect a pregnancy at 3–4 weeks (corresponding to β-hCG concentrations of 1500–2500 mIU/ml). By 7 weeks, the embryo should be visualized by all techniques and cardiac activity detected.

INITIAL ANTENATAL EVALUATION

After the diagnosis of pregnancy has been established, a prenatal appointment is made, at which time a comprehensive history is taken, focusing on previous pregnancy outcome and any medical or surgical conditions that may affect pregnancy. The details of a recommended history (Fig. 5.1) include a history of past pregnancies, past medical history with specific attention to issues that may affect pregnancy, information pertinent to genetic screening, and information about the course of the current pregnancy. Special attention is also given to diet and the use of tobacco, alcohol, medication, and substance abuse. Routine laboratory studies are ordered (Table 5.1 and Fig. 5.2) and the patient is given instruc-

Patient Addressograph

ACOG ANTEPARTUM RECORD

DATE _____

NAME _____
LAST · FIRST · MIDDLE

ID # _____ HOSPITAL OF DELIVERY _____

NEWBORNS PHYSICIAN _____ REFERRED BY _____

BIRTHDATE	AGE	RACE	MARITAL STATUS	ADDRESS:			
MO DAY YR		W B O	S M W D SEP				
OCCUPATION ☐ HOMEMAKER ☐ OUTSIDE WORK _____ ☐ STUDENT _____ Type of Work			EDUCATION (LAST GRADE COMPLETED)	ZIP: PHONE: MEDICAID # / INSURANCE			
EMERGENCY CONTACT:					RELATIONSHIP:		PHONE:

TOTAL PREG	FULL TERM	PREMATURE	ABORTIONS INDUCED	ABORTIONS SPONTANEOUS	ECTOPICS	MULTIPLE BIRTHS	LIVING

PAST PREGNANCIES (LAST SIX)

DATE MO / YR	GA WEEKS	LENGTH OF LABOR	BIRTH WEIGHT	TYPE DELIVERY	ANES.	PLACE OF DELIVERY	PERINATAL MORTALITY YES / NO	TREATMENT PRETERM LABOR YES / NO	COMMENTS / COMPLICATIONS

PAST MEDICAL HISTORY

	O Neg + Pos.	DETAIL POSITIVE REMARKS INCLUDE DATE & TREATMENT			
DIABETES			RH SENSITIZED		
HYPERTENSION			TUBERCULOSIS		
HEART DISEASE			ASTHMA		
RHEUMATIC FEVER			ALLERGIES (DRUGS)		
MITRAL VALVE PROLAPSE			GYN SURGERY		
KIDNEY DISEASE / UTI			OPERATIONS / HOSPITALIZATIONS (YEAR & REASON)		
NERVOUS AND MENTAL			ANESTHETIC COMPLICATIONS		
EPILEPSY			HISTORY OF ABNORMAL PAP		
HEPATITIS / LIVER DISEASE			UTERINE ANOMALY		
VARICCSITIES / PHLEBITIS			INFERTILITY		
THYROID DYSFUNCTION			IN UTERO DES EXPOSURE		
MAJOR ACCIDENTS			STREET DRUGS		
HISTORY OF BLOOD TRANSFUSION			OTHER		
USE OF TOBACCO		# CIGS / DAY PRIOR TO PREG _____ # CIGS / DAY NOW _____ AGE ONSET SMOKING _____ YEARS	USE OF ALCOHOL		# DRINKS / WK PRIOR TO PREG _____ # DRINKS / WK NOW _____ AGE ONSET DRINKING _____ YEARS

INFECTION SCREENING	YES	NO			
HIGH RISK AIDS?			PATIENT OR PARTNER HAVE HISTORY OF GENITAL HERPES?		
HIGH RISK HEPATITIS B?			RASH OR VIRAL ILLNESS SINCE LAST MENSTRUAL PERIOD?		
LIVE WITH SOMEONE WITH TB OR EXPOSED TO TB?			HISTORY OF STD, GC, CHLAMYDIA, HPV, SYPHILIS?		
			OTHER?		

Figure 5.1. ACOG Antepartum Record (Part 1: Initial evaluation).

GENETICS SCREENING
INCLUDES PATIENT, BABY'S FATHER, OR ANYONE IN EITHER FAMILY WITH:

	YES	NO		YES	NO
1. PATIENT'S AGE ≥ 35 YEARS?			10. HUNTINGTON CHOREA?		
2. ITALIAN, GREEK, MEDITERRANEAN, OR ORIENTAL BACKGROUND (MCV < 80)?			11. MENTAL RETARDATION?		
3. NEURAL TUBE DEFECT (MENINGOMYELOCELE, OPEN SPINE, OR ANENCEPHALY)?			IF YES, WAS PERSON TESTED FOR FRAGILE X?		
4. DOWN SYNDROME (MONGOLISM)?			12. OTHER INHERITED GENETIC OR CHROMOSOMAL DISORDER?		
5. JEWISH (TAY SACH'S)?			13. PATIENT OR BABY'S FATHER HAD A CHILD WITH BIRTH DEFECT NOT LISTED ABOVE, ≥ 3 FIRST TRIMESTER SPONTANEOUS ABORTIONS, OR A STILLBIRTH?		
6. SICKLE CELL DISEASE OR TRAIT?					
7. HEMOPHILIA?			14. MEDICATIONS OR STREET DRUGS SINCE LAST MENSTRUAL PERIOD?		
8. MUSCULAR DYSTROPHY?			IF YES, AGENT(S)		
9. CYSTIC FIBROSIS?					

COMMENTS _____

_____

_____

_____

PRESENT PREGNANCY

	O Neg + Pos.	DETAIL POSITIVE REMARKS INCLUDE DATE & TYPE RX.			
1. VAGINAL BLEEDING			5. HEADACHE		
2. VAGINAL DISCHARGE/ODOR			6. ABDOMINAL PAIN		
3. VOMITING			7. URINARY COMPLAINTS		
4. CONSTIPATION			8. FEBRILE EPISODE		
			9. OTHER		

COMMENTS _____

_____

_____ INTERVIEWER'S SIGNATURE_____

INITIAL PHYSICAL EXAMINATION

DATE _____ / _____ / _____   PRE-PREGNANCY WEIGHT _____   HEIGHT _____   BP _____

1. HEENT	☐ NORMAL	☐ ABNORMAL	12. RECTUM	☐ NORMAL	☐ ABNORMAL	
2. FUNDI	☐ NORMAL	☐ ABNORMAL	13. VULVA	☐ NORMAL	☐ CONDYLOMA	☐ LESIONS
3. TEETH	☐ NORMAL	☐ ABNORMAL	14. VAGINA	☐ NORMAL	☐ INFLAMMATION	☐ DISCHARGE
4. THYROID	☐ NORMAL	☐ ABNORMAL	15. CERVIX	☐ NORMAL	☐ INFLAMMATION	☐ LESIONS
5. BREASTS	☐ NORMAL	☐ ABNORMAL	16. UTERUS	☐ NORMAL	☐ ABNORMAL	☐ FIBROIDS ____WEEKS
6. LUNGS	☐ NORMAL	☐ ABNORMAL	17. ADNEXA	☐ NORMAL	☐ MASS	
7. HEART	☐ NORMAL	☐ ABNORMAL	18. DIAGONAL CONJUGATE	☐ REACHED	☐ NO	_____ CM
8. ABDOMEN	☐ NORMAL	☐ ABNORMAL	19. SPINES	☐ AVERAGE	☐ PROMINENT	☐ BLUNT
9. EXTREMITIES	☐ NORMAL	☐ ABNORMAL	20. SACRUM	☐ CONCAVE	☐ STRAIGHT	☐ ANTERIOR
10. SKIN	☐ NORMAL	☐ ABNORMAL	21. ARCH	☐ NORMAL	☐ WIDE	☐ NARROW
11. LYMPH NODES	☐ NORMAL	☐ ABNORMAL	22. PELVIC TYPE	GYNECOID	☐ YES	☐ NO

COMMENTS (Number and explain abnormals) _____

_____

_____

_____

_____

_____ EXAM BY: _____

Figure 5.1. ACOG Antepartum Record (Part 1: Initial evaluation).

Patient Addressograph

ACOG ANTEPARTUM RECORD

DATE _____

NAME _____
LAST   FIRST   MIDDLE

ID # _____

PROBLEMS / PLANS (DRUG ALLERGY:)	MEDICATION LIST: Start date Stop date
1.	1.
2.	2.
3.	3.
4.	4.

EDD CONFIRMATION

INITIAL EDD:
LMP   ___/___/___   = EDD ___/___/___
INITIAL EXAM   ___/___/___ = ___ WKS. = EDD ___/___/___
ULTRASOUND   ___/___/___ = ___ WKS. = EDD ___/___/___
INITIAL EDD   ___/___/___   INITIALED BY _____

LMP ☐ DEFINITE   MENARCHE_____ (AGE ONSET)
    ☐ NORMAL AMOUNT / DURATION   MENSES MONTHLY   ☐ YES ☐ NO
    ☐ APPROXIMATE (MONTH KNOWN)   FREQUENCY Q _____ DAYS
    ☐ UNKNOWN   PRIOR MENSES _____ DATE
                     ON BCP'S AT CONCEPTION   ☐ NO ☐ YES

HCG − ___/___/___   HCG + ___/___/___

18-20 WEEK EDD UPDATE:

QUICKENING   ___/___/___ + 22 WKS. = ___/___/___
FUNDAL HT. AT UMBIL.   ___/___/___ + 20 WKS. = ___/___/___
FHT W / FETOSCOPE   ___/___/___ + 20 WKS. = ___/___/___
ULTRASOUND   ___/___/___ = ___ WKS. = ___/___/___

FINAL EDD   ___/___/___   INITIALED BY _____

32-34 WEEK EDD - UTERINE SIZE CONCORDANCE

± 4 OR MORE CMS. SUGGESTS THE NEED FOR ULTRASOUND EVALUATION

VISIT DATE (YEAR _____)												
WEEKS GEST. BEST EST.												
HT FUNDUS (CM.)												
PRESENTATION - VTX, BR, TRANSVERSE												
FHR PRESENT: F=FETOSCOPE O =ABSENT D=DOPTONE												
FETAL MOVEMENT: +=PRESENT D=DECREASED O =ABSENT												
PREMATURITY: SIGNS / SYMPTOMS: VAGINAL BLEEDING												
MUCUS SHOW / DISCHARGE												
+ PRESENT CRAMPS / CONTRACTIONS												
O ABSENT DYSURIA												
PELVIC PRESSURE												
CERVIX EXAM (DIL. / EFF. / STA.)												
BLOOD PRESSURE INITIAL												
REPEAT												
EDEMA + PRESENT O ABSENT												
WEIGHT												
CUMULATIVE WEIGHT GAIN												
URINE: (GLUCOSE / ALBUMIN / KETONES)												
NEXT APPOINTMENT												
PROVIDER												
TEST REMINDERS	8-18 WEEKS CVS / AMNIO / MSAFP		24-28 WEEKS GLUCOSE SCREEN / RhIG									

Figure 5.2. ACOG Antepartum Record (Part 2: Antepartum visits).

GUIDELINES: EDUCATION AND LABORATORY

INITIAL LABS	DATE	RESULT	REVIEWED	COMMENTS/ADDITIONAL LAB
BLOOD TYPE	/ /	A B AB O		
RH TYPE	/ /	+ / –		
ANTIBODY SCREEN	/ /	– / +		
HCT / HGB	/ /	_____ % _____ gm/dl		
PAP SMEAR	/ /	NORMAL / ABNORMAL / _____		
RUBELLA	/ /	– / +		
VDRL	/ /	– / +		
GC	/ /	– / +		
URINE CULTURE / SCREEN	/ /	– / +		
HB S AG	/ /	– / +		

8 - 18 WEEK LABS (WHEN INDICATED)	DATE	RESULT		
ULTRASOUND	/ /			
MSAFP	/ /	_____ MOM		
AMNIO / CVS	/ /	– / +		
KARYOTYPE	/ /	46, XX OR 46, XY / OTHER _____		
ALPHA-FETOPROTEIN	/ /	NORMAL _____ ABNORMAL _____		

24 - 28 WEEK LABS (WHEN INDICATED)	DATE	RESULT		
HCT / HGB	/ /	_____ % _____ gm/dl		
DIABETES SCREEN	/ /	1 HR. _____		
GTT (IF SCREEN ABNORMAL)	/ /	____ FBS ____ 1 HR. ____ 2 HR. ____ 3 HR.		
RH ANTIBODY SCREEN	/ /	– / +		
RhIG GIVEN (28 WKS)	/ /	SIGNATURE _____		

32 - 36 WEEK LABS (WHEN INDICATED)	DATE	RESULT		
ULTRASOUND	/ /	– / +		
VDRL	/ /	– / +		
GC	/ /	– / +		
HCT / HGB	/ /	_____ % _____ gm/dl		

OPTIONAL LAB (HIGH RISK GROUPS)	DATE	RESULT		
HIV	/ /			
HGB ELECTROPHORESIS	/ /	AA AS SS AC SC AF		
CHLAMYDIA	/ /	– / +		

PLANS / EDUCATION

	COUNSELED YES NO		COUNSELED YES NO
TOXOPLASMOSIS PRECAUTIONS (CATS/RAW MEAT)_____		TUBAL STERILIZATION_____	
CHILDBIRTH CLASSES_____		VBAC COUNSELING_____	
PHYSICAL ACTIVITY_____		CIRCUMCISION_____	
PREMATURE LABOR SIGNS_____		TRAVEL_____	
NUTRITION COUNSELING_____		**REQUESTS** _____	
METHOD OF ANESTHESIA_____			
BREAST OR BOTTLE FEEDING_____		**OTHER** _____	
NEWBORN CAR SEAT_____			
POSTPARTUM BIRTH CONTROL_____		**TUBAL STERILIZATION** DATE INITIALS	
ENVIRONMENTAL/WORK HAZARDS_____		CONSENT SIGNED ____ / ____ / ____ _____	

Figure 5.2. ACOG Antepartum Record (Part 2: Antepartum visits).

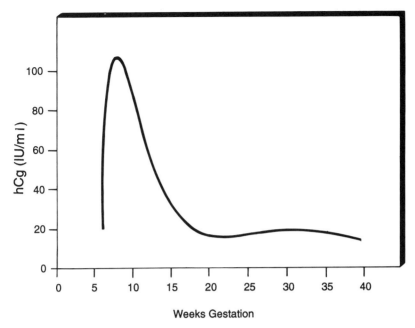

Figure 5.3. hCG concentrations in pregnancy.

tions concerning routine prenatal care, warning signs of complications, whom to contact with questions or problems, and nutritional and social service information. A complete physical examination is performed, including a Pap test and a cervical culture for *Neisseria gonorrhoeae* and *Chlamydia*.

If medical or obstetric problems are identified during the initial assessment or at any subsequent visit, the pregnancy is designated "at risk" and appropriate specific management initiated.

Initial Assessment of Gestational Age: the EDC

Every effort is made to accurately assess gestational age from which the *EDC or "due date"* (or the new term, *estimated date of delivery (EDD)*) is calculated (Fig. 5.2). This information is crucial to obstetric management, as it is needed to identify situations such as possible preterm labor or postdates pregnancy. Initial assessment of gestational age is made by obtaining a thorough *menstrual history*. "Normal" pregnancy lasts 40 ±2 weeks calculated from the 1st day of the last normal

menses (*menstrual age*). In a patient with an idealized 28-day menstrual cycle, ovulation occurs on day 14, so that the *fertilization age* or *conception age* of the normal pregnancy is actually 38 weeks. The use of the first day of the last menses as a starting point for gestational age assignment is standard and menstrual age is most commonly used.

To establish an *accurate menstrual age*, the date of onset of the last normal menses is crucial. A light bleeding episode should not be mistaken for a normal menstrual period. A history of irregular periods or taking medications that alter cycle length such as oral contraceptives, other hormonal preparations, and psychoactive medications can confuse the menstrual history. If sexual intercourse is infrequent or timed for conception based on basal body temperature readings, a patient may know when conception is most likely to have occurred, thus facilitating an accurate calculation of gestational age.

Pelvic examination by an experienced examiner is accurate in determining gestational age within 1–2 weeks until the second trimester, at which time the lower uterine segment begins to form, thereby making clinical

Table 5.1
Routine Obstetric Laboratory Tests

Test	Discussion
Initial laboratory tests	
ᵩ Complete blood count	To determine hematologic status
ᵊ Urinalysis and urine culture and sensitivity	To evaluate for UTI and renal function[a]
ᵛ Blood group, Rh	To determine blood type and Rh status; risk of isoimmunization
ᵝ Antibody screen	To detect antifetal antibodies, which may damage fetus or make procurement of compatible blood for transfusion more difficult. The antibody screen is usually negative. Anti-I and anti-Lewis are seen in about 1% of patients and are of no consequence to the fetus.
	Serologic test for syphilis RPR, VDRL; to detect previous/current infection; if positive, follow-up tests required, e.g., FTA-ABS
Hepatitis B surface antigen	To detect for carrier status or possibly active disease; if positive, further testing indicated
ᵈ Rubella titer	85% of mothers have evidence of prior infection. If patient is seronegative, special precautions are needed to avoid infection, which can severely affect fetus, and vaccination is required postpartum.
ᵊ Pap smear	To screen for cervical dysplasia/cancer
ᵒ Cervical culture for *N. gonorrhoeae, Chlamydia*	To screen for infection; both can cause neonatal conjunctivitis and have been associated with premature labor and postpartum endometritis.
Sickle cell test	To detect hemoglobinopathy. Patients with sickle cell trait (SA) are at higher risk for UTI; with SS disease, for multiple obstetric complications.
Glucose screening (usually 1 h Glucola)	To screen for glucose intolerance
Subsequent assessments	
Serum α-fetoprotein (AFP)	Screening test at 15–18 weeks. Initially for neural tube defects only; now known that both high and low levels are potentially associated with other adverse outcomes.
Hematocrit at approximately 28 weeks	To screen for anemia
Glucose screening at approximately 28 weeks	To screen for glucose intolerance

[a]UTI, urinary tract infection; RPR, rapid plasma reagin; VDRL, venereal disease research laboratory test; FTA-ABS, fluorescent antibody treponemal absorbed test.

estimation of gestational age less accurate. From 16–18 weeks gestation until 36 weeks gestation, the fundal height in centimeters is roughly equal to the number of weeks of gestational age in normal singleton pregnancies.

Obstetric ultrasound examination is the most accurate measurement available in the determination of gestational age. In the first trimester, transvaginal or transabdominal techniques allow gestational age determination with ±1–2 weeks accuracy by combination measurements of the gestational sac and embryo/fetus. In the second trimester, accuracy is still high, in the ±2-week range. In the latter portions of the third trimester, however, accuracy decreases to ±2–3 weeks.

SUBSEQUENT ANTENATAL EVALUATION

For a patient with a normal pregnancy, *periodic antepartum visits* at 4-week intervals are usually scheduled until 32 weeks, at 2-week intervals between 32 and 36 weeks, and weekly thereafter. Patients with high risk pregnancies or those with ongoing complications are usually seen more frequently depending on the clinical circumstances. At each visit, patients are asked about how they are feeling and if they are having any problems, such as vaginal bleeding, nausea/vomiting, dysuria, or vaginal discharge. After quickening, patients are asked if they continue to feel fetal movement and if it is the same or less since the last antepartum visit. Decreased fetal movement is a warning sign requiring further evaluation of fetal well-being.

The only routine laboratory test performed at every prenatal visit is *determination of glucosuria and proteinuria.* A trace of glucosuria is a normal finding in pregnancy and requires no further evaluation. More marked glucosuria requires further evaluation, especially if there is a family history or previous obstetric history of glucose intolerance. Anything other than the presence of trace proteinuria should be considered abnormal and should result in further evaluation.

Maternal physical findings measured at each prenatal visit include blood pressure, weight, and assessment for edema. *Blood pressure* generally declines in midpregnancy, rising again in later pregnancy. Compared to baseline levels, however, any increase in the systolic pressure of more than 30 mm Hg or any increase in the diastolic pressure of more than 15 mm Hg suggests pregnancy-associated hypertension. The *maternal weight* is compared to the pregravid weight and to the generally prescribed recommendation of a 25–30-pound weight gain through the course of pregnancy. There is usually a 3–4-pound increase between monthly visits. Significant deviation from this trend may require nutritional assessment and further evaluation. The presence of significant *edema* in the lower extremities and/or hands is very common in pregnancy and, by itself, is not abnormal. Fluid retention can be associated with hypertension, however, so that blood pressure, as well as weight gain and edema, must be evaluated in conjunction before the findings are presumed to be innocuous.

Obstetric physical findings made at each visit include measurement of the uterine size by pelvic examination or fundal height measurement, documentation of the presence and rate of fetal heart tones, and assessment of the presentation of the fetus. Until approximately 18–20 weeks, the *uterine size* is generally stated as "weeks size," such as 12 weeks size, 15 weeks size, etc. Beginning at 18–20 weeks gestation (when the fundus is palpable at or near the umbilicus) the uterine size can be assessed with the use of a tape measure: *fundal height measurement.* In this procedure, the top of the uterine fundus is identified and the zero end of the tape measure is placed at this uppermost part of the uterus. The tape is then carried anteriorly across the pregnant uterus to the level of the symphysis pubis. Until 36 weeks, the number of weeks gestation corresponds quite closely with the fundal height in centimeters in the normal singleton pregnancy. Thereafter, the fetus moves downward into the pelvis beneath the symphysis pubis ("lightening"), and fundal height measurement is less reliable. If the fundal height measurement is significantly greater than expected, i.e., "large for dates," possible etiologies include incorrect assessment of gestational age, multiple pregnancy, macrosomia (large fetus), hydatidiform mole, and excess accumulation of amniotic fluid (hydramnios). A fundal height measurement less than expected, i.e., "small for dates," suggests the possibility of incorrect assessment of gestational age, hydatidiform mole, fetal growth retardation, inadequate amniotic fluid accumulation (oligohydramnios), or even intrauterine fetal demise.

Fetal heart activity should be verified at every visit, by direct auscultation or by the use of a fetal Doppler device. The normal fetal heart rate is 120–160 bpm; the maternal pulse may also be detected with the Doppler device, so that simultaneous palpation of maternal pulse and auscultation of fetal pulse may be necessary to differentiate the two. Deviation from the normal rate or occasional arrhythmias must be evaluated carefully.

Several determinations concerning the fetus can be made by *palpation of the pregnant uterus*. The most important of these is the *presentation* or "presenting part" of the fetus, i.e., what part of the fetus is entering the pelvis first. This is especially important after 34 weeks. Before that time, breech, oblique, or transverse presentations are not uncommon, nor are they significant, as they are quite variable from day to day. *As term approaches, over 95% of fetuses will be in the cephalic presentation* ("head down"), *with other presentations rather uncommon: breech* ("bottom first") *about 3½% and shoulder less than 1%.* Unless the fetus is in a transverse lie (the long axis of the fetus is not parallel with the mother's long axis), the presentation will be either the head (vertex, cephalic) or the breech (buttocks). *The head is hard and well-defined by ballottement, the physical examination finding the head freely mobile in the fluid-filled uterus;* the breech is softer and therefore more difficult to outline. If a breech presentation is noted between 34 and 37 weeks, the option of external cephalic version (ECV) must be entertained and discussed with the patient. This procedure involves turning of the fetus from the breech presentation to a vertex presentation, thereby avoiding the potential adverse consequences of a vaginal breech delivery.

SPECIFIC TECHNIQUES OF FETAL ASSESSMENT

Evaluation of the fetus can be conveniently categorized as assessment of: (*a*) fetal growth, (*b*) fetal well-being, and (*c*) fetal maturity. The appropriate interpretation of these tests in light of the natural course of any antenatal problem provides a firm base upon which decisions are made.

Assessment of Fetal Growth

Fetal growth can be assessed by fundal height measurement and ultrasonography. The increase in fundal height through pregnancy is predictable. Deviation of more than 2 cm in fundal height measurement from that expected at a particular gestational age between 18 and 36 weeks should prompt repeat measurement and may lead to further evaluation. A deviation of 4 cm or more requires further evaluation including ultrasound in most cases.

Ultrasonography is most valuable in assessing fetal growth. In early pregnancy, determination of the gestational sac diameter and the crown-rump length correlate very closely with gestational age. Later in pregnancy, measurement of the biparietal diameter of the skull, the abdominal circumference, the femur length, and the cerebellar diameter can be used to assess gestational age and, using various formulae, estimate fetal weight. The range of normal values for these measurements increases significantly as pregnancy advances so that a specific assessment of gestational age in the third trimester may be ±3 weeks of the actual age. Earlier in pregnancy there is less deviation in normal values and the information derived is of greater accuracy. Measurements in the late first and early second trimesters are most reliable, generally ±1–2 weeks.

Assessment of Fetal Well-Being

Assessment of *fetal well-being* includes maternal perception of fetal activity and several tests employing electronic fetal monitors and ultrasonography. Tests of fetal well-being have a wide range of uses including the *assessment of fetal status at a particular time* and *prediction of fetal status for varying time intervals* depending on the test and the clinical situation.

An active fetus is generally a healthy fetus, so that *quantification of fetal activity* is a common test of fetal well-being. A variety of methods can be used to quantify fetal activity, including the time necessary to achieve a certain number of movements each day, an average of the number of fetal movements in a given period of time repeated several times a day, or counting the number of movements in a given hour. If, for example, the mother

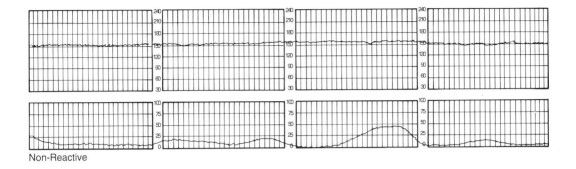

Non-Reactive

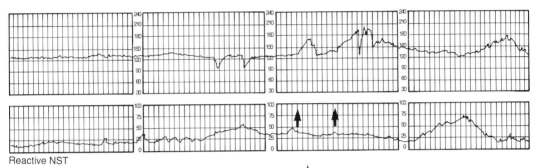

Reactive NST

Figure 5.4. Non-stress testing, ⬆, fetal movement.

detects greater than four fetal movements while lying comfortably and focusing on fetal activity for 1 hour, the fetus is considered to be healthy. This type of testing has several advantages—it is reliable, inexpensive, and it involves the patient in her own care. For these reasons, fetal movement testing is frequently a part of routine obstetric care late in pregnancy or earlier if high risk conditions warrant.

Techniques using *electronic fetal monitoring* and *ultrasonography* are more costly but also provide more specific information. The most common tests utilized are the non-stress test, the contraction stress test (called the oxytocin challenge test if oxytocin is used), and the biophysical profile.

The *non-stress test (NST)* measures the response of the fetal heart rate to fetal movement. With the patient in the left lateral position and the electronic fetal monitor transducer placed on her abdomen to record the fetal heart rate, the patient is asked to note fetal movement, usually accomplished by pressing a button, which records such notation on the fetal monitor strip. The interpretation of the non-stress test rests on the reaction of the fetal heart rate to fetal movement. A *normal or reactive NST* occurs when the fetal heart rate increases by at least 15 bpm over a period of 15 sec following a fetal movement. Two such accelerations in a 20-min span is considered reactive or normal. The absence of these accelerations in response to fetal movement is a *nonreactive NST*. Examples of reactive and nonreactive tests are illustrated in Figure 5.4. A reactive NST is generally reassuring in the absence of other indicators of fetal stress. Depending on the clinical situation, the test is repeated every 3–4 days or weekly. A nonreactive NST must be immediately followed with further assessment of fetal well-being.

Whereas the non-stress test evaluates the fetal heart rate response to fetal activity, the *contraction stress test (CST)* measures the response of the fetal heart rate to the stress of a uterine contraction. With uterine contractions, uteroplacental blood flow is temporarily reduced. *A healthy fetus is able to compensate for this intermittent decreased blood flow, whereas a fetus who is compromised is unable to do so, demonstrating abnormalities such as fetal heart rate decelerations.* To perform a CST, a tocodynamometer is placed on the maternal abdomen along with a fetal heart rate transducer. If contractions are occurring spontaneously, the test is known as a contraction stress test; if oxytocin infusion is required to elicit contractions, the test is called an *oxytocin challenge test (OCT)*. The normal fetal heart rate response to contractions is for the baseline fetal heart rate to remain unchanged and for there to be no fetal heart rate decelerations. Decelerations, especially of the late variety (see Chapter 17, "Intrapartum Fetal Distress"), are nonreassuring. Repetitive decelerations following each contraction when three contractions are occurring in a 10-minute window constitute a positive or abnormal CST or OCT. This is usually an indication for delivery.

Tests of fetal well-being carry a significant risk of *false-positive results*, that is, where the test suggests the fetus is in jeopardy but the fetus is actually healthy. For this reason, these tests must be interpreted together with other assessments and are often repeated within 24 hours to verify the results. In addition, interpretation of the NST and CST are often combined. Because positive OCTs are common, fetal heart rate reactivity can have a significant impact on the final interpretation of the tests (see Chapter 17, "Intrapartum Fetal Distress," for discussion of reactivity). If an OCT is positive, evidence for "reactivity" is sought. If the NST is reactive, the OCT result may be interpreted as a false-positive result. If, however, the positive OCT is accompanied by a nonreactive NST, the combination is considered especially worrisome and fetal distress is likely when labor begins.

The *biophysical profile* is a series of five assessments of fetal well-being, each of which is given a score of 0 or 2 (Table 5.2). The parameters include a reactive non-stress test, the presence of fetal breathing movements, the presence of fetal movement of the body or limbs, the finding of fetal tone (flexed extremities as opposed to a flaccid posture), and an adequate amount of amniotic fluid volume. Perinatal outcome can be correlated with the score derived from these five parameters. A score of 8–10 is considered normal, a score of 6 is equivocal requiring further evaluation, and a score of 4 or less is abnormal, usually requiring immediate intervention.

The importance of adequate *amniotic fluid volume* is well established. Diminished amniotic fluid is thought to represent decreased fetal urinary output caused by chronic stress and shunting of blood flow away from the kidneys. The decreased amniotic fluid provides less support for the umbilical cord, which may be more frequently compressed, resulting in chronic fetal stress. Changes in tone, breathing movements, and fetal movements are more likely to be signs of acute stress to the central nervous system.

Assessment of Fetal Maturity

In some high risk obstetric situations, the maternal or fetal status is so grave that immediate delivery is required regardless of gestational age; in others, a decision must be made as to whether the mother and fetus are at greater risk by continued antepartum management or whether delivery is best. If the pregnancy is viable but less than 36 weeks, the question becomes in part, "How premature is the pregnancy?" and more specifically, "Will the risk of prematurity-associated problems such as respiratory distress syndrome (RDS) be greater than those of continued intrauterine life?"

Because the respiratory system is the last fetal system to mature functionally, many of the *tests available to assess fetal maturity* focus on this organ system. Such tests, termed *direct tests* if they specifically measure substances associated with lung maturity, are routinely employed, although not all tests are utilized in all hospitals. Other tests measure parameters from which the likelihood of ma-

Table 5.2
Biophysical Profile

Biophysical variable	Score	Explanation
Fetal breathing movements (FBM)	Normal = 2	≥1 FBM ≥30 sec duration in 30 min
	Abnormal = 0	No FBM ≥30 sec duration in 30 min
Gross body movement	Normal = 2	≥3 discrete body/limb movements in 30 min
	Absent = 0	≥2 discrete body/limb movements in 30 min
Fetal tone	Normal = 2	≥1 episode active extension with return to flexion of fetal limbs/trunk or opening/closing of hand
	Absent = 0	Either slow extension with return to partial flexion or movement of limb in full extension or absent fetal movement
Reactive fetal heart rate	Normal = 2	Reactive NST
	Absent = 0	Nonreactive NST
Qualitative amniotic fluid volume	Normal = 2	≥1 pocket of amniotic fluid ≥1 cm in two perpendicular planes
	Absent = 0	No amniotic fluid or no pockets of fluid >1 cm in two perpendicular planes

turity can be estimated; these are termed *indirect tests*, the most common being ultrasonography.

Neonatal RDS is the inability of the newborn to successfully ventilate due to immaturity of the newborn lungs. RDS results from lack of a group of phospholipids, collectively known as *surfactant*, which decrease the surface tension within alveolar sacs and thereby promote easy ventilation by maintaining patency of these sacs. In utero, production of these phospholipids remains low until 32–33 weeks, after which production increases. There is a great variation in this process. Gestational age alone does not reliably predict surfactant production or lung maturity. The disorder of RDS is manifest by signs of respiratory failure — grunting, chest retractions, nasal flaring, and hypoxia, possibly leading to acidosis and death. Management consists of skillful support of ventilation and correction of associated metabolic disturbances until the neonate can ventilate successfully without assistance. Recently, administration of synthetic or semisynthetic surfactant to the neonate has been under investigation and offers additional hope for an improved outcome for these infants.

The fetus breathes in utero and phospholipids enter the amniotic fluid where they can be obtained by amniocentesis and measured. Direct tests that measure components of surfactant are listed in Table 5.3. Use of fluid obtained vaginally after spontaneous rupture of membranes is not as common, although such fluid can be used for certain tests in some instances.

Ultrasonographic determination of gestational age and estimated fetal weight are commonly performed indirect tests to help assess maturity. Unfortunately, the correlation between fetal size and maturity is not sufficient that adequate reliability can be given to this parameter, especially in the marginal maturational period between 28 and 35 weeks gestation.

Performed correctly, any test that indicates fetal maturity is associated with the subsequent development of RDS in 2% or less of cases. The predictive value of these tests is much less helpful. Overall, only 50% of infants delivered shortly after an immature fetal maturity test result will develop RDS.

OTHER CONSIDERATIONS AND COMMON QUESTIONS IN PREGNANCY
Employment

In normal pregnancy there are few restrictions concerning work, although it is benefi-

Table 5.3
Tests of Fetal Lung Maturity

Tests	Endpoint for maturity	Comment
Lecithin/sphingomyelin ratio (L/S ratio)	≥2.0	Lecithin is the major component of surfactant; this test measures its production compared to sphingomyelin, a substance with constant production throughout pregnancy. The L/S ratio was the first reliable test of fetal lung maturity; the method is involved methodologically and labor intensive. It has been replaced by less costly tests in many laboratories.
Phosphatidylglycerol	Present	A minor phospholipid that "appears" late in pregnancy; can be measured several ways, therefore results are reported in different ways.
Foam stability index	≥47	Measures the ability of amniotic fluid surfactant to maintain foam at the meniscus of a solution of amniotic fluid and alcohol.

cial to moderate activity to allow for additional periods of rest. Strenuous work should be avoided. A physician's note asking employers to transfer pregnant patients to less physically demanding activities is often needed.

The traditional time designated for *maternity leave* is approximately 1 month prior to the expected date of delivery and extending until 6 weeks after birth. This may be modified depending upon complications of pregnancy, the work involved, the employer attitude, the rules of the health care system under which the patient receives care, and the wishes of the patient.

Exercise

Moderate exercise programs can be continued during pregnancy. Overly strenuous exercise, especially for prolonged periods, should be avoided. Patients unaccustomed to regular exercise should not undertake vigorous new programs during pregnancy.

Tobacco

Smoking should be prohibited during pregnancy because of the established risks to both mother and newborn. In addition to the adverse maternal effects, metabolites from burning tobacco and paper covering are quickly transferred from the patient to her fetus. Infants born to women who smoke weigh less than those born to nonsmokers. Even exposure to passive smoking is associated with high levels of tobacco metabolites. At times, the gastrointestinal discomforts of early pregnancy are associated with a decreased interest in cigarette smoking. The patient should take advantage of this opportunity to cease smoking.

Sexual Intercourse

Sexual activity is not restricted during a normal pregnancy. It may be restricted or prohibited under certain circumstances where it is known to have special risks, e.g., placenta previa, premature rupture of membranes, and preterm labor.

Travel

Travel is not prohibited during pregnancy, although it is customary for patients to avoid distant travel in the last month of pregnancy. This is not because of substantial risk to either mother or fetus, but rather because of the likelihood that labor will ensue away from home and customary health care providers. When traveling, patients are advised to avoid long periods of immobilization such as sitting. Walking every 1–2 hours, even for short periods, promotes circulation, especially in the lower legs, and decreases the risk of thromboembolic problems.

Headaches

Headaches are common in early pregnancy and may be severe. The etiology of such headaches is not known. Treatment with acetaminophen in usual doses is recommended.

Nausea and Vomiting

The majority of pregnant women experience some degree of upper gastrointestinal symptoms in the first trimester of pregnancy. Classically, these symptoms are worse in the morning (the so called "morning sickness"). However, patients may experience symptoms at other times or even throughout the day. Treatment consists of frequent small meals, avoidance of an "empty stomach" by ingesting crackers or other bland carbohydrates, and patience. Medication specifically for nausea and vomiting during pregnancy (Bendectin) was removed from the market of the manufacturer several years ago because of growing litigation concerning congenital anomalies. This occurred even though the safety of the drug had actually been well established. Components of that drug, pyridoxine (vitamin B_6) and an antihistamine, have been used successfully. A variety of other antinausea agents are sometimes used in patients unresponsive to conservative treatment.

Fatigue

In early pregnancy, patients often complain of extreme fatigue that is unrelieved by rest. There is no specific treatment, other than adjustment of the patient's schedule to the extent possible to accommodate this temporary lack of energy. Patients can be reassured that the symptoms disappear in the second trimester.

Leg Cramps

Leg cramps, usually affecting the calves, are common during pregnancy. A variety of treatments including oral calcium supplement have been proposed over the years, none of which is especially successful. Massage and rest are often advised.

Back Pain

Achy lower back pain is common, especially in late pregnancy. The altered center of gravity caused by the growing fetus places unusual stress on the lower spine and associated muscles and ligaments. Treatment focuses on heat, massage, and analgesia. A specially fitted girdle may also help.

Varicose Veins and Hemorrhoids

Varicose veins are not *caused* by pregnancy but often first appear during the course of gestation. Besides the disturbing appearance to many patients, varicose veins can cause an aching sensation, especially when patients stand for long periods of time. Support hose can help diminish the discomfort, although they have no effect on the appearance of the varicose veins. Popular-brand support hose do not provide adequate relief from this aching that prescribed elastic hose can. *Hemorrhoids* are varicosities of the hemorrhoidal veins. Treatment consists of sitz baths and local preparations. Varicose veins and hemorrhoids regress postpartum, although neither condition may abate completely. Surgical correction of varicose veins or hemorrhoids should not be undertaken for about the first 6 months postpartum, to allow for the natural involution to occur.

Vaginal Discharge

The hormonal milieu of pregnancy often causes an increase in normal vaginal secretions. These normal secretions must be distinguished from vaginitis, where symptoms of itching and malodor are present, and spontaneous rupture of membranes, where thin clear fluid appears.

OBSTETRIC STATISTICS

The rates of maternal and fetal mortality are of importance in evaluating the natural history of disease and in the quality of obstetric care. Four statistics are commonly used for this purpose. *Maternal death* occurs during pregnancy, and is *direct* if the cause of death is an obstetric disease, *indirect* if the cause of death is a disease coexisting with pregnancy, and *nonmaternal* if an accident. The *maternal death rate* is the number of deaths of obstetric cause per 100,000 live births. *Fetal death* is synonymous with *stillbirth* and is the number of infants born without any signs of life, expressed as the *fetal death rate* or *stillbirth rate* per 1000 infants born. *Neonatal death* refers to an infant's death within the first 7 days of life, expressed as the *neonatal mortality rate* per 1000 live births. *Perinatal death* is fetal plus neonatal deaths, expressed as the *perinatal mortality rate* per 1000 total births.

More pleasant statistics are the *birth rate*, expressed as the number of births per 1000 population, and the *fertility rate*, expressed as the number of live births per 1000 female population ages 15 through 45 years.

FURTHER READINGS

Creasy RK, Resnick R. Maternal-fetal medicine: principles and practice. 2nd ed. Philadelphia: WB Saunders, 1989.
———. Chapter 10. Maternal nutrition. 171–180.
———. Chapter 11. Effects of chemical and environmental agents. 181–194.
———. Chapter 12. General principles and application of ultrasound. 195–253.
———. Chapter 14. Fetal breathing and body movement. 268–288.
———. Chapter 17. Fetal heart rate. 314–344.
———. Chapter 19. Fetal biophysical assessment by ultrasound. 357–362.
———. Chapter 24. Amniotic fluid tests of fetal lung maturity. 414–426.

SELF-EVALUATION

Case 5-A

A 38-year-old G1 presents for her first prenatal visit. She is unsure of her LMP, saying "it was sometime about 7 or 8 months ago." She is found to have chronic hypertension for which she has declined treatment and she also smokes. On physical examination her fundal height is found to be 30 cm.

Question 5-A-1

Which of the following evaluations should be performed initially to help determine the patient's gestational age?
A. NST
B. OCT
C. biophysical profile
D. amniocentesis
E. ultrasonography

Answer 5-A-1

Answer: E

Discussion: NST, OCT, and biophysical profile (BPP) are tests of fetal well-being, not of gestational age. They may be needed in this patient, as there may be evidence of a pregnancy that is small for gestational age. Lecithin/sphingomyelin ratio (L/S) and phosphatidylglycerol determination via amniocentesis are tests for fetal lung maturity. They may be needed if fetal or maternal indications necessitate timely delivery.

Question 5-A-2

How accurate will a single ultrasound be in determining gestational age in this patient?
A. completely accurate
B. ±1 week
C. ±2 weeks
D. ±3 weeks

Answer 5-A-2

Answer: C

Discussion: Several variables will determine how accurate an ultrasonographic determination of gestational age can be in this patient. In general, however, late ultrasound is relatively inaccurate, about ±2 weeks. Since the patient's menstrual history is unclear, the ultrasound results will need to be interpreted in the context of other findings. Serial ultrasound evaluations may be needed.

Question 5-A-3

For further consideration: What are the possible additional problems associated with the patient's chronic hypertension and smoking? What are the fetal effects and how do they relate to fetal age estimation by ultrasonography?

Case 5-B

A 19-year-old G2P0010 is followed for normal antepartum care. On her visit at 39 weeks gestational age, she reports the baby seems to be moving less than during the previous week.

Question 5-B-1

Which of the following tests are most appropriate at this time?

A. NST
B. OCT
C. biophysical profile
D. amniocentesis for L/S and phosphatidyl-glycerol determinations
E. ultrasonography

Answer 5-B-1

Answer: A

Discussion: At term, the perception of decreased fetal movement may merely be associated with engagement of the fetal head and increased fetal size. An NST is the least invasive test of fetal well-being and, if reassuring, is sufficient in a normal pregnancy. OCT is too invasive and has a high false-positive rate. Biophysical profile is not invasive, but is too costly and time consuming for an initial evaluation of decreased fetal movement in a normal pregnancy. At 38 weeks, amniocentesis will provide no useful information as fetal lung maturity is reasonably assured.

Question 5-B-2

In this case, the NST is found to be reactive.

For further consideration: Is further evaluation indicated? If so, what? Is biophysical profile determination warranted? Are kick counts useful at this gestational age?

chapter 6

MEDICAL AND SURGICAL CONDITIONS OF PREGNANCY

Virtually any maternal medical or surgical condition can complicate the course of a pregnancy and/or be affected by pregnancy. Accordingly, physicians providing obstetric care must have a thorough understanding of the effect of pregnancy on the natural course of a disorder, the effect of the disorder on a pregnancy, and the change in management of the pregnancy and/or disorder caused by their coincidence. In this chapter, selected common medical and surgical complications that may be encountered during the course of obstetric care are discussed. Only a small portion of possible medical-surgical disorders are discussed; more detailed and inclusive discussions are the province of texts of maternal-fetal medicine, medicine, and surgery.

The following 17 disorders are discussed:

1. Anemias
2. Urinary tract disease
3. Renal disease
4. Respiratory disease
5. Cardiac disease
6. Glucose intolerance and diabetes
7. Endocrine disease
8. Infectious disease
9. Thromboembolic disorders
10. Neurologic disease
11. Gastrointestinal disease
12. Genital disease
13. Hepatobiliary diseases
14. Abdominal surgical conditions
15. Substance abuse
16. Coagulation disorders
17. Cancer

(1.) ANEMIAS IN PREGNANCY

The plasma and cellular composition of blood changes significantly during the course of pregnancy because of an expansion of plasma volume proportionally greater than that of the red blood cell mass. Since the hematocrit reflects the proportion of blood made up of primarily red blood cells, the hematocrit demonstrates a "physiologic" decrease during pregnancy (the so-called "*physiologic anemia of pregnancy*"). This decrease in hematocrit is not actually an anemia. *Anemia in pregnancy is generally defined as a hematocrit less than 30% or a hemoglobin of less than 10 g/ dl.* Because of monthly blood loss with menstrual flow and contemporary dietary practices, which lack sufficient iron and protein, women often enter pregnancy with a lowered iron store and sometimes a lowered hematocrit. When faced with the expansion of the maternal red cell mass and fetal iron needs, additional demands on the mother for iron outstrip the iron stores that are available; the result: iron deficiency anemia. It is for these reasons that supplemental iron is appropriately prescribed for pregnant women. *Iron deficiency anemia* is by far the most frequent type of anemia seen in pregnancy, accounting for 90% or more of all cases.

Because iron deficiency is the most common form of anemia in pregnancy, extensive evaluation of anemic pregnant patients should be delayed until an empiric trial of iron therapy is given and the effect observed. If the presumed iron deficiency anemia is severe, the classic findings are small, pale erythrocytes manifest on blood smears (microcytic, hypochromic) and red cell indices indicating a low MCV (mean corpuscular volume) and MCHC (mean corpuscular hemolytic concentration). Further laboratory studies usually demonstrate a decreased serum iron, an increased total iron binding capacity, and a decrease in serum ferritin. A recent dietary history is also highly suggestive, especially if there exists the consuming of nonedible substances (*pica*) such as starch. Such dietary indiscretion may contribute to iron deficiency by decreasing the amount of nutritious food and iron consumed.

Iron therapy is generally given in the form of ferrous sulfate taken two times a day. Each 325-mg tablet provides approximately 60 mg of elemental iron. A response to therapy is first seen as an increase in the reticulocyte count approximately 1 week after the institution of iron therapy. Because of the plasma expansion associated with pregnancy, the hematocrit may not increase significantly, but rather stabilizes or increases only slightly.

The second most common form of anemia seen in pregnancy is *folate deficiency*. Although folate is found in green, leafy vegetables, the demands of fetal and maternal growth during pregnancy require folate supplementation. Folate deficiency is especially likely in multiple gestation and when patients are taking medications such as penytoin (Dilantin). Folate deficiency on blood smear is characterized by hypersegmented neutrophils and indices suggesting large cell volume (macrocytic anemia). Treatment of folate deficiency anemia is 1 mg of folate orally on a daily basis, the amount generally found in most prenatal vitamin supplements.

With a *mixed iron and folate deficiency anemia*, the microcytic changes of iron deficiency negate the megaloblastic changes of folate deficiency, resulting in a normocytic and normochromic anemia. In such cases, treatment with either iron or folate alone will not be followed by a rise in red cell production.

Thalassemia trait may also present as microcytic, hypochromic anemia, but unlike iron deficiency anemia, the serum iron and total iron binding capacity are normal. In addition, the hemoglobin A_2 is elevated.

The direct fetal consequences of anemia are minimal, although infants born to mothers with iron deficiency may have diminished iron stores as neonates. The maternal consequences of anemia are those associated with any adult with anemia. If the anemia is corrected, the woman with an adequate red cell mass enters the labor and delivery process with *additional* protection against the need for transfusion.

The *sickle cell diseases* may be grouped into those with minimal maternal and fetal morbidity (sickle cell trait, S-A; sickle cell-β-thalassemia, S-β-thal) and those with considerable maternal morbidity and occasional mortality (sickle cell disease, S-S; sickle cell-hemoglobin C, S-C). Patients with S-A disease (defined as less than 40% Hgb-S on quantitative hemoglobin electrophoresis) are inclined to maternal urinary tract infections, particularly asymptomatic bacteriuria. Otherwise the pregnancies of patients with S-A and S-β-thal are generally unaffected. Patients with S-S and S-C disease, in contrast, may suffer vaso-occlusive episodes ("crisis") with acute episodes of uteroplacental insufficiency and morbidity, such as prematurity and intrauterine growth retardation. Although prophylactic maternal red cell transfusions have been popular, the risks of multiple blood transfusions and the general improvement in outcome in patients with hemoglobinopathies without transfusion have shifted the therapeutic emphasis to conservative management. Transfusions are, for the most part, reserved for complications of hemoglobinopathies such as congestive heart failure, sickle cell disease crises, and severely low levels of hemoglobin. Careful antenatal assessment using standard techniques is an important part of managing patients with hemoglobinopathies.

2. URINARY TRACT DISEASE IN PREGNANCY

Urinary tract infections are common in pregnancy. Approximately 8% of all women (pregnant and nonpregnant) will have greater than 10^5 colonies of a single bacteria on a midstream culture. Many nonpregnant women are asymptomatic (asymptomatic bacteriuria), whereas during pregnancy, symptoms are more likely, as are cystitis and pyelonephritis. *Asymptomatic bacteriuria* during pregnancy is thought to be due to pregnancy-associated urinary stasis and glucosuria. This relative urinary stasis in pregnancy is a result of decreased ureteral tone and motility, mechanical compression of the ureters at the pelvic brim, and compression of the bladder and ureteral orifices. It is standard care to obtain a urine culture at the onset of prenatal care and to treat patients with asymptomatic bacteriuria. A 7–10 day course of ampicillin or nitrofurantoin is quite effective in most cases, as the most common organism is *Escherichia coli*. Approximately 25% of patients not treated for asymptomatic bacteriuria will proceed to symptomatic urinary tract infection. Suppressive antimicrobial therapy is indicated if there are repetitive urinary tract infections during pregnancy.

Patients with *cystitis* complain of urinary frequency, urgency, dysuria, and bladder discomfort. Occasionally, hematuria is also seen. Fever is unlikely, and its presence should suggest upper urinary tract infection. The treatment of cystitis is the same as that of asymptomatic bacteriuria.

Patients with *pyelonephritis* are acutely ill, with fever, costovertebral tenderness, general malaise, and often dehydration. It occurs in 2% of all pregnant patients and is one of the most common medical complications of pregnancy requiring hospitalization. After obtaining a urinalysis and urine culture, patients are treated with intravenous hydration and antibiotics, commonly a first generation cephalosporin. Uterine contractions may accompany these symptoms; if uncontrolled, preterm labor may ensue. Contractions usu-

ally cease but specific tocolytic therapy may be required. It is known that *E. coli* can produce phospholipase A, which in turn can promote prostaglandin synthesis, resulting in an increase in uterine activity. Fever is also known to induce contractions so that antipyretics are required for a temperature greater than 100°F. Attention must be paid to the patient's response to therapy and her general condition; sepsis can occur in 2–3% of patients with pyelonephritis. If improvement does not occur within 48–72 hours, urinary tract obstruction or urinary calculus should be considered along with a reevaluation of antibiotic.

The organisms most commonly cultured from the urine of symptomatic pregnant patients are *E. coli* and other Gram-negative aerobes. Follow-up can be with either frequent urine cultures or empiric antibiotic suppression with an agent such as nitrofurantoin.

Recurrent symptoms or failure to respond to usual therapy suggests another etiology for the findings of concurrent urinary tract disease. In these patients, a complete urological evaluation 6 weeks after pregnancy may be warranted.

Urinary calculi are occasionally identified in patients during pregnancy although pregnancy per se does not promote stone development. A persistently alkaline urine also is frequently associated with patients with urinary calculi as is urinary tract infection with *Proteus* species. Symptoms similar to those of pyelonephritis but without fever are suggestive of urinary calculi. Although typically renal colic pain may be found, it is seen less frequently in pregnancy than in the nonpregnant state. Usually, hydration and expectant management, along with straining of urine in search of stones, will suffice as management. Occasionally, however, the presence of a stone can lead to infection and/or complete obstruction, which may require drainage by either ureteral stent or percutaneous nephrostony. When the diagnosis of urinary calculi is uncertain, a limited exposure intravenous pyelogram may be obtained.

3. RENAL DISEASE IN PREGNANCY

Pregnancy in patients with preexisting renal disease is encountered frequently, as treatment such as dialysis and transplantation allow these patients health sufficient to support ovulation and pregnancy. *During preconception counseling*, these patients are best advised to avoid pregnancy unless their blood creatinine levels are 2 mg % or less and their diastolic blood pressure is less than 90 mm Hg.

Pregnancy often has no adverse effect on patients with chronic renal disease. In general, patients with mild renal impairment (serum creatinine less than 1.4 mg/dl) have relatively uneventful pregnancies provided other complications of pregnancy are absent. Patients with moderate renal impairment (serum creatinine greater than 1.4 mg/dl) have a more guarded prognosis with an increased incidence of deterioration of renal function. In about 1/2 of patients with renal disease, proteinuria manifests. An increase in proteinuria during pregnancy is not, by itself, a serious consequence. A brief review of the effect of pregnancy on common chronic renal disease is presented in Table 6.1. The presence of hypertension prior to pregnancy or the development of hypertension through the course of pregnancy is a more worrisome finding with respect to both the course of the patient's renal disease and to the pregnancy.

Chronic renal disease is associated with an increased risk of first trimester spontaneous abortion. When pregnancy continues, there is an increased incidence of intrauterine growth retardation so that serial assessment of fetal well-being and growth is recommended in most cases. Pregnancy following renal transplantation is generally associated with a good prognosis if at least 2 years have lapsed since the transplant was performed and thorough renal assessment reveals no evidence of active disease or rejection.

Table 6.1
Effect of Pregnancy on Common Chronic Renal Diseases

Renal disease	Effects
Chronic pyelonephritis	No effect on renal lesion Increased incidence symptomatic urinary tract injection (UTI)
Urolithiasis	No direct effect on renal lesion UTI more frequent in some cases
Diabetic nephropathy	No effect on renal lesion Increased incidence UTI, preeclampsia
Chronic glomerulonephritis	No effect on renal lesion in the absence of hypertension Increased incidence UTI
Systemic lupus erythematosus (SLE)	Often no effect on renal lesion although about 1/3 patients show some worsening of renal function Prognosis improves if SLE is in remission more than 6 months
Polycystic disease	No effect on renal lesion
Scleroderma	Unusual association with pregnancy because onset of disease more common in 4th and 5th decades No effect on preexisting renal lesion Disease may be fulminant if onset during pregnancy; postpartum exacerbation common
Periarteritis nodosa	Maternal and neonatal mortality rates high because of frequent association with malignant hypertension; poor prognosis; therapeutic abortion should be presented as an option of management

4. RESPIRATORY DISEASE IN PREGNANCY

The mechanical and hormonal changes associated with pregnancy alter the functional characteristics of the respiratory system. Most women experience *dyspnea of pregnancy* in the latter half of pregnancy because of changes, such as increased abdominal pressure, causing decreased diaphragmatic excursion. Reassurance and advice to sleep in a semisitting position usually suffice for this problem.

Upper Respiratory Infections (URIs) and Pneumonia in Pregnancy

The incidence and severity of the viral *common cold (URI)* is unchanged in pregnancy. After appropriate diagnosis excluding more serious problems, supportive care emphasizing hydration, rest, good diet, and mild antipyretics such as acetaminophen usually suffice. *Pneumonia* is an uncommon but serious complication in pregnancy. The most common causative organisms are *Streptococcus pneumoniae* and *Mycoplasma pneumoniae*. Beyond routine diagnostic steps, which may and should include chest radiographs, blood gas determinations are important to exclude maternal hypoxia, which may adversely affect the fetus. Management includes hydration, antipyretics, antibiotic therapy, respiratory toilet and oxygen supplementation if needed, and evaluation of fetal well-being.

Asthma

Bronchial asthma is encountered in approximately *1% of pregnant patients*, approximately 15% of whom will have one or more severe asthma attacks during pregnancy. The *effect of asthma on pregnancy* is variable, but includes increased risks of chronic hypoxia, intrauterine growth retardation, and rarely intrauterine fetal demise. Because of these associations, the management of asthma in pregnancy is directed toward minimizing the likelihood of exacerbations coupled with prompt treatment of any acute respiratory symptoms and serial assessment of fetal well-being.

Patients with *infrequent, mild asthmatic exacerbations* may be followed with minimal evaluation or treatment. These patients should be encouraged to avoid undue physical exertion and to obtain adequate rest, to avoid dehydration and exposure to allergins, and to seek immediate medical evaluation if symptoms of respiratory infection develop.

Patients with more *severe asthma* should be maintained on their prepregnancy medical regimens. A rapid response to inhalers containing β-adrenergic receptor stimulants such as epinephrine and isoproterenol (Isuprel) may be expected. The addition of a xanthine preparation such as theophylline, which inhibits phosphodiesterase, increasing cyclic AMP and controlling bronchospasm, or a β_2-receptor stimulator such as terbutaline are often helpful to reduce the frequency and severity of exacerbations. Baseline pulmonary function tests and a chest radiograph are prudent. These patients should observe the same life-style recommendations as patients with less severe disease.

Patients with severe asthma should be managed by a medical team including an obstetrician and pulmonologist. These patients often require glucocorticoids and frequent hospitalization. Glucocorticoids cross the placental barrier and are associated with intrauterine growth retardation, a risk already exacerbated by the chronic hypoxia of severe asthma. Serial fetal evaluation for growth and acute monitoring for fetal well-being during exacerbations are essential.

Tuberculosis in Pregnancy

Tuberculosis is uncommon in pregnancy in the United States, and less than 200 cases of congenital tuberculosis have been reported. The causative agent *Mycobacterium tuberculosis* is acquired primarily by inhalation of droplets produced by infected individuals. Inactive infection (positive skin test and negative chest x-ray) is treated by isoniazid for 1 year. Active

Table 6.2
Reproductive Effects of Smoking

Decreased fertility
Increased risk of spontaneous abortion
Increased risk of ectopic pregnancy
Decreased birth weight (average ½ pound)
Increased risk of preterm delivery (preterm labor, premature rupture of membranes)
Increased risk of abruptio placentae and placenta previa
Increased risk of sudden infant death syndrome (SIDS)
Increased risk of developmental problems

Table 6.3
New York Heart Association Functional Classification of Heart Disease

Class I	No cardiac decompensation
Class II	No symptoms of cardiac decompensation at rest
	Minor limitations of physical activity
Class III	No symptoms of cardiac decompensation at rest
	Marked limitations of physical activity
Class IV	Symptoms of cardiac decompensation at rest
	Increased discomfort with any physical activity

infection (positive cultures, symptomatic infection) is treated by isoniazid plus rifampin as well as pyridoxine to combat the neuropathy often associated with isoniazid.

Smoking in Pregnancy

It is estimated that 1/3 of pregnant women smoke despite vigorous public education programs explaining the risks to the smoker (cancer, heart disease, etc.). Pregnant smokers also place their infants at increased risk of decreased birth weight, intrauterine growth retardation, abruptio placentae, and perhaps long-term neurologic abnormalities (Table 6.2). Patients should be counseled to stop or significantly reduce smoking during pregnancy.

5. CARDIAC DISEASE IN PREGNANCY

In the past, most pregnant patients with cardiac disease had rheumatic heart disease; patients with congenital heart disease usually died before reaching reproductive age. Presumably, modern treatment of congenital and acquired heart disease allows many patients to reach their reproductive years and become pregnant. As a result, patients with rheumatic heart disease and acquired infectious valvular heart disease (associated with drug use) comprise only one half of pregnant cardiac patients. Considering that pregnancy is associated with cardiac output increases of 40%, the risks to mother and fetus are often profound. Ideally, cardiac patients should

have preconceptional care directed at maximizing cardiac function. They should also be counseled about the risks their particular heart disease poses in pregnancy. Some patients may choose to avoid pregnancy; others may choose to terminate a pregnancy rather than assume the risks to themselves and/or their fetus; still others may choose to continue pregnancy under intense medical and obstetric management.

The *classification of heart disease* of the New York Heart Association is useful to evaluate all types of cardiac patients with respect to pregnancy. It is a functional classification, which is independent of type of heart disease (Table 6.3). Patients with septal defects, patent ductus arteriosus, and mild mitral and aortic valvular disorders often are in classes I or II and do well throughout pregnancy. Primary pulmonary hypertension, uncorrected tetralogy of Fallot, Eisenmenger syndrome, and certain other conditions are associated with a much worse prognosis (frequently death) through the course of pregnancy. For this reason, patients with such disorders are advised not to become pregnant.

General management of the pregnant cardiac patient consists of avoiding conditions that add additional stress to the workload of the heart beyond that already imposed by pregnancy, including prevention and/or correction of anemia, prompt recognition and treatment of any infections, a decrease in physical activity and strenuous work, and proper weight gain.

A low sodium diet and resting in the lateral decubitus position to promote diuresis are especially helpful interventions. Adequate rest is essential. For patients with class I or II heart disease, increased rest at home is advised. In more severe classes, hospitalization and treatment for cardiac failure are often required. Coordinated management between obstetrician, cardiologist, and anesthesiologist is necessary for patients with significant cardiac dysfunction.

The fetuses of patients with functionally significant cardiac disease are at increased risk for low birth weight and prematurity.

The *antepartum management of pregnant cardiac patients* includes serial evaluation of maternal cardiac status as well as fetal well-being and growth. Anticoagulation, antibiotic prophylaxis for subacute bacterial endocarditis, invasive cardiac monitoring, and even surgical correction of certain cardiac lesions during pregnancy can be all accomplished if necessary. The *intrapartum and postpartum management of pregnant cardiac patients* includes consideration of the increased stress of delivery and postpartum physiological adjustment. Labor in the lateral position to facilitate cardiac function is often desirable. Every attempt is made to facilitate vaginal delivery given the increased cardiac stress of cesarean section. Because cardiac output rises by 40–50% during the second stage of labor, shortening this stage by the use of forceps is often advisable. Conduction anesthesia to reduce the stress of labor is also recommended. Even with patients who are stable at the time of delivery, it must be remembered that an additional rise in cardiac output is manifest in the puerperium because of the additional 500 ml added to the maternal blood volume as the uterus contracts to a nonpregnant configuration. Indeed, the majority of obstetric patients who die with cardiac disease do so following delivery.

Rheumatic heart disease remains a common cardiac disease in pregnancy. As the severity of the associated valvular lesion increases, these patients are at higher risk for thromboembolic disease, subacute bacterial endocarditis, cardiac failure, and pulmonary edema. A high rate of fetal loss is also seen in these patients. About 90% of these patients have mitral stenosis whose associated mechanical obstruction worsens as cardiac output increases during pregnancy. Mitral stenosis associated with atrial fibrillation has an especially high likelihood of congestive failure.

Maternal cardiac arrhythmias are occasionally encountered during pregnancy. Paroxysmal atrial tachycardia is the most commonly encountered maternal arrhythmia and is usually associated with too strenuous exercise. Underlying cardiac disease such as mitral stenosis should be suspected when atrial fibrillation and flutter are encountered.

Peripartum cardiomyopathy is rare but an especially severe pregnancy-associated cardiac condition. It occurs in the last month of pregnancy or the first 6 months following delivery and is difficult to distinguish from other cardiomyopathies except for its association with pregnancy. A myocarditis is responsible for some of these cases, whereas in other cases no apparent etiology can be determined. A classic patient at increased risk for peripartum cardiomyopathy is one who is black, multiparous, over 30 years of age, and with a history of twins or preeclampsia. Management includes bed rest, digoxin, diuretics, and, in some cases, anticoagulation. The mortality rate is high. The best clinical sign related to prognosis is cardiac size 6 months after diagnosis. In patients with persistent cardiomegaly, the risk of death in the near future is great. In patients in whom the heart size has returned to normal, the prognosis is better, although recurrence in a subsequent pregnancy is likely. Counseling the patient about the benefits of sterilization is warranted.

6. GLUCOSE INTOLERANCE AND DIABETES MELLITUS IN PREGNANCY

Approximately 2% of pregnancies are complicated by diabetes that either develops during pregnancy or was antecedent to preg-

Table 6.4
Classifications of Diabetes in Pregnancy

ADA Classification

Type I diabetes	Diagnosed in childhood, often brittle and difficult to control
Type II diabetes	Adult-onset glucose intolerance
Gestational diabetes	Glucose intolerance identified during pregnancy

The diabetic status is then described, for example, type II diabetes with mild vascular disease.

White Classification

A. Gestational diabetes, onset in pregnancy
B. Onset after age 20
   Duration less than 10 years
   No vascular disease
C. Onset between ages 10–19
   Duration 10–19 years
   No vascular disease
D. Onset under age 10
   Duration greater than 20 years
   Some vascular disease: retina, legs
E. Pelvic arteriosclerosis by x-ray
F. Vascular nephritis
R. Proliferative retinopathy
T. Transplantation

nancy. In either case, diabetes has significant implications for pregnancy and, conversely, pregnancy significantly affects diabetes.

Classification of Diabetes Mellitus

The White classification was used for many years to group cases of diabetes during pregnancy on the basis of age at onset of diabetes, duration of diabetes, and complications such as vascular disease. In recent years, the simpler *Diabetes Classification of the American Diabetic Association* (ADA) has become more commonly used. In the ADA classification, three forms of glucose intolerance are identified. *Type I diabetes* refers to diabetes diagnosed in childhood and is often brittle and difficult to control. It is thought to result from an immunologic destruction of beta cells of the pancreas. Diabetic ketoacidosis is common in patients with this type of diabetes. *Type II diabetes* refers to the patient who has adult-onset glucose intolerance. These

patients are frequently overweight and can often be controlled with a carefully followed diet. This type of diabetes is thought to result from exhaustion of the beta cells rather than their destruction. *Gestational diabetes* refers to a new glucose intolerance identified during pregnancy. In most patients it is a reversible condition, although glucose intolerance in subsequent years occurs more frequently in this group of patients. These classifications are summarized in Table 6.4.

Interrelationships between Pregnancy and Diabetes Mellitus

Effects of Pregnancy upon Glucose Metabolism/Diabetes

Dietary habits are frequently changed during pregnancy, most notably with a decrease in food intake early in pregnancy because of nausea and vomiting and altered food choices. Several pregnancy-associated hormones also have a major effect on glucose metabolism. Most notable of these is the hormone *human placental lactogen (hPL)*, which is produced in abundance by the enlarging placenta. hPL affects both fatty acid and glucose metabolism. It promotes lipolysis with increased levels of circulating free fatty acids and causes a decrease in glucose uptake and gluconeogenesis. In this manner, hPL can be thought of as an antiinsulin. The increasing production of this hormone as pregnancy advances generally requires ongoing changes to be made in insulin therapy to adjust for this effect. Other hormones that have demonstrated lesser effects include: *estrogen and progesterone*, which interfere with the insulin-glucose relationship; and *insulinase*, which is produced by the placenta and degrades insulin to a limited extent. These effects of pregnancy upon glucose metabolism make the management of pregnancy-associated diabetes difficult. Diabetic ketoacidosis (DKA), for example, is more common in pregnant patients.

Effects of Glucose Metabolism/Diabetes upon the Gravida

With increased renal blood flow, the simple diffusion of glucose in the glomerulus increases beyond the ability of tubular reabsorption, resulting in a normal *glucosuria* of pregnancy, commonly of about 300 mg/day. With diabetics this may be much higher, but, because of poor correlation with blood glucose concentrations, using glucose is of little value in glucose management during pregnancy. This glucose-rich urine is an excellent environment for bacterial growth so that pregnant diabetics have a twofold incidence of *urinary tract infection* compared to nondiabetics.

In addition to the added difficulties in glucose management and the increased risk of diabetic ketoacidosis during pregnancy, diabetics have a twofold increase in the incidence of pregnancy-induced hypertension *(PIH) or preeclampsia*, over nondiabetics, and thereby for the risks associated with these hypertensive states. Diabetic *retinopathy* worsens in about 15% of pregnant diabetics, some proceeding to proliferative retinopathy and loss of vision if the process remains untreated by laser coagulation.

Effects of Glucose Metabolism/Diabetes upon the Neonate

3x risk · anomalies

Infants of diabetic mothers (IDM) are at a threefold increased risk of *congenital anomalies* over the 1–2% baseline risk of all patients. The most commonly encountered anomalies are cardiac and limb deformities. Sacral agenesis is a unique but rare anomaly for this group. *Excessive fetal growth* or *macrosomia,* usually defined as a fetal weight in excess of 4500 g, is more common in diabetic pregnant patients because of the fetal metabolic effects of increased glucose transfer across the placenta. This excessive neonatal size can lead to problems with fetopelvic disproportion requiring cesarean section or causing shoulder dystocia at the time of attempted vaginal delivery.

CPD -

The *neonatal hypoglycemia* often encountered in these neonates is thought to result from the sudden change in the steady-state arrangement wherein increased glucose crossing the placenta was countered in the fetus by an increase in insulin levels. Once separated from the maternal supply of glucose, the higher level of insulin causes a significant neonatal hypoglycemia, In addition, these neonates are subject to an increased incidence of *neonatal hyperbilirubinemia, hypocalcemia, and polycythemia.*

Another complication of pregnancy in diabetic patients is an amniotic fluid volume increased above 2000 ml, a condition known as *hydramnios or polyhydramnios*. Encountered in about 10% of diabetics, this increase in amniotic fluid volume and uterine size is associated with an increased risk of abruptio placentae and preterm labor. It is also a predisposing factor for postpartum uterine atony.

The risk of *spontaneous abortion* is similar in well-controlled diabetics and nondiabetics, whereas the risk is significantly increased if glucose control is poor. There is also an increased risk of *intrauterine fetal demise* and *stillbirth*, especially when diabetic control is inadequate.

IDM also tend to have a five- to sixfold increased frequency of *respiratory distress syndrome*. The usual tests of lung maturity are often poorly predictive for these infants (Table 6.5).

Laboratory Diagnosis of Glucose Intolerance/Diabetes in Pregnancy

Approximately *1% of all pregnant patients are known diabetics prior to pregnancy*. For these patients, obstetric diabetic management ideally begins prior to conception with the goal of optimal glucose control before and during pregnancy. Although there is controversy as to whether or not this causes a reduction in the risk of congenital anomalies, other maternal and neonatal benefits make it clear that a diabetic woman entering pregnancy

Table 6.5
Maternal and Fetal Complications of Pregnancy Associated with Maternal Diabetes

Maternal effects
  Hyperglycemia and glucosuria
  Diabetes ketoacidosis
  Increased incidence of urinary tract infection
  PIH/preeclampsia
  Retinopathy
Neonatal effects
  Congenital anomalies
  Macrosomia
  Hypoglycemia
  Hyperbilirubinemia
  Hypocalcemia
  Polycythemia
  Hydramnios
  Intrauterine fetal demise/spontaneous abortion

Table 6.6
Glucose Tolerance Tests in Pregnancy

1-Hour Glucola screening test
  50-g glucose challenge with no glucose preparation with sampling at 1 hour postchallenge
  Normal: <140 mg % plasma glucose
3 Hour glucose tolerance test
  100-g glucose challenge after 3 days glucose preparation with sampling as shown
  Normal values:

	Less than stated mg % at:			
Time in hours	Fasting	1	2	3
Plasma glucose	105	190	165	145
Blood glucose	90	165	145	125

should be at optimum glucose control if at all possible.

Gestational diabetes is usually identified by prenatal screening of all pregnancy patients, although it may be suspected in patients with known *risk factors* for gestational diabetes, including a history of giving birth to a infant weighing more than 4000 g, a history of repeated spontaneous abortions, a history of unexplained stillbirth, a strong family history of diabetes, obesity, or persistent glucosuria. *One half of patients identified as having gestational diabetes do not, however, have such risk factors. This is the rationale for universal glucose screening in pregnancy.*

The most commonly used screening test for glucose intolerance during pregnancy does not require the patient to be in a fasting state. One hour after consuming 50 g of glucose solution (Glucola), blood is drawn for plasma glucose determination. The currently recognized upper limit of normal for the *1-hour Glucola* test is 140 mg %. Patients whose glucose value exceed this limit generally require a *3-hour glucose tolerance test*. After adequate carbohydrate loading for 3 days (generally, 150 g of carbohydrate/day), the first step in a 3-hour glucose tolerance test is a fasting plasma glucose sample. Thereafter, the patient consumes 100 g of glucose in the form of Glucola and has blood drawn at 1, 2, and 3 hours thereafter for determination of plasma glucose levels. The upper limits of normal for the 3-hour Glucola at 0, 1, 2, and 3 hours are, respectively, 105, 190, 165, and 145 mg % plasma (or for blood glucose, 90, 165, 145, and 125 mg %, respectively). Two or more abnormal values make the diagnosis of gestational diabetes. One abnormal value is considered suspicious and testing is repeated in 4–6 weeks depending on the gestational age at the time of the initial test. These standards are summarized in Table 6.6.

In patients lacking any risk factors, the *1-hour Glucola screening is usually performed between 24 and 28 weeks gestation*, since glucose intolerance is generally manifest after that time. In patients with factors suggesting possible glucose intolerance, the testing is performed at the onset of prenatal care and, if normal at that time, repeated as the third trimester commences. Using this screening method, approximately 15% of patients will have an abnormal screening test. Of those patients who then proceed to have the standard 3-hour oral glucose tolerance test, approximately 15% will be diagnosed as having gestational diabetes.

Management of Diabetes during Pregnancy

Often overlooked in the overall management of a patient whose pregnancy is complicated by diabetes mellitus is the importance of *patient education*. The long-standing diabetic should realize that much tighter control of her glucose levels is advised during pregnancy, with greater attention and more frequent glucose monitoring. The impact of pregnancy on diabetes and vice versa must also be emphasized to the pregnant diabetic patient. The newly diagnosed diabetic should receive general diabetic counseling along with information on the unique features of the combination of diabetes and pregnancy. With either type of patient, intense management may be quite stressful and all those involved with obstetric care should be mindful of the need for extra attention that many of these patients share.

The overall goal of management is to control glucose values within fairly circumscribed limits, to serially evaluate fetal well-being, and to time delivery to maximize outcome for both mother and fetus/neonate. *The mainstay of diabetes management is nutritional counseling about an appropriate diet*. Although the recommended increase in daily caloric intake has been proposed as 30 kcal/kg of ideal body weight, most pregnant diabetics end up on a daily caloric recommendation of 2300–2400 cal, composed of approximately 25% fat, 25% protein, and 50% complex carbohydrates. With careful attention to diet, most gestational diabetics do not require insulin.

Patients are generally followed with morning fasting and 2-hour postbreakfast plasma glucose determinations, optimally obtained the morning of their office visit. For "ideal" control, the fasting plasma glucose should be maintained in the 90–100 mg % range and the 2-hour postbreakfast plasma glucose maintained at less than 120 mg %, although values up to 140 mg % may be acceptable in selected circumstances. Home glucose monitoring is now widely available with convenient kits requiring a level of sophistication that most patients can achieve.

For patients in whom no exogenous insulin is necessary, the perinatal outcome is good. Pregnancy is allowed to continue to term with delivery planned at that time. Careful evaluation of fetal weight by ultrasonography is important, as the incidence of macrosomia remains increased in these patients.

Insulin therapy is required for the patient whose plasma glucose values exceed the limits noted for glucose tolerance testing or which exceed the "ideal" levels for dietary management. Insulin does not cross the placenta and therefore does not directly affect the fetus. Instead, enough insulin is given to maintain normal blood glucose levels since glucose does cross the placenta and in excessive concentration can harm the fetus. A mixture of short- and long-acting insulin is given in morning and evening injections so that there is insulin activity at all times, thus maintaining a uniform blood glucose level. A common method is to administer two thirds of the dose in the AM and one third in the PM. The insulin requirements of a pregnant patient are expected to increase due to increased "insulin resistance" as pregnancy progresses.

Once the patient has begun insulin therapy, plasma glucose values are obtained four times a day, typically at 7:00 AM, 11:00 AM, 4:00 PM, and 10:00 PM. Insulin doses are adjusted to maintain a fasting level under 100 mg % and other levels under 140 mg %. Understanding the duration of action of each type of insulin will provide a logical framework for adjusting insulin doses if needed. The fasting glucose reflects the dose of NPH insulin given prior to dinner on the evening before. The 11 AM plasma glucose value reflects the morning regular insulin received 3–4 hours earlier. The 4 PM plasma glucose value reflects the morning NPH, and the 10 PM plasma glucose value reflects the evening doses of regular insulin. Incremental changes in glucose administration should be about 1–3 units at a time in order to avoid rapid changes in glucose values.

A fraction of hemoglobin known as hemoglobin A_{1c} reflects glucose values over the preceding 6–8 weeks. This test has been used to monitor glucose control and to predict the likelihood of congenital anomalies in diabetics early in pregnancy. Overall, the value of this test has been disappointing in clinical use. Fructosamine, which reflects glucose values on a shorter term interval of 2–3 weeks, also has limited clinical value.

Pregnant diabetics, especially type I diabetics, are prone to diabetic ketoacidosis. This serious complication can usually be avoided with frequent monitoring of blood glucose levels, attention to diet, careful insulin administration, and the avoidance of infections. Management of diabetic ketoacidosis is not different from management of DKA in nonpregnant patients and consists of adequate fluids, insulin, glucose, and electrolyte stabilization. Fetal death can accompany DKA, so electronic fetal monitoring of the fetus is essential until the maternal metabolic status is stabilized. At the other end of the spectrum, hypoglycemia is encountered at times, especially early in pregnancy, when nausea and vomiting interfere with caloric intake. Although hypoglycemia does not have untoward effects on the fetus, the symptoms and potential trauma that the patient may experience should be avoided.

Infections are more frequently encountered in pregnant diabetics. Periodic urine cultures should be obtained to detect asymptomatic bacteriuria, as the risk of urinary tract infection and pyelonephritis is twice that of the nondiabetic gravida. Patients should also be told to promptly report any other symptoms that suggest infection, so that aggressive treatment can be initiated.

Because of the risk of progressive retinopathy, pregnant diabetics should have an initial ophthalmologic evaluation and serial examinations during their pregnancies.

Fetal Assessment in Diabetic Pregnancy

Beginning at about 30–32 weeks gestation, various measures to evaluate the fetal growth and well-being are undertaken. *Daily fetal kick counts* are an inexpensive and reliable screening test. Serial *non-stress testing and/or biophysical profile* measurements are also initi-

ated, usually on a once or twice weekly schedule, but more frequently if clinical indicators warrant. Serial *ultrasonography* is performed to detect fetal anomalies and developing polyhydramnios and to follow fetal growth. Both intrauterine growth retardation and macrosomia are seen in IDM. When the estimated fetal weight by *ultrasound* is greater than 4500 g, macrosomia is diagnosed; when greater than 5000 g, cesarean section for delivery is recommended to avoid the risk of shoulder dystocia and similar birth trauma.

Delivery in Diabetic Pregnancy

In general, the goal is for the pregnant diabetic to deliver a healthy child vaginally. The adequacy of glucose control, the well-being of the infant, estimated fetal weight by ultrasound, the presence of hypertension or other complications of pregnancy, the gestational age, the presentation of the fetus, and the status of the cervix are all factors involved in decisions regarding delivery. *In the well-controlled diabetic with no complications, induction at term (38–40 weeks) is often undertaken.*

If an *earlier delivery* is deemed necessary for either fetal or maternal indications, fetal maturity studies are performed prior to effecting delivery. To avoid the potential delivery of an infant who might suffer respiratory distress syndrome, some clinicians require that two or more tests indicate fetal lung maturity, as opposed to a single test in nondiabetics. Ideally, the presence of phosphatidylglycerol confirms the presence of fetal lung maturity, but this phospholipid might not be present in detectable amounts even late in pregnancy.

The route of delivery is influenced by the estimated fetal weight. If the estimated fetal weight is greater than 4500 g, cesarean section rather than attempted vaginal delivery may be considered depending on maternal factors such as pelvic size. When the estimated fetal weight is greater than 5000 g, the risk of birth trauma is significantly increased and cesarean delivery is recommended.

Whether the patient's labor begins spontaneously or is induced, *intrapartum glucose control* is generally managed by a constant glucose infusion of 100 ml of 5% dextrose/hour with frequent plasma glucose assessments. Short-acting insulin may be administered if needed, either by constant infusion or by intermittent injection. Somewhat surprisingly, patients whose glucose has been difficult to control through pregnancy often have very satisfactory levels of glucose when so managed.

Postpartum Management in Diabetic Pregnancy

With delivery of the placenta, the source of the "antiinsulin" factors is removed. Human placental lactogen has a short half-life and its effect on plasma glucose is evident within hours. Many patients do not require any insulin whatsoever in the first several days postpartum, and routine management generally consists of frequent glucose determinations using a sliding scale approach with minimal insulin injections. For patients with gestational diabetes, no further insulin is required postpartum. In patients with preexisting diabetes, insulin is generally resumed at one half of the prepregnant dose once a patient is taking a normal diet. Thereafter, insulin can be adjusted over the ensuing weeks with requirements usually reaching the prepregnancy level.

Over 95% of gestational diabetics will return to a completely normal glucose status postpartum. Glucose tolerance screening is advocated 2–4 months postpartum for these patients to detect the 3–5% who remain diabetic and require treatment.

Diabetic women are best advised to have their pregnancies early in their reproductive lives before serious vascular complications arise. *Contraception* is best accomplished by barrier methods of intrauterine devices, as oral contraceptives may adversely affect maternal blood vessels.

7. ENDOCRINE DISEASE IN PREGNANCY

Thyroid Disease in Pregnancy

Thyroid function in pregnancy remains normal although some clinical manifestations of pregnancy, e.g., warm skin, palpations, etc., may mimic thyroid dysfunction. The diagnosis of thyroid disease in pregnancy is dependent on the interpretation of laboratory tests. Total thyroxine (T_4) and triiodothyronine (T_3) serum concentrations are elevated and the triiodothyronine resin uptake (T_3RU) lowered during pregnancy because of estrogen-induced increases in thyroxine-binding globulin (TBG). Free T_4 and T_3 concentrations are unchanged, however. Calculation of the index for free T_3 and T_4 aids in the diagnosis since a high value is consistent with hyperthyroidism and a low value, with hypothyroidism. Thyroid-stimulating hormone (TSH) concentration is unchanged in pregnancy.

Hyperthyroidism complicates about 0.2% of pregnancies and in 85% of cases is associated with Graves disease, with the remainder of cases associated with acute and subacute thyroiditis, chronic lymphocytic thyroiditis (Hashimoto's disease), toxic nodular goiter, and hydatidiform mole and choriocarcinoma. Diagnosis is suspected with the classic stigmata of hyperthyroidism with or without goiter and confirmed by elevated thyroid function studies. Treatment with the antithyroid medication Propylthiouracil (PTU) blocks intrathyroid synthesis of T_4 as well as peripheral conversion of T_4 to T_3 and has the additional advantage of lessened placental transfer to the fetus as compared with the other common medicine methimazole (Tapazole). Neonatal hypothyroidism may result from suppression of the fetal thyroid with PTU. Radioactive iodine is contraindicated during pregnancy because of its effect on the fetal thyroid. Infants of hyperthyroid mothers are at increased risk for low birth weight. Surgical therapy is rarely warranted during pregnancy.

Hypothyroidism is rarely encountered in pregnancy, as it is associated with anovulation and infertility. Diagnosis is suspected with the classic stigmata of hypothyroidism with or without goiter and confirmed by lowered thyroid function studies. Management with replacement thyroxine (Synthroid) is indicated.

Parathyroid Disease in Pregnancy

Hyperparathyroidism is exceedingly rare in pregnancy but associated with significant perinatal morbidity and mortality. Neonates are often low birth weight, and over 50% develop neonatal tetany when the maternal calcium supply is removed. Parathyroid surgery is the treatment of choice.

Hypoparathyroidism, even rarer than hyperparathyroidism in pregnancy, is usually associated with inadvertent removal of the parathyroids during thyroid surgery. Treatment includes vitamin D and calcium supplementation.

Other Endocrinopathies in Pregnancy

Adrenocortical insufficiency (Addison's disease), Cushing's syndrome, congenital adrenal hyperplasia, and hyper- and hypopituitarism are exceedingly rarely associated with pregnancy. *Diabetes insipidus* is also rarely encountered and has no direct effect on pregnancy. Patients with *pituitary tumors* are now being seen because of effective medical treatment of prolactinomas with bromocriptine. Bromocriptine may be discontinued in pregnancy and the patient followed closely for evidence of tumor growth (headache, changes in visual field), at which time surgical therapy may be indicated on an individual basis.

8. INFECTIOUS DISEASES IN PREGNANCY

Group B Streptococcus

The group B β-hemolytic streptococci are important causes of perinatal infections. Asymptomatic cervical colonization occurs in up to 30% of pregnant women, but cultures may be positive only spasmodically even in the same patient. Approximately 50% of infants exposed to the organism in the lower genital tract will become colonized. For most of these infants, such colonization is of no consequence, but for about 1–4 infants per 1000 live births, clinical infection occurs.

Early onset infection is manifest as septicemia, pneumonia, and/or meningitis. Such an infection is much more likely in premature infants than in term gestations. The mortality rate is 50%. Late onset infection occurs up to 4 weeks after delivery. Meningitis is the most common specific infection and the mortality is approximately 25%. Prematurity is not a factor for late onset infection.

Routine cervical culture of patients and treatment for cultures possible for group B streptococcus have failed because of the ubiquitous nature of this organism. A common method of management of group B streptococcus infections involves frequently obtaining cultures from patients in whom premature delivery is likely, i.e., those with premature rupture of membranes or those with preterm labor. While awaiting culture results, empiric treatment with penicillin or ampicillin is generally prescribed. Some centers recommend treatment of patients with positive cultures even at term.

In the mother, postpartum endometritis may be due to infection with group B streptococcus. The onset is often sudden and within 24 hours of delivery. Significant fever and tachycardia are present; sepsis may follow.

Syphilis

Syphilis is caused by the motile spirochete *Treponema pallidum*, which survives only in vivo. The spirochete is transmitted by direct contact, invading intact mucus membranes or areas of abraded skin.

Abortion, stillbirth, and neonatal death are more frequent in any untreated patient, whereas neonatal infection is more likely in primary or secondary rather than latent syphilis. Infants with congenital syphilis may be asymptomatic or have the classic stigmata of the syndrome, although most infants do not develop evidence of disease for 10–14 days after delivery. Early evidence of disease includes a maculopapular rash, snuffles, mucous patches on the oropharynx, hepatosplenomegaly, jaundice, lymphadenopathy, and chorioretinitis. Later signs include Hutchinson's teeth, mulberry molars, saddle nose, and saber shins.

Serologic testing is the mainstay of diagnosis. Nontreponemal tests identify antibodies developed in response to nonspecific antigens from the immunologic inflammatory response to the spirochete. Test results are reported in quantitative titers, e.g., 1:8; the higher the titer, the greater the inflammatory response. Because false-positive VDRL or RPR tests can be seen in chronic diseases such as leprosy, autoimmune diseases (e.g., lupus), and in drug addiction, treponemal-specific tests are used to confirm infection and identify antibody specific against *T. pallidum*. A positive result indicates either active diseases or previous exposure. Darkfield microscopy can be used to identify the spirochete directly.

Treatment consists of a single 2.4 million unit IM benzathine penicillin injection for primary and secondary infection or latent disease of less than 1-year duration. For latent disease of greater than 1-year duration, three injections are given at weekly intervals. A fourfold rise in serologic titer indicates inadequate treatment or reinfection and treatment is indicated in either case. Response to therapy is evaluated by following serologic titers.

Gonorrhea

Routine screening for *Neisseria gonorrhoeae* is universal. Recovery rates vary from 1 to 8%, depending on the population screened. Infection of the uterus (including the fetus) and the fallopian tubes is rare after the first weeks of pregnancy. At delivery, however, infected mothers may transmit the organism, causing gonococcal ophthalmia in the neonate. In the past, such infection was a prominent cause of blindness, but nowadays routine prophylactic treatment of the newborn's eyes with silver nitrate or tetracycline is very effective in preventing neonatal gonorrhea.

Genital Herpes

Herpes simplex virus (HSV) is a DNA virus that poses significant risk to the fetus/neonate. Herpes infections are categorized as either primary or recurrent; it is the primary form that poses the greatest risk to the fetus. Delivery through a lower genital tract with primary herpes virus infection is associated with neonatal infection in 50% or more of cases, a neonatal mortality of approximately 50% of those infected, and serious neurologic sequelae in many survivors. The risk of neonatal infection is much lower with recurrent infections, presumably because of a decreased inoculum size.

The diagnosis of HSV infections is suspected when clinical examination shows the characteristic tender vesicles with ulceration followed by crusting. Confirmation is by cell culture, with most positive results reported within 72 hours. Multinucleated giant cells can be seen on Pap smears or with use of a Tzanck test in roughly half the cases.

If herpes virus is suspected during the course of pregnancy, a culture from a lesion is generally obtained to confirm the diagnosis. In such patients, or any patient with a history of herpes virus infection, careful visualization of the lower genital tract is important at the onset of labor or when rupture of membranes occurs. If no lesions are identified, vaginal delivery is deemed safe. Cesarean delivery is recommended if herpes lesions are identified on the cervix, in the vagina, or on the vulva at the time of labor or spontaneous rupture of membrane (SROM). This is true whether or not the lesions are associated with primary or recurrent infection. Despite this, 1 of 20 infants delivered by cesarean section for this reason develop HSV infection. Acyclovir is used if symptoms are serious, although its safety in pregnancy has not been assured.

Cytomegalovirus

Cytomegalovirus (CMV) infection affects 1% of births in the United States and is the *most common congenital infection*. A DNA virus, which may be transmitted in saliva, semen, cervical secretions, breast milk, blood, or urine, CMV infection is often asymptomatic, although it can cause a short febrile illness. Like the herpes virus to which it is related, CMV may have a latency period, only to reactivate at a later time.

Either primary or recurrent maternal infection is associated with a *0.5–1.5% risk of intrauterine infection*, although severely affected infants are more often associated with primary seroconversion during pregnancy. About 10% of infected infants will demonstrate congenital defects of varying severity, including microcephaly with or without intracranial calcifications, intrauterine growth retardation, or hepatosplenomegaly. About 10% of asymptomatic CMV-infected infants will subsequently develop sensoneural hearing loss, chorioretinitis, mild neurologic effects, and dental defects.

The *diagnosis* is clinical and by exclusion. There is no reliable serologic testing presently available.

There is *no treatment* for maternal or neonatal CMV infection. Prevention of infection by habits emphasizing personal cleanliness and selectivity of personal contacts is important. Unlike herpes, active lower genital tract infection is not associated with increased risk to the neonate and is not an indication for cesarean section.

Rubella

Rubella ("German" or "3-day" measles) is an RNA virus with important perinatal impact if infection occurs during pregnancy. Approximately *15% of reproductive-aged women lack immunity* to this virus and are susceptible to infection. The virus is spread by airborne droplets, with an incubation period of 14–21 days postexposure. Clinical disease is associated with communicability from approximately 7 days prior to rash development through 4 days after the onset of rash. Once infection occurs, immunity is lifelong.

If a woman develops *rubella infection in the first trimester*, there is an increased risk of both *spontaneous abortions* and *congenital rubella syndrome*. Although 50–70% of babies with congenital rubella appear normal at birth, many subsequently develop signs of infection. Common defects associated with the syndrome include congenital heart disease including patent ductus arteriosus, mental retardation, deafness, and cataracts. The risk of congenital rubella is related to the gestational age at the time of infection such that up to 9/10 of babies acquire the syndrome if infection occurs at less than 11 weeks; 1/3 at less than 11–12 weeks; 1/4 at less than 13–14 weeks; 1/10 at less than 15–16 weeks; and 1/20 in the third trimester. Primary infection can be diagnosed using acute and convalescent sera for IgM and IgG antibodies.

Young women should be aware of their rubella status and should be *vaccinated remote from pregnancy* if they are found to be susceptible. For this reason, prenatal screening for IgG rubella antibody is routine. It is recommended that pregnancy be delayed 3 months following immunization, as the vaccine utilizes a live attenuated rubella virus that induces antibodies in more than 95% of vaccinations. Because there is a 5% failure rate, the patient should be rechecked 6 weeks after vaccination to assure antibody response. In women identified as lacking antibody during pregnancy, vaccination at the time of hospital discharge postpartum is recommended. Such management poses no risk to the newborn or other children; breastfeeding is not contraindicated.

There is no effective *treatment* for a pregnant patient who is infected with rubella. Human immune γ-globulin will not prevent or lessen the effect of infection. No antiviral therapy is available. Maternal treatment is supportive.

Toxoplasmosis

Infection with the *intracellular parasite Toxoplasma gondii* occurs primarily through ingestion of the infectious tissue cysts in raw or poorly cooked meat or through contact with feces from infected cats, which contain infectious sporulated oocytes. The latter may remain infectious in moist soil for more than a year. Only cats who hunt and kill their prey are reservoirs for infection, not those who exclusively eat prepared foods. Asymptomatic infection is common. One third of reproductive-aged women have antibodies to toxoplasmosis.

Infection in the first trimester causes more severe fetal disease than infection in the third trimester, but, conversely, the rates of infection are less in the first than in the third trimester. Sixty percent of infants whose mothers are infected during pregnancy have serologic evidence of infection. Of these, 75% show no gross evidence of infection at birth. However, congenital disease can cause severe mental retardation with chorioretinitis, blindness, epilepsy, intracranial calcifications, and hydrocephalus.

Because infection is usually asymptomatic, *diagnosis* is dependent on serologic testing. Unfortunately, these tests cannot predict the time of infection with accuracy so that the routine screening of patients is not recommended. Further, such testing is of limited value in specific clinical situations. Fetal blood testing is possible when infection is likely to have occurred.

Treatment for suspected *first trimester* infection focuses on counseling about the risks of serious congenital infection and the possibility of therapeutic pregnancy termination. Treatment for these patients where pregnancy termination is not an option or for those suspected of being infected in *later pregnancy* is a combination of sulfadiazine and pyrimethamine. However, pyrimethamine is teratogenic in laboratory animals in the first

trimester so that its use is not recommended during this time.

Prevention of infection would be an important part of prenatal care, including the suggestion that all meats should be thoroughly cooked and that cats should be kept indoors and fed only store-bought foods. If a cat is kept outside, others should feed and care for the cat and its wastes.

Acquired Immunodeficiency Syndrome (AIDS)

Human immunodeficiency virus (HIV) is a *retrovirus*, which converts its own RNA into DNA by means of the specific enzyme, reverse transcriptase. The virus has a marked propensity for invasion of the T4 (helper/inducer) cells whose continued destruction results in depletion of the lymphocyte population, a reversal of the T4 (helper)/T8 (suppressor) ratio of lymphocytes, and finally, clinically significant defects in cell-mediated immunity.

Live virus has been isolated from blood, semen, urine, breast milk, and vaginal secretions, as well as from most body tissues. Transmission is by direct contact with infected material, especially blood and "genital" secretions. Most HIV patients fall into three groups at this time: homosexual/bisexual males, IV drug users, and recipients of blood products. Two other groups growing in numbers are infants with perinatal infection and heterosexuals who encounter infected individuals sexually. Present evidence suggests that HIV is not transmitted through household and other routine contacts, close personal contact except sexual, or animal vectors.

HIV infection does cause antibody formation (seroconversion). However, the antibody provides no protection for the patient or others; seroconversion means the patient has live virus that may be transmitted. The "seroconversion" incubation period is from weeks to years with a suggested mean time of 4 months. Perinatal incubation times are estimated at 1–80 months with a mean of 10 months. The risk of HIV transmission from HIV-positive mothers to their infants is presumably estimated at 30%.

Infected patients may have a mononucleosis-like syndrome but are usually asymptomatic. *Diagnosis is based on serologic enzyme-linked immunosorbent assay (ELISA) testing for HIV antibody and confirmation with a Western blot (electrophoresis). A positive ELISA and Western blot confirm HIV infection.* Newborns may have antibody for some time, which is passively acquired from their infected mother. After several months, this dissipates unless the infant is also infected.

The mean interval between serovonversion (acquisition of the HIV virus) and development of AIDS exceeds 7 years. There is presumably no effective treatment for HIV infection. AZT (zidovudine) has provided some promise for some patients and other drugs are under development. Treatment is centered on prevention of opportunistic, life-threatening infections such as *Pneumocystis carinii* and other protozoal and fungal infections and the early detection of neoplasms such as Kaposi's sarcoma and non-Hodgkin's lymphoma.

Prevention is a major focus. This includes safe sexual practices, abstinence from IV drug use or at least the use of clean, nonshared needles, and appropriate protective measures for patients and medical staff in health care settings. Infected women should avoid becoming pregnant.

9. THROMBOEMBOLIC DISORDERS IN PREGNANCY

An increase in key coagulation factors and venous stasis as a result of relaxed vasculature contribute to the development of thromboembolic disorders during pregnancy and the puerperium. This group of disorders includes phlebitis, both superficial and deep vein, and pulmonary embolism.

With superficial phlebitis, redness and tenderness are accompanied by palpable veins in the involved area, usually the calves. It is of little consequence if treated with elevation of the legs, rest, heat, and mild analgesics.

The risk of deep venous thrombosis, although increased in pregnancy, is even further increased in the several weeks following delivery. The clinical presentation may be varied, depending upon the level of involvement in the lower extremities. Calf pain with tenderness to manipulation and edema can be present in differing degrees. Popliteal tenderness may be noted. Various techniques of diagnosis are available, none of which is entirely satisfactory. The gold standard is venography, but Doppler examination and impedance plethysmography can be helpful.

Treatment of deep venous thrombosis is with heparin anticoagulation. Coumadin is reserved for the postpartum state, since it can be teratogenic in early pregnancy and may cause fetal bleeding later in pregnancy. With heparin, rest, and analgesia, symptoms of deep venous thrombosis subside in approximately a week but heparin is continued well into the postpartum period.

Septic pelvic thrombophlebitis occurs postpartum, the result of bacterial infection in the uterus, with spread to the right ovarian veins. Patients under treatment for pelvic infection may have persistent fever spikes despite improvement in other evidence of infection, such as uterine tenderness. In some cases, a palpable and tender mass representing the right uterine vein can be identified. Response to heparinization is prompt, although spontaneous resolution can also occur.

Deep venous thrombosis is generally a forerunner of pulmonary embolism (PE), although the initial presentation can be pulmonary in nature. Unfortunately, clinical findings of tachypnea, shortness of breath, ECG changes, and other so-called "classic" signs may be misleading. When a pulmonary embolus is suspected, arterial blood gases should be obtained. PaO_2 less than 80 mm Hg suggests pulmonary embolism. Regardless of cause, patients with a diminished PaO_2 need oxygen therapy. The ventilation/perfusion lung scan is helpful in diagnosing pulmonary embolism. Results are often given as "low" or "high" probability for PE; at times, pulmonary angiography is necessary to confirm the diagnosis.

If the PE occurred during pregnancy, full anticoagulation is continued well into the puerperium. If the PE is first diagnosed following delivery, anticoagulation with coumadin can be accomplished after initial heparinization.

10. NEUROLOGIC DISEASE IN PREGNANCY

Epilepsy in Pregnancy

Epilepsy occurs in approximately 0.5% of pregnant women and is characterized by paroxysmal changes in sensory, cognitive, emotional, or psychomotor function as a result of disordered brain function. Epilepsy may be caused by neurological injury, brain lesions, or idiopathic dysfunction. During pregnancy, elevated estrogen levels excite seizure foci, whereas elevated progesterone levels counteract this effect. As a result, epileptic activity is unchanged in 50% of patients, increased in 40% of patients, and decreased in 10% of patients. Prepregnancy frequency of seizures is the best predictor of seizure activity during pregnancy.

Patients with epilepsy appear to have a three- to fourfold increased risk (6–10%) of bearing children with congenital anomalies. However, because many standard anticonvulsants also have teratogenic effects, the cause and effect relationships are uncertain. There is also an increased incidence of seizure disorders in the offspring of epileptic mothers (1/30). During a seizure, there is the additional risk of acute uteroplacental insufficiency.

Phenytoin (Dilantin) has been the standard anticonvulsant for the management of epilepsy. Its use during pregnancy is associated with the fetal hydantoin syndrome, which includes microcephaly, facial clefts and dysmorphism, limb malformations, and distal phalangeal and nail hypoplasia. Phenobarbital is also associated with cleft lip and palate,

albeit at a reduced frequency. Because of these concerns for teratogenesis, the most commonly used anticonvulsant in pregnancy is carbamazepine (Tegretol), which appears to be relatively safe with respect to congenital anomalies. Most anticonvulsants also cause bone marrow suppression and depression of vitamin K-dependent clotting factors so that there is a higher risk of fetal and neonatal hemorrhage. Supplemental folate and neonatal administration of vitamin K are indicated.

Cerebrovascular Accidents in Pregnancy

During pregnancy, the 4 per 100,000 incidence of cerebrovascular accidents (CVAs) in patients under age 35 and 25 per 100,000 in patients age 35–45 is increased 13-fold. Resulting from several abnormalities such as aneurysms or vascular malformations, cerebral embolism, or central venous thrombosis, CVAs are usually of sudden onset with headache and visual disturbance followed by seizure or loss of consciousness and cardiovascular instability.

Diagnosis is suspected from history and physical examination and confirmed by imaging studies including computed tomography and arterial angiography.

General treatment includes cardiorespiratory support for the mother and evaluation of fetal well-being when pregnancy is at a viable gestational age.

Specific treatment depends on the etiology of the CVA. Vascular aneurysms are often silent until rupture and more common after 30 years of age. The most common of these congenital defects of the media elastica of the vessels is the "berry aneurysm," which occurs at the circle of Willis. Aneurysms are more likely to rupture as pregnancy advances. Treatment is supportive and surgical if needed. Arteriovenous shunts are usually recognized in younger patients; treatment is surgical. Cerebral embolism is the most common cause of stroke in pregnancy. Predisposing factors include mitral stenosis with atrial fibrillation or cardiomyopathy with mural thrombi, cerebral vasculitis, thrombotic thrombocytopenic purpura, polycythemia, and sickle cell disease. Treatment is identification and treatment of the underlying cause.

Myasthenia Gravis in Pregnancy

Myasthenia gravis is an autoimmune disease characterized by muscular weakness and easy fatigability as a result of circulating antibodies to acetylcholine receptors. The course of this uncommon complication of pregnancy (about 1/20,000 patients) is variable during pregnancy with a tendency for exacerbation postpartum. Treatment consists of anticholinesterases such as neostigmine or pyridostigmine and avoiding neuromuscular blocking agents that might precipitate a crisis, especially magnesium sulfate. About 10% of infants will have transient myasthenic symptoms due to placental transport of maternal antibodies.

Multiple Sclerosis in Pregnancy

Multiple sclerosis is an autoimmune demyelination disease seen in about 5/10,000 pregnancies and characterized by a variable course during pregnancy and a threefold relapse rate in the postpartum period. Treatment is supportive. Infants of multiple sclerosis victims have a 3% lifetime risk of developing the disease as compared to a 0.1–0.5% lifetime risk for the general population.

11. GASTROINTESTINAL DISEASE IN PREGNANCY

Nausea and Vomiting in Pregnancy and Hyperemesis Gravidarum

The majority of women experience some degree of nausea and vomiting in the first trimester of pregnancy. Classically, symptoms are predominately present in the morning ("morning sickness"), but they may occur throughout the day and evening. A variety of causes have been suggested for these symptoms, although none has been clearly determined. Frequent small feedings and avoidance of foods that are unpleasant to the pa-

tient will usually relieve symptoms to a manageable level. Prenatal vitamin supplements, may aggravate these gastrointestinal symptoms and can be withheld.

A variety of antiemetics can be prescribed if the above measures fail to provide adequate relief.

Hyperemesis gravidarum (intractable emesis during pregnancy) is a more severe form of nausea and vomiting in pregnancy associated with severe symptoms as well as weight loss, dehydration, ketosis, and electrolyte disturbances. Hospitalization and treatment with balanced crystalloid solutions and necessary electrolytes and "NPO status" will generally eliminate symptoms and correct metabolic disturbances in a short time. Diet can then be reinstituted slowly and progressively. Recurrences sometimes necessitate repeat hospitalizations.

Symptoms of nausea and vomiting in early pregnancy should not be presumed to be "morning sickness." It is necessary to rule out other more serious causes of such symptoms. Fortunately, nausea and vomiting in pregnancy is short-lived and most patients can look forward to cessation of symptoms as the second trimester begins.

Gastroesophageal Reflux in Pregnancy

At least one half of patients experience gastroesophageal reflux in the third trimester of pregnancy. It does not alter the course of pregnancy nor is it detrimental to the fetus, but it is uncomfortable for the patient. The cause is a combination of decreased intraabdominal space and increased pressure due to the enlarging uterus and the effect of progesterone to decrease lower esophageal sphincter tone.

Treatment includes reassurance, elevating the head of the patient's bed, small more frequent meals, and liberal use of antiacids at bedtime and after meals.

Ptyalism in Pregnancy

Ptyalism or excessive salivation is especially annoying for a small number of patients, sometimes approaching a liter production per day. Medical treatment with tincture of belladonna or atropine alter ptyalism only slightly so that reassurance of the time-limited nature of the problem is a mainstay of management.

Pancreatitis in Pregnancy

Pancreatitis complicates less than 0.1% of pregnancies, usually in the third trimester during the peak rise in plasma triglycerides or in patients with cholelithiasis, alcohol abuse, severe pregnancy-induced hypertension, and preexisting liver disease. There is considerable maternal morbidity (congestive heart failure, pulmonary effusion, hypotension, hyperglycemia, acidosis) and mortality (estimated at 10%) and a perinatal mortality rate of 11–38%.

The diagnosis is suspected in patients with nausea, emesis, and epigastric pain radiating to the back. Laboratory confirmation includes a transient rise in serum amylase and lipase levels as well as hypocalcemia. Treatment include supportive care, nothing by mouth to suppress pancreatic secretions, nasogastric suction, intravenous fluid therapy, and analgesia. Antibiotics are indicated if there is a fever. Vigorously treated, pancreatitis is usually self-limited in pregnancy.

Appendicitis in Pregnancy

Appendicitis complicates about 0.1% of pregnancies and is the most common surgical emergency in pregnancy. Maternal mortality is 2% in the first and second trimesters and approaching 10% in the third trimester as compared to 0.25% in nonpregnant patients. The increases mortality is due primarily to delay in diagnosis and to a doubling in the rate of perforation during pregnancy. Premature labor is the most common perinatal complication.

The diagnosis is suspected with nausea and vomiting preceded by anorexia and associated with periumbilical or right lower quadrant pain. The gravid uterus may mask the diagnosis by altering the position of the appendix and sequestering inflammatory exudate. Appendectomy with or without vigorous antibiotic therapy is necessary. Electronic fetal monitoring during and after surgery is essential.

12. DENTAL DISEASE IN PREGNANCY

Pregnancy-associated gingivitis is encountered in about 1/2 of pregnancies. The gums are hypertrophied, red, and inflamed due to the hormonal changes of pregnancy. They are uncomfortable, bleed easily, and are more susceptible to poor dental hygiene. Pregnancy-associated gingivitis is related to poor dental hygiene combined with the hormonal changes of pregnancy. Occasionally an inflammatory growth will appear in the papilla area between the teeth. Misnamed "pregnancy tumor," this is simply a pyogenic granuloma exacerbating pregnancy-associated gingivitis. Good dental hygiene and astringent mouthwashes offer some relief to this problem, which regresses with the end of pregnancy.

Emergency and routine *dental care* can be provided as usual, although many dentists try to minimize intervention during pregnancy. Local anesthetics without epinephrine offer little risk. Other modalities such as nitrous oxide are best avoided during pregnancy.

13. HEPATOBILIARY DISEASES IN PREGNANCY
Hepatitis

Hepatitis is the major cause of jaundice (bilirubin >4 mg/dl) during pregnancy. Viral hepatitis takes several forms, including the more common, hepatitis A (HAV), hepatitis B (HBV), and hepatitis C (HVC; parenterally transmitted non-A, non-B hepatitis), and the less common hepatitis D (HDV, formerly the δ agent) and hepatitis E (HEV, formerly known as epidemic or water-borne non-A, non-B hepatitis). Hepatitis A is spread by ingestion of contaminated food or water and by fecal-oral transmission and accounts for approximately 10% of cases of hepatitis in pregnancy. Its symptoms and signs are often vague after an incubation period of 15–50 days, and there is little, if any, effect on pregnancy. Pregnant women exposed to hepatitis A can be given γ-globulin following guidelines for nonpregnant adults. Hepatitis C often follows transfusion with blood or blood components with an incubation period of approximately 50 days. It can also spread through sexual contact. Many cases of hepatitis C are mild with similar but much less severe effects on pregnancy as compared to hepatitis B. Hepatitis D is uncommon but often associated with a fulminant hepatitis. Hepatitis E is clinically similar to hepatitis A but milder, except in pregnancy where maternal mortality may be quite high. Hepatitis C, D, and E combined account for approximately 10% of cases of hepatitis in pregnancy.

Hepatitis B is the most common hepatitis in pregnancy, accounting for approximately 80% of cases. It is spread by infected blood or serous body products via percutaneous or permucosal routes and has an incubation period of 15–50 days. Groups at special risk for HBV include intravenous drug users, homosexuals, health care workers and others who come in contact with potentially infected materials on a regular basis, individuals with multiple sexual partners or whose partners include high risk individuals, and hemophiliacs and others receiving blood components regularly.

The course of hepatitis B infection is not significantly affected by pregnancy. There is a wide range of clinical presentation, from asymptomatic illness through a mild episode with low grade fever and nausea to hepatic failure, coma, and death in unusual circumstances. Serum chemistry abnormalities include elevated serum transaminase levels, often above 1000 milliunits/ml, and an increased serum albumin. Most patients recover completely within 3–6 months, and less than 10% develop chronic infection with circulating HBV antigens.

Vertical transmission to the fetus at delivery is now recognized to pose significant danger to the neonate. Untreated, the majority of infants who are infected become chronic carriers capable of transmitting the infection to others. Hepatic carcinoma and cirrhosis are other unusual sequelae. These adverse outcomes have led to the recent institution of universal screening of all pregnant patients for the presence of the hepatitis B surface antigen (HBsAg). Women so identified should also undergo testing for antibodies and for the presence of the "e" antigen. The presence of the envelope ("e") antigen is associated with an 80% risk of fetal transmission and of the infant becoming a chronic carrier.

If its mother is identified as a carrier or develops hepatitis B during pregnancy, the neonate should receive both active immunization for hepatitis (hepatitis B vaccine) and passive immunization with hepatitis B immunoglobulin (HBIG). Hepatitis B recombinant vaccine is recommended for pregnant women who are at high risk for contracting HBV. HBIG should be given to susceptible pregnant women within 48 hours of exposure to HBV.

During pregnancy, the diagnosis of hepatitis is made on the basis of liver function studies and the presence or absence of antigens and corresponding antibodies as depicted in the accompanying figure. Treatment is supportive with hospitalization usually recommended until patients are capable of maintaining good nourishment.

Cholestasis in Pregnancy

Cholestasis of pregnancy (pruritus gravidarium) occurs in less than 0.1% of pregnancies and is the second most common cause of jaundice in pregnancy. It usually occurs in the third trimester although it is encountered throughout pregnancy. The etiology is unclear but probably involves an increased hepatic sensitivity to estrogen resulting in cholestasis without the hepatocellular damage seen in cholecystitis or cholelithiasis.

Patients present with generalized, often intense, pruritus associated with fatigue, jaundice, and often dark urine. Laboratory evaluation reveals serum bile acid levels elevated to 10–100 times normal, elevated serum alkaline phosphatase to 10 times normal, and bilirubin levels elevated up to 5 mg/ml.

The main effect of cholestasis of pregnancy is the discomfort of intense pruritis. Occasional coagulation abnormalities due to decreased vitamin K absorption have been reported.

Treatment consists of antipruritics such as diphenhydramine hydrochloride (Benadryl) or hydroxyzine hydrochloride (Vistaril), topical skin preparations containing lanolin as a base, and reassurance. Cholestyramine may decrease the bile acid levels but is associated with gastrointestinal disturbances. Phenobarbital may be tried if cholestyramine is not effective in inducing hepatic microsomal function. Recurrence in future pregnancies and with oral contraceptive use is likely.

Cholelithiasis in Pregnancy

Cholelithiasis occurs at the same incidence of 0.1% in pregnancy as without pregnancy. Properly treated, maternal and fetal outcomes are uncompromised, whereas failure to treat effectively is associated with an increased fetal mortality rate. The pathogenesis and pathophysiology in pregnancy is also unchanged, with supersaturation of bile with cholesterol, followed by crystallization and formation of gallstones, uncomfortable distention of the gallbladder and blockage of the cystic duct causing biliary colic and jaundice. An association with fatty food intake is noted. In pregnancy, increased estrogen/progesterone concentrations may increase the concentration of cholesterol and the rate of stone formation.

The clinical history of food-associated colic and laboratory evidence of elevated liver enzymes and bilirubin is confirmed by ultrasonography of the gallbladder.

Asymptomatic cholelithiasis in pregnancy requires no treatment except admonitions about fatty food intake. Biliary colic is treated with nasogastric suction, hydration, analgesia, and antibiotics if needed. Lack of improvement or the development of pancreatitis is usually indication for cholecystectomy.

Acute Fatty Liver of Pregnancy

Acute fatty liver of pregnancy is a rare complication of pregnancy, but its severity and maternal mortality rate of 30% make its timely diagnosis and treatment of importance. Acute fatty liver usually occurs late in pregnancy in primigravidas and is characterized by vague gastrointestinal symptoms becoming worse over several days time. Thereafter headache, mental confusion, and epigastric pain may ensue, and if untreated, there may be rapid development of coagulopathy, coma, multiple organ failure, and death. Laboratory findings include an initial modest elevation in bilirubin and an elevation of transaminase levels, but the magnitude of these elevations is not great and the disease may be misdiagnosed as being minor in nature. Treatment of this serious complication is correction of coagulopathy and electrolyte imbalances, cardiorespiratory support, and delivery as soon as feasible, by the vaginal route if possible.

14. ABDOMINAL SURGICAL CONDITIONS IN PREGNANCY

Careful management of patients with surgical conditions should provide optimal care for the mother and enhance perinatal outcome. Any pregnant patient presenting with a potential surgical condition should be fully evaluated regardless of her pregnant status, i.e., necessary radiographic or other studies should not be avoided just because the patient is pregnant. For procedures such as x-rays of the chest, an abdominal shield may be used to avoid unnecessary exposure to the fetus. In general, exposure to low doses of radiation are considered safe for the fetus, especially when compared to the misdiagnosis of a serious surgical condition. The fetus should be monitored as thoroughly as possible consistent with the stage of gestation and need for intervention. For a viable pregnancy this means electronic fetal monitoring for fetal heart tones and the possibility of uterine activity. The supine position should be avoided, if at all possible, to avoid supine hypotensive syndrome. Oxygen administration may be helpful and is certainly not harmful. In general, those caring for these patients should be constantly aware of both maternal and fetal considerations. For example, in pregnancy the residual lung volume is diminished, providing less reserve for respiratory function. As another example, delayed gastric emptying makes aspiration more likely should surgery be necessary.

Abdominal trauma, regularly encountered in pregnancy, is most commonly associated with automobile accidents. Wearing of seat belts (both lap and shoulder harness) should be encouraged during pregnancy. A special type of trauma that must be kept in mind is physical abuse. This may occur in up to 10% of pregnant patients and may not be divulged by the patient. Frequently, a variety of somatic complaints, including abdominal symptoms, may be offered or excuses given for obvious signs of trauma.

From an obstetric viewpoint, *the most important consideration about abdominal trauma is the possibility of abruptio placentae.* Direct trauma to the uterus is not necessary for a shearing effect on the placenta to occur. Patients whose pregnancies have proceeded beyond the point of viability must be monitored for several hours following abdominal trauma to detect possible fetal heart rate abnormalities resulting from diminished oxygenation due to the abruption. Monitoring for vaginal bleeding is important, although the bleeding may be concealed. Uterine tenderness may be a sign of abruption. A test to detect fetal-maternal hemorrhage, such as the Kleihauer-Betke test, should be performed. In some cases, coagulation studies are obtained to detect subtle changes associated with placental abruption. Tetanus toxoid should be administered to pregnant patients following the same guidelines as those for nonpregnant patients.

15. SUBSTANCE ABUSE IN PREGNANCY

Use of a variety of legal and illicit drugs during pregnancy has climbed at an alarming rate in recent years. Management of patients involved in substance abuse is compounded by a variety of social problems, frequently inadequate prenatal care and poor nutrition. Despite these frustrations, help and encouragement to these patients must be given at every opportunity, as the consequences are so significant to the mother and her offspring.

Smoking

The decrease in smoking has occurred more slowly in women than in men, and regrettably, young women now appear to be initiating smoking at an earlier age than in years past. A variety of adverse pregnancy outcomes have been associated with cigarette smoking, as seen in Table 6.2. These complications result from the effects of carbon monoxide and altered placental perfusion due to vasoconstriction induced by nicotine. The pregnant woman who smokes endangers not only herself but also her unborn child. For some women, pregnancy provides a unique opportunity to cease or at least reduce smoking, an incentive that may be aided by the diminished appetite and nausea seen in pregnancy.

Alcohol

Consumption of excessive alcohol can have disastrous consequences on pregnancy. The fetal alcohol syndrome has been described in the offspring of heavy drinkers. Growth retardation and distinct facial characteristics are seen in these children, along with cardiovascular and limb defects. The perinatal mortality rate is excessive and one third or more of survivors may have mental retardation. Whereas this constellation of findings is seen in half of women who consume the equivalent of six drinks a day, various stigmata may be seen in women who consume as little as two to three drinks a day. As the safe level of alcohol consumption in pregnancy is not known, any significant alcohol use in pregnancy should be discouraged. The risk of spontaneous abortion is also increased in patients consuming alcohol.

Cocaine

In some populations, up to 25% of pregnant women use cocaine. This local anesthetic causes intense vasoconstriction, tachycardia, and hypertension. It crosses the placenta easily. The likelihood of both growth retardation and preterm birth are increased in cocaine users. An increased risk of intestinal atresia and genitourinary malformations has been reported in fetuses born to cocaine users. The most significant and specific risk in pregnancy is that of placental abruption, which often occurs after the acute ingestion of cocaine. Infants of cocaine users can be quite irritable in the days following delivery. These infants are subsequently at increased risk for sudden infant death syndrome (SIDS).

16. COAGULATION DISORDERS IN PREGNANCY

Thrombocytopenia in Pregnancy

Thrombocytopenia is generally diagnosed when the platelet count is less than 100,000/mm^3, although thrombocytopenia-associated bleeding usually occurs at platelet concentrations of less than 20,000/mm^3. While leukemia and other neoplastic processes may be responsible for thrombocytopenia, these conditions are fortunately quite rare in obstetric patients. Drugs are common causes of thrombocytopenia. The list of drugs that cause thrombocytopenia is extensive, including acetaminophen and a variety of antibiotics. Because pregnant women consume various drugs, it may be difficult to assign the cause of thrombocytopenia to a specific drug, and an empiric withdrawal of medications may be required to make a diagnosis of drug-associated disease.

Immune thrombocytopenic purpura (ITP) is an autoimmune disorder characterized by the development of an antiplatelet antibody.

Bone marrow aspiration reveals megakaryocyte hyperplasia. Treatment of ITP is initially with steroids. If unsuccessful, γ-globulin may be administered instead of performing a splenectomy, which formerly was the second-line treatment for this disorder.

Systemic lupus erythematosus (SLE) can have thrombocytopenia as one of its manifestations. Patients with low platelet counts should be evaluated for this autoimmune disorder. Thrombocytopenia is also seen in the hypertensive-associated HELLP syndrome.

Disseminated intravascular coagulopathy (DIC) in obstetrics is associated with placental abruption, retention of a dead fetus, sepsis, preeclampsia, and amniotic fluid embolism. Patients with these conditions must be carefully monitored for evidence of DIC. Findings include prolonged bleeding, decreased clotting factors, and elevated fibrin degradation products.

Lupus anticoagulant refers to immunoglobulins that interfere with phospholipid-related coagulation tests that were initially discovered in patients with SLE. Subsequently, it has been found that some patients with this clotting inhibitor lack other evidence of the more commonly seen SLE. The problem in these patients is that abnormal intravascular clotting occurs in the arterial system. Paradoxically, the activated partial thromboplastin time (aPTT) is prolonged, owing to the interference in this test by the immunoglobulins. Patients with lupus anticoagulant have a rate of reproductive wastage in excess of 90%. Spontaneous abortions and growth retardation are commonly seen. Second or third trimester fetal loss without apparent etiology may be associated with this antiphospholipid syndrome. Screening of patients with poor reproductive histories includes the aPTT and a test for anticardiolipin antibodies, which have been shown to be associated with this clinical picture. Treatment of patients with these disorders includes steroids and low dose aspirin.

17. CANCER IN PREGNANCY

About 1 in 1000 pregnancies are complicated by cancer. The most common malignancies include cervical cancer, breast cancer, melanoma, ovarian cancer, leukemia/lymphoma, and colorectal cancer. Management must balance the maternal risks of the cancer and its treatment against the perinatal risks of treatment or lack thereof.

Cervical Dysplasia and Carcinoma in Pregnancy

Abnormal cervical cytology is encountered in 3% of pregnant women. Its colposcopic evaluation is essentially the same as in the nonpregnant patient with the exception that endocervical curettage (ECC), with its risk of iatrogenic rupture of membranes, and biopsy, with its increased bleeding, are used more sparingly. Treatment of cervical dysplasia is expectant during the pregnancy, usually deferred until 6–8 weeks after delivery, at which time reevaluation is undertaken.

Carcinoma in situ of the cervix is evaluated as with dysplasia, i.e., serial Pap smear and colposcopies are used to rule out progression of disease. Treatment is then based on the evaluation during the postpartum period.

Microinvasive cervical carcinoma is evaluated by conization in the second or third trimester to exclude the possibility of invasive cervical cancer.

The management of invasive cervical cancer will depend on extent of diseases, gestational age, fetal lung maturity, and ultimately the desires of the patient and her family.

Breast Cancer in Pregnancy

About 0.3 per 1000 pregnancies are complicated by breast cancer. The relationship between breast cancer and pregnancy is uncertain. Diagnosis of breast cancer during pregnancy is made difficult by the change of breast size and consistency. To date, the stage-for-stage survival rates for breast cancer are unaffected by pregnancy.

Treatment of breast cancer must be individualized. Pregnancy termination has no recognized advantage in the treatment of breast cancer. Chemotherapeutic agents can be administered to the pregnant patient. There is no evidence that breast cancer adversely affects the pregnancy.

Ovarian carcinoma is quite rare in pregnancy, seen in about 1 of every 10,000–20,000 pregnancies. Although ovarian carcinoma must be considered in the differential diagnosis of an adnexal mass in pregnancy, more common causes are corpus luteum cysts or benign neoplasms. Surgical intervention for a mass is best deferred until the second trimester to avoid potential adverse surgical and/or anesthetic effects during the first trimester.

FURTHER READINGS

Creasy RK, Resnick R, eds. *Maternal-fetal medicine: principles and practice*. Philadelphia: WB Saunders, 1991.

SELF-EVALUATION

Case 6-A

A 23-year-old G1 is seen at 8 weeks gestational age for obstetric care. Her mother is an insulin-dependent diabetic.

Question 6-A-1

Which, if any, of the following laboratory studies should be performed?

A. fasting blood sugar at initial prenatal testing
B. fasting blood sugar at 28 week laboratory testing
C. 1-hour Glucola at initial prenatal testing
D. 1-hour Glucola at 28 week laboratory testing
E. 3-hour glucose tolerance test (GTT) at initial prenatal testing
F. 3-hour GTT at 28 week laboratory testing

Answer 6-A-1

Answer: C

Discussion: Given the patient's family history of diabetes, testing before 28 weeks is indicated. The most commonly performed test would be a 1-hour Glucola. A fasting blood sugar would be less desirable, as it might miss an early glucose intolerance. Glucose tolerance testing is inappropriate as an initial screening test.

Question 6-A-2

The 1-hour Glucola is reported as 181 mg %. Appropriate management steps include:

A. a 2500-cal American Diabetes Association (ADA) diet
B. 1-hour Glucola at 28 week laboratory testing
C. 3-hour GTT
D. 3-hour GTT at 28 week laboratory testing
E. routine obstetric care

Answer 6-A-2

Answer: A, C

Discussion: The 1-hour Glucola is above the 140 mg % screening limit so that glucose tolerance testing is required. Delay to 28 weeks is inappropriate, as the effects of glucose intolerance/diabetes are additive over time and, perhaps, more profound in early pregnancy. For this reason, the presumptive addition of an ADA diet is an excellent precaution.

Question 6-A-3

For further consideration: A 3-hour GTT is performed and the results in mg % are 150, 199, 256, and 199. What will your management plan include? Will you seek consultation with specialists, and if so, whom and for what reason? What will you counsel the patient and her husband about the risks to herself and her child?

Case 6-B

A 19-year-old G2P1001 at 35 weeks gestational age complains of a backache following an automobile accident. While driving to work, her automobile was hit from behind, buffeting her against the restraints of her lap/shoulder harness. Her abdomen hit the steering wheel lightly.

Her antepartum course has heretofore been unremarkable. She notes nothing amiss except a sore back and a bruise over the lower part of her abdomen.

Physical examination is entirely normal except for the bruise she has mentioned. Her cervix is closed and there is no vaginal bleeding.

Question 6-B-1

Appropriate management includes:

A. obstetric ultrasound within 1 week
B. obstetric ultrasound at this time
C. electronic fetal monitoring within 1 week
D. electronic fetal monitoring at this time
E. amniocentesis

Answer 6-B-1

Answer: B, D

Discussion: Abruptio placentae and preterm labor may manifest some hours after trauma to the gravid abdomen. Monitoring for uterine and fetal status is necessary, perhaps for 24 hours according to some authorities. Ultrasound examination for abruptio placentae and biophysical profile are useful.

Question 6-B-2

For further consideration: How long will you monitor this patient? What will you tell her about the risks to her and her child? Are any other laboratory tests useful?

chapter 7

PREMATURE RUPTURE OF MEMBRANES

Beginning early in pregnancy, amniotic fluid is produced continuously as the result of fetal urine production, fetal pulmonary effluent, passage of fluid across the fetal membranes, and passage of fluid across the skin. Amniotic fluid provides protection against infection, protects the fetus from trauma, and provides a space wherein the umbilical cord may float. It also allows for free fetal movement and provides the tracheobronchial fluid which allows intrauterine fetal breathing and in turn full fetal respiratory development. Decreased or absent amniotic fluid can lead to compression of the umbilical cord and decreased placental blood flow. Disruption (rupture) of these fetal membranes is associated with loss of protective effects of amniotic fluid.

Premature rupture of membranes (PROM) is defined as rupture of the chorioamniotic membrane prior to the onset of labor. PROM occurs in approximately 10–15% of all pregnancies. There are a number of associated complications, including infection (chorioamnionitis), prolapsed umbilical cord, and abruptio placentae. About 5% of patients with PROM will, in addition, be preterm. The consequences of PROM differ dramatically depending upon the gestational age at the time of rupture. Accordingly, some use the classification *preterm* PROM to signify patients whose infants face the additional consequences of prematurity, including respiratory distress syndrome.

The *cause of PROM* is not clearly understood. Sexually transmitted diseases (STDs) play a role, since such *infections* are more commonly found in women with premature rupture of membranes than in those without STD. The idea that intact fetal membranes and normal amniotic fluid protect the fetus from infection is becoming more questionable because it appears that subclinical intraamniotic infection may be responsible for PROM in certain cases. Metabolites produced by bacteria may either weaken the fetal membranes or initiate uterine contractions through stimulating prostaglandin synthesis.

The *relationship between PROM and preterm contractions also is unclear.* It is theorized that preterm contractions may cause dilation of the cervix, thereby exposing the fetal membranes to infective agents, which may then cause spontaneous rupture of the membranes. This *triad of PROM, preterm labor, and infection* remains an important clinical consideration but requires further research.

There is also uncertainty about the impact of gestational age and the length of time since membrane rupture on the likelihood of *intrauterine infection.* Chorioamnionitis poses a major threat to the mother and to the fetus as the cause of fetal sepsis. Patients with intraamniotic infection can experience significant fever (generally, greater than 100.5°F), tachycardia (maternal and fetal), and uterine tenderness. Purulent cervical discharge is usually a very late finding. The maternal white blood cell count is generally elevated, but this finding may be misleading for two reasons: the white blood cell (WBC) count rises somewhat in normal pregnancy, with an upper limit of normal of 12,000–13,000/mm³; and the WBC normally rises with uterine contractions and labor, at times to a level exceeding 20,000/mm³. Patients with chorioamnionitis often enter spontaneous and often tumultuous labor. Once the diagnosis of chorioamnionitis is made, treatment consists of

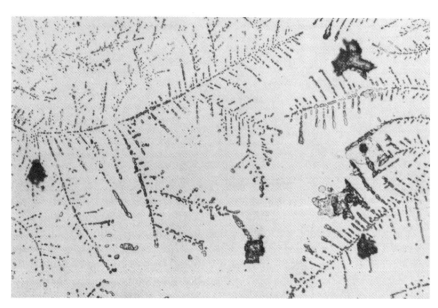

Figure 7.1. Ferning.

antibiotic therapy and prompt delivery by induction or augmentation of labor if spontaneous labor does not ensue promptly.

DIAGNOSIS

Fluid passing through the vagina must be presumed to be amniotic fluid until a full evaluation has ruled out this possibility. At times, patients will describe a "gush" of fluid, whereas at other times there is a history of steady leakage of small amounts of fluid. *Intermittent urinary leakage* is common during pregnancy, especially near term, and this can be confused with PROM. Likewise, the normally increased vaginal secretions in pregnancy, as well as perineal moisture (especially in hot weather), may be mistaken for amniotic fluid.

The Nitrazine test is used to distinguish amniotic fluid from urine or vaginal secretions. The *Nitrazine test* is based on the fact that amniotic fluid is quite alkaline, with a pH between 7.1 and 7.3, whereas vaginal secretions in pregnancy usually have pH values of less than 4.5 and 6.0. To perform the Nitrazine test, a sample of fluid obtained from the vagina during a speculum examination is placed on a strip of Nitrazine paper. The paper turns dark blue in response to amniotic fluid. Cervical mucus and blood and semen are both sources of false-positive results.

The *"fern test"* is named from the pattern of arborization that occurs when amniotic fluid is placed on a slide and is allowed to dry 5–7 min in room air. This pattern, which resembles a fern plant, is due to the sodium chloride content of the amniotic fluid (Fig. 7.1). The ferning pattern from amniotic fluid is fine with multiple branches as shown, whereas that of cervical mucus is thick with much less branching. This test is considered more indicative of ruptured membranes than the Nitrazine test but, as with any test, it is not 100% reliable.

Ultrasound can be very helpful in evaluating the possibility of rupture of membranes. If ample amniotic fluid is visible on ultrasound examination, the diagnosis of PROM must be questioned; however, small amounts of amniotic fluid leakage can occur and sufficient amniotic fluid will still be visible on scan. When there is less than the expected amount of fluid seen on ultrasound, the differential diagnosis of oligohydramnios must also be considered.

EVALUATION AND MANAGEMENT

Patients with PROM are *hospitalized for their initial evaluation* and further management. In the hospital environment, evaluations may proceed quickly and efficiently so that delivery may be accomplished if needed. *Factors to be considered in the management of the patient with premature rupture of membranes include:* the gestational age at the time of rupture, the presence of uterine contractions, the likelihood of chorioamnionitis, the amount of amniotic fluid around the fetus, and the degree of fetal maturity.

The patient's *history,* as well as the management factors listed above, must be carefully evaluated for information relevant to the diagnosis. *Abdominal examination* includes palpation of the uterus for tenderness as well as fundal height measurement for evaluation of gestational age and fetal lie.

A pelvic examination with a sterile speculum is performed to assess the liklihood of vaginal infection and to obtain *cervical cultures* for *Neisseria gonorrhoeae,* β-hemolytic streptococcus, and possibly *Chlamydia.* The cervix is visualized for its degree of dilation as well as for the presence of free-flowing amniotic fluid. Fluid is obtained from the vaginal vault for Nitrazine and/or fern testing. If there is fluid pooled in the vaginal vault, it is sent for *fetal maturity testing.* The test for phosphatidylglycerol (PG) is considered the most reliable indicator of fetal lung maturity, since PG is not found in vaginal secretions or blood. *Because of the risk of infection, intracervical digital examination should be avoided unless and until the patient is in active labor.*

Ultrasound examination can be helpful in determining gestational age, verifying the fetal presentation, and assessing the amount of amniotic fluid remaining within the uterine cavity. It has been shown that labor is less likely to occur when an adequate volume of amniotic fluid remains within the uterus.

If the gestational age is thought to be in the transitional time of fetal maturity, i.e., from 34 to 36 weeks, or if there is clinical suspicion for the presence of uterine infection, amniotic fluid may be collected by *amniocentesis* from any pocket of fluid located on ultrasound. Fluid can be assessed by Gram staining and culture, and tests of fetal maturity performed. The presence of bacteria on Gram stain is a better predictor of infection than the presence of white blood cells.

If the assessment just described suggests *intrauterine infection,* antibiotic therapy and delivery are indicated. The antibiotic prescribed should have a broad spectrum of coverage because of the polymicrobial nature of the infection. Delivery is usually accomplished by induction of labor or, if the infant is a preterm breech, possibly by cesarean delivery. If the patient is beginning to have uterine contractions or if the cervix is dilated beyond about 3 cm, labor is usually allowed to proceed. As in labor not related to PROM, oxytocin augmentation may be necessary later. Persistent contractions after PROM may be a manifestation of infection, possibly subclinical, so that most clinicians do not attempt to inhibit labor when such contractions begin spontaneously.

If the fetus is significantly preterm and in the absence of infection, expectant management is generally chosen: patients are assessed carefully on a daily basis for uterine tenderness as well as maternal or fetal tachycardia. WBC counts are obtained frequently, usually daily for several days. Frequent ultrasound assessment helps to determine amniotic fluid volumes since amniotic fluid may reaccumulate around the fetus. Daily fetal movement monitoring by the mother can also be helpful to assess fetal well-being. In the absence of sufficient amniotic fluid to buffer the umbilical cord from external pressure, compression of the cord can lead to fetal heart rate decelerations. If these are frequent and severe, there should be early and expeditious delivery to avoid fetal damage or death. Electronic fetal monitoring is used frequently during the initial evaluation period to search for any fetal heart rate decelerations.

There is inconclusive evidence supporting the use of *steroids to enhance fetal pulmonary maturity* in patients with PROM. Some clinicians give an agent such as betamethasone, whereas others do not. Despite the immunosuppresive property of steroids, they do not seem to present a major risk of infection.

At times the leakage of amniotic fluid will cease and the fetal membranes are said to "seal over." Should this occur, patients can be monitored at home, with careful attention to temperature and uterine tenderness as noted above. Unfortunately, this sealing over is unlikely. Much more common is the onset of uterine contractions and frank labor in the first week following rupture of membranes. For this reason, it is the exceptional patient who can expect to be discharged home with premature rupture of membranes.

Premature rupture of membranes at very early gestational ages, such as prior to 25–26 weeks gestation, presents additional problems. In addition to the risks of prematurity and infection already discussed, the very premature fetus faces the additional hazards of *pulmonary hypoplasia* and the *amniotic band syndrome.* The relationship of PROM with both of these entities is both interesting and important. For normal fetal lung development to occur, it is necessary that fetal breathing movements take place. During intrauterine life, the fetus normally inhales and exhales amniotic fluid. This adds substances generated in the respiratory tree to the amniotic fluid pool, including the phospholipids that form the basis for many of the fetal maturity tests. If rupture of fetal membranes occurs prior to 25–26 weeks gestation, the absence of amniotic fluid interferes with this normal breathing process and, therefore, with pulmonary development. The end result is a failure of normal growth and differentiation of the respiratory tree. If severe, the fetus is said to have *pulmonary hypoplasia.* Neonatal death then occurs because of an inability to maintain ventilation. The development of pulmonary hypoplasia is not necessarily an all-or-none phenomenon, but rather represents a spectrum of disordered development. The *amniotic band syndrome* refers to a constellation of findings associated with entanglement of fetal parts with the amniotic membranes that can collapse around the fetus once rupture of membranes occurs. These bands may cause virtually any type of deformity, including amputation of extremities or fingers, as well as a number of other anatomic disruptions. Patients with ruptured membranes early in pregnancy assume these additional risks if expectant management is chosen. On the brighter side, PROM that occurs early in pregnancy, sometimes following genetic amniocentesis, has a greater likelihood of "sealing over" with reaccumulation of amniotic fluid.

FURTHER READINGS

Garite TJ. Premature rupture of membranes. In: Scott JR, DiSaia PJ, Hammond CB, Spellacy WN, eds. Danforth's obstetrics and gynecology. 6th ed. Philadelphia: JB Lippincott, 1990:Chapter 18.

Main DM, Main EK. Preterm birth. In: Gabbe SG, Niebyl JR, Simpson JL, eds. Obstetrics, normal and problem pregnancies. 2nd ed. New York: Churchill Livingstone, 1991:Chapter 25.

SELF-EVALUATION

Case 7-A

A 25-year-old G1 at 30 weeks gestational age by menstrual history and early pelvic and ultrasound examinations presents with a history of "water leaking from my vagina" for the last 4 hours. Her pregnancy has been unremarkable except for a positive cervical *Chlamydia* culture at the time of her initial obstetric visit at 8 weeks gestational age. The infection was treated and a repeat culture was negative.

Question 7-A-1

Which of the following should be included in the initial evaluation of this patient?

A.   sterile speculum examination
B.   sterile vaginal examination
C.   external electronic fetal monitoring
D.   cervical cultures for *N. gonorrhoeae* and *Chlamydia*
E.   transabdominal ultrasonography
F.   amniocentesis

Answer 7-A-1

Answer: A, C, D, E

Initial evaluation should be to determine if PROM has occurred. Thus, a sterile speculum examination to look for fluid is appropriate, but not a bimanual examination, which may increase the risk of infection. Fern and Nitrazine (pH) determinations can be made on the fluid, and at the same time cultures from the cervix taken, especially important in this patient with a previous history of *Chlamydia* infection. Similarly, external fetal monitoring (EFM) and ultrasonography are valuable and offer no risk, whereas amniocentesis is unnecessarily invasive at this time.

Question 7-A-2

Examination shows no fluid coming from the os nor in the vaginal vault. The Nitrazine test is negative. Ultrasound shows adequate fluid. EFM shows a reassuring fetal heart rate (FHR) pattern without evidence of uterine activity.

Which of the following are likely explanations of "fluid" coming from this patient's vagina?

A. involuntary urination
B. normally increased vaginal secretions in pregnancy
C. perineal moisture (especially in hot weather)
D. patient anxiety

Answer 7-A-2

Answer: A, B, C, D

All of the reasons for fluid leakage from the vagina are commonly encountered in pregnancy.

Case 7-B

A 36-year-old infertility patient, who conceived after being administered clomiphene citrate, is now G1 at 26 weeks gestational age based on last menstrual period (LMP) and early physical examination and ultrasonography. She presents with the history of a gush of fluid from her vagina 1 hour ago. She is now feeling "little twinges" in her uterus, a new and disturbing sensation. She is very frightened.

Speculum examination shows fluid coming from the cervical os, which is Nitrazine and fern positive. The patient's cervix appears to be about 1 cm dilated. On EFM the fetal heart rate is 170 and there are occasional uterine contractions. The patient is afebrile and her uterus is not tender. Her WBC is found to be 16,000/mm.

Question 7-B-1

Which of the following are likely problems in this case?

A. premature labor
B. intrauterine infection
C. pulmonary hypoplasia
D. amniotic band syndrome

Answer 7-B-1

Answers: All of these are serious clinical considerations for this patient and her fetus.

Question 7-B-2

For further consideration: Obviously, this patient has gone to great lengths to be pregnant. Now she is faced with difficult decisions and your advice is important. Will you recommend tocolysis if uterine activity increases? Will you recommend steroids to help with pulmonary maturity? Will you place her on antibiotic therapy? What will you tell her about her chances of continuing the pregnancy for a week? For 6 weeks? To maturity?

25-26 wks
pulm hypoplasia
amniotic band

eu cont = 30 sec!
reg contractions [illegible] <10 min apart 20·36 wks

PRETERM LABOR AND PRETERM BIRTH

Since *preterm birth* resulting from preterm labor (PTL) is the most common cause of perinatal morbidity and mortality, its prevention, when possible, and treatment are major concerns in obstetric care. The *consequences of preterm labor and preterm birth* occur with increasing severity and frequency the earlier the gestational age of the newborn. Besides perinatal death in the very young fetus, common complications of PTL include respiratory distress syndrome (hyaline membrane disease), intraventricular hemorrhage, necrotizing colitis, sepsis, and seizures. Long-term morbidity associated with preterm labor and delivery includes bronchopulmonary dysplasia and developmental abnormalities. The significant impact of preterm birth is best summarized by this fact: *the 10% of babies born prematurely account for over 50% of all perinatal morbidity and mortality in the United States.*

In the consideration of the consequences of preterm delivery, it is important to *separate the concepts of low birth weight and prematurity.* Prematurity reflects gestational age, whereas low birth weight is based on the single parameter of weight, usually 2500 g or less. For example, a growth-retarded fetus of a hypertensive patient may weigh well under 2500 g at 40 weeks gestation. Such an infant is a low birth weight infant but not preterm, and will suffer the consequences associated with low birth weight and maternal hypertension, but not of premature birth. Likewise, an infant of a diabetic mother may be delivered before term, weigh in excess of 2500 g, and still have the significant perinatal morbidities of preterm birth.

Many preterm births are the result of deliberate intervention for a variety of pregnancy complications and hence are unavoidable perinatal complications. A major cause of preterm birth, however, is preterm labor. *Preterm labor* (PTL) is defined as the presence of *regular uterine contractions, occurring with a frequency of 10 min or less between 20 and 36 weeks gestation, with each contraction lasting at least 30 sec. This uterine activity is accompanied by cervical effacement, cervical dilation, and/or descent of the fetus into the pelvis.* However, variations of this definition are commonly used, so it is often difficult to know when a patient is really in PTL. This presents a problem because treatment appears to be more effective when initiated early in the course of preterm labor; waiting for cervical changes to occur to establish a definitive diagnosis may limit successful therapy.

ETIOLOGY AND PREVENTION OF PRETERM LABOR

A number of *causes and associated factors* have been implicated in PTL. These are presented in Table 8.1. Unfortunately, in most cases, preterm labor is "idiopathic," in that no cause can be identified.

Recently, increased attention has been given to developing mechanisms of *identifying patients at high risk for preterm labor* and to educating patients and physicians about the early signs and symptoms of PTL. Such recognition will allow the physicians to prevent or treat PTL before it progresses to the point that preterm birth is inevitable. Several risk scoring systems have been utilized that com-

Table 8.1
Factors Associated with Preterm Labor

Idiopathic
Dehydration
Premature rupture of membranes (PROM)
Incompetent cervix
  Primary
  Secondary to surgery, e.g., cone biopsy of cervix
Infections
  Urinary
  Cervical (β-hemolytic streptococcus especially)
  Intraamniotic
Excessive uterine enlargement
  Hydramnios
  Multiple gestation
Uterine distortion
  Leiomyomas
  Septate uterus
Placental abnormalities
  Abruptio placentae
  Placenta previa
Maternal smoking (strong implications)
Substance abuse
Coitus
Iatrogenic: indicated induction of labor

Table 8.2
Risk Assessment of Preterm Labor

Risk factors	Points assigned
Socioeconomic conditions	
8 years or less completed education	3
Less than 16 years old	4
Heavy physical or stressful work	3
2 or more children at home	1
Past history	
Second trimester spontaneous abortion	5
Pyelonephritis	4
Less than 1 year since last birth	1
Premature labor, treated with tocolytic therapy	10
Current history	
Second trimester bleeding	4
Dilation of internal cervical os	4
large uterine fibroids	3
Total weight gain 8 pounds or less by 26 weeks	2
Assessment performed at beginning of prenatal care; score updated at 24–28 weeks	
Risk of preterm delivery	
High: 10 or greater	Risk 20–25%
Medium: 6–9	
Low: 5 or less	

Table 8.3
Symptoms and Signs of Preterm Labor

Menstrual-like cramps
Low, dull backache
Abdominal pressure
Pelvic pressure
Abdominal cramping (with or without diarrhea)
Increase or change in vaginal discharge (mucous, watery, light blood discharge)
Uterine contractions, often painless

bine information available at the initial obstetric interview with information obtained throughout pregnancy. These scoring systems probably are of some benefit, but their success in predicting PTL has been relatively low. In patients with high risk scores, the likelihood of preterm labor is about 25%. For multiparas, the most important etiologic factor for PTL is a history of preterm labor in a previous pregnancy. Elements of some risk assessment schemes are shown in Table 8.2.

Patient and physician education has focused on *recognition of the signs and symptoms that suggest PTL* (Table 8.3). Patients with such symptoms should be strongly advised to seek medical attention, and physicians and nurses providing obstetric care must carefully evaluate all such patients. There are indicators that often precede PTL. Patients destined to develop frank preterm labor have increased uterine irritability and more frequent contractions in the weeks before the actual diagnosis of labor. They also often experience an increased sensation of pelvic pres-

sure. In patients at high risk for preterm labor, ambulatory electronic fetal monitoring (periodic monitoring at home along with frequent contact with personnel trained in recognition of preterm labor) has been suggested as being beneficial. The value of this procedure has not been universally accepted, and its cost is considerable.

As *early and often asymptomatic dilation and effacement of the cervix seems to be associated with an increased likelihood of preterm labor*, a pelvic examination between 24 and 28 weeks gestation is now a common part of prenatal care. For patients at higher risk for preterm labor, evaluations are performed earlier in pregnancy and more frequently through the second half of gestation.

EVALUATION OF A PATIENT IN SUSPECTED PRETERM LABOR

Once a patient describes symptoms and signs suggestive of preterm labor, evaluation should be prompt. Application of an *external electronic fetal monitor* may help to quantify the frequency and duration of contractions; the intensity of uterine contractions is assessed very poorly on an external monitor, but abdominal palpation by experienced personnel can prove helpful. The *status of the cervix* should be determined, either by visualization with a speculum or by gentle digital examination. Changes in cervical effacement and dilation on subsequent examinations are important in the evaluation of both the diagnosis of PTL and the effectiveness of management. Subtle changes are often of great clinical importance so that serial examinations by the same examiner are optimal although not always practical.

Because urinary infections can predispose to uterine contractions, a careful *urinalysis and urine culture* should be obtained. At the time of speculum examination, *cervical cultures* should be taken for group B β-streptococcus and, when indicated by history or physical examination findings, for *Chlamydia* and *N. gonorrhoeae*. *Chlamydia* has been implicated in some cases of preterm labor.

Ultrasound examination can be useful in assessing the gestational age of the fetus, estimation of the amniotic fluid volume (spontaneous rupture of membranes with fluid loss may precede preterm labor and may be unrecognized by the patient), fetal presentation, and placental location. The technique also can reveal the existence of fetal congenital anomalies. Because placenta previa and placental abruption may lead to preterm contractions, patients should also be monitored for bleeding.

Because either clinical or subclinical infection of the amniotic cavity is thought to be associated with preterm labor in some cases, *amniocentesis* may be performed. The presence of bacteria in amniotic fluid is correlated with the subsequent development of infection, as well as preterm labor, which is less responsive to therapy. The presence of white cells in the amniotic fluid increases the likelihood of infection developing. Antibiotic therapy before delivery is of limited value because of difficulty establishing sufficient antibiotic levels in the fetoplacental unit. At the time of amniocentesis, additional amniotic fluid may be obtained for pulmonary maturity studies, which could have bearing on subsequent management. Tocolysis, the suppression of uterine contractions by pharmacologic means, may not be appropriate if there is indication of fetal lung maturity.

MANAGEMENT OF PRETERM LABOR

The purpose in treating preterm labor is to delay delivery, if possible, until fetal maturity is attained. Management involves *two broad goals*: first, the *detection and treatment of disorders associated with preterm labor* and, second, *therapy for the preterm labor* itself. Although it is fortunate that over 50% of patients with preterm contractions have spontaneous resolution of abnormal uterine activity, this complicates the evaluation of treatment. First, one may not know whether there was actual preterm labor or simply normal preterm uterine activity. It may be difficult to know whether it was the treatment that stopped the preterm labor or whether it would have stopped without therapy.

Because dehydration has been known to lead to uterine irritability, *therapy often begins with intravenous hydration*. In a significant number of patients, this therapy alone will cause cessation of uterine contractions.

Various *tocolytic therapies* have been utilized in the management of preterm labor. These are summarized in Table 8.4. Differ-

Table 8.4
Agents Used in Treating Preterm Labor

Class (example) and action	Comments
Magnesium sulfate Competes with calcium for entry into cells	High degree of safety. Often used as first agent. May cause flushing or headaches. At high levels may cause respiratory depression (12–15 mg/dl) or cardiac depression (>15 mg/dl).
β-Adrenergic agents (ritodrine, terbutaline) Increases cyclic AMP in cell, which decreases free calcium	β-Receptors are of two types: $β_1$ predominate in heart, intestines; $β_2$ predominate in the uterus, lungs, and blood vessels. Side effects include hypotension, tachycardia, anxiety, chest tightening or pain, ECG changes; also increased pulmonary edema very infrequently but possible, especially with fluid overload.
Prostaglandin synthetase inhibitors (indomethacin) Decrease prostaglandin (PG) production by blocking conversion of free arachidonic acid to PG	Premature constriction of ductus arteriosus possible especially after 34 weeks; bradycardia, growth retardation hypoglycemia reported earlier, but concern has decreased with broader experience.
Calcium channel blockers (nifedipine) Prevent calcium entry into muscle cells	Newest tocolytic; possible decrease in uteroplacental blood flow, fetal hypoxia, hypercarbia. More experience needed.

ent treatment regimens address specific mechanisms involved in the maintenance of uterine contractions, and each, therefore, may be best suited for certain patients.

Typically, *patients diagnosed as having preterm labor receive one form of therapy, with the addition or substitution of other forms should the initial treatment be unsuccessful.* As noted in Table 8.4, adverse effects, at times serious and even life threatening to the mother, can occur. These possibilities must be taken into account in selecting a therapy. The maturity of the fetus is a consideration in deciding how aggressively to pursue therapy, and, in general, the vigor with which therapy is undertaken diminishes as the gestational age of the fetus increase. One might be more willing to accept potential adverse effects for a patient in preterm labor at 26 weeks as opposed to 35 weeks. It is customary to stop therapy at 36 weeks. Treatment sequences may vary from hospital to hospital depending upon the individual hospital experience and the success rate with various therapeutic regimens.

Contraindications to tocolysis include advanced labor, a mature fetus, an anomalous fetus, intrauterine infection, significant vaginal bleeding, conditions where the adverse effects of tocolysis may be marked, and a variety of obstetric complications that contraindicate delay in delivery.

Relatively early in the third trimester, such as 28–32 weeks, management may include administration of certain *steroids* such as betamethasone, *which may enhance pulmonary maturity.* While a common practice, the results of recent evaluations of the efficacy of steroids have been disappointing. Whether steroid administration places the patient at higher risk for infection is another question that has not been clearly answered. In some patients with severe adverse effects of tocolytic therapy, such as pulmonary edema, it has been noted that steroids given to promote fetal lung maturity may have contributed to the maternal respiratory problems. This is another factor that should be considered when steroid use is contemplated.

FURTHER READINGS

Anderson HF, Merkatz IR. Preterm labor. In: Scott JR, DiSaia PJ, Hammond CB, Spellacy WN, eds. Danforth's obstetrics and gynecology. 6th ed. Philadelphia: JB Lippincott, 1990:Chapter 17.

Main DM, Main EK. Preterm birth. In: Gabbe SG, Niebyl JR, Simpson JL, eds. Obstetrics, normal and problem pregnancies. 2nd ed. New York: Churchill Livingstone 1991:Chapter 25.

SELF-EVALUATION

Case 8-A

A 26-year-old G2P0101 presents with complaints of vaginal discharge, urinary frequency, and a sensation of pelvic pressure. She says she may be contracting sometimes, but she isn't sure. She is at 28 weeks gestational age by dates and early ultrasound examination. Her first child was delivered by cesarean section at 29 weeks gestational age after tocolysis with magnesium sulfate and terbutaline had failed and the fetus was found to be breech. Her past medical history includes three episodes of chlamydia, the last in the first trimester of this pregnancy. Her antenatal course during this pregnancy has been otherwise unremarkable.

Question 8-A-1

Based on this history, which of the following evaluations are indicated at this time? (Choose all that apply.)

A. urinalysis (UA), culture and sensitivity (C&S)
B. obstetric ultrasound
C. cervical evaluation
D. amniocentesis
E. cervical cultures for *Chlamydia, N. gonorrhoeae*, and group B β-streptococcus

Answer 8-A-1

Answers: A, C, E

With a history of urinary frequency and previous *Chlamydia* infection, urinalysis and appropriate cultures are important initial steps. Cervical evaluation is crucial in determining if this patient wiht a previous preterm labor and delivery is again in preterm labor, for which she is at high risk. Obstetric ultrasound is useful, but not immediately. Evaluation for uterine activity by electronic fetal monitor is appropriate to assess for the presence of significant uterine contractions. Finally, amniocentesis is not indicated in the initial evaluation, since at this time the patient is not known to be in preterm labor.

Question 8-A-2

The patient is found to have a long, closed cervix and irregular uterine contractions that resolve with hydration. The fetal heart rate pattern is reassuring. UA shows 40 WBC per high power field (HPF).

For further consideration: What therapy is appropriate? Is tocolysis indicated on a prophylactic basis? Is amniocentesis indicated to rule out intrauterine infection? Based on the additional data, how would you assess the patient's risk for preterm labor and birth?

Case 8-B

A 29-year-old G4P2103 presents complaining of painful uterine contractions for 2 hours and a sensation of pelvic fullness. She is 30 weeks gestational age based on LMP and two ultrasound examinations. She has had three uneventful vaginal deliveries, two at term and one at 35½ weeks.

Cervical examination shows she is 3 cm dilated and 90% effaced, membranes intact, a cephalic part at zero station. On EFM she is having uterine contractions every 4 min, which the nurse evaluates as moderate to strong in intensity; the fetal heart pattern is reassuring.

Question 8-B-1

Which interventions are required at this time? (Choose all that apply.)

A. IV fluids
B. ultrasound to evaluate for fetal anomalies
C. tocolysis with magnesium sulfate
D. UA, C&S, and cervical cultures
E. amniocentesis

Answer 8-B-1

Answers: A, B, C, D

Immediate intravenous hydration and tocolysis with magnesium sulfate are indicated. Urinalysis and cultures are important information for future management and can be easily obtained. After tocolytic therapy has been started, ultrasound is appropriate. If tocolysis is successful, consideration for amniocentesis may then be in order.

Question 8-B-2

Tocolysis with intravenous fluids and magnesium sulfate is successful, with cervical changes arrested for the time at 3 cm dilation and 90% effacement.

For further consideration: What will you tell the patient about the risks and benefits of steroid therapy in her situation? Will you use the same or different agents if uterine contractions reoccur? Will you consider discharge if uterine contractions do not reoccur? If so, will you send the patient home on a tocolytic? Is electronic ambulatory fetal monitoring warranted in this patient?

chapter 9

OBSTETRIC HEMORRHAGE

An estimated 5% of women will describe bleeding of some extent during pregnancy. At times, the amount of bleeding is hardly more than "spotting," whereas at other times profuse hemorrhage can lead to maternal death in a matter of minutes. In most cases, bleeding is minimal spotting, often following sexual intercourse, and is thought to be related to trauma to the friable ectocervix. Small polyps on the cervix can also cause small amounts of bleeding. Table 9.1 lists causes of bleeding in the second half of pregnancy. A previous Pap test and examination of the lower genital tract should eliminate the likelihood of lower genital tract neoplasms in most cases. At times, patients may mistake bleeding from hemorrhoids for vaginal bleeding, but the difference is easily distinguished by examination.

The two causes of antepartum hemorrhage in the second half of pregnancy that require greatest attention, because of the as-

Table 9.1
Causes of Bleeding in the Second Half of Pregnancy

Vulva
  Varicose veins
  Tears or lacerations
Vagina
  Tears or lacerations
Cervix
  Polyp
  Glandular tissue (normal)
  Cervicitis
  Carcinoma
Intrauterine
  Placenta previa
  Abruptio placentae
  Vasa previa

sociated maternal and fetal morbidity and mortality, are placenta previa and abruptio placentae. Various characteristics of these entities are compared in Table 9.2.

PLACENTA PREVIA

Placenta previa refers to an abnormal location of the placenta over or in close proximity to the internal cervical os. Placenta previa can be categorized as *complete or total* if the entire cervical os is covered, *partial* if the margin of the placenta extends across part but not all of the internal os, *marginal* if the edge of the placenta lies adjacent to the internal os, and *low lying* if the placenta is located near but not adjacent directly to the internal os (Fig. 9.1). The *etiology* of placenta previa is not understood, but abnormal vascularization has long been proposed as a mechanism for this abnormal placement of the placenta. In some cases, such as in twin pregnancy, or if the placenta is hydropic, it may extend to the region of the internal cervical os because of its size alone. Increasing maternal age, increasing parity, and previous cesarean delivery are factors commonly associated with placenta previa, although recent evidence suggests that age alone is not an important factor.

The *incidence* of placenta previa varies with gestational age, usually reported as about 1/250 pregnancies. With common use of ultrasonography examinations, it has been shown repeatedly that the placenta may cover the internal cervical os in about 5% of pregnancies when examined at midpregnancy, a finding seen even more frequently earlier in

119

gestation. Because of subsequent growth of both the upper and lower uterine segments, the placenta appears to "migrate" away from the internal os in the majority of cases. The likelihood of this apparent movement diminishes as the gestational age at first detection increases.

The average gestational age at the time of the first bleeding episode is 29–30 weeks. Although the bleeding may be substantial in amount, it

Table 9.2
Features of Placenta Previa and Abruptio Placentae

	Placenta previa	Abruptio placentae
Magnitude of blood loss	Variable	Variable
Duration	Often ceases within 1–2 h	Usually continues
Abdominal discomfort	None	Can be severe
Fetal heart rate pattern on electronic monitoring	Normal	Tachycardia, then bradycardia Loss of variability Decelerations frequently present Intrauterine demise not rare
Coagulation defects	Rare	Associated, but infrequent DIC often severe when present[a]
Associated history	None	Cocaine use Abdominal trauma Maternal hypertension Multiple gestation Polyhydraminos

[a]DIC, disseminated intravascular coagulation.

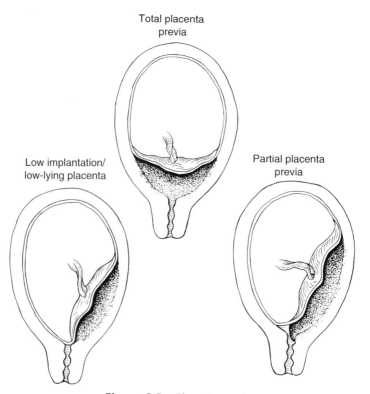

Figure 9.1. Placenta previa.

almost always ceases spontaneously, unless digital examination or other trauma occurs. The bleeding is caused by separation of part of the placenta from the lower uterine segment and cervix, possibly in response to mild uterine contractions. The blood that is lost is usually maternal in origin. The patient often describes a sudden onset of bleeding without any apparent antecedent signs. There is no pain associated with placenta previa in most cases, unless coincidental uterine contractions occur.

Ultrasonography has been of enormous benefit in localizing the placenta. If the placenta lies in the posterior portion of the lower uterine segment, its exact relationship with the internal os may be difficult to ascertain. In most cases, though, ultrasonography examination can accurately diagnose placenta previa (Fig. 9.1) or, by illustrating the placenta location away from the cervix and lower uterine segment, exclude it as a cause for bleeding.

The basic *management* of patients with placenta previa includes hospitalization with hemodynamic stabilization, followed by expectant management until fetal maturity has occurred. Bleeding episodes may or may not occur, but continued hospitalization provides ready access to prompt care, especially transfusions and rapid delivery. If the fetus is thought to be mature by gestational age criteria or by amniocentesis for fetal lung maturity testing, there is little benefit to be gained by a delay in delivery. The further from term that bleeding from placenta previa occurs, the more important it is to delay delivery to allow for further fetal growth and maturation. The degree of bleeding and the maturity of the fetus must be constantly weighed in managing these patients. Fetal maturity is usually assessed at approximately 36 weeks, with cesarean delivery performed once the fetus is deemed mature.

In some cases, when the location of the placenta cannot be accurately determined by ultrasound, the route of delivery is determined by a "double set-up" examination. This procedure involves careful evaluation of the cervix in the operating room with full preparations for rapid cesarean delivery. If placental tissue is seen or palpated at the internal cervical os, prompt cesarean with delivery is performed. If the placental margin is away from the internal os, artificial rupture of the membranes and oxytocin induction of labor may be performed in anticipation of vaginal delivery. Prior to the widespread utilization of ultrasound, this procedure was done more frequently than it is in modern obstetrics; nonetheless, it is still an important tool in selected cases.

Abnormal placental location can be further complicated by abnormal growth of the placental mass into the substance of the uterus, a condition termed *placenta accreta*. At the time of delivery, sustained and significant bleeding may ensue, often requiring hysterectomy.

ABRUPTIO PLACENTAE

Whereas placenta previa refers to the abnormal location of the placenta, *abruptio placentae, often called placental abruption, refers to the premature abnormal separation of the placenta from the uterine wall.* While it shares some clinical features with placenta previa, particularly vaginal bleeding, other characteristics serve to distinguish abruptio placentae from placenta previa, the most important of which are abdominal discomfort and painful uterine contractions (Table 9.2).

Placental abruption occurs when there is hemorrhage into the decidua basalis, leading to premature placental separation and further bleeding. The cause for this bleeding is not known. Placental abruption is associated with maternal hypertension and sudden decompression of the uterus in cases of rupture of membranes in a patient with excessive amniotic fluid (hydramnios) or after delivery of the first of multiple fetuses. A more recent and serious association involves cocaine use by the mother that leads to intense vasoconstriction and, in some cases, sudden separation of the placenta from the uterine wall. Placental abruption can also occur following

Partial separation

Marginal separation

Complete separation,
concealed hemorrhage

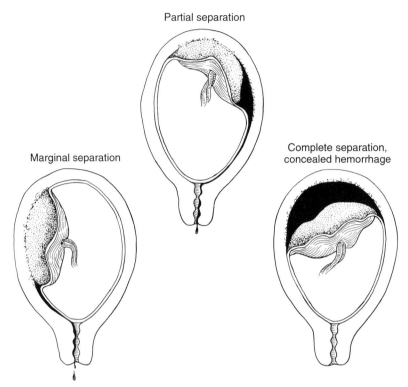

Figure 9.2. Relationship between vaginal bleeding and placental abruption.

trauma, even when the extent of injury is not considered serious. For example, pregnant women involved in motor vehicle accidents can sustain placental abruption even though lap belts and shoulder strap restraints are used. Moreover, direct trauma to the abdomen is not required, as sudden force applied elsewhere to the body can result in coup and contrecoup injury.

The anatomic relationship between vaginal bleeding and placental abruption is shown in Figure 9.2. If the bleeding and subsequent separation of a placenta permits access to the cervical os, vaginal bleeding will be apparent. If the placental location is higher in the uterus, or if the bleeding is more central and the margins of the placenta remain attached to the underlying uterus, blood may not escape into the vagina. Thus, the amount of vaginal bleeding is extremely variable, from none to heavy. The bleeding into the basalis stimulates the uterine muscle

to contract and the uterus will be painful to the patient and tender to touch. Unusually painful uterine contractions are frequent and the uterus may feel constantly tense. At times, the bleeding can penetrate the uterine musculature to such an extent that, at the time of cesarean delivery, the entire uterus has a purplish or bluish appearance, owing to such extravasation of blood (Couvelaire uterus). Despite its unusual appearance, no treatment is required, as spontaneous resolution of the condition will occur postpartum.

Because the separation of the placenta from the uterus interferes with oxygenation of the fetus, *fetal distress is quite common* in cases of significant placental abruption. Thus, in any patient in whom placental abruption is suspected, electronic fetal monitoring should be included in the initial management. Fetal death owing to deprivation of oxygen is, unfortunately, not rare with placental abruption.

Coagulation abnormalities may also be found, thereby compounding the patient's already compromised status. Placental abruption is the most common cause of consumptive coagulopathy in pregnancy and is manifested by hypofibrinogenemia as well as by increased levels of fibrin degradation products. The platelet count can also be decreased, and prothrombin time and partial thromboplastin time can be increased also. This coagulopathy is a result of intravascular and retroplacental coagulation. The intravascular fibrinogen is converted to fibrin by way of the extrinsic clotting cascade. Not only, then, is serum fibrinogen decreased, but platelets and other clotting factors are thereby also depleted. Transfusion with crystalloid and whole blood should be implemented as soon as possible for those patients who require either volume replacement or oxygen-carrying capacity. Whole blood helps to replace not only volume, but also oxygen-carrying capacity. Whole blood may also contain some clotting factors, including fibrinogen. Many experts recommend component therapy (e.g., packed red cells, platelets, fresh frozen plasma, etc.) rather than whole blood therapy. The extent of placental abruption is generally categorized as the proportion of the maternal surface of the placenta on which a clot is detected at the time of delivery, e.g., "50% abruption."

Ultrasound is of little benefit in diagnosing placental abruption, except to exclude placenta previa as a cause for the hemorrhage. Relatively large retroplacental clots may be detected on ultrasound examination, but the absence of ultrasonographically identified retroplacental clots does not rule out the possibility of placental abruption and, conversely, a retroplacental echogenic area can be seen in patients without placental abruption. The diagnosis rests on the "classic" clinical presentation of vaginal bleeding, a tender uterus, and frequent uterine contractions with some evidence of fetal distress. The extravasation of blood into the uterine muscle causes contractions such that the resting intrauterine pressure, when measured with an intrauterine pressure catheter, is often elevated; this sign can be helpful in making the diagnosis.

Management of a patient with placental abruption when the fetus is mature is hemodynamic stabilization and delivery. Careful attention to blood component therapy is critical and the coagulation status must be followed carefully. Unless there is evidence of fetal distress or hemodynamic instability, vaginal delivery by oxytocin induction of labor is preferable to a cesarean delivery, although the maternal or fetal status may require that abdominal delivery be performed. Where the fetus is not mature and the placental abruption is limited and not associated with premature labor or fetal or maternal distress, observation with close monitoring of both fetal and maternal well-being may be considered while awaiting fetal maturity.

VASA PREVIA

Although rarely encountered, *vasa previa* presents significant risk to the fetus. In *vasa previa, the umbilical cord inserts into the membranes of the placenta* (rather than into the central mass of the placental tissue), and one such vessel lies below the presenting fetal part in the vicinity of the internal os. Should this vessel rupture, fetal bleeding will occur. Because of the low blood volume of the fetus, seemingly insignificant amounts of blood may place the fetus in jeopardy. A small amount of vaginal bleeding associated with fetal tachycardia may be the clinical presentation. A test to distinguish fetal blood from maternal blood, such as the Kleihauer-Betke or the APT test, can be of value when such a condition is suspected. Such tests distinguish between maternal and fetal blood on the basis of the marked resistance to pH changes in fetal red cells compared to the friable nature of adult red cells in the presence of strong bases.

APPROACH TO A PATIENT WITH VAGINAL BLEEDING IN THE SECOND HALF OF GESTATION

In any woman with vaginal bleeding during the second half of pregnancy, fetal and maternal status should be evaluated promptly. At the same time that a search is undertaken for the cause of the bleeding, attention must be directed toward stabilization of the maternal hemodynamic state. The approach is not unlike that for any hemorrhaging patient and includes ready access for fluid replacement through one or more large bore intravenous catheters, serial complete blood counts, type and cross-match of ample amounts of blood, and, if the condition is unstable, intracardiac monitoring. Attention to urinary output is a simple and important reflection of the volume status of a patient. Because normal antepartum blood volume expansion is substantial, pregnant women may lose considerable amounts of blood before vital sign changes are apparent.

In more than half of the cases of significant vaginal bleeding in pregnancy, no specific cause can be discovered despite careful evaluation. In general, patients with significant bleeding should remain hospitalized until delivery, although in some cases minimal bleeding will cease, and the patient will appear normal in every way. Caution is advised, however, as patients with bleeding of undetermined etiology can be at greater risk for preterm delivery, intrauterine growth retardation, and fetal distress than patients with bleeding of known cause.

SELF-EVALUATION

Case 9-A

A 26-year-old G1 at 29 weeks gestational age by LMP has phoned the hospital saying she had an episode of bright red vaginal bleeding without other symptoms about 2 hours ago. You have not seen her previously.

Question 9-A-1

Your best instruction to her is:

A. Have the patient call back if there is another episode of bleeding.
B. Have the patient come in for evaluation.
C. Have the patient make an office appointment.
D. Have the patient make an appointment in radiology for ultrasound evaluation.

Answer 9-A-1

Answer: B

Immediate evaluation of fetal and maternal status is required. Placenta previa may present in this manner and, although the first bleeding episode may have been self-limited, the second may be much more profuse. Although there are no reported symptoms, abruptio placentae is still a possibility with the associated need for prompt fetal evaluation.

Question 9-A-2

The patient arrives at the hospital and is found to have stable vital signs. Further history includes a fall, hitting her abdomen about 6 hours before the bleeding episode. The patient's physical examination includes a very mildly tender uterus over the area of the fall, minimal vaginal spotting, and speculum examination showing no cervical dilation nor evidence of rupture of membranes.

Immediate management should include:

A. IV fluids
B. electronic fetal monitoring
C. ultrasound evaluation
D. amniocentesis
E. Kleihauer-Betke test

Answer 9-A-2

Answer: A, B, C, E

Since the mother is hemodynamically stable, immediate evaluation of fetal status using electronic fetal monitoring and ultrasound are indicated, as you have not established a cause of the bleeding. Ultrasound examination is often advised before any vaginal examination, although a careful speculum examination is advocated before ultrasound examination by some authorities. Venous access is indicated in the event of further bleeding. Amniocentesis may be needed in the future, but at present is too invasive for the information to be obtained.

Question 9-A-3

For further consideration: What do you expect to find on ultrasound examination? Does the history of trauma affect your differential diagnosis? What is the purpose of the Betke-Kleihauer test? The patient's husband wants to know how long to expect his wife to be in the hospital. What will you tell him?

Case 9-B

A 26-year-old G6P5005 presents for her routine antepartum visit at 18 weeks gestational age. She is most distressed because at her ultrasound visit the day before, she was told by the technician that her placenta was partly over the opening of her womb.

Question 9-B-1

Which of the following would you tell the patient?

A. She has a placenta previa and will definitely require cesarean section.
B. She has a vasa previa and will definitely require cesarean section.
C. She has a placental abruption and will definitely require cesarean section.
D. She has a placenta previa and may require cesarean section.
E. She has a vasa previa and may require cesarean section.
F. She has a placental abruption and may require cesarean section.

Answer 9-B-1

Answer: D

The ultrasound is consistent with a partial placenta previa. Since the growth of the upper and lower uterine segments may result in the placenta "migrating away" from the cervical os, it is too early to be certain that cesarean will be required.

Question 9-B-2

For further consideration: The patient and her husband are quite upset about this news after five normal pregnancies and deliveries. They ask what caused this problem and how likely is a cesarean section. How will you answer them?

chapter 10

HYPERTENSION IN PREGNANCY

Hypertensive disorders are among the most common and yet serious conditions seen in obstetrics. These disorders cause substantial morbidity and mortality for both mother and fetus despite improved prenatal care. The etiology of hypertension unique to pregnancy remains unknown.

Hypertension in pregnancy is generally defined as a diastolic blood pressure of 90 mm Hg or greater, or a systolic blood pressure at or above 140 mm Hg, or as *a rise in the diastolic blood pressure of at least 15 mm Hg or in the systolic blood pressure of 30 mm Hg or more* when compared to previous blood pressures. This definition requires that the increased blood pressures be present on at least two separate occasions, 6 hours or more apart. Although this definition seems quite clear, its use in clinical practice is difficult because of various problems in obtaining a reliable assessment of blood pressure. The position of the patient influences blood pressure. It is lowest with the patient lying in the lateral position, highest when standing, and at an intermediate level when sitting. The choice of the correct size blood pressure cuff also influences blood pressure readings. Also, in the course of pregnancy, blood pressure typically declines slightly in the middle trimester, only to rise to prepregnant levels as gestation nears term. If a patient has not been seen previously, there is no baseline blood pressure upon which to compare new blood pressure determinations, thereby making the diagnosis of pregnancy-related hypertension more difficult.

CLASSIFICATION OF HYPERTENSIVE DISEASE IN PREGNANCY

Various classifications of hypertensive disorders in pregnancy have been proposed. Table 10.1 presents the commonly used classification of the American College of Obstetricians and Gynecologists (ACOG). Since hypertensive disorders in pregnancy represent a spectrum of disease, classification systems should not be considered as rigid markers on which all management decisions are made.

Preeclampsia is defined as *the development of hypertension with proteinuria or edema (or both), induced by pregnancy, generally in the second half of gestation.* Preeclampsia is more common in women who have not carried a previous pregnancy beyond 20 weeks and is more frequent at the extremes of the reproductive years. Preeclampsia is classified as *severe* if there is a blood pressure above 160/110 mm Hg, marked proteinuria (generally greater than 1 g/24-h urine collection, or 2+ or more on dipstick of a random urine), oli-

Table 10.1
Hypertensive Disorders in Pregnancy[a]

Pregnancy-induced hypertension
  Preeclampsia
    Mild preeclampsia
    Severe preeclampsia
  Eclampsia
Chronic hypertension preceding pregnancy (any etiology)
Chronic hypertension (any etiology) with superimposed pregnancy-induced hypertension
  Superimposed preeclampsia
  Superimposed eclampsia

[a]Classification of the American College of Obstetricians and Gynecologists.

guria, cerebral or visual disturbances such as headache and scotomata, pulmonary edema or cyanosis, epigastric or right upper quadrant pain, evidence of hepatic dysfunction, or thrombocytopenia. These myriad changes illustrate the multisystem alterations associated with preeclampsia during pregnancy. *Eclampsia* is the presence of convulsions, not caused by neurologic disease, in a woman whose condition also meets the criteria of preeclampsia. *Chronic hypertension* is defined as hypertension present prior to the 20th week of gestation or beyond 6 weeks postpartum. Chronic hypertension can be due to a variety of causes, although the majority of cases are deemed essential hypertension. The greatest risk to a woman with chronic hypertension during pregnancy is the development of superimposed preeclampsia or eclampsia, which occurs in approximately 25% of cases. At times, it is difficult to distinguish between preeclampsia and chronic hypertension when a patient is seen late in pregnancy with an elevated blood pressure. In such cases, it is always wise to assume that the findings represent preeclampsia and treat accordingly. Finally, *preeclampsia or eclampsia superimposed upon chronic hypertension* is defined as the development of preeclampsia or eclampsia in a patient with preexisting chronic hypertension.

Not mentioned in the ACOG classification is the finding of hypertension in late pregnancy in the absence of other findings suggestive of preeclampsia. Such a condition has been termed *transient hypertension of pregnancy or gestational hypertension*. Although isolated hypertension is certainly seen in late pregnancy and in the first day or two postpartum, caution should be taken in assuming that these patients have hypertension alone.

PATHOPHYSIOLOGY OF HYPERTENSION IN PREGNANCY

Hypertension in pregnancy affects the mother and newborn to varying degrees depending on the severity of disease. Given the characteristic multisystem effects, it is clear that several pathophysiologic mechanisms are involved. Unfortunately, present understanding of these mechanisms lags behind the ability to describe the clinical manifestations. One common pathophysiologic finding in hypertension in pregnancy, especially when there is progression to preeclampsia, is *vasospasm*. Although numerous theories ranging from poor nutrition to climate changes have been proposed to explain this vascular phenomenon, the etiology of the vasospasm remains unknown. Interestingly, it has been shown that women with uncomplicated pregnancies are extraordinarily resistant to the effects of the potent pressor angiotensin II, while those patients destined to develop preeclampsia do not demonstrate the decreased peripheral resistance normally seen in pregnancies. Hepatocellular dysfunction, coagulopathy, and renal dysfunction are also encountered, more commonly in severe cases of the disease.

Presumably because of vasospastic changes, placental size and function are decreased. The results are progressive fetal hypoxia and malnutrition, as well as an increase in the incidence of intrauterine growth retardation, oligohydramnios, and dysmaturity. With the stress of uterine contractions during labor, the placenta is often incapable of supporting the fetus, resulting in intrapartum fetal distress with progressive hypoxia and acidosis.

EVALUATION OF HYPERTENSION IN PREGNANCY

The history and physical examination are directed toward detection of pregnancy-associated hypertensive disease and its stigmata. A review of current obstetric records, if available, is especially helpful to ascertain changes or progression in findings. *Visual disturbances*, especially scotomata (spots before the eyes), or unusually severe or persistent *headaches* are indicative of vasospasm. *Right upper quadrant (RUQ) pain* may indicate liver involvement, presumably involving distention of the liver capsule. Any history of *loss of consciousness or seizures*, even in the patient with a known seizure disorder, may be significant.

The patient's weight is compared with her pregravid weight and with previous weights during this pregnancy, with special attention to excessive or too rapid weight gain. Peripheral edema is common in pregnancy, especially in the lower extremities; however, persistent edema unresponsive to resting in the supine position is not normal, especially when it also involves the upper extremities and face. Indeed, the puffy-faced, edematous hypertensive pregnant woman is the classic picture of severe preeclampsia. Careful blood pressure determination in the sitting and supine positions is necessary. Fundoscopic examination may detect vasoconstriction of retinal blood vessels, presumably indicative of similar vasoconstriction of other small vessels. Tenderness over the liver attributed in part to hepatic capsule distension may be associated with complaints of RUQ pain. The patellar and Achilles deep tendon reflexes should be carefully elicited and hyperreflexia noted. The demonstration of clonus at the ankle is especially worrisome.

The maternal and fetal laboratory evaluations for pregnancy complicated by hypertension are presented in Table 10.2 and demonstrate by the wide range of tests the multisystem effects of hypertension in pregnancy. Maternal liver and renal dysfunction and coagulopathy are a concern and require serial evaluation. Evaluation of fetal well-being with ultrasonography, NST/OCT, and/or biophysical profile is crucial.

MANAGEMENT OF HYPERTENSION IN PREGNANCY

The goal of management of hypertension in pregnancy is to balance the management of both fetus and mother to optimize each outcome. In general, maternal blood pressure should be monitored and the mother should be observed for the sequelae of the hypertensive disease. Intervention for maternal indications should occur when the risk of permanent disability or death for the mother without intervention outweighs the risks to the fetus caused by intervention. For the fetus, there should be regular evaluation of fetal well-being and fetal growth, with intervention becoming necessary if the intrauterine environment provides more risks to the fetus than delivery with subsequent care in the newborn nursery.

MANAGEMENT OF PREECLAMPSIA

The severity of the preeclampsia and the maturity of the fetus are the primary considerations in the management of preeclampsia. Care must be individualized, but these are well-accepted general guidelines.

The mainstay of patients with *mild preeclampsia* and an immature fetus is *bed rest*, preferably with as much of the time as possible spent in a lateral decubitus position. In this position, cardiac function and uterine blood flow are maximized and maternal blood pressures in most cases are normalized. This improves uteroplacental function, allowing normal fetal growth and metabolism. For a patient with mild preeclampsia who has access to medical care and is motivated to care for herself, bed rest at home with daily weighing (if possible), fetal movement count records, and home blood pressure determinations (if available) will usually suffice. The patient is instructed to recognize signs and symptoms indicating worsening of the preeclampsia and to notify her physician in such an event. In the absence of significant changes in condition, such care will allow the fetus to grow and become more functionally mature. In addition, induction of labor, if needed, is more likely to be successful as gestational age approaches term.

Hospitalization is recommended if the patient lacks either transportation for frequent prenatal visits or motivation to maintain bed rest, or for the patient in whom expectant management at home does not result in normalization of blood pressure. The same regimen is used in the hospital, but better compliance is assured in this more controlled environment.

Table 10.2
Laboratory Assessment of Pregnant Hypertensive Patients

Tests or procedures	Rationale
Maternal studies	
Complete blood count	Increasing hematocrit may signify worsening vasoconstriction and decreased intravascular volume
Platelet count	Thrombocytopenia and coagulopathy are associated with worsening
Coagulation profile (PT, PTT)ª	PIH
Fibrin split products	
Liver function studies	Hepatocellular dysfunction is associated with worsening PIH
Serum creatinine	Decreased renal function is associated with worsening PIH
24-h urine for	
Creatinine clearance	
Total urinary protein	
Uric acid	
Fetal studies	
Ultrasound examination	To assess for pregnancy-associated hypertension effects on the fetus:
Fetal weight and growth	IUGR
Amniotic fluid volume	Oligohydramnios
Placental status	Chronic fetal stress/distress
NST/OCT	
Biophysical profile	

ªPT, prothrombin time; PTT, partial thromboplastin time; PIH, pregnancy-induced hypertension; IUGR, intrauterine growth retardation.

For the patient with *worsening preeclampsia* or the patient who has *severe preeclampsia* or *eclampsia*, stabilization with magnesium sulfate, antihypertensive therapy as indicated, monitoring for maternal and fetal well-being, and delivery by induction or cesarean section is required. A 24-hour delay in delivery to allow steroid administration to enhance fetal pulmonary maturity may be indicated in some cases.

For over half a century, *magnesium sulfate* has been used to prevent convulsions. It has virtually no effect on blood pressure. Other anticonvulsants such as diazepam or phenytoin are infrequently used in obstetrics. Magnesium sulfate may be administered by intramuscular or intravenous routes, although the latter is more common. An initial 4-g loading dose is given intravenously over 20–30 min, followed by a constant infusion of 1–3 g/h. In 98% of cases, convulsions will be prevented. Therapeutic levels are 4–7 mEq/L, with toxic concentrations having predictable consequences: loss of deep tendon reflexes at 7–10 mEq/L, depression of respirations at 10–15 mEq/L, and cardiac arrest at about 30 mEq/L. Frequent evaluations of the patient's patellar reflex and respirations are necessary to monitor for manifestations of toxic serum magnesium concentrations. In addition, because magnesium sulfate is excreted solely from the kidney, maintenance of urine output at greater than 25 ml/h will avoid accumulation of the drug. Reversal of the effects of excessive magnesium concentrations is accomplished by the slow intravenous administration of 10% calcium gluconate along with oxygen supplementation and cardiorespiratory support if needed.

Antihypertensive therapy is indicated if the diastolic blood pressure is repeatedly above 110 mm Hg. *Hydralazine* (Apresoline) is the initial antihypertensive of choice, given in 5-mg increments intravenously until acceptable blood pressures are obtained. A 10–15-min response time is usual. The goal of such therapy is to reduce the diastolic pressure to the 90–100 mm Hg range. Further reduction of the blood pressure may impair uterine blood flow to rates dangerous to the fetus. Other antihypertensive agents may be used if hydralazine is not effective.

Once anticonvulsant and antihypertensive therapy is established, attention is directed toward *delivery*. Induction of labor is often attempted, although cesarean delivery may be needed if either induction is unsuccessful or not possible, or because of worsening maternal or fetal status. At delivery, blood loss must be closely monitored because patients with preeclampsia or eclampsia have significantly reduced blood volumes. *After delivery*, patients are kept in the labor and delivery area for 24 hours for close observation of their clinical progress and further administration of magnesium sulfate to prevent postpartum eclamptic seizures. Approximately one quarter of all preeclamptic patients who have eclamptic seizures will have them prior to labor, about one half during labor, and about one quarter after delivery. Usually the vasospastic process begins to reverse itself in the first 24–48 hours, as manifest by a brisk diuresis.

The management of patients with *chronic hypertension in pregnancy* involves closely monitoring maternal blood pressure and watching for the superimposition of preeclampsia or eclampsia and following the fetus for appropriate growth and fetal well-being. Also, the patient should be encouraged to increase the amount of time she rests. Medical treatment of milder forms of chronic hypertension has been disappointing in that no significant improvement in pregnancy outcome has been demonstrated. Antihypertensive medication is generally not given unless the diastolic blood pressure exceeds 110 mm Hg. Methyldopa is the most commonly used antihypertensive medication for this purpose. It was formerly taught that diuretics were contraindicated during pregnancy, but diuretic therapy is no longer discontinued in the patient who is already on such therapy prior to becoming pregnant.

HELLP SYNDROME

HELLP is an acronym for a specific set of hypertensive patients with: **h**emolysis, **l**iver dysfunction, and **l**ow **p**latelets. Recently described as a distinct clinical entity, patients with this syndrome are often multiparous, somewhat older than the average obstetric patient, and somewhat less hypertensive than many preeclamptic patients. The liver dysfunction may be manifest as right upper quadrant pain and is all too commonly misdiagnosed as gallbladder disease or indigestion. The maternal and fetal mortality for patients with HELLP is significant, making accurate diagnosis imperative. Treatment consists of cardiovascular stabilization, correction of coagulation abnormalities, and delivery. These very sick patients are best cared for in a high risk obstetric center.

FURTHER READINGS

Cunningham FG, MacDonald PC, Gant NF. Williams obstetrics, 18th ed. East Norwalk, CT: Appleton & Lange, 1989:653–691.

Gabbe SG, Niebyl JR, Simpson JL. Obstetrics: normal and problem pregnancies. 2nd ed. New York: Churchill Livingstone, 1991:993–1056.

Roberts JM. Pregnancy-related hypertension. In Creasy RK, Resnik R, eds. Maternal-fetal medicine: principles and practice, Philadelphia: WB Saunders, 1989: 777–823.

SELF-EVALUATION

Case 10-A

A 38-year-old G2P1001 presents for prenatal care at 10 weeks gestational age by good dates and initial pelvic examination. Her obstetric history includes a normal pregnancy and delivery at age 17. Four years ago she was diagnosed as having essential hypertension and placed on a diuretic and methyldopa; she says her blood pressure "runs about 140/90 most of the time."

On physical examination the patient weighs 280 pounds. A blood pressure taken with a large cuff is 135/85 supine and 140/95 sitting. She has mild arteriolar narrowing on fundoscopic examination, a normal cardiovascular examination, a 10-week size uterus, normal deep tendon reflexes (DTRs), and 1+ lower extremity peripheral edema. Her urine sample "dipstick" shows 1+ protein and trace glucose.

Question 10-A-1

Your initial diagnosis is:

A. pregnancy-induced hypertension
B. mild preeclampsia
C. severe preeclampsia
D. eclampsia
E. chronic hypertension
F. chronic hypertension with superimposed pregnancy-induced hypertension

Answer 10-A-1

Answer: E

This patient's hypertension precedes her pregnancy. Although her status nears the definition of mild preeclampsia, which would give her the diagnosis of chronic hypertension with superimposed mild preeclampsia, her stable history precludes this diagnosis at her initial visit.

Question 10-A-2

Your initial management should include:

A. discontinue the diuretic and methyldopa
B. recommend strict bed rest at home
C. recommend therapeutic abortion
D. hospitalize for the remainder of pregnancy
E. none of these

Answer 10-A-2

Answer: E

Initial management should be to maximize rest, but strict bed rest at home is too much restriction at this time. Modern obstetric practice is to not change the antihypertensive medications of chronic hypertensive patients who become pregnant. Instead, the regimen is continued while maternal and fetal evaluations commence. There is no indication for hospitalization nor for therapeutic abortion.

Case 10-B

A 19-year-old G1 has had an unremarkable antepartum course since her first prenatal visit at 8 weeks. At the start of her 32nd week she complains of swollen hands and feet and "puffy eyes," which have been getting worse for the last 2 days.

Her blood pressure is 150/95 compared to her usual blood pressure of 130/70. After resting for 30 min, her blood pressure is 145/85. Her "dipstick urinary protein" is 1–2+. She reports daily fetal movement that has not changed and denies headache, abdominal pain, or dizzy spells.

Question 10-B-1

Your initial diagnosis is:

A. pregnancy-induced hypertension
B. mild preeclampsia
C. severe preeclampsia
D. eclampsia
E. chronic hypertension
F. chronic hypertension with superimposed pregnancy-induced hypertension

Answer 10-B-1

Answer: B

This patient has mild preeclampsia. Her 1–2+ proteinuria is disconcerting, but her rapid improvement in blood pressure with 30 min of rest is reassuring, as is her history of an active fetus.

Question 10-B-2

Which of the following evaluations are indicated at the present time?

A. obstetric ultrasound
B. non-stress test (NST)
C. oxytocin challenge test (OCT)
D. amniocentesis for fetal lung maturity determination
E. pelvic examination
F. biophysical profile
G. complete blood count (CBC), coagulation profile, liver function studies
H. 24-h urine collection for total protein and creatinine clearance

Answer 10-B-2

Answer: A, B, E, F, G, H

Because there is no need to deliver the fetus at this time, fetal lung maturity is not an issue. Without evidence of fetal stress, OCT is not warranted unless the NST is not reassuring.

Ultrasound can evaluate amniotic fluid volume and provide the biophysical profile. The chemical evaluations of maternal status are indicated, if for no other reason than to serve as a baseline evaluation if the mother's condition deteriorates. A pelvic examination is a wise precaution at this time to evaluate the favorability of the cervix as the potential for induction exists if the maternal or fetal status worsens.

chapter 11

ISOIMMUNIZATION

Isoimmunization refers to *the development of antibodies to red blood cell antigens following exposure to such antigens from another individual.* In pregnancy, *the "other individual" is the fetus,* one half of whose genetic makeup is derived from the father. If the mother is exposed to fetal red cells during pregnancy or at delivery, she may develop antibodies to fetal cell antigens. Later in that pregnancy, or more commonly with the subsequent pregnancy, the antibodies can cross the placenta and hemolyze fetal red cells, leading to fetal anemia. In a pregnancy complicated by isoimmunization, the manufacture of maternal antibody that destroys fetal red cells is countered by the ability of the fetus to manufacture sufficient red cells to permit survival and growth.

NATURAL HISTORY OF ISOIMMUNIZATION

For a clear understanding of this complication of pregnancy, the natural history of the disorder must be fully appreciated. Isoimmunization can involve many of the *several hundred blood group systems.* This disorder is frequently referred to as Rh isoimmunization since this is the system most frequently involved. For the sake of this discussion, the Rh system will be used as an example, although it should be remembered that isoimmunization can and does develop with many other blood systems such as Kell, Duffy, Kidd, and others.

Within the Rh system, there are several specific antigens, the one most commonly associated with hemolytic disease being the "D" antigen. If a fetus is Rh positive, having received the genes for the Rh antigen from its father, and the mother lacks the Rh antigen, that is, she is Rh negative, the conditions exist for the development of isoimmunization. In the first such pregnancy, the infant typically has no complications. At the time of delivery, however, exposure of the mother's blood to fetal red cells, even in miniscule amounts, can lead to the development of antibodies to this antigen. Antibody development will occur in about 15% of cases of an Rh-negative mother and Rh-positive fetus. In a subsequent pregnancy, passage of minute amounts of fetal blood across the placenta, which occurs quite frequently, can lead to an *anamnestic response* of maternal antibody production. If the type of antibody produced is of the IgM variety, the large size of the molecule prevents passage across the placenta. However, in the case of the Rh factor, the antibody produced is predominantly the smaller IgG, which freely crosses the placenta and enters the fetal circulation. Once in the fetal vascular system, the antibody attaches to the Rh-positive red blood cells and hemolyzes them. The bilirubin produced in this hemolytic process is transferred back across the placenta to the mother and metabolized. *The condition of the fetus is determined by the amount of maternal antibody transferred across the placenta and the ability of the fetus to replace the red blood cells that have been destroyed.*

In the first affected pregnancy, the infant may be anemic at delivery and may soon develop elevated levels of bilirubin, since hemolysis continues after birth and the newborn must now rely on its own, somewhat immature, liver to metabolize the bilirubin.

135

Table 11.1
Risk of Sensitization

Obstetric/medical event	Chance of sensitization
	%
Ectopic pregnancy	<1
Full-term pregnancy	1–2
Amniocentesis	1–3
Spontaneous abortion	3–4
Induced abortion	5–6
Full-term delivery, ABO compatible or incompatible	14–17
Mismatched blood transfusion	90–95

In subsequent pregnancies, with an Rh-positive fetus, the process of antibody production and transfer may be accelerated, leading to the development of more significant anemia. In such cases, the fetal liver can manufacture additional red cells. However, this activity reduces the amount of proteins manufactured by the fetal liver. In turn, the reduced protein production can lead to a decreased oncotic pressure within the fetal vascular system, resulting in fetal ascites and subcutaneous edema. At the same time, the severe fetal anemia can lead to high output cardiac failure. This combination of findings is referred to as *hydrops fetalis*.

The tendency is for each subsequent baby to be more severely affected, but this is not always the case. The level of fetal disturbance may remain the same or, occasionally, may even be less than in the previous pregnancy. If subsequent fetuses are Rh negative, which is commonly the case if the father is a heterozygote, the fetus will not be affected at all (Table 11.1).

DIAGNOSIS

Isoimmunization can often be diagnosed on the basis of *history*. A woman with a previous diagnosis of isoimmunization or with a previous birth where the neonatal course was consistent with this disorder is at risk for recurrence. As part of routine antenatal *laboratory evaluation*, maternal blood is tested for the presence of a variety of antibodies that may cause significant disturbances in the fetus. Any significant antibodies are further evaluated for the strength of antibody response, which is reported in a titer format (e.g., 1:4, 1:16, etc.). During this testing process, other antibodies may be discovered that do not cause significant fetal/neonatal problems. The two most common of these are the anti-Lewis and anti-I. When these antibodies are found, titers are not reported because of their lack of clinical importance.

MANAGEMENT

Antibody titers as described above would seem to be a good marker of maternal antibody production, but in fact, such titers are of limited usefulness. In the first sensitized pregnancy, titers do seem to be helpful, but thereafter, they are of virtually no value since they do not reflect the current fetal condition. Even in the initial sensitized pregnancy, the greatest value is in distinguishing those pregnancies where antibody production is so low as to be nonthreatening to the fetus from those which there are likely to be significant consequence. *A titer of 1:16 or greater is generally considered the critical point* where there is sufficient risk of fetal jeopardy to warrant additional evaluation.

Amniotic fluid assessment is of great value in managing the isoimmunized patient. Practical use of amniotic fluid analysis became a reality about 1960, when Liley found that *the level of bilirubin in the amniotic fluid accurately reflects the condition of the fetus*. The mechanism by which bilirubin enters the amniotic fluid from the fetal compartment is still not understood. However, in the second half of normal pregnancy, the level of bilirubin normally decreases progressively. The level of bilirubin in an affected, isoimmunized patient can be evaluated in relationship to natural decline. The level of bilirubin in the amniotic fluid is determined using a spectrophotometer. Normal amniotic fluid subjected to spectrophotometric analysis has a characteristic curve, as shown in Figure 11.1. The

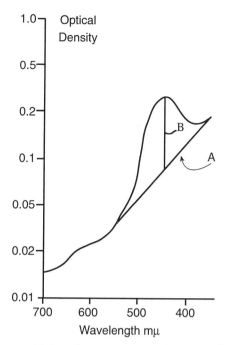

Figure 11.1. Absorption curve of amniotic fluid by spectrophotometer in a patient with isoimmunization. A, anticipated curve for normal amniotic fluid. B, deviation of curve due to bilirubin in amniotic fluid; expressed as ΔOD_{450}.

presence of bilirubin causes a characteristic deviation in this curve, at 450 nm. This degree of deviation is refered to as the ΔOD_{450}. Following the pioneering work of Liley and others, normal OD values have been determined and are shown in Figure 11.2. Experience has shown how ΔOD_{450} relates to the severity of fetal problems, as shown in the figure.

Amniotic fluid is obtained from the patient by amniocentesis at periodic intervals between the 20th and 30th week of pregnancy, depending on the history of previous pregnancies. OD values are then plotted on a curve, as shown in Figure 11.2, which allows estimation of the degree of severity of the anemia in the fetus. Based upon this level of severity, in conjunction with the gestational age, a decision about expected management, transfusion of the fetus, or delivery can be made. *Markedly elevated ΔOD_{450} values indicate a severely affected fetus, intermediate values indicate a moderately affected fetus, and low values represent a fetus not or only mildly affected.*

Assessment of the affected fetus by *periodic ultrasonography* can be very helpful in detecting severe signs of the hemolytic process, namely subcutaneous edema and ascites. Under ultrasound guidance, the umbilical cord can be sampled directly (percutaneous umbilical blood sampling (PUBS)) and fetal blood taken for hematocrit determination to assess the severity of anemia. Later in pregnancy, general tests of fetal well-being are utilized in the isoimmunized patient, as the ability of an affected fetus to withstand the stresses of pregnancy and labor may be compromised.

TRANSFUSIONS

Transfusion of Rh-negative red blood cells to the fetus *is indicated when*, on the basis of the above assessment, it is determined that *the fetus is in significant jeopardy* for hydrops or fetal death. Traditionally, blood was transfused into the fetal abdominal cavity where absorption takes place over subsequent days. More recently, direct fetal transfusions into the umbilical cord (PUBS) under ultrasonography guidance are being utilized more frequently, with positive results. Physicians experienced and skilled in this technique are critical to its success. The procedure carries with it a risk of fetal death of up to 3%, a risk that must be weighed against the predicted future course for the fetus in utero and the potential adverse consequences of preterm delivery. The quantity of red blood cells to be transferred can be calculated using the gestational age and size of the fetus and the fetal hematocrit. As the transferred cells are Rh negative, they are not affected by the transplacental maternal antibody. Timing of subsequent transfusions can be determined based on the severity of disease and the predicted life span of the transfused cells.

PREVENTION

Maternal exposure and subsequent sensitization to fetal blood usually occurs at delivery,

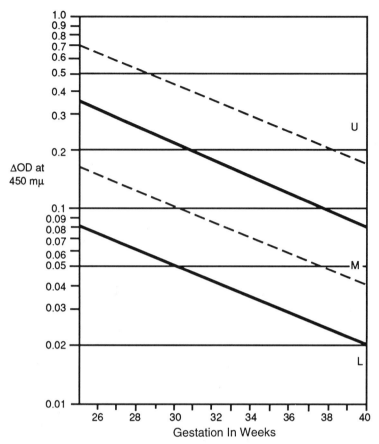

Figure 11.2. Liley curve. ΔOD_{450}, obtained as in Figure 11.1, is plotted by gestational age. Condition of fetus can be estimated by the zone (lower (L), middle (M), upper (U),) in which the ΔOD_{450} is plotted. In the upper zone, the fetus is severely affected; in the middle zone, moderately affected; and, in the lower zone, minimally affected or not affected.

and much less commonly during pregnancy. In the late 1960s, it was determined that the antibody to the "D" antigen of the Rh system could be prepared from donors previously sensitized to the antigen. Subsequently, it was found that *administration of this antibody (Rh immune globulin) soon after delivery could, by passive immunization, prevent an active antibody response by the mother in most cases.* Rh immune globulin is effective only for the D antigen of the Rh system. No similar preparations are available for patients sensitized with the many other possible antigens. It is now standard practice for Rh-negative patients who deliver Rh-positive infants to receive an intramuscular dose of 300 μg of this Rh immune globulin (RhoGAM) within 72 hours

of delivery. With this practice, the risk of subsequent sensitization decreases from approximately 15% to approximately 2%. This residual 2% was determined to be the result of sensitization occurring *during the course of pregnancy* (as opposed to at delivery), usually in the third trimester. Administration of a 300-μg dose of Rh immune globulin to Rh-negative patients at 28 weeks was found to reduce the risk of sensitization to about 0.2%.

Prophylaxis with Rh immune globulin in Rh-negative women is not necessary if the father of the pregnancy is *known with certainty* to be Rh negative. While testing of the father can be done, *if there is any question as to the paternity, prophylactic administration of Rh im-*

Table 11.2
Indications for Rh Immune Globulin Administration in an Unsensitized Rh-Negative Patient[a]

At about 28 weeks pregnancy
Within 3 days of delivery of an Rh-positive infant
At the time of amniocentesis
After positive Kleihauer-Betke test
After an ectopic pregnancy
After a spontaneous or induced abortion

[a]Unless the father of the pregnancy is known to be Rh negative.

mune globulin should be given as described, since the risk is negligible and the potential benefits are considerable.

In summary, Rh-negative pregnant patients who have no antibody on initial screening are retested at 28 weeks (to detect the rare patient sensitized earlier in pregnancy). If no sensitization has occurred, they are given Rh immune globulin to protect them from antibody formation for the remainder of pregnancy. If the father is known to be Rh negative, this practice is not necessary. After delivery, the child's blood type and Rh status are determined, and if the child is Rh positive, a second dose of Rh immune globulin is given to the new mother.

There are other situations where Rh immune globulin should be administered (Table 11.2). Because the amount of fetal red cells required to elicit an antibody response is minute, about 0.01 ml, *any circumstance in pregnancy where fetomaternal hemorrhage can occur warrants Rh immune globulin administration*. Furthermore, as fetal red cell production begins with 6 weeks of conception, sensitization can occur in patients who have a spontaneous or scheduled pregnancy termi-

nation. Because the dose of antigen in such situations is low, a reduced dose of 50 μg of Rh immune globulin can be utilized to prevent sensitization. Amniocentesis and other trauma (such as resulting from an auto accident) during pregnancy are other indications for the standard 300-μg dose of Rh immune globulin. In cases of trauma or bleeding during pregnancy, the extent, if any, to which fetomaternal hemorrhage has occurred can be evaluated using the Kleihauer-Betke test or similar test that allows the identification of fetal cells in maternal circulation. In the test, a sample of maternal blood is subjected to a strong base such as KOH. Maternal cells are very sensitive to changes in pH and, therefore, promptly lyse and become "ghost" cells. Fetal cells are much more resistant to such agents and remain intact. A ratio of fetal to maternal cells can be assessed by counting a thousand or more total cells under the microscope and determining how many cells retain the dark appearance representing fetal cells. Then the maternal blood volume is calculated and, using the ratio just described, the total amount of fetomaternal hemorrhage is derived. Since a standard 300-μg dose of Rh immune globulin will effectively neutralize 15 ml of fetal red blood cells, the appropriate dose can then be administered.

FURTHER READINGS

Bowman JM. Hemolytic disease (erythroblastosis fetalis). In: Creasy RK, Resnik R, eds. Maternal-fetal medicine: principles and practice. Philadelphia: WB Saunders, 1989:613–649.

Cunningham FG, MacDonald PC, Gant NF. Williams obstetrics. 18th ed. East Norwalk, CN: Appleton Lange, 1989:461–476.

chapter 12

MULTIPLE GESTATION

At first glance, twin pregnancy is often considered a novelty, with pleasant images of identical children dressed alike. In fact, pregnancies with multiple fetuses pose significant medical risks for both the mother and her offspring and special care is necessary to achieve an optimal outcome. Caring for two or more infants likewise challenges even the most devoted parents. This chapter will provide an overview of twin pregnancy—its diagnosis, antepartum, intrapartum, and postpartum care—with reference to pregnancies with three or more fetuses when relevant. In general, all potential complications with twin pregnancies are somewhat more frequent and more serious as the number of fetuses increases.

INCIDENCES OF MULTIPLE GESTATION

The overall incidence of recognized twins in the United States is approximately 1 in 90, slightly higher in blacks and slightly lower in whites. Twin gestations can be characterized as dizygotic (fraternal) or monozygotic (identical). Dizygotic twins occur when two separate ova are fertilized by two separate sperm and, in fact, represent two siblings who happen to be born at approximately the same time. Monozygotic twins represent division of the fertilized ovum at various times after conception. There is a marked difference in the incidence of twinning in various populations, almost exclusively due to the incidence of dizygotic twinning. The *incidence of monozygotic twinning* is fairly constant around the world *at approximately 1 in 250 pregnancies*, whereas *dizygotic* twinning occurs as fre-

quently as *1 in 20 pregnancies* in certain African countries. Increasing age and increasing parity are independent factors for dizygotic twinning. A familial factor is present in twinning that follows the maternal lineage. Ultrasonography, which allows early detection and serial evaluations, has provided valuable information concerning the outcome of twin pregnancies. Only about one half of twin pregnancies detected in the first trimester result in the delivery of viable twins, with the remaining associated with death and resorption of one fetus with eventual delivery of a single fetus. Both spontaneous abortions and congenital anomalies occur more frequently in multiple pregnancies than in singleton pregnancies.

The likelihood of twinning is increased significantly if *fertility agents* or *other assisted reproductive technologies* are utilized. With clomiphene citrate induction of ovulation, the twinning rate is about 6–8%. With the use of exogenous gonadotropin therapy, the rate increases to about 25–35%. As in vitro fertilization programs typically insert several fertilized ova into the uterine cavity, multiple fetuses would be expected to occur in some instances; in fact, the rate of two or more fetuses is about 35–40%.

NATURAL HISTORY

As the number of fetuses increases, the expected *duration of pregnancy* diminishes. Compared to singleton pregnancies, which deliver at 40 weeks, twins deliver at an average of 37 weeks, triplets at 33 weeks, and quadruplets at an average of 29 weeks. Thus, with each additional fetus, the length of ges-

141

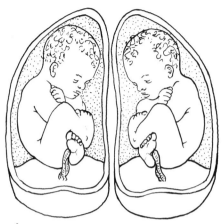

A Two placentas, two amnions, two chorions — dichorionic diamniotic

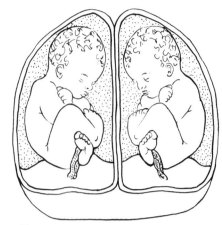

B One placenta, two amnions, two chorions — dichorionic diamniotic

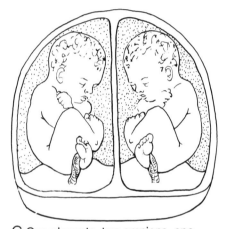

C One placenta, two amnions, one chorion — monochorionic diamniotic

Figure 12.1. Development of the amnion and chorion in twin pregnancies.

tation is decreased by about 4 weeks. Although all twins face certain risks, *monozygotic twins face additional risks related to the time when twinning occurs*. The developmental sequence associated with this separation of the conceptus into twins explains the basis for these problems, as well as explaining the configuration of the fetal membranes at delivery. If division of the conceptus occurs within 3 days of fertilization, each fetus will be surrounded by an amnion and chorion, and the membranes are termed diamniotic/dichorionic. If division occurs between the 4th and 8th day following fertilization, the chorion has already begun to develop, whereas the amnion has not. Therefore, each fetus will be surrounded by an amnion, but a single chorion will surround both twins, a condition termed diamniotic/monochorionic. Division from day 9 to day 12 takes place after development of both the amnion and the chorion, and the twins will share a common sac, a condition termed monoamniotic/monochorionic (Fig. 12.1). Division thereafter is incomplete, resulting in the development of conjoined twins, which may be fused in any of a multitude of ways, but usually at the chest and/or abdomen. Further development can result in various vascular anastomoses between the fetuses which, in turn, can lead to a condition known as *twin-twin transfusion syndrome*. In this circumstance, blood flow of the fetuses mixes such that there is net flow from one twin to another, at times with disastrous consequences. The so-called donor twin can have impaired growth, anemia, hypovolemia, and other problems. On the other hand, the recipient twin can develop hypervolemia, hypertension, polycythemia, and congestive heart failure as a result of this abnormal transfusion. A secondary manifestation involves the amniotic fluid dynamics. Because of transudate across the skin or, probably more importantly, increased urinary output owing to its hypervolemia, the recipient produces abundant amniotic fluid, whereas the donor twin may in fact have oligohydramnios. The hydramnios in one twin further compounds the risk of preterm labor in multifetal pregnancies.

DIAGNOSIS OF MULTIPLE GESTATION

Twin pregnancy is usually *suspected when the uterine size is excessively large for the calculated gestational age*. Although there is a variation in fundal height measurements in singleton pregnancies, a discrepancy of 4 cm between the weeks gestation and the carefully measured fundal height should prompt evaluation to either detect twins, reassign gestational age, diagnose hydramnios, or provide other explanation for the discrepancy. In modern obstetrics, the diagnosis of twins or multiple gestation *is usually made by obstetric ultrasonography*.

Once the diagnosis of twin pregnancy has been made, subsequent antenatal care addresses each of the *potential concerns* for mother and fetus listed in Table 12.1. Although the maternal blood volume is greater with a twin gestation than with singleton pregnancy, the anticipated blood loss at delivery is also greater. *Anemia* is more common in these patients and a balanced diet with iron, folate, and possibly other micronutrients is important. Although the value of bed rest in prolonging gestation is controversial, it is generally advised that a woman limit her activity after 24–26 weeks to avoid *premature labor*, which is more common in twin gestations. Careful attention to detection of uterine contractions is important and the patient should be cautioned about signs of preterm labor, such as low back pain, a thin vaginal discharge, and diarrhea. Cervical examinations to detect early effacement and dilation are usually done every 1–2 weeks. At these visits, evidence suggesting pregnancy-induced hypertension is also gathered, which includes careful measurement of blood pressure and testing for protein in the urine. Beginning at 30–32 weeks, daily fetal kick counts are usually begun to help assess *fetal well-being*. Although somewhat surprising, patients can almost always distinguish movements of different fetuses. Non-stress tests or other fetal monitor testing is begun as the pregnancy approaches term. Fortunately, fetal lung maturity is achieved somewhat earlier in twin pregnancies when compared with singleton pregnancies.

The chief antenatal assessment in twin pregnancy remains the periodic ultrasonography examination, which is done every 4 weeks after 20 weeks gestation. At each examination, growth of each fetus is assessed and an estimate of amniotic fluid volume made. If growth is discordant, usually defined as a 20% difference in weight (difference in weight/weight of larger fetus ≥20%), ultrasonography may be performed more often and tests of fetal well-being (such as non-stress test, kick counts) are begun at 30–32 weeks. Fetal breathing and body movements, as well as body tone (elements of the biophysical profile), can also be determined with ultrasonography.

INTRAPARTUM MANAGEMENT

Intrapartum management is largely *determined by the presentation of the twins*. In gen-

Table 12.1
Antenatal Management of Twin Pregnancies

Concern	Action
Adequate nutrition	Balanced diet; additional increase in daily caloric intake; multivitamin and mineral supplements (e.g., Fe)
Increased blood loss at delivery	Prevent anemia (see above)
Fetal growth	Bed rest beginning at 24–26 weeks—value unclear, but also decreases preterm labor
Preterm labor	Educate patient on signs of labor; increase bed rest; cervical examinations every 1–2 weeks; home monitoring in select cases
Pregnancy-induced hypertension	Frequent blood pressure determinations; frequent urinary protein assessment
Fetal growth, discordant growth	Periodic ultrasonography examinations

eral, if the first (presenting) twin is in the cephalic (vertex) presentation, labor is allowed to progress to vaginal delivery, whereas if the presenting twin is in a position other than cephalic, cesarean delivery is often performed. During labor, the heart rate of both fetuses is monitored separately. Approaches to the delivery of twins will vary depending on gestational age, presentation of the twins, and the experience of the attending physicians. Regardless of the delivery plan, access to full obstetric anesthetic and pediatric services is mandatory, in that cesarean delivery may be required on short notice.

If vaginal delivery of the first twin is accomplished and the second twin is also cephalic, delivery of the second twin generally proceeds smoothly. With proper monitoring of the second twin, there is no urgency in accomplishing the second delivery. If the second twin is presenting in any way other than cephalic, there are two primary manipulations that may effect vaginal delivery. The first is *external cephalic version* whereby, using ultrasonographic visualization, the fetus is gently guided into the cephalic presentation by abdominal massage and pressure. The second maneuver is *internal podalic version*, in which the physician reaches a hand into the uterine cavity, identifies the lower extremities of the fetus, and gently delivers the infant via breech delivery. The possibility of a prolapsed umbilical cord must always be borne in mind when delivery of twins is to be ac-

complished. Postpartum, the overdistended uterus may not contract normally, leading to uterine atony and postpartum hemorrhage.

FURTHER READINGS

Chitkara U, Berkowitz R. Multiple gestations. In Gabbe SG, Neibyl JR, Simpson JL, eds. Obstetrics, normal and problem pregnancies. 2nd ed. New York: Churchill-Livingstone, 1991:881.

Cunningham FG, MacDonald PC, Gant NF. Multifetal pregnancy. In: Williams Obstetrics. 18th ed. East Norwalk, CN: Appleton & Lange, 1989:629–651.

SELF-EVALUATION

Case 12-A

A 21-year-old G0 with a family history of twins seeks your opinion about ovulation induction proposed by her reproductive endocrinologist. She is especially interested in risks of having twins and some of the possible complications.

Questions 12-A-1 through 12-A-4

Match the following clinical situations with the corresponding incidence.

1. monozygotic twins
2. dizygotic twins
3. twinning with ovulation induction
4. twinning with in vitro fertilization

A. 1 of 3 pregnancies
B. 1 of 20 pregnancies
C. 1 of 250 pregnancies
D. 1 of 12 pregnancies

Answers 12-A-1 through 12-A-4

1. C
2. B
3. D
4. A

Questions 12-A-5 through 12-A-8

Match the time twinning occurs with the corresponding arrangement of fetal membranes.

5. division within 3 days of fertilization
6. division between 4 and 8 days of fertilization
7. division between 9 and 12 days of fertilization
8. division 12 days after fertilization

A. conjoined twins
B. monoamniotic/monochorionic
C. diamniotic/dichorionic
D. diamniotic/monochorionic

Answers 12-A-5 through 12-A-8

5. C
6. D
7. B
8. A

Case 12-B

At 32 weeks gestation, a 35-year-old G1P0 with known twins is noted to have a fundal height not commensurate with gestational age. Her weight gain and blood pressure are normal as are her antenatal laboratory studies. She says the babies are moving normally and that she feels well although "rather large."

Question 12-B-1

Which of the following interventions, if any, are indicated?

A. oxytocin challenge test (OCT)
B. ultrasound
C. non-stress test (NST)
D. induction of labor if cephalic/cephalic presentation

Answer 12-B-1

Answers: B, C

Intrauterine growth retardation and discordant growth are both common in twin pregnancies. Measurements of each fetus for comparison may reveal abnormal development. If found, further testing with possible delivery is indicated. Evaluation of fetal well-being at the time of obstetric ultrasound and NST are noninvasive tests that yield valuable information. Given the risk of premature labor, OCT is less commonly used and would best be reserved if the NST is not reassuring. Delivery should be contemplated only if one or both fetuses is compromised.

chapter 13

INTRAUTERINE GROWTH RETARDATION

The term intrauterine growth retardation (IUGR) is used to describe infants whose weights are much lower than expected for their gestational age. *A fetus/infant whose weight lies in the lowest 10% of the normal population is designated as having IUGR*, a determination based upon standard weight/gestational age tables. By definition then, the prevalence of IUGR will be 10%. As opposed to "low birth weight" it is important to remember that IUGR is based on weight for a *specific gestational age*. Thus, careful assessment of gestational age is crucial to diagnosing, and therefore managing, patients with IUGR.

The fetus with IUGR is best viewed as fragile, that is, potentially lacking adequate reserves for continued intrauterine stress or neonatal adaptation. Such infants are at greater risk for intrauterine fetal death or neonatal death, asphyxia, and fetal distress prior to or during labor, and once delivered, they are at risk for meconium aspiration, hypoglycemia, hypothermia, respiratory distress, and many other potential problems. Because of these risks, it is important to identify such babies in utero, maximize the quality of their intrauterine environment, time and implement their delivery using the safest means possible, and provide superb care in the neonatal period.

ETIOLOGY OF INTRAUTERINE GROWTH RETARDATION

For a fetus to thrive in utero, an adequate number of fetal cells must be present and differentiated properly. In addition, adequate foodstuffs, other nutrients, and oxygen must

Table 13.1
Causes of Intrauterine Growth Retardation

Maternal	Fetal
Behavior	Infections
Smoking	Rubella
Drugs	Cytomegalovirus
Alcohol	(CMV)
Nutritional deficiencies	Anomalies
Maternal disease	Chromosomal
Hypertension	Other genetic
Cyanotic heart disease	
Others	

be available via an adequately functioning uteroplacental unit. Although a number of *causes of intrauterine growth retardation* have been recognized (Table 13.1), a definite cause of IUGR cannot be identified in approximately 50% of all cases. Therefore, IUGR must be suspected at every visit in every patient. Causes of IUGR can be conveniently grouped into maternal and fetal origins. Maternal smoking has been known for many years to be associated with decreased birth weight, to a magnitude of roughly one half pound at term. Since maternal habits are important causes of growth retardation, if such behavior is modified, there will be resultant improvement in the fetal outcome.

The recommended maternal *weight gain* during pregnancy is about 30 pounds. If there are marked nutritional deficiencies, however, a decrease in fetal weight has been demonstrated. In studies performed during World War II, severe famine and marked caloric restriction resulted in decreased birth weights of $\frac{1}{2}$ to 1 pound, depending upon the nutritional status of the women prior to the onset of nutritional deprivation. It is difficult to define the role of less severe forms of nutritional deficiencies on fetal growth. In pregnancies with multiple fetuses, even normal nutrition may not be enough to provide adequate nutrition for all fetuses, resulting in growth retardation.

The most common known maternal factor associated with intrauterine growth retardation is *hypertensive disease*. Vasospasm diminishes uteroplacental blood flow and hence the ability of the mother to provide adequate nutrition to the fetus through the placenta. From 25 to 30% of all cases of IUGR are associated with maternal hypertensive disease. Other maternal disorders may likewise interfere with fetal growth, notably *cyanotic heart disease* and *hemoglobinopathies*.

Fetal causes of intrauterine growth retardation include congenital infections and congenital anomalies. The most clearly understood *fetal infections* that interfere with growth are due to rubella and cytomegalovirus infections, especially at early gestational ages. These infections may be manifest only as mild "flu-like" illnesses, but their occurrence should be noted. Damage to the fetus during organogenesis can result in a decreased cell number, which is manifest by diminished growth later in gestation. Probably 5% or less of all cases of IUGR are related to early infection with these or other viral agents. Bacterial infections have not been implicated in IUGR. *Congenital anomalies* account for up to 15% of all cases of IUGR. Chromosomal anomalies such as trisomy 21, 18, and 13 are typically associated with diminished fetal growth. Other genetic abnormalities, such as certain congenital heart defects and a variety of dysmorphic syndromes likewise result in smaller than expected infants.

EVALUATION AND MANAGEMENT

The diagnosis of IUGR is suspected from the *history*. A patient with a history of having a child with intrauterine growth retardation is at increased risk for a recurrence of this problem. Personal habits such as smoking and use of alcohol or other drugs of abuse such as cocaine should be part of the routine obstetric history obtained at the onset of prenatal care. Recognition of such elements in the history is important so every effort can be made to discourage such behavior. A medical history of disorders potentially interfering with fetal growth, primarily hypertension, should be obtained at the onset of prenatal care.

Physical examination is limited in usefulness in diagnosing IUGR, but it serves as an important *screening test* for abnormal fetal growth. Maternal size and weight gain throughout pregnancy have a limited utility, but access to such information is readily available and a low maternal weight or little or no weight gain through pregnancy can suggest IUGR. Between approximately 15 and 36 weeks gestation, *fundal height measurement* should advance in centimeter increments in close parallel with gestational age in weeks. Thus, a patient at 28 weeks gestation would be expected to have a fundal height of close to 28 cm. Serial measurements, especially by the same examiner, can serve as an effective screening test for IUGR, since an increase in fundal height less than expected may suggest the diagnosis of IUGR and raise the need for additional testing. Clinical estimations of fetal weight are not very helpful in diagnosing IUGR, except when fetal size is grossly diminished.

Ultrasonography has provided an important obstetric tool to diagnose and assess intrauterine growth retardation. Measurements of various fetal structures can be compared to standardized tables that reflect normal growth. The measurement of the biparietal diameter, head circumference, abdominal circumference, and femur length are among the measurements usually obtained. Ratios of these measurements and equations can provide useful information with respect to fetal size. The diameter of the cerebellum appears to be unaltered by a number of the factors that lead to growth retardation. Accordingly, in patients with uncertain gestational age, measurement of the diameter of this structure may prove helpful.

By the use of ultrasonography, IUGR can be distinguished as asymmetric or symmetric. *Asymmetric IUGR* refers to an unequal decrease in the size of structures. For example, the abdominal circumference may be low but the biparietal diameter at or near normal. Such asymmetry can be seen with severe nutritional deficiencies or with hypertension, where fetal access to nutrients is compromised. In *symmetrical IUGR*, all structures are approximately equally diminished in size with a relative sparing of fetal brain and heart compared to asymmetric IUGR. Congenital anomalies or early intrauterine infection can alter cell number and lead to this type of IUGR. This distinction is not always clear, but it does serve as a guide in seeking the etiology of IUGR.

In patients at increased risk for intrauterine growth retardation, a *baseline ultrasonography* examination should be obtained early in prenatal care and usually repeated periodically. As growth retardation is related to gestational age, all patients whose length of pregnancy is uncertain should be assessed with physical examination and ultrasonography to establish an accurate gestational age as early in pregnancy as possible. Ultrasonography also can identify the amount of amniotic fluid present. The combination of oligohydramnios (diminished amniotic fluid volume) and intrauterine growth retardation is especially worrisome because it is associated with severe disease and/or worsening outcome. The mechanism is thought to be decreased fetal blood volume, which diminishes renal blood flow, which in turn leads to a reduction of urine output, a primary source of amniotic fluid in the second half of pregnancy.

Direct studies of the fetus are useful in selected patients with IUGR. Fetal tissue can be obtained via amniocentesis (fetal fibroblasts floating in the amniotic fluid), chorionic villus sampling (CVS, biopsy of placenta), direct blood sampling, percutaneous umbilical blood sampling (PUBS), or removal of fetal plasma and cells. PUBS also permits immunoglobin studies and viral cultures to be obtained in patients with suspected viral infections as a cause of IUGR. Moreover, the level of oxygenation and the acid-base status can be assessed with this technique. PUBS and to some extent CVS are less widely available than ultrasound-directed amniocentesis.

Once intrauterine growth retardation has been diagnosed, *the goal is to deliver the healthiest possible infant at the optimal time.* This involves a balance between the degree of prematurity estimated at the time of diagnosis with the degree of suspected fetal compromise. Initial management consists of a comprehensive attempt to determine a cause for the IUGR. If a correctable etiology is found, corrective action should be taken. Management of the patient with IUGR can be categorized as antepartum, intrapartum, and postpartum (or neonatal) (Table 13.2). *Antepartum management* consists of efforts to determine the cause of the IUGR, promote growth, and monitor carefully for fetal compromise. Ultrasonography by experienced personnel can usually identify congenital anomalies that may be associated with IUGR. Measurements of amniotic fluid volume of fetal structures can be made on a serial basis. The degree of IUGR can then be followed in the ensuing weeks. Bed rest, or at least limited activity, is often prescribed for patients for IUGR, since limitation of activity, especially with the patient lying in the left-lateral position, maximizes uterine blood flow. This has a salutory effect on fetal growth.

Determination of fetal activity by the so-called kick counts is a useful way of assessing *fetal well-being*. Various electronic fetal monitoring tests, such as the non-stress test or contraction stress test, or electronic fetal monitoring combined with ultrasound (the biophysical profile) can be utilized once or twice weekly, or even more frequently, to assess the condition of the fetus. Although these tests can be helpful if the results are normal, the high false-positive rate must be considered when management decisions

Table 13.2
Assessment and Management of Patient with Intrauterine Growth Retardation

Antepartum	Intrapartum	Postpartum (neonatal)
Eliminate cause, if possible	Electronic fetal monitoring	Pharyngeal suction
Bed rest, frequent fetal movement counts	Preparation for cesarean delivery Amnioinfusion	Effective neonatal resuscitation as needed
Serial sonography	Oxygen therapy	Avoid hypoglycemia
Non-stress test, contraction stress test, biophysical profile	Neonatal/anesthesia consultation	Avoid hypothermia
Doppler ultrasound		Oxygen therapy if needed
Amniocentesis for maturity studies		
PUBS		

covering delivery are made. Use of these tests in combination may reduce this false-positive rate. Examination of the blood flow through the umbilical cord with Doppler ultrasound may be useful in patients with IUGR, although reports about the value of this test are inconclusive. In selected patients with IUGR of uncertain cause, fetal blood aspirated directly through PUBS can be sent for viral antibody titer, chromosome analysis, and other parameters reflecting fetal oxygenation and acid-base status. Amniocentesis for tests of fetal lung maturity may provide information helpful in selecting the timing of delivery.

The decision regarding proper *time for delivery* is based on a combination of factors. The fetus who is thought to be in marked jeopardy may be delivered by scheduled cesarean section without a trial of labor if its ability to withstand labor is questionable and an induced labor is likely to be lengthy. If induction of labor is undertaken, however, constant electronic fetal monitoring to detect signs suggestive of fetal jeopardy is important. Preparations for cesarean delivery should be made since rapid deterioration of the fetus may occur. Consultation with anesthesia and neonatology personnel is important for optimal care of the patient and her newborn infant. Amnioinfusion (instillation of warmed normal saline via transcervical catheter) may be helpful if fetal heart rate decelerations thought to be due to diminished amniotic fluid volume are present. Maternal oxygen therapy may be beneficial throughout the course of labor.

Expert *neonatal care* is critical because of the reduced capacity of the fetus/infant to adapt and adjust to extrauterine life. Due to the frequent passage of meconium prior to delivery, the mouth and nasopharynx must be suctioned, usually with direct visualization of the vocal cords. These infants are prone to other complications such as respiratory distress, hypoglycemia, and hypothermia. Fortunately, infants who survive the neonatal period have a generally good prognosis.

FURTHER READINGS

Creasy RK, Resnick R. IUGR in maternal-fetal medicine. Philadelphia: WB Saunders, 1990.
Cunningham FG, MacDonald PC, Grant NF., in IUGR, Williams obstetrics. 18th ed. East Norwalk, CT: Appleton & Lange, 1989:615–616, 764–773.

SELF-EVALUATION

Case 13-A

A 36-year-old G2P0010 is seen for her first prenatal visit at 8 weeks. Her medical history includes essential hypertension, smoking, and poor dietary habits. She had three hospitalizations for pelvic inflammatory disease and one for a cone biopsy of the cervix. Her family history includes a sister with Down syndrome, a mother and grandmother with insulin-dependent diabetes, and a sister with carcinoma of the breast.

On physical examination, the patient's blood pressure is 160/95 and she has 1 + proteinuria. She weighs 200 pounds and is 5 feet 1 inch tall. Her general physical examination is normal with the following specific findings: (a) normal breast examination; (b) 2/6 holosystolic murmur without radiation or extra sounds; (c) obese abdomen without masses; (d) cervix consistent in appearance with her history; (e) retroverted 14-week sized uterus, which is slightly irregular in shape; and (f) 2 + dependent edema and normal DTRs.

Question 13-A-1

This patient is at increased risk for a growth-retarded infant. Of the several risk factors mentioned, which pose the most likely threats?

A. obesity
B. poor nutrition
C. hypertension
D. smoking
E. status post cone biopsy
F. history of STDs or infectious disease
G. family history of Down syndrome
H. family history of diabetes
I. family history of breast carcinoma
J. cardiac murmur
K. uterus with irregular shape
L. uterus whose size is greater than expected by LMP dates

Answer 13-A-1

Answers: B, C, D, F, G, H

Obesity per se is not a direct risk factor for IUGR, although it may contribute to general health concerns such as hypertension and the risk of glucose intolerance. Poor nutrition is a risk, although the maternal-fetal unit is able to compensate for considerable dietary inadequacy. This patient's hypertension and smoking are major risk factors, both having great potential for diminution of placental function. A family history of Down syndrome in a 36-year-old woman is of concern, as a genetically abnormal baby may also be growth retarded. Diabetes may be associated with abnormal fetal growth, both growth retardation and macrosomia. Although a family history of

breast cancer places the patient at higher risk for breast cancer, it has no direct relationship to IUGR risks. A systolic murmur is common in pregnancy and with hypertension in pregnancy, but any underlying cardiac dysfunction may be an increased risk factor for IUGR. A size/dates disparity must be resolved and accurate dating established so that fetal growth may be evaluated, but this disparity is itself not a risk factor of IUGR. The irregular uterine shape suggests a fibroid uterus, but does not pose an independent risk for IUGR.

Question 13-A-2

Of the following prenatal evaluations/initial managements, which are of special relevance to this patient's risks for IUGR, and why?

A. nutrition consultation
B. social service consultation
C. ECG
D. echocardiogram
E. 24-h urine for creatinine clearance (CCr) and total protein
F. glucose screening
G. genetics counseling with genetic amniocentesis
H. STD screening: cultures, infective titers
I. mammography
J. obstetric (OB) ultrasound
K. Pap smear
L. colposcopy
M. counseling about smoking

Answer 13-A-2

Answers: A, B, E, F, G, J, M

The antenatal evaluations and initial interventions address risk factors for IUGR seen in this patient. Mammography is not indicated in this pregnant patient with a negative physical examination, but should be scheduled for the postpartum period. Colposcopy will not be necessary as long as the Pap smear is normal. ECG and echocardiogram would only be warranted if the heart murmur is felt to be clinically significant. Routine STD screening is appropriate but extensive evaluation is not warranted.

Case 13-B

A 28-year-old G2P1001 at 32 weeks gestational age has a fundal height lagging behind growth gestational age with a 5 cm discrepancy at this time. A late first trimester ultrasound had been consistent with her gestational age by dates. Her first baby was delivered by cesarean section for fetal distress. The baby was reportedly "too small" and had not "grown right." The baby is well, at home, but is suffering some difficulty in school.

Question 13-B-1

An ultrasound performed at this time should provide what information?

A. biophysical profile
B. evaluation of fetal growth
C. evaluation for fetal anomalies
D. evaluation of amniotic fluid volume
E. PUBS for genetic evaluation

Answer 13-B-1

Answers: A, B, C, D

The first four choices address the issues of fetal growth and fetal well-being, both of which require assessment at this time. PUBS has a place in the evaluation of the growth-retarded fetus, but only after the diagnosis of IUGR has been made and then under specific conditions when the risk of the procedure outweighs the risk of not obtaining the information from the test. It is not yet apparent that PUBS is indicated.

For further consideration: Ultrasonographic evaluation shows concordant growth of fetal head and trunk, but an overall growth in the 20th percentile for the estimated gestational age. Biophysical profile is reassuring (10 of 10).

How should this patient be managed? What tests will be used and how often are they to be done?

chapter 14

POSTTERM PREGNANCY

Term pregnancy lasts from 38 to 42 weeks, i.e., the due date or estimated date of confinement is the projected EDC ±2 weeks. *A patient who has not delivered by the completion of the 42nd week* (294 days from the 1st day of the last normal menstrual period) *is said to be postterm* (a common synonym is postdates). This condition occurs in about 8–10% of pregnancies and carries with it an increased risk of adverse outcome, although the majority of infants delivered after 42 weeks are healthy. The increased morbidity and mortality in a small percent of cases, however, warrants careful evaluation of all postterm pregnancies. In addition, postterm pregnancies can create significant stress for the patient, her family, and those caring for her. Therefore, the physician should "reassure" the patient and discuss with her the options for management.

ETIOLOGY OF POSTTERM PREGNANCY

The actual cause of postterm pregnancy is not known. Because fetal anencephaly often leads to postterm pregnancy, it is hypothesized that there may be a dysfunction in the fetal pituitary-adrenal axis, which is needed for the initiation of normal labor. Uterine contractility has been shown to be diminished in some cases of postterm pregnancy, suggesting a cause intrinsic to the myometrium. Whatever the etiology, there is a tendency for recurrence of postterm pregnancy. About 50% of patients having one postterm pregnancy will experience prolonged pregnancy with their next gestation.

EFFECTS OF POSTTERM PREGNANCY

The morbidity and mortality for the postterm fetus increases severalfold compared with term pregnancies. This is due to several reasons. Approximately one fifth of postterm newborns demonstrate *dysmaturity*, or *postmaturity syndrome*. Dysmature infants often are growth retarded and have loss of subcutaneous fat, giving the child a classic wizened, elderly appearance. Integumentary changes are also seen, including long nails, scaling epidermis, and meconium staining of the nails, skin, and umbilical cord. About one fourth of prolonged pregnancies result in a *macrosomic infant* (that is, greater than 4500 g). These infants may demonstrate altered glucose and bilirubin metabolism. They also have an increased incidence of birth trauma, especially shoulder dystocia and associated brachial plexus injury during vaginal delivery, as well as of cesarean section resulting from fetopelvic disproportion. In fetal macrosomia, there can also be maternal trauma, with lacerations of the maternal perineum or, in the case of cesarean delivery, of the uterus and other pelvic organs.

The *diminished amniotic fluid volume, or oligohydramnios*, associated with postterm pregnancy is largely responsible for the *increased fetal stress and distress* seen in the antepartum and intrapartum periods. Amniotic fluid volume reaches its maximal amount of about 1 L at 36–37 weeks gestation and thereafter diminishes to an average of less than half that at 42 weeks. The umbilical cord normally floats freely in the amniotic fluid. The loss of significant fluid volume means a loss in protection for the umbilical cord so that impingement on the cord can occur.

Increasingly severe *placental dysfunction* with decreased transfer of water, electrolytes, glucose, amino acids, and oxygen can occur in postterm pregnancy. Two fifths of placentas from postterm pregnancies demonstrate placental infarcts, calcification, and fibrosis consistent with decreased functional capability. This intrauterine nutritional and respiratory deprivation may contribute to fetal stress and to the development of postmaturity syndrome.

Another special concern in postterm pregnancies is meconium passage and the possibility of aspiration of meconium (*meconium aspiration syndrome*), which can lead to severe respiratory distress from mechanical obstruction of both small and large airways, as well as meconium chemical pneumonitis. Meconium passage is not limited to postterm pregnancies; it is seen in 13–15% of all term pregnancies. The incidence of meconium passage rises as pregnancy becomes prolonged. Since diminished amniotic fluid volume is also present in postterm pregnancy, the neonate is more likely to aspirate more concentrated solutions of this toxic, particulate meconium.

DIAGNOSIS OF POSTTERM PREGNANCY

The diagnosis of postterm pregnancy rests upon establishment of the correct gestational age. Every effort should be made to accurately assess gestational age as early as possible in pregnancy when the parameters used for this purpose are most discriminating and reliable. With improved access to prenatal care and the greater importance placed upon accurate gestational age assessment, the percentage of patients in whom postterm pregnancy is "suspected" but whose dates are uncertain has diminished. Nonetheless, an alarmingly high number of patients do not seek prenatal care early in pregnancy or do not have an accurate gestational age determination. Physicians should be suspicious of the presumed

due date of any patient who first appears for prenatal care late in pregnancy who might be "1 or 2 months overdue." Care should be taken to properly evaluate her fetus for the stigmata of postterm pregnancy.

MANAGEMENT OF POSTTERM PREGNANCY

The first step in management of postterm pregnancy is a careful review of the information used to establish the gestational age to be as certain as possible that is correct. Once the diagnosis of postterm pregnancy is established, the *management options are either to induce labor or to continue surveillance of fetal well-being until spontaneous labor occurs.*

If gestational age is felt to be firmly established, factors that influence the decision of whether to deliver or not rest with the patient's concerns and desires, the assessment of fetal well-being, and the status of the cervix. Induction of labor is appropriate if the cervix is favorable, that is, softened, effaced, and somewhat dilated, and if the patient prefers labor induction. If the cervix is not favorable or the patient does not wish induction of labor, fetal well-being is monitored while awaiting spontaneous labor or a change in the cervix so that induction is appropriate. A variety of management schemes have been devised for this "waiting period," none of which is clearly superior. Daily fetal movement counting is included in most management plans, along with nonstress testing or oxytocin challenge testing once or twice weekly and frequent assessments of amniotic fluid volume by ultrasound. A biophysical profile done twice weekly is also widely used.

If the gestational age is not well established, the clinician utilizes whatever information is available to determine the "best" date. Amniocentesis is not especially helpful, as fetal lung maturity is rarely a question in the postterm evaluation. When the best date is selected, a management plan similar to that for a postterm pregnancy with well-established dates is used.

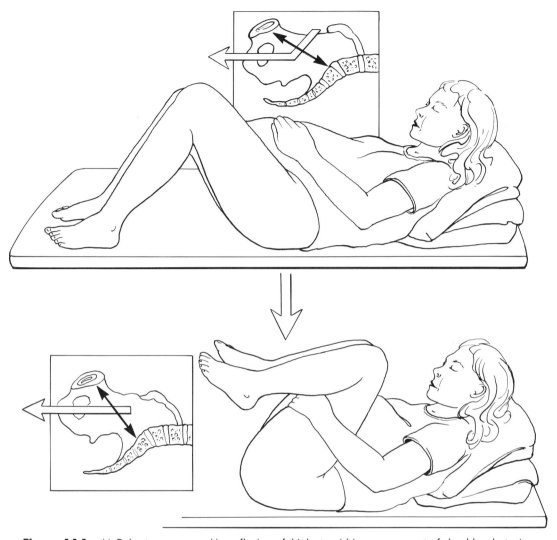

Figure 14.1. McRoberts maneuver: Hyperflexion of thighs to aid in management of shoulder dystocia.

Although there is no absolute time within which labor must be induced, many believe that delivery should be effected by either 42 or 43 weeks. Induction of labor can be attempted using intravenous Pitocin (oxytocin) or prostaglandin vaginal suppositories (Prostin (carboprost tromethamine)). In some patients, if the cervix is quite unfavorable, cesarean section without attempted induction may be performed. Proponents of such "cutoff" dates are said to favor "aggressive management," citing increased morbidity and mortality after 42 or 43 completed weeks gestation. Modern methods for surveillance of fetal well-being make it less logical to be dogmatic about mandatory induction at a given gestational age. Proponents of "expectant management" allow pregnancy to continue for some time as long as there is evidence of fetal well-being. In any case, if the cervix is unfavorable and induction is required, attempts can be made to "ripen" the cervix by the use of prostaglandin E_2 gel or by insertion of laminaria, a hydrophylic device, which, with time, begins to dilate the cervix.

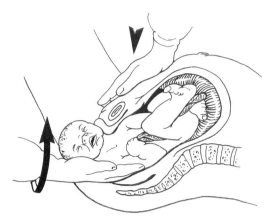

Figure 14.2. Rotation plus suprapubic pressure to aid in management of shoulder dystocia.

Because of the risk of macrosomia-associated birth trauma, ultrasonographic estimation of fetal weight should be obtained before any induction of labor in a postterm pregnancy. If the estimated fetal weight is greater than 4500–5000 grams, cesarean section is the appropriate mode of delivery.

Patients with postterm pregnancies should be advised to come promptly to the hospital when labor pains commence. Once the onset of regular contractions occurs, careful electronic fetal monitoring should be employed throughout labor because of the risk of fetal stress/distress. Intrapartum management includes the artificial rupture of membranes, when possible, to allow detection of meconium and to allow the placement of a fetal scalp electrode and intrauterine pressure catheter. Because of the increased risk of cesarean delivery for fetal stress and because of the potential problems associated with meconium, both anesthesia and pediatric personnel should be alerted that a postterm patient is in labor.

At the time of delivery, special precautions are taken. If meconium passage has been noted, the infant's naso- and oropharynx should be suctioned prior to delivery of the shoulders, since compression of the chest has forced fluid within the chest upward to the pharynx. Pediatric support should be in the delivery room in order to provide prompt visual examination of the infant's airway to a level beneath the larynx and to suction any meconium material. This infant management significantly decreases, but does not eliminate, the likelihood of meconium aspiration syndrome. Because of the risk of macrosomia, the physician performing the delivery should be familiar with the techniques used to treat shoulder dystocia such as exaggerated flexion of the thighs (Figure 14.1) and suprapubic pressure (Figure 14.2).

FURTHER READINGS

Eden RA. Postdate pregnancy. In: Eden RD, Boehm FH, eds. Assessment and care of the fetus. East Norwalk, CN: Appleton & Lange, 1990:Chapter 54.

SELF-EVALUATION

Case 14-A

A 35-year-old G1P0 patient presents on June 6 for prenatal care, saying that her previous doctor said she was due "about now." The prenatal records she brings include the notation of a "light LMP" on September 20, a "period" on August 25, fetal movement "sometime just before Christmas," a first pelvic examination on November 1, which showed an anteverted 10–11 week-size uterus, an ultrasound on January 4 consistent with a 15-week gestation and another in May 15 consistent with a "term" pregnancy. The patient says the baby is moving as much this week as during the previous 2 weeks. The patient has no obstetric risk factors. Physical examination is completely normal. The fundal height is 38 cm and the cervix is closed and uneffaced with the vertex at −1 station. The patient asks to be induced and delivered now.

Question 14-A-1

She should be told that:

A. Another ultrasound should be obtained to clarify her gestational age.

B. No action by the physician is needed.

C. Induction is appropriate at this time.

D. Further evaluation is needed before a course of management can be recommended.

Answer 14-A-1

Answer: D

The patient's gestational age requires clarification before a rational management can be formulated. In addition, induction without indication poses undue risks to mother and fetus, especially with an unfavorable cervix as depicted in this case. Ultrasound is most useful in determination of gestational age in late first and second trimesters, but only relatively precise (±2–3 weeks) in the third trimester.

Question 14-A-2

Based on the information given, the best estimate of this patient's gestational age is:

A. 38 weeks
B. 39 weeks
C. 40 weeks
D. 41 weeks
E. 42 weeks
F. 43 weeks

Answer 14-A-2

Answer: D

The LMP of 9/20 was "light," whereas that of 8/25 was "normal." Although this is insufficient to establish dates, the "normal" LMP of 8/25 is consistent with the first pelvic examination and midtrimester ultrasound and not inconsistent with the late trimester ultrasound. Thus, setting a gestational age of 41 weeks is appropriate.

Question 14-A-3

Which of the following studies are appropriate at this time?

A. ultrasound to establish gestational age
B. ultrasound to evaluate amniotic fluid volume
C. biophysical profile
D. electronic fetal monitoring of the fetus (non-stress or stress test)
E. amniocentesis to determine fetal lung maturity

Answer 14-A-3

Answer: B, C, D

Ultrasound is relatively imprecise in the last trimester for gestational age measurement, although it is useful for evaluation of amniotic fluid volume and for biophysical profile measurement. Likewise, electronic fetal monitoring, e.g., non-stress test to assess the fetal status is appropriate. Amniocentesis is not needed, as fetal lung maturity is not an issue.

Question 14-A-4

All the studies performed on this patient were reassuring as to maternal and fetal status. One week later, on 6/13 the patient reports that the baby is still moving well, although she feels more pelvic pressure and has been having cramps. On physical examination, the fundal height is unchanged and the cervix is 90% effaced, 3 cm dilated, with the vertex at zero station with intact membranes. The patient again requests induction of labor.

She should now be told that:

A. Another ultrasound to determine gestational age is necessary.
B. She should not worry; she will deliver when she is ready.
C. Induction of labor is appropriate.
D. Further studies are necessary before a course of management can be recommended.

Answer 14-A-4

Answer: C

The patient's cervical examination has now changed to one favorable for induction, which is now the least risky management for mother and fetus. If the cervical examination had been unchanged, continued evaluation of fetal well-being would have been appropriate. Delivery would be indicated if there were evidence of fetal distress or at 42 or 43 weeks, depending on the physician's attitude toward the maximum allowable duration of gestation.

Case 14-B

A patient G1P0 at 41 weeks confirmed by first trimester ultrasound has had an unremarkable pregnancy. Fetal well-being studies are normal. The fundal height is 41 cm. On pelvic examination, the cervix is uneffaced and closed and the cephalic part is at −3 station. After a week of expectant management, the patient reports good fetal movement and some mild contractions. On examination, fundal height is 40 cm. FHRs are 140 bpm, and pelvic examination shows the vertex at −3 station, intact membranes, and a cervix dilated to 4 cm and 90% effaced. The patient requests induction of labor.

Question 14-B-1

The patient should be told that:
A. Another ultrasound will be ordered for clarification of gestational age.
B. She should not worry; she will deliver when she is ready.
C. Labor will be induced now.
D. She is in labor.

Answer 14-B-1

Answer: D

The duration of pregnancy is clear and no further studies are needed. A patient in early labor at 42 weeks gestation should proceed to delivery.

Question 14-B-2

Which of the following studies are appropriate at this time for this patient?
A. ultrasound to estimate fetal weight
B. electronic fetal monitoring of the fetus
C. amniocentesis to determine fetal lung maturity
D. artificial rupture of the membranes

Answer 14-B-2

Answer: A, B

The fundal height and pelvic examination suggest the possibility of macrosomia. If macrosomia is discovered by ultrasonographic estimation of fetal weight, a clinical decision whether to try for a vaginal delivery or to proceed with cesarean section must be made based on the estimated fetal weight, the clinical pelvimetry, the status of the fetus, and the informed wishes of the parents. Electronic monitoring of the postterm fetus during labor is important because of the higher risk of uteroplacental insufficiency. Artificial rupture of the membranes will allow direct fetal heart monitoring via fetal scalp electrode and allow assessment for the presence of meconium, but this should be done when the presenting part is sufficiently into the pelvis. At −3 station, the risk of cord prolapse is higher than if the presenting part were applied to the cervix.

chapter 15

NORMAL LABOR AND DELIVERY

Labor is the process by which products of conception (fetus, placenta, cord, and membranes) are expelled from the uterus. It is defined as the progressive effacement and dilation of the uterine cervix resulting from contractions of the uterine musculature. Cervical dilation that occurs without uterine contractions is not considered true labor. Uterine contractions without effacement and dilation of the cervix occur normally in the third trimester of pregnancy and are termed Braxton Hicks contractions or "false labor."

CHANGES PRIOR TO THE ONSET OF LABOR

Eighty-five percent of patients will undergo spontaneous labor between 37 and 42 weeks gestation. It is impossible to predict when labor will commence, but several events frequently occur prior to the onset of labor. As the patient approaches term, the uterus undergoes an increasing number of uterine contractions of greater intensity. Although spontaneous uterine contractions occur throughout pregnancy, toward the latter part of pregnancy they attain the intensity and frequency that patients perceive to be those of true labor. These uterine contractions are not associated with progressive dilation of the cervix, however, and therefore do not fit the definition of labor. They are *Braxton Hicks contractions, or "false labor."* It is frequently difficult for the patient to distinguish these often uncomfortable contractions from those of true labor, and, as a result, it is difficult for the physician to determine the true onset of labor by history taking alone. Braxton Hicks contractions are typically shorter in duration and less

intense than true contractions, with the discomfort characterized as over the lower abdomen and groin areas. It is not uncommon for these contractions to resolve with ambulation. True labor, on the other hand, is associated with contractions that the patient feels over the uterine fundus, with radiation of discomfort to the low back and low abdomen. These contractions become increasingly intense and frequent. The ultimate test as to whether or not contractions are those of true labor is whether or not they are associated with cervical effacement and dilation.

Another event that occurs late in pregnancy is termed *"lightening,"* in which the patient reports a change in the shape of her abdomen, the result of the fetal head descending into the pelvis. Not only does the abdomen change shape, but the patient reports that the baby is "dropping." The patient often notices that the lower abdomen is more prominent, the upper abdomen is more flat, and there may be more frequent urination as the bladder is compressed by the fetal head. The patient may also report an easier time breathing, as there is less pressure on the diaphragm.

Patients often report the passage of blood-tinged mucus late in pregnancy. This *"bloody show"* results as the cervix begins thinning out (*effacement*) with the concomitant extrusion of mucus from the cervical glands. Cervical effacement is common prior to the onset of true labor, as the internal os is slowly drawn into the lower uterine segment. Therefore, the cervix is often significantly effaced prior to the onset of labor, particularly in the nulliparous patient.

EVALUATION FOR LABOR

Instruction as to when to report to the hospital when labor is suspected is a routine part of antepartum care. *Patients are instructed to come to the hospital for any of the following reasons:* if their contractions occur approximately every 5 minutes for at least 1 full hour; if there is a sudden gush of fluid or a constant leakage of fluid (suggesting spontaneous rupture of membranes); if there is significant bleeding; or if there is significant decrease in fetal movement. At the time of initial evaluation at the hospital, the *prenatal records* are reviewed by the physician in order to: (*a*) identify complications of pregnancy up to that point; (*b*) confirm gestational age in order to differentiate preterm labor from labor in a term pregnancy; and (*c*) review pertinent laboratory information. A *focused history* by the physician helps in determining the nature and frequency of the patient's contractions, the possibility of spontaneous rupture of membranes or significant bleeding or changes in maternal or fetal status. A *limited general physical examination* is performed (with special attention to vital signs) as well as the abdominal and pelvic examinations. If contractions occur during this physical examination, they may be palpated for intensity and duration by the examining physician. Auscultation of the fetal heart tones is also of critical importance, particularly following a contraction, in order to determine the possibility of any fetal heart rate deceleration.

The *initial abdominal examination* is helpful in determining fetal lie and presentation. *Lie* is the relationship of the long axis of the fetus with the maternal long axis. It is longitudinal in 99% of cases, occasionally transverse, and rarely oblique (where the axes cross at a 45° angle, usually converting to a transverse or longitudinal lie). *Presentation* is determined by the "presenting part," i.e., that portion of the fetus lowest in the birth canal, palpated during the abdominal examination and when a vaginal examination is performed. For example, in a longitudinal lie, the presenting part is either breech or cephalic. The most common cephalic presentation is the one in which the head is sharply flexed onto the fetal chest such that the occiput or vertex "presents." The abdominal examination may be accomplished utilizing *Leopold's maneuvers* (Fig. 15.1), a series of four palpations of the fetus through the abdominal wall that helps accurately determine fetal presentation, lie, and *position* (the relationship of the fetal presenting part to the right and left side of the maternal pelvis) (Fig. 15.2). The four Leopold's manuevers illustrated in Figure 15.1 include the following:

1. Determining what occupies the fundus. In a longitudinal lie, the fetal head is differentiated from the fetal breech, the latter being larger and less clearly defined.
2. Determining location of small parts. Using one hand to steady the fetus, the fingers on the other hand are used to palpate either the firm, long fetal spine or the various shapes and movements indicating fetal hands and feet.
3. Identifying descent of the presenting part. Suprapubic palpation identifies the presenting part as the fetal head, which is relatively mobile, or a breech, which moves the entire body. The extent to which the presenting part is felt to extend below the symphysis suggests the station of the presenting part.
4. Identifying the cephalic prominence. As long as this cephalic prominence is easily palpable, the vertex is not likely to have descended to 0 station.

As part of the abdominal examination, palpation of the uterus during a contraction is helpful in determining the intensity of that particular contraction. The uterine wall is not easily indented with firm palpation during a true contraction, but it is easily indented during a Braxton Hicks contraction.

The *vaginal examination* should be performed using an aseptic technique. If it is unclear whether or not membranes have been ruptured, a sterile speculum examination should be performed prior to any digital examination of the cervix to ascertain if spontaneous rupture of the membranes has occurred (see Chapter 7, "Premature Rupture of Membranes"). Visualization of the cervix

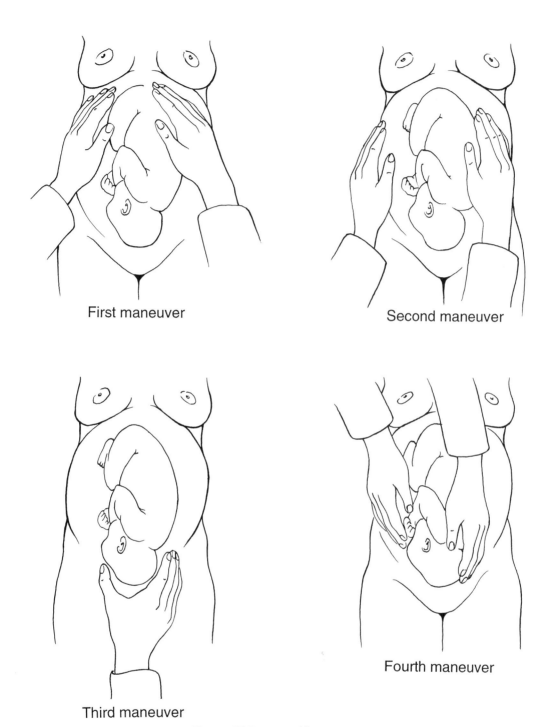

First maneuver

Second maneuver

Third maneuver

Fourth maneuver

Figure 15.1. Leopold maneuvers.

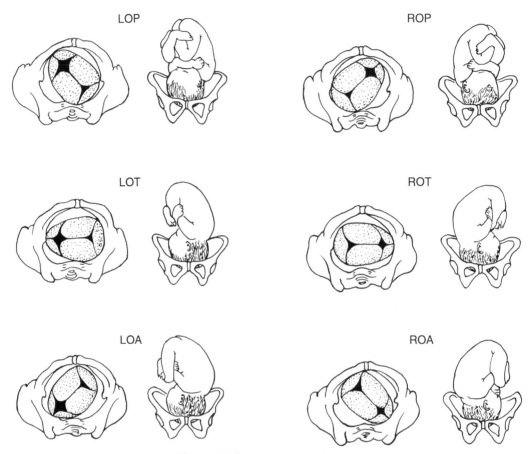

LOP   ROP

LOT   ROT

LOA   ROA

Figure 15.2. Vertex presentations.

through the speculum also allows for better identification of the source of any bleeding (see Chapter 9, "Obstetric Hemorrhage," the heading Third Trimester Bleeding). The digital portion of the vaginal examination allows the examiner to determine the degree of *cervical effacement* (expressed as percent effacement, i.e., a cervix that is thinned to one half of its original 2 cm length is termed 50%, whereas a cervix that is virtually totally thinned is described as 100% effaced), as well as the consistency (firm or soft) of the cervix (Fig. 15.3). A cervix that is not effaced, but is softened, is more likely to undergo spontaneous labor sooner than a cervix that remains firm, as it is earlier in pregnancy. If the cervix is not significantly effaced, it may also be evaluated for its relative position, i.e., anterior, midposition, or posterior in the vagina.

A cervix that is palpable anterior in the vagina is more likely to undergo spontaneous onset of labor sooner than one found in the posterior portion of the vagina. The cervix is also palpated for cervical dilation, described as centimeters of dilation. The individual examiner uses one or two fingers to identify the diameter of the opening of the cervix. The presenting part of the fetus can usually be palpated by vaginal examination. *Fetal station* is also determined by identifying the relative level of the foremost part of the fetal presenting part relative to the level of the ischial spines. If the presenting part has reached the level of the ischial spines, it is termed "0 station." The distance between the ischial spines to the pelvic inlet above as well as from the spines to the pelvic outlet below is divided into thirds, and these measurements

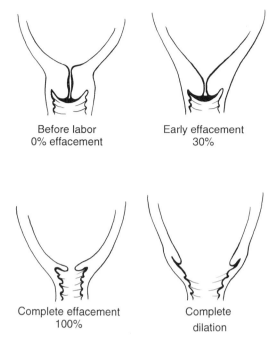

Before labor
0% effacement

Early effacement
30%

Complete effacement
100%

Complete
dilation

Figure 15.3. Effacement and dilation.

are used to further define station. If the presenting part is palpable at the pelvic inlet, it is called " – 3", if it has descended one third of the way to the ischial spines, it is called " – 2 station", etc. Descent of the fetal presenting part below the spines is similarly defined as + 1 station, + 2 station, etc. (Fig. 15.4). The clinical significance of the fetal head presenting at 0 station is that this suggests that the biparietal diameter of the fetal head, the greatest transverse diameter of the fetal skull, has negotiated the pelvic inlet.

If the patient is found not to be in active labor, i.e., less than 3–4 cm dilated, and there is no confounding medical or obstetric problems, she is sent home to await the onset of true labor. If there is a question as to whether or not true labor has commenced, the patient may be reevaluated after approximately 1 hour. In some cases, patients are encouraged to ambulate in order to differentiate Braxton Hicks contractions from true labor. If the patient is in labor, she is admitted to the labor area of the hospital and active management of labor is undertaken.

STAGES OF LABOR

Although labor is a continuous process, it is divided into three functional stages. The *first stage* is the interval between the onset of labor and full cervical dilation. The first stage is further divided into two phases. The *latent phase* encompasses cervical effacement and early dilation. The second is the active phase during which more rapid cervical dilation occurs, usually beginning at approximately 3–4 cm. The *second stage* encompasses complete cervical dilation through the delivery of the infant. The *third stage* begins immediately after delivery of the infant and ends with the delivery of the placenta. The *fourth stage* of labor is defined as the immediate postpartum period of approximately 2 hours after delivery of the placenta during which time the patient undergoes significant physiologic adjustment. Table 15.1 outlines the duration of various stages of labor as defined by Friedman.

MECHANISM OF LABOR

The mechanism of labor (also known as the cardinal movements of labor) refers to the changes of the position of the fetus as it passes through the birth canal. The fetus usually descends in a fashion whereby the occipital portion of the fetal head is the lowermost part in the pelvis and rotates towards the largest pelvic segment. This vertex presentation occurs in 95% of term labors. As a result, the cardinal movements of labor are defined relative to this presentation. How a fetus in the breech presentation accommodates to the birth canal would be significantly different. In order to accommodate to the maternal bony pelvis, the fetal head must undergo several movements as it passes through the birth canal. These movements are accomplished by means of the forceful contractions of the uterus. These *cardinal movements of labor* do not occur as a distinct series of movements, but do describe in total how the fetal head adapts to the bony pelvis. These are: (*a*) engagement, (*b*) descent, (*c*) flexion,

164

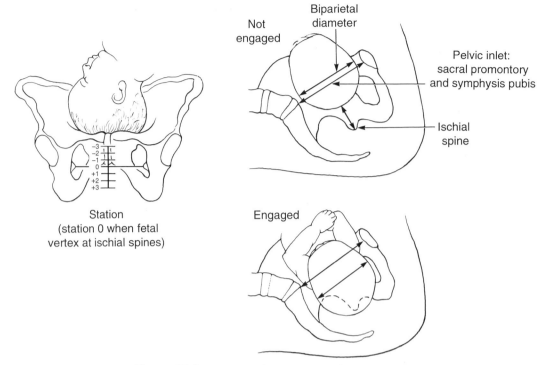

Figure 15.4. Station and engagement of the fetal head.

Table 15.1
Mean Duration of the Various Phases and Stages of Labor with Their Distribution Characteristics

	Latent phase h	Active phase h	Maximum dilation cm/h	Second stage h
Nulliparas				
Mean	6.4	4.6	3.0	1.1
Limit[a]	20.1	11.7	1.2	2.9
Multiparas				
Mean	4.8	2.4	5.7	0.39
Limit[a]	13.6	5.2	1.5	1.1

[a]5th or 95th percentile.

(*d*) internal rotation, (*e*) extension, (*f*) external rotation, and (*g*) expulsion (Fig. 15.5).

Engagement is defined as descent of the biparietal diameter of the head below the pelvic inlet, diagnosed clinically by palpation of the presenting part below the level of ischial spines. The importance of this event is that it demonstrates to some extent that the bony pelvis is adequate to allow significant descent of the fetal head. It is not uncommon for the fetal head to become engaged prior to the onset of true labor, particularly in nulliparous patients. *Descent of the presenting part* is a necessity for the successful completion of passage through the birth canal. The greatest rate of descent occurs during the latter portions of the first stage of labor and during the second stage of labor. Figure 15.6 is a graphic demonstration of fetal descent and dilation of the cervix. *Flexion of the fetal head* allows for the smaller diameters of the fetal head to present to the maternal pelvis. *Internal rotation*, like flexion, facilitates presentation of the optimal diameters of the fetal head to the bony pelvis. *Extension of the fetal head* occurs as it reaches the introitus. To accommodate to the upward curve of the birth canal, the flexed head now extends. *External rotation* occurs after delivery of the head as the head rotates to "face forward" relative to its shoulders. *Expulsion* is the final delivery of the fetus from the birth canal.

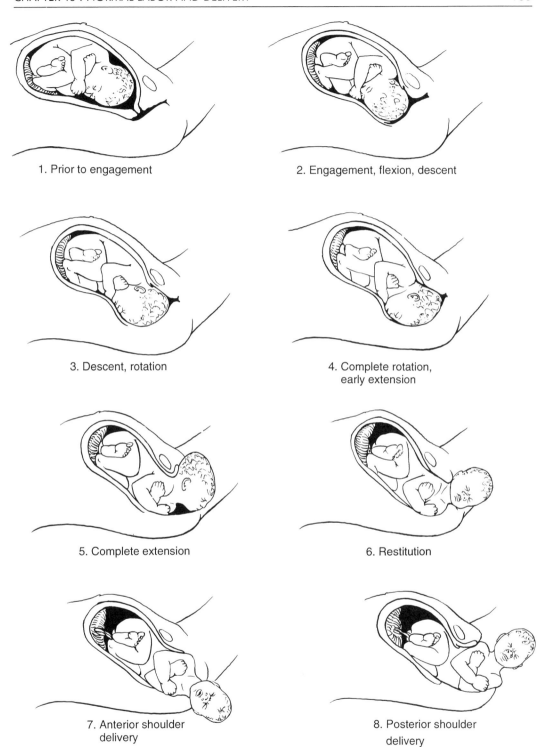

1. Prior to engagement

2. Engagement, flexion, descent

3. Descent, rotation

4. Complete rotation, early extension

5. Complete extension

6. Restitution

7. Anterior shoulder delivery

8. Posterior shoulder delivery

Figure 15.5.   Cardinal movements of labor.

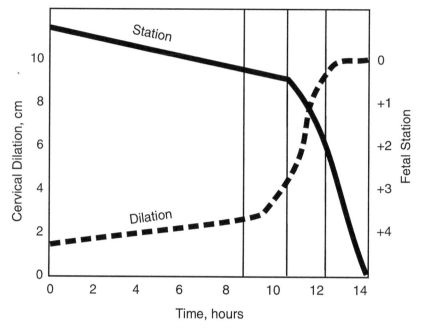

Figure 15.6. Graphic presentation of cervical dilation and station during labor.

MANAGEMENT OF LABOR

Although the patient may have undergone some education regarding the labor and delivery process, it is important to realize that the patient has significant fears that remain. The patient should not be left unattended for any significant length of time, and a "support person" may be allowed to remain with the patient throughout the labor and delivery process in most cases. Maternal vital signs should be taken at least every 30 minutes. The patient should be given nothing by mouth except for small sips of water, ice chips, or hard candies. Laboratory information, including hematocrit, type and screen, platelet count, and urinalysis for glucose and protein, are obtained when the patient is admitted to the hospital. An intravenous line is frequently inserted in order to provide hydration and immediate access to the intravascular space should medications be necessary. As the gastrointestinal tract significantly slows in its functions during labor, hydration by means of the intravenous line is optimal.

During the course of labor, descent of the fetus causes the bladder to be elevated relative to the lower uterine segment and cervix. This often results in the patient having difficulty voiding. The patient should, therefore, be encouraged to void frequently. Catheterization may become necessary if the bladder becomes distended.

Depending on individual institutional limitations, the patient may be allowed to labor in any of several positions. Typically, the patients are kept at bed rest in a sitting or reclining position. The lateral recumbent position is more comfortable for some patients whereas other patients choose to ambulate or sit in a rocking chair during the first stage of labor. At all times, close monitoring of the fetal heart rate must be available. *Electronic fetal monitoring* is very common and often routine, but it is probably not necessary for the low risk term pregnancy. If routine monitoring is not undertaken, auscultation of the fetal heart rate should be performed at least every 15 minutes immediately after uterine contractions. During the second stage of labor, fetal heart rate auscultation should be performed after each uterine contraction. If electronic fetal monitoring is undertaken, either as routine or for patients who are considered at risk, an external tocodynamometer is initially used to assess uterine activity. As this provides information regarding only the frequency and duration of contractions, internal pressure monitoring using an intrauterine catheter can be performed to more accurately measure intensity of contractions. This internal form of fetal monitoring requires rupture of the membranes, and therefore can usually not be accomplished until the cervix is at least 1–2 cm dilated. Fetal heart rate can be monitored externally by Doppler ultrasound or internally using a direct fetal electrocardiogram, which is obtained by applying a scalp electrode. The latter technique allows for more detailed evaluation of subtle changes in fetal heart rate pattern (see Chapter 17, "Intrapartum Fetal Distress"). Whenever artificial rupture of the membranes is to be performed, the presenting part must be well-applied to the cervix. This minimizes the risk of an iatrogenic umbilical cord prolapse.

Because the latent phase of labor may be affected by *analgesic and anesthetic agents*, these should generally not be employed until the active phase of labor. There is no evidence that either analgesics or anesthetics significantly affect the active phase of labor. Many patients have prepared for labor using childbirth education classes, during which time they are taught techniques of relaxation to deal with the pain of labor contractions. Some of these patients, however, find the use of narcotic analgesics to be helpful adjuncts to these measures. In the doses typically given during labor, neonatal depression is not a major concern, although theoretically possible. Any anesthetic technique used during the labor and delivery process should take into account those sensory pathways involved. During the first stage of labor, pain results from contraction of the uterus and dilation of the cervix. This pain travels along the visceral afferents, which accompany sympathetic nerves entering the spinal cord at T-

10, T-11, T-12, and L-1. As the head descends, there is also distention of the lower birth canal and perineum. This pain is transmitted along somatic afferents that comprise portions of the pudendal nerves that enter the spinal cord at S-2, S-3, and S-4. The anesthetic technique that provides pain relief during labor is the epidural block. The advantage of this technique is its ability to provide analgesia during labor as well as excellent anesthesia for delivery. It can also be used in either vaginal or abdominal deliveries. Spinal anesthetic can be used for vaginal or abdominal delivery also, but is typically given just prior to delivery. A pudendal block can be administered easily at the time of delivery to provide perineal anesthesia for a vaginal delivery (Fig. 15.7).

Epidural anesthesia is superior to spinal anesthesia in that it can be left as a continuous source of analgesia and anesthesia during both the labor and delivery process. It avoids the risk of spinal headache in the mother and reduces the risk of sympathetic blockade, which could lead to hypotention. There is also less motor blockade than with spinal anesthesia. Although the pudendal block is the easiest to perform and also has the least potential risk to the mother and fetus, its utility is also the most limited. *General anesthesia* is reserved only for cesarean sections in selected cases. The potential risk of complications such as maternal aspiration reduces its more widespread utility.

Evaluation of the patient's progress of labor is accomplished by means of a series of pelvic examinations. The number of examinations should be minimized in order to avoid increasing significantly the risk for chorioamnionitis. At the time of each vaginal examination, the perineum is cleansed and a sterile lubricant is used. Each examination should identify cervical dilation, effacement, station, and the status of the membranes. These findings should be noted graphically on the hospital record in order that abnormalities of labor may be identified. During the latter portions of the first stage of labor, patients may report the urge to push. This may signify significant de-

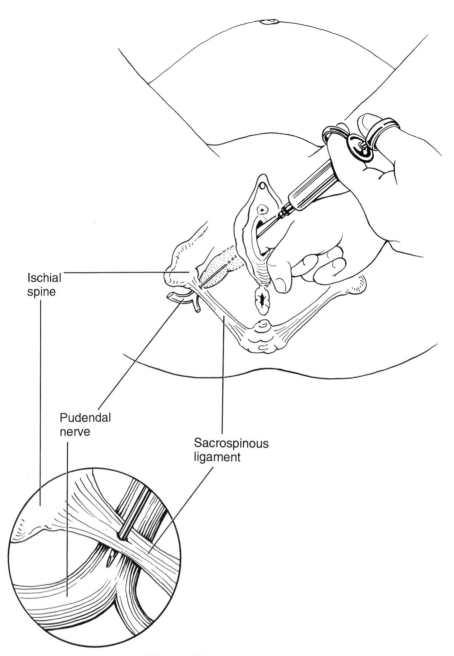

Figure 15.7. Pudendal block.

Ischial spine

Pudendal nerve

Sacrospinous ligament

scent of the fetal head with pressure on the perineum. More frequent vaginal examinations during this time may be necessary. Similarly, in case of significant fetal heart rate decelerations, more examinations may be necessary to determine whether or not the umbilical cord is prolapsed or if delivery is imminent.

In addition to rupturing the membranes to insert an intrauterine pressure catheter or a fetal scalp monitor, *artificial rupture of membranes* may be beneficial in other ways. The

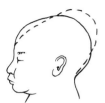 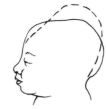

Figure 15.8. Molding of head.

presence or absence of meconium can be identified. Blood in the amniotic fluid may also have significance (see Chapter 9, "Obstetric Hemorrhage," the heading Third Trimester Bleeding). Rupture of the membranes does, however, carry some risk, as the incidence of infection may be increased if labor is prolonged or umbilical cord prolapse may occur if rupture of the membranes is undertaken prior to engagement of the presenting fetal part. *Spontaneous rupture of membranes* has similar risks. The fluid should be observed for meconium and blood. Fetal heart tones should be assessed after membranes spontaneously rupture.

Once the *second stage of labor* has been reached (i.e., "complete" or 10 cm of cervical dilation), maternal effort ("pushing") can be added to the involuntary contractile forces of the uterus in order to facilitate delivery of the fetus. With the onset of each contraction, the mother is encouraged to inhale, hold her breath, and perform an extended Valsalva maneuver. This abdominal pressure aids in fetal descent through the birth canal. It is during this time that the fetal head may undergo further alterations. If identified prior to the second stage of labor, these changes should be noted on the pelvic examination and may indicate a significant problem in negotiation of the birth canal. *Molding* is an alteration in the relationship of the fetal cranial bones, even resulting in partial bone overlap. Some minor degree is common as the fetal head adjusts to the bony pelvis. The greater the disparity between the fetal head and the bony pelvis, the greater the amount of molding (Fig. 15.8). *Caput succedaneum* is the edema of the fetal scalp caused by pressure on the fetal head by

the cervix. Extended second stages may last as long as 2–3 hours, and the prolonged resistance encountered by the fetal vertex may prevent appropriate identification of fontanels and sutures. Both caput and molding resolve in the first few days of life.

DELIVERY

The patient should be prepared for a well-controlled delivery of the fetal head. In general, the nulliparous patients take a greater amount of time than the multiparous patients to deliver once the second stage of labor has started. The position of the patient for delivery most preferred by physicians is the dorsal lithotomy position. This allows the physician to have better control of delivery with better exposure for both the delivery and subsequent surgical repair, if needed. Other positions are preferred by some patients. With each successive contraction, the maternal force as well as uterine contractions cause more of the fetal scalp to be visible at the introitus. If necessary, an *episiotomy* should be performed only after the perineum has been thinned considerably by the descending fetal head (Fig. 15.9). By enlarging the vaginal outlet, an episiotomy facilitates delivery and is indicated in cases of instrumental delivery and/or protracted or arrested descent. The role of routine prophylactic episiotomy is unclear and is therefore best left to the individual doctor and patient. If used, episiotomies are usually cut midline or occasionally laterally as a mediolateral episiotomy. Advantages of the former include less pain, ease of repair, and less blood loss. The primary disadvantage is greater risk of extension into a third or fourth degree laceration.

As the fetal head "crowns," i.e., distends the vaginal opening, it is delivered by extension in order to allow the smallest diameter of the fetal head to pass over the perineum. This decreases the likelihood of laceration or extension of episiotomy. To facilitate this, the physician performs a modified *Ritgen's maneuver*. In this, one hand is placed over the vertex while the other exerts pressure

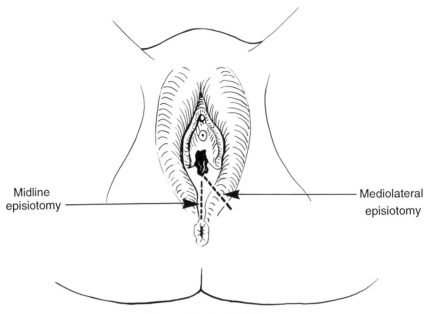

Midline episiotomy

Mediolateral episiotomy

Figure 15.9. Episiotomy.

through the perineum onto the fetal chin. A sterile towel is utilized to avoid contamination of this hand. The chin can then be delivered slowly, with control applied by both hands. After the head is delivered, nasal and oral suction is performed with a bulb syringe. If meconium has been present, suctioning of the pharynx is also accomplished. The neck should then be evaluated for the possible presence of a nuchal cord, which should be reduced over the fetal head if present. If the cord is tight, it may be doubly clamped and cut (Fig. 15.10). After delivery of the head, the shoulders descend and rotate to a position in the anteroposterior diameter of the pelvis. The attendant's hands are placed on the chin and vertex, applying downward pressure, thus delivering the anterior shoulder. To avoid injury to the brachial plexus, care is taken not to put excessive force on the neck. The posterior shoulder is then delivered by upward traction on the fetal head (Fig. 15.11). Delivery of the body now occurs easily. The fetus is then cradled in the attendant's arms, with the head down to maximize drainage of secretions to the oropharynx. Further suctioning is accomplished prior to clamping of the umbilical cord. To avoid significant heat loss, the newborn should not be exposed to significant periods of ambient room temperature without being completely dry. The infant should be taken to the warmer, where further care can be undertaken.

THIRD STAGE OF LABOR

Immediately after delivery of the infant, the uterus significantly decreases in size. Delivery of the placenta is imminent as the uterus rises in the abdomen, indicating that the placenta has separated and has entered the lower uterine segment. A gush of blood may follow, with the cord lengthening. If the placenta does not separate spontaneously, excess traction on the cord should be avoided. Instead, the physician may choose to manually explore the uterus and remove the placenta by using the side of his or her hand to form a cleavage plane between the placenta and the uterine wall. The placenta can then be manually removed. Blood from the umbilical cord should be obtained and sent for type and Rh testing. In some instances, cord pH arterial blood gases are obtained prior to placental separation. The

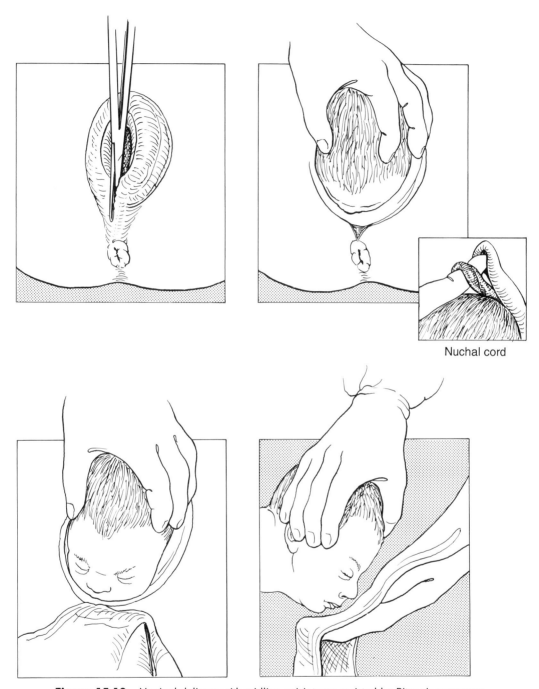

Nuchal cord

Figure 15.10. Vaginal delivery with midline episiotomy assisted by Ritgen's maneuver.

cord should also be evaluated for the presence of the expected two umbilical arteries and one umbilical vein.

After the placenta has been removed, the uterus should be palpated to ensure that it has reduced in size and become firmly contracted. Excessive blood loss at this or any subsequent time should suggest the possibility of uterine atony. The use of uterine massage as well as oxytoxic agents such as oxyto-

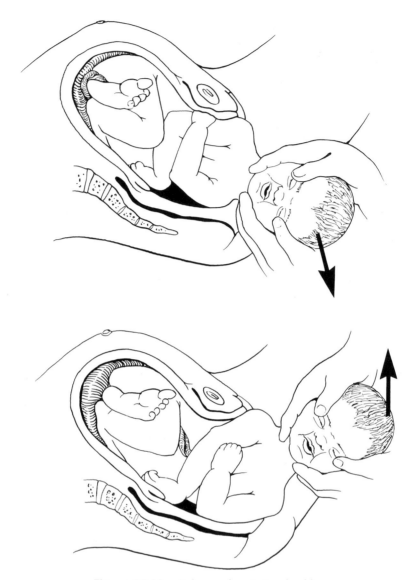

Figure 15.11. Delivery of posterior shoulder.

cin, Methergine (methylergonovine maleate), or prostaglandins may be routinely used.

Inspection of the birth canal should be accomplished in a systematic fashion. The introitus and vulvar areas, including the periurethral area, should be evaluated for lacerations. Ring forceps are commonly used to hold and evaluate the cervix.' Lacerations, if present, are most commonly found at 3 o'clock and 9 o'clock on the cervix. Lacerations of the vagina and/or perineum, as well as extensions of the episiotomy, are also evaluated. Repair is accomplished with an absorbable suture. Obstetric lacerations are classified in Table 15.2.

INDICATIONS FOR OPERATIVE DELIVERY

Techniques of operative delivery include obstetric forceps, vacuum extraction, and cesarean section. Forceps are primarily utilized to supply traction to the fetal head

Table 15.2
Classification of Obstetric Lacerations

First degree	Involves the vaginal mucosa or perineal skin, but not the underlying muscle
Second degree	Involves the underlying fascia or muscle, but not the rectal sphincter or rectal mucosa
Third degree	Extends through the rectal sphincter but not into the rectum
Fourth degree	Extends into the rectal mucosa

Table 15.3
Conditions for Forceps Application

Cervix	Fully dilated
Membranes	Ruptured
Position and station of fetal head	Known and engaged
Anesthesia	Adequate for maternal comfort
Maternal pelvis	Evaluated and found appropriate

Table 15.4
Forceps Classification

Outlet forceps. The fetal skull has reached the perineal floor, the scalp is visible between contractions, the sagittal suture is in the anteroposterior diameter or in the right or left occiput anterior or posterior position, but not more than 45° from the midline.
Low forceps. The leading edge of the skull is station +2 or more. Rotations are divided into 45° or less and more than 45°.
Midforceps. The head is engaged but the leading edge of the skull is above +2 station.

when the mother's voluntary efforts in conjunction with uterine contractions are insufficient to deliver the infant. Occasionally, forceps are used to rotate the fetal head prior to traction to complete the vaginal delivery. In addition, forceps may be used to control delivery of the fetal head, thereby avoiding any potentially precipitous delivery of the fetal head. Proper application of obstetric forceps by an experienced clinician is necessary to avoid the potential

risk of trauma to both maternal and fetal parts. Table 15.3 is a list of conditions necessary to apply forceps, and Table 15.4, the types of forceps applications.

Vacuum extraction is sometimes used in lieu of obstetric forceps. Because traction is applied only to the instrument, some believe that the delivery is more physiologic and has less potential for trauma than forceps.

Cesarean section now accounts for up to 40% of births in some obstetrical units. The rate of cesarean section was stable at less than 5% until 1965. Cesarean section rates have increased since that time for various reasons. One of the major reasons often cited is the ready availability of neonatal intensive care units, in which infants have a significantly greater survival rate than what was once the case. Another factor in the increase in the rate of cesarean sections is accounted for by the abdominal delivery for breech presentations. Cesarean sections are also performed for three other indications: fetal distress, dystocias, and as a repeat procedure. An increasing number of cesarean sections are being done for dystocia and uterine inertia. In addition, increased sophistication for fetal surveillance provides more information about the possibility of fetal distress. As a result, more cesarean sections can be attributed to cases of fetal distress. Approximately 20% of the increase in the rate of cesarean sections is due to repeat cesarean births. For many years, it was felt that a previous cesarean section mandated that all future deliveries would also have to be abdominal. With the increasing tendency to attempt vaginal birth after cesarean section (VBAC), fewer cesarean sections are now being performed for this indication alone.

Deciding on cesarean delivery is significant, as the maternal mortality associated with cesarean delivery is two to four times that of a vaginal birth, i.e., 1 per 2500 to 1 per 5000 operations. Cesarean section can be performed through various incisions in the uterus. An incision through the thin lower uterine segment allows for subsequent trials

Table 15.5
Apgar Scoring System

Sign	Score		
	0	1	2
Heart rate	Absent	Below 100	Over 100
Muscle tone	Limp	Some flexion of extremities	Active motion
Respiratory effort	Absent	Slow, irregular	Good cry
Reflex activity response to stimulation	No response	Grimace	Cough, sneeze, or crying
Color	Blue or pale	Body pink and extremities blue	Completely pink

at VBAC. An incision through the thick, muscular upper portion of the uterus, a "classical" cesarean section, carries a greater risk for subsequent uterine rupture if labor occurs so that repeat cesarean sections for these patients is still recommended.

FOURTH STAGE OF LABOR

For the first hour or so after delivery, the likelihood of serious postpartum complications is the greatest. Postpartum uterine hemorrhage occurs in approximately 1% of patients, whereas infection in the form of endometritis is seen in approximately 5% of patients. The patient should have been closely evaluated to rule out episiotomy extension with or without laceration, uterine atony, or uterine perforation. Immediately after the delivery of the placenta, the uterus is palpated to ascertain that it is firm. Uterine palpation through the abdominal wall is repeated as frequent intervals during the immediate postpartum period in order to ascertain uterine atony. Perineal pads are applied and the amount of blood on these pads as well as pulse and pressure are monitored closely for the first several hours after delivery in order to identify excessive blood loss.

CARE OF THE NEWBORN

Once the newborn has been delivered, it is transported to the warming unit, which is equipped with a radiant heat source. The neonate is dried well in order to minimize the loss of core temperature. The nose and oropharynx are suctioned once again as the infant is placed in the supine position with the head lowered and turned to one side. The newborn is expected to both breathe and cry within the first 30 seconds. Suctioning as well as mild stimulation of the infant by rubbing the back or slapping the feet help to stimulate this.

The initial evaluation of the infant is carried out at 1 and 5 minutes using the Apgar scoring system (Table 15.5). In general, a low 1-minute Apgar identifies the newborn who requires particular attention, whereas the 5-minute Apgar can be utilized to evaluate the effectiveness of any resuscitative efforts that have been undertaken.

Apgar scores of 7–10 are indicative of an infant who requires no active resuscitative intervention; scores of 4–7 are considered indicators of mildly to moderately depressed infants. The severely depressed infants with Apgar scores of less than 4 rarely require a full evaluation using the Apgar score. Instead, immediate resuscitative efforts are started, which may include endotracheal intubation and suctioning with the possible use of positive pressure oxygen.

The Apgar score was designed as a quick assessment of the newborn and should not be used to define birth asphyxia. These scores should not be utilized to identify the cause of the newborn's depression, nor can they be used to predict long-term neurologic outcome.

SELF-EVALUATION

Case 15-A

A 21-year-old G1 at term presents with regular uterine contractions occurring every 3–4 minutes. Pelvic examination reveals 100% effacement and 5 cm dilation, membranes intact, with a vertex presentation at −1 station.

Question 15-A-1

What is the best description of this patient's labor?

A. first stage, latent phase
B. first stage, active phase
C. second stage
D. third stage
E. fourth stage

Answer 15-A-1

Answer: B

Question 15-A-2

Labor continues for 5 hours with the same contraction pattern. Electronic fetal heart rate monitoring is reassuring of fetal well-being. Pelvic examination shows complete dilation and effacement with a markedly molded caput at 0 station.

For further consideration: What is the significance of the station at this time? What is the significance of the "markedly molded caput?" What interventions are indicated: Internal pressure monitor? A trial at "pushing"? Forceps- or vacuum-assisted vaginal delivery? Cesarean section?

Case 15-B

A 25-year-old G1 at term complains of intermittent painful uterine contractions, which are especially painful in the lower abdomen and wax and wane in "strength." There is no history of loss of fluid per vaginam nor vaginal bleeding.

Question 15-B-1

The most likely diagnosis based on history alone is:

A. Braxton Hicks contractions
B. true labor
C. urinary tract infection
D. placental abruption

Answer 15-B-1

Answer: A

The description of the contractions suggests Braxton Hicks rather than true labor contraction. Neither urinary tract infection nor placental abruption is likely, but should be kept in mind in the differential diagnosis of patients presenting with lower abdominal pain.

Question 15-B-2

What maneuver(s) may help determine whether these pains represent true labor contractions?

A. waiting to ascertain if the contractions become more regular
B. having the patient walk to see if the contractions lessen or worsen in severity
C. performing a pelvic examination
D. performing electronic fetal heart evaluation

Answer 15-B-2

Answer: A, B, C

The initial step in management should be a pelvic examination. If the cervix is not effaced and dilated, the patient may be in the latent phase of labor or not in labor at all. Reexamination after approximately 1 hour or after a period of walking can help determine if cervical changes have occurred.

chapter 16

ABNORMAL LABOR

Abnormal labor, or *dystocia* (literally meaning difficult labor or childbirth), results when anatomic or functional abnormalities of the fetus, the maternal bony pelvis, the uterus and cervix, and/or a combination of the above interfere with the normal course of labor and delivery. The diagnosis and management of dystocia is a major health care issue since more than one fourth of all cesarean sections are performed for this indication. Since the goal of modern obstetrics is a safe, healthy delivery for both mother and fetus, minimizing the morbidity and mortality of the labor process continues to be a primary focus of clinical attention.

Abnormal labor describes complications of the normal labor process: *slower-than-normal progress (protraction disorder)* or a *cessation of progress (arrest disorder)*. The patterns of abnormal labor are summarized in Table 16.1. Less specific terms have also been applied to abnormal labor patterns. "Failure to progress" describes lack of progressive cervical dilation and/or descent of the fetus and is similar to the arrest disorders. "Cephalopelvic disproportion" is a disparity between the size or shape of the maternal pelvis and the fetal head, preventing vaginal delivery, and is similar to an arrest disorder. This may be due to the size or shape of the pelvis and/or the fetal head, or a relative disparity due to malpresentation of the fetal head.

CAUSES OF ABNORMAL LABOR

Correct diagnosis and management of abnormal labor requires evaluation of the mechanisms of labor: the "power," the "passenger," and the "passage," otherwise referred to as the uterine contractions, the fetal presentation, and the maternal pelvis, respectively.

Evaluation of the "Power"

The "power," or uterine contractions, may be evaluated both qualitatively and quantitatively. Frequency and duration of contractions can be subjectively evaluated by *manual palpation of the gravid abdomen during a contraction.* Strength of uterine contractions is

Table 16.1
Abnormal Labor Patterns

Type of abnormal labor	Definition
Prolonged latent phase	No progress from latent to active phase of labor For nulligravidas: in >20 h For multiparas: in >14 h
Protraction disorders	Prolonged active phase of labor such that: Cervical dilation proceeds at less than 1.2 cm/h for nulligravidas or 1.5 cm/h for multiparas Descent of the presenting part proceeds at less than 1 cm/h for nulligravidas or 1.5 cm/h for multiparas
Arrest disorders	Secondary arrest of dilation; No progress in the active phase of labor No cervical dilation for more than 2 hours for nulligravida or multipara No progress in the second stage of labor (*arrested descent*): No descent of the presenting part in more than 1 hour

often judged by how much the uterine wall can be "indented" by an examiner's finger during a contraction: strong contraction, no indentation; moderate contraction, some indentation; mild contraction, considerable indentation. Although subjective, such determinations by an experienced examiner are of value. The frequency and duration of uterine contractions may be measured more quantitatively utilizing a *tocodynamometer* while performing external electronic fetal monitoring. The actual pressure generated within the uterus cannot, however, be directly measured without the use of an *internal pressure catheter*. For cervical dilation to occur, each contraction must generate at least 25 mm of mercury of pressure, with 50–60 mm Hg being considered the optimal intrauterine pressure. The frequency of contractions is also important in generating a normal labor pattern, with a minimum of three contractions in a 10-minute window usually considered adequate. During the first stage of labor, therefore, arrest of labor should not be diagnosed until the cervix is at least 4 cm dilated, i.e., the latent phase of labor has been completed, and a pattern of uterine contractions that is adequate both in frequency and intensity has been established.

During the *second stage of labor*, the "powers" include both the uterine contractile forces and the voluntary maternal expulsive efforts. Conditions such as maternal exhaustion, excessive anesthesia, or other medical conditions such as cardiac disease or neuromuscular disease may affect these combined forces so that they are insufficient to facilitate delivery. Forceps-assisted vaginal delivery or cesarean section may then be required.

Evaluation of the "Passenger"

Evaluation of the "passenger" includes estimation of fetal weight and clinical evaluation of fetal lie, presentation, position, and attitude. If a fetus has an estimated weight greater than 4500 g, the incidence of dystocias, including shoulder dystocia or cephalopelvic disproportion, is greater. Because ultrasound estimations of fetal weight are often inaccurate by as much as 500–1000 g, care must be taken to use the information in conjunction with the entire clinical assessment.

If the fetal head is asynclitic (turned to one side) or if the fetal head is extended, a larger cephalic diameter is presented to the pelvis, also increasing the possibility of dystocia. A brow presentation will typically convert to either a vertex or face presentation, but if persistent, causes dystocia requiring cesarean section. Likewise, a face presentation requires cesarean section in most cases, although a mentum anterior presentation (chin towards mother's abdomen) may be delivered vaginally in some instances. Persistent occiput posterior positions are also associated with longer labors, approximately 1 hour in multiparous patients and 2 hours in nulliparous patients. Occasionally, delivery from the occiput posterior position is not possible, and the vertex must be rotated to the occiput anterior position. The fetal head can be rotated manually or, if necessary, with forceps or vacuum. When dystocia due to the fetal position cannot be corrected either manually or with instruments, cesarean section is appropriate.

Fetal anomalies, including hydrocephaly and soft tissue tumors, may also cause dystocia. The use of prenatal ultrasound significantly reduces the incidence of unexpected dystocia for this reason.

Evaluation of the "Passage"

Unfortunately, measurements of the bony pelvis are relatively poor predictors of ultimate successful vaginal delivery. Clinical pelvimetry, i.e., manual evaluation of the diameters of the pelvis, cannot predict whether a fetus can successfully negotiate the birth canal, except in rare circumstances when the pelvic diameters are so small as to render the pelvis "completely contracted." X-ray pelvimetry or other imaging techniques are also of no clinical utility when determining whether or not a patient will require cesarean section for dystocia. Before assuming that the bony pelvis is preventing vaginal delivery, adequate contractions must be assured. In addition to the bony pelvis, there are soft tissue etiologies of dystocia, e.g., a distended bladder or colon, an adnexal mass, or a uterine fibroid. In some instances, epidural anesthesia may contribute to dystocia by decreasing the tone of the pelvic floor musculature.

EVALUATION OF ABNORMAL LABOR

Graphic demonstration of cervical dilation and effacement facilitates assessing a patient's progress in labor and identifying any type of abnormal labor pattern that may develop. Throughout labor, maternal and fetal well-being are continuously assessed along with the progress in labor. The mother, in particular, should be provided moral support and encouragement as the possibility of prolonged labor is faced and the various interventions are considered. Keeping the patient and support person fully apprised of the situation is an important aspect of the management of potentially abnormal labor.

Each *vaginal examination* should provide the following information: dilation of the cervix in centimeters, percentage effacement of cervix, station of the presenting part, presence of caput or molding of the fetal head, and position of the presenting part. The results of each examination are compared to previous examinations and any changes noted. In cases of failure of descent of the fetus, clinical reevaluation of the bony pelvis and its relationships to the fetus helps to identify the potential need for operative vaginal delivery or cesarean section.

Uterine contractions can be assessed by manual palpation or by electronic fetal monitor as previously discussed. The uterine contraction pattern and/or the force of the contractions may be inadequate, either causing the abnormal labor pattern or resulting from a mechanical disorder.

In the past, *x-ray pelvimetry* was utilized to aid in the evaluation of the maternal pelvis during labor. It was felt that the size and

shape of the pelvis could be visualized, as could fetal position and station. Unfortunately, this radiologic approach to managing dystocia has been shown not to be of benefit.

PATTERNS OF ABNORMAL LABOR

Abnormal labor, or dystocia, is divided into prolongation disorders and arrest disorders. These abnormal labor patterns are demonstrated graphically in Figure 16.1.

A latent phase of labor exceeding 20 hours in a primigravid patient or 14 hours in a multigravid patient is abnormal. The causes of such a *prolonged latent phase* of labor include abnormal fetal position, unripe cervix when labor commences, administration of excess anesthesia, fetopelvic disproportion, and dysfunctional/ineffective uterine contractions. The presence of a prolonged latent phase does not necessarily herald an abnormal active phase of labor. In addition, some patients who are initially thought to have a prolonged latent phase turn out only to have false labor. Although certainly of concern, particularly to the patient, a prolonged latent phase does not in and of itself pose a danger to the mother or fetus.

A *prolonged active phase* in the primigravid patient lasts longer than 12 hours or has a rate of cervical dilation of less than 1.2 cm/h; for a multipara, 1.5 cm/h. Causes of a prolonged active phase include fetal malposition, fetopelvic disproportion, excess use of sedation, inadequate contractions, and rupture of the fetal membranes prior to the onset of active labor. Risks associated with a prolonged active phase include increased rates of operative vaginal deliveries or cesarean section, and an associated increased risk of fetal compromise. In the absence of fetal distress, slow cervical dilation poses no threat to mother or fetus and can be allowed to progress, albeit slowly. On the other hand, *secondary arrest of dilation* should be assessed promptly and acted upon. Secondary arrest of dilation occurs when cervical dilation during the active phase of labor stops for 2 or more hours and is demon-

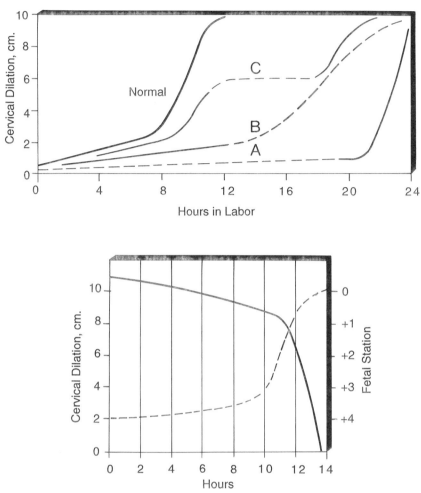

Figure 16.1. Abnormal labor. *Top*, Examples of labor patterns: A, prolonged latent phase. B, prolonged active phase. C, arrest of active phase. *Bottom*, Relationship of descent of presenting part of fetus (*solid line*) and progressive dilation of cervix (*broken line*).

strated by a flattening of the labor curve. Dilation ceases either because uterine contractions are no longer sufficient to maintain the progress of labor or labor arrests in spite of adequate uterine contractions, usually associated with too large an infant, fetal lie/position/attitude that disallows progress in labor, or a too small or abnormally shaped pelvis. Since ineffective contractions can be associated with mechanical factors such as disproportion and malpresentation, careful evaluation of all factors is necessary.

In the multiparous patient, a prolonged active phase is defined as lasting more than 6 hours. Cervical dilation should occur at a rate of at least 1.5 cm/h. Although a prolonged active phase is much less common in multiparous patients, the physician cannot be lulled into a false sense of security by the history of previous successful vaginal birth(s). Careful evaluation of all the factors is no less important in the multiparous patient than in the primiparous patient.

Active descent of the presenting part should occur progressively beginning late in the first stage and throughout the second stage of labor. An "arrest of descent" over a 2-hour period is suggestive of either cephalo-

Table 16.2
Differentiating Contractions of True and
False Labor (Braxton Hicks)

True labor	False labor
Regular intervals, gradually increasing	Irregular intervals and duration
Intensity increasing	Intensity unchanged
Cervical dilation occurs	No cervical dilation
Back and abdominal discomfort	Lower abdominal discomfort
No relief from sedation	Relief from sedation

pelvic disproportion or ineffective uterine contractions.

MANAGEMENT OF ABNORMAL LABOR

Induction of labor is the stimulation of uterine contractions, prior to the spontaneous onset of labor, with the goal of achieving delivery. The incidence of prolongation of the first stage of labor can be minimized by avoiding unnecessary intervention, i.e., labor should not be induced when the cervix is not well-prepared ("ripe"). Prolonged first stage of labor can be correctly diagnosed by accurately differentiating true labor from false labor, the latter being best treated with rest and sedation (Table 16.2).

A *prolonged latent phase* can be managed by either *rest* or *augmentation of labor* with intravenous oxytocin once mechanical factors have been ruled out. If the patient is allowed to rest, one of the following will occur: she will cease having contractions, in which case she is discharged from the hospital; she will go into active labor; or she will continue as before, in which case oxytocin may be administered to augment the uterine contractions. The use of amniotomy, or artificial rupture of membranes, is also advocated for patients with prolonged latent phase. Although it is unclear how this works, it is felt that the fetal head provides a better dilating force than does the intact bag of waters. In addition, there may be a release of prostaglandins, which could aid in augmenting the force of contractions. Before amniotomy

is performed, the presenting part should be firmly applied to the cervix so as to minimize the risk of causing an umbilical card prolapse. The fetal heart rate should be evaluated both before and immediately after rupture of the membranes.

During the *active phase of labor*, mechanical factors such as fetal malpositions and malpresentations as well as fetopelvic disproportion must be considered prior to augmentation of uterine contractions with oxytocin. In cases where the fetus fails to descend in the face of adequate contractions, disproportion is likely and cesarean section warranted. If no disproportion is present, oxytocin can be used if uterine contractions are judged to be inadequate. In cases of maternal exhaustion resulting in secondary arrest of dilation, rest followed by augmentation with oxytocin is often effective. If not already ruptured, artificial rupture of the membranes is also recommended.

Should fetal or maternal distress occur, prompt intervention is warranted. If this happens during the second stage of labor with the vertex low in the pelvis, forceps or vacuum can be used to effect a vaginal delivery. If the presentation is breech, cesarean section should be carried out. Distress of either mother or baby in the first stage of labor mandates cesarean delivery.

MANAGEMENT OF PROLONGED SECOND STAGE

In the past, a 2-hour second stage was considered indication for cesarean section or operative vaginal delivery. Data now show that if the fetal heart rate is reassuring, it is safe to allow the mother to continue pushing in an attempt to accomplish vaginal delivery. As long as both mother and baby are doing well, the second stage of labor does not have to be concluded in any specific time frame. Should disproportion exist, cesarean section is necessary. If not, oxytocin may be used to improve the frequency and/or strength of contractions. Because this is the one phase of labor over which the patient has some control, emotional support and encouragement are of great importance. Bearing down efforts by the patient in conjunction with the uterine contractions help bring about delivery. In some cases, the use of an episiotomy may provide relief from the perineum that has resisted delivery. Similarly, forceps or vacuum extraction may be used to bring about the necessary descent and rotation of the fetus, resulting in vaginal delivery.

RISKS OF PROLONGED LABOR

Prolonged labor can have deleterious effects on both fetus and mother. Maternal risks include infection, maternal exhaustion, lacerations, and uterine atony with possible hemorrhage. In addition, there are the attendant risks of any operative delivery. Fetal risks include asphyxia, trauma from difficult deliveries, infection, and possibly cerebral damage due to prolonged pressure to the head.

FURTHER READINGS

Cunningham FG, MacDonald PC, Gant NF. Williams obstetrics, 18th ed. East Norwalk, CN: Appleton & Lange, 1989.

———. Chapter 18. Dystocia caused by anomalies of the expulsive forces. 341–348.

———. Chapter 19. Dystocia caused by abnormalities in presentation, position, or development of the fetus. 349–376.

———. Chapter 20. Dystocia caused by pelvic contraction. 377–384.

———. Chapter 21. Dystocia from other abnormalities of the reproductive tract. 385–392.

Eden RD, Boehm FH. Assessment and care of the fetus. East Norwalk, CN: Appleton & Lange, 1990.

———. Chapter 54. Eden RD. Postdate pregnancy. 767–778.

———. Chapter 55. Collea JV. Malpresentation. 779–790.

SELF-EVALUATION

Case 16-A

A 19-year-old G1 at 41 weeks gestational age presents complaining of uterine contractions. Her antepartum course has been unremarkable; her baby is active. Her fundal height is 45 cm and her uterine contractions are occur-

ring every 6 minutes and judged to be mild in intensity; fetal heart tones are normal without deceleration. Pelvic examination shows the cervix to be 50% effaced, 3 cm dilated, with a cephalic part at −2 station, and membranes intact.

Question 16-A-1

Which of the following are appropriate managements at this time?

A. monitored labor
B. ultrasound for fetal weight determination
C. amniotomy
D. cesarean section for fetopelvic disproportion
E. patient discharged home with reassurance

Answer 16-A-1

Answer: A, B

Discussion: The patient may or may not be in labor. Monitoring will help evaluate the pattern of uterine activity and the fetal heart rate. Ultrasound for fetal weight may be helpful, as there is information to suggest macrosomia. Amniotomy is not advisable with a high presenting part. There is no indication for operative delivery nor is it appropriate to send the patient home until it is known whether she is in labor and whether her baby is well.

Question 16-A-2

The patient develops regular, more intense uterine contractions and progresses to 6 cm dilation and 100% effacement with the vertex descending to −1 station. Thereafter, uterine contractions become somewhat less intense and there is no further dilation for 2½ hours.

For further consideration: Is cesarean section indicated, and if so, for what diagnosis? If not, is augmentation indicated? If so, are there further data needed before augmentation is appropriate?

Case 16-B

A 31-year-old G2P1001, who delivered an 8½-pound son vaginally 8 years ago, presents at term in active labor and progresses rapidly to complete dilation. She then begins to push. After 2 hours of monitored labor, the vertex has progressed from −1 station to +1 station but with a prominent caput succedaneum noted. The fetal heart rate pattern is reassuring.

Question 16-B-1

Which of the following are appropriate next steps in this patient's management?

A. forceps delivery
B. cesarean section
C. continued monitored labor
D. augmentation with oxytocin

Answer 16-B-1

Answer: C

Discussion: After this patient has had a second stage of labor prolonged beyond the tradi-tional 2-hour limit, there has been some de-scent from −1 to +1 station. Continued moni-tored labor is appropriate if clinical evalua-tion indicates that the baby is not macrosomic or malformed, or there is not obvious fetopel-vic disproportion. If either is the case, cesar-ean section would be appropriate. Augmenta-tion of the contractions would be appropriate if they were inadequate in frequency or inten-sity. Forceps delivery would be appropriate if either maternal or fetal condition warranted delivery *and* the fetus were in a position to be so delivered. In this case, at +1 station with caput succedaneum present, it is unlikely to be deliverable via forceps.

chapter 17

INTRAPARTUM FETAL DISTRESS

Intrapartum fetal distress occurs in 5–10% of pregnancies when the function of the maternal-fetal physiologic unit is so altered during labor that fetal death or serious injury is likely to occur. It is the task of the obstetric team to recognize this situation and to intervene to avoid or minimize injury to the fetus. The decision to intervene is often difficult because fetal heart rate monitoring and fetal acid-base measurement are sometimes difficult to interpret. To help interpret these indirect measures of fetal compromise, the obstetric team correlates the intrapartum status with the patient's antepartum information, including historical risk factors (e.g., hypertension, maternal smoking), physical examination information (e.g., hypertension, fetal size), laboratory information (e.g., glucose tolerance data, ultrasound examinations), and dynamic testing information (e.g., biophysical profile determinations, NST/OCT testing). When interpreting this information, the obstetric team is especially alert for items that are known to predispose to the three *categories of causes of fetal distress*: uteroplacental insufficiency, umbilical cord compression, and fetal conditions/anomalies (Table 17.1).

The *uteroplacental unit* provides oxygen and nutrients to the fetus while receiving carbon dioxide and wastes, the products of the normal aerobic fetal and placental metabolisms. *Uteroplacental insufficiency* occurs when the uteroplacental unit starts to fail at this task. Initial fetal responses include fetal hypoxia (anoxia); shunting of blood flow to the fetal brain, heart, and adrenal glands; and transient variable or late decelerations of the fetal heart rate in an attempt to decrease oxygen consumption. *If the cause of the fetal hy-poxia is not recognized and corrected, a fetal respiratory and then metabolic acidosis will ensue. These patterns of fetal distress are usually reversible by either altering the conditions of uteroplacental function or by rapid delivery of the baby.* If delivery occurs promptly, the 1-minute Apgar score may be low, but the 5-minute score is usually high. Apgar scores are a measure of fetal reactions after delivery and are scored on a 0–10 scale. If, however, the fetus continues to experience hypoxia, the

Table 17.1
Causes of Fetal Distress

Category	Examples of specific etiologies
Uteroplacental insufficiency	Placental edema
	Maternal diabetes
	Hydrops fetalis
	Rh isoimmunization
	Placental "accidents"
	Abruptio placentae
	Placenta previa ± accreta
	Postdatism
	Intrauterine growth retardation (IUGR)
	Uterine hyperstimulation
Umbilical cord compression	Umbilical cord accidents
	Umbilical cord prolapse or entanglement (gross, occult)
	Umbilical cord knot
	Abnormal umbilical cord insertion
	Anomalous umbilical cord
	Oligohydramnios (from any cause)
Fetal conditions/ anomalies	Sepsis (maternal/fetal; chorioamnionitis)
	Fetal congenital anomalies
	IUGR
	Prematurity
	Postdatism

time will come when the fetus will progressively switch over to anaerobic glycolysis, shunt more blood flow to vital organs, and progressively develop a metabolic acidosis superimposed on the respiratory one. Lactic acid accumulates as this process continues and progressive damage to vital organs occurs, especially the fetal brain and myocardium. At delivery, both the 1- and 5-minute Apgar scores are usually depressed, and if the intervention was not timely, serious and possibly permanent damage (and sometimes even death) result. Fortunately, deleterious fetal acid-base changes are usually preceded by hypoxia manifest in fetal heart rate changes, which can be recognized by electronic monitoring or intermittent auscultation. Timely intervention is then usually possible once fetal distress has been identified. The techniques of intrapartum monitoring are designed to discover this process as early as possible.

INTRAPARTUM MONITORING
Fetal Heart Rate Monitoring
Methods of Fetal Heart Rate Evaluation

Prior to the popular use of electronic fetal monitoring (EFM), intermittent auscultation of the fetal heart rate after contractions was the technique used to assess intrapartum fetal well-being. With the use of EFM, fetal heart rate patterns have been identified and associated with various fetal conditions and prognoses. In the last few years, the now generalized use of these monitors has come into question. Continuous EFM of "high risk patients" who have a predictable increased risk of intrapartum fetal distress is usually not questioned. The value of EFM is questioned in "low risk patients" whose risk of intrapartum fetal distress is known to be small, yet it is interesting that it is in this group of patients that the risk of unexpected fetal distress is highest. Given the present widespread use of EFM, the debate will be long and vigorous with the ultimate pattern of use of both EFM and intermittent fetal heart rate auscultation uncertain.

Fetal Heart Rate

EFM fetal heart rates are described by rate and by pattern of variability. The techniques are described in Chapter 15, "Normal Labor and Delivery." The *baseline fetal heart rate* ("normal fetal heart rate") at term is defined as 120–160 beats per minute (bpm), with slightly higher rates in preterm fetuses. *Baseline fetal tachycardia* is defined as greater than 160 bpm for 10 or more minutes. Fetal tachycardia may be transient (generally less than 10 minutes) and without significance, although it is sometimes associated with situations that may require various interventions to avoid permanent fetal damage. *Baseline fetal bradycardia* is defined as less than 120 bpm for 10 or more minutes and is sometimes associated with conditions that may require attention (Fig. 17.1). Two other heart rate patterns are defined. A *sinusoidal heart rate pattern* is where the rate is 120–160 bpm, but there is a smooth undulating pattern of 5–10 bpm in amplitude (very reminiscent of a sine wave) and shortened short-term variability. The cause of this pattern is unknown, although it has been associated with fetal anemia and Rh isoimmunization. It is felt to be ominous, requiring intervention. *Fetal arrhythmias* are usually transient and are diagnosed by fetal ECG. If they persist, evaluation of the fetus for inherent pathology (especially hydrops and congenital anomalies) is indicated, as some treatment may be needed upon delivery, or, rarely, intrapartum.

Fetal Heart Rate Variability

Fetal heart rate (FHR) variability is the most reliable single EFM indicator of fetal status (fetal well-being). FHR variability results from a complex interplay of cardioinhibitory and cardioaccelerator centers in the fetal brain, which, in turn, are extremely sensitive to the fetal biochemical status (oxygenation and acid-base status). The presence of good variability is highly suggestive of adequate fetal central nervous system (CNS) oxygenation. Two types of variability are described (Fig. 17.1). *Short-term variability* is the varia-

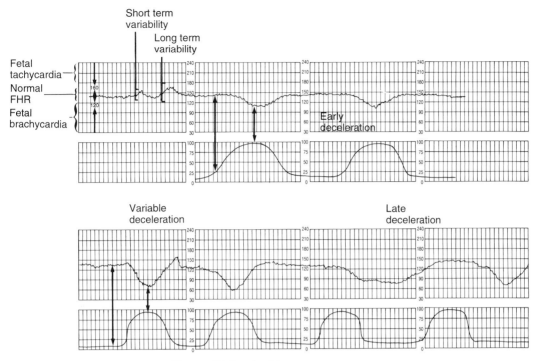

Figure 17.1. Fetal heart rate patterns.

tion in amplitude seen on a beat-to-beat basis, normally 3–8 bpm; *long-term variability* is an irregular, crude "wave-like" pattern with a cycle of 3–5 cycles per minute and an amplitude of 5–15 bpm. These patterns are normally encountered after approximately 28 weeks gestation, but they are difficult to interpret (especially their absence) prior to this gestational age. Short-term variability is measurable only with the use of an internal fetal scalp electrode (FSE), whereas long-term variability may be measured, albeit not as well as with FSE, by Doppler measurement. Decreased variability is associated with fetal hypoxia and/or acidemia, drugs that may depress the fetal CNS (e.g., maternal narcotic analgesia), fetal tachycardia, fetal CNS and cardiac anomalies, prolonged uterine contractions (uterine hypertonus), prematurity, and fetal sleep. Care must be taken in the interpretation of decreased variability when a transient cause such as fetal sleep may be involved, lest an unnecessary intervention be considered.

Periodic Fetal Heart Rate Changes

The FHR may vary with uterine contractions by slowing or accelerating in periodic patterns. These changes in FHR are in response to two mechanisms: (*a*) intrinsic reflex fetal heart rate control, especially responses to hypoxia and acidemia as well as normal reflex responses, and (*b*) fetal myocardial hypoxia. Periodic FHR changes are classified into patterns based on their shape, magnitude (in beats per minute (bpm)), and relationship to the same parameters of the uterine contractions with which they are associated. These patterns have prognostic value for the intrapartum evaluation of the fetus (Fig. 17.1).

Accelerations of the FHR are associated with an intact fetal mechanism unstressed by hypoxia and acidemia, and hence are viewed as reassuring and generally indicative of fetal well-being. Stimulation of the fetal scalp by digital examination will usually engender a heart rate acceleration in the uncompromised, nonacidotic fetus and is used by some

Table 17.2
Baseline Fetal Heart Rates

Fetal heart rate	Description	Associated causes
bpm >160 for >10 minutes	Fetal tachycardia	Maternal fever and infection Fetal infection Fetal anemia Maternal thyrotoxicosis Fetal tachyarrhythmias Maternal treatment with β_2-sympathomimetic or parasympatholytic (e.g., atropine) drugs Fetal immaturity Fetal hypoxia
120–160	Normal FHR	Normal function of maternal-fetal unit
<120 for >10 minutes	Fetal bradycardia	Maternal treatment for β-blockers (e.g., propranolol) Fetal congenital heart block (as in systemic lupus erythematosus (SLE) where an antibody may be produced that crosses the placenta and damages the conduction system of the fetus) Fetal anoxia

obstetricians as a test of fetal well-being. External sound/vibration stimulation, also termed acoustic stimulation, is also used for this purpose.

Early FHR decelerations are slowings of the FHR (never below 100 bpm), which begin as the uterine contraction begins, reach their nadir at the peak of the uterine contraction, and return to the baseline FHR with the end of the uterine contraction, i.e., mirror images of the uterine contraction. These early decelerations are due to *pressure on the fetal head* from the birth canal, causing a reflex response via the vagus nerve with acetylcholine release at the fetal sinoatrial node. This response may be blocked with vagolytics such as atropine.

Variable FHR decelerations are slowings of the FHR, which may start before, during, or after the uterine contraction starts, but are characterized by a rapid fall in the FHR, often to below 100 bpm, and then a rapid return to baseline after a few seconds at its nadir, i.e., also an "almost mirror image" out of phase in time and in shape. These variable decelerations are also reflex mediated, usually associated with *umbilical cord compression* and

mediated via the vagus nerve with sudden and often erratic release of acetylcholine at the fetal sinoatrial node, resulting in the characteristic sharp deceleration slope of these decelerations. Umbilical cord compression may result from wrapping of the cord around parts of the fetus, anomalies, or even knots in the umbilical cord and is especially associated with oligohydramnios where the buffering space for the umbilical cord created by the amniotic fluid is lost. These variable decelerations are the most common periodic FHR pattern. They are often correctable by changes in the maternal position to relieve pressure upon the umbilical cord. Infusion of fluid unto the amniotic cavity (amnioinfusion) has also been used effectively to relieve pressure on the umbilical cord. If the FHR falls below 100 bpm, a sterile vaginal examination is indicated to check for a prolapsed umbilical cord, a rare but emergent cause of the sudden development of this usually benign periodic FHR pattern. If the FHR falls below 60–70 bpm for more than 30 seconds, repetitive variable decelerations will often have a summative effect on fetal well-being, with the development of hypoxia, acidemia,

Table 17.3
Grading of Periodic FHR Patterns

Pattern/grade	Fall	Duration
	bpm	sec
Variable		
Mild	Any value	<30
Moderate	<70	>30, <60
Severe	<70	>60
Late		
Mild	<15	Any duration
Moderate	15–45	Any duration
Severe	>45	Any duration

and distress. If the FHR falls below 60 bpm, transient loss of fetal SA node function has been noted with transient "fetal cardiac arrest." These decelerations below 60–70 bpm require careful evaluation as to cause and intervention if indicated. Variable and late decelerations have been classified as mild, moderate, and severe, with the assertion that the risk of fetal hypoxia and acidosis increases with the degree of deceleration (Table 17.2 and 17.3).

Late FHR decelerations are slowings of the FHR that start after the uterine contraction starts, reach their nadir after the peak of the uterine contraction, and resolve to baseline after the uterine contraction is over, i.e., also a mirror image but "late" relative to the entire uterine contraction. These late decelerations are viewed as ominous, especially if repetitive, and are *sometimes associated with uteroplacental insufficiency* with decreased intervillous exchange of oxygen and carbon dioxide and *progressive fetal hypoxia and acidemia.* They are associated with causes of uteroplacental insufficiency, including postdatism, placental abruption, maternal hypertension, maternal diabetes, maternal anemia, maternal sepsis, and problems with uterine contractions such as hyperstimulation or hypertonia. Intervention is usually required, the nature and timing depending on full evaluation of the maternal and fetal status. Certainly, the need to intervene increases with the progression of fetal compromise. One evaluation that is often used to help guide interventions is direct measurement of fetal acid-base status.

Measurement of Fetal Acid-Base Status

When the uteroplacental unit is functioning normally, even with the stress of uterine contractions, which cause a transient decrease in placental intervillous perfusion, fetal acid-base status is easily maintained in normal ranges. *Normal fetal acid-base status* is mirrored in the normal umbilical cord blood gas values at term seen in Table 17.4. When there is *uteroplacental insufficiency*, inadequate fetal oxygenation causes a switch from fetal aerobic to fetal anaerobic metabolism, resulting in the production of lactate and progressive fetal acidosis, compounding the deleterious effects of fetal hypoxia. Initially, the fetus responds by shunting blood flow to the brain and heart from other organs. With progressive hypoxia, late decelerations develop and, with the addition of acidosis, loss of beat-to-beat variability. Brain and myocardial damage follow, with subsequent high risk of other end organ damage. When there are indicators of such an ominous situation (e.g., persistent late decelerations on EFM and decreased beat-to-beat variability) direct measurement of the fetal acid-base status is an option. The most common methods are fetal scalp capillary blood gas or blood pH measurement.

FETAL SCALP pH/BLOOD GAS EVALUATION

The chorioamnion must be ruptured and the presenting part descended so as to allow access to the presenting fetal part through the cervical os, which must be dilated at least 2–3 cm. Given access to the fetal part, either head or breech, a plastic or metallic cone is inserted through the os and pressed against the fetal scalp. The scalp surface is thoroughly cleaned and the cone held with enough pressure to avoid dilution of the blood with amniotic fluid. A thin layer of silicone gel is often applied to the surface, serving to provide a smooth uniform surface upon which the

Table 17.4
Normal Umbilical Cord and Fetal Scalp Blood Gas Values

Umbilical cord		Values	Fetal scalp
Venous	Arterial		
7.34 ± 0.15	7.28 ± 0.15	pH	7.25 to 7.40
30 ± 15	15 ± 10	PO_2	15 ± 10
35 ± 8	45 ± 15	PCO_2	45 ± 15
5 ± 4	7 ± 4	Base deficit	7 ± 4

blood droplet may form. A small incision is then made in the fetal scalp with a specialized lancet, and the drops of blood that form are collected in a heparinized capillary tube and analyzed. Pressure is applied to the incision site through one or two uterine contractions, until bleeding stops. Care must be taken not to make the incision over a fontanel or suture line. A caput succedaneum will not alter the pH information obtained.

Scalp blood samples are often difficult to interpret because absolute parameters that mandate specific interventions do not exist. Instead, as with other measures of fetal well-being, the information obtained must be correlated with the aggregate understanding of the status of the maternal-fetal unit at the time of the measure. Some general guidelines based on the scalp pH are often used. A scalp pH that is greater than 7.25 is generally considered reassuring, requiring no further scalp sampling unless other measures of fetal well-being worsen, giving new indication for fetal scalp sampling. If the scalp pH is in the range between 7.20 and 7.24, concern about the possible development of fetal hypoxia/acidemia exists and, generally, repeat scalp measurements are made within 15–30 minutes. If, however, the scalp pH is less than 7.19, fetal hypoxia and acidemia are demonstrated, and generally interventions are required on an immediate basis to ameliorate the cause of the fetal distress or to affect delivery. Although a rare situation, maternal acidosis may complicate the evaluation of scalp pH results. A free-flowing maternal venous sample may be evaluated for pH, as the fetal sample will usually be approximately 0.1 pH unit below the maternal value.

MANAGEMENT

Interpretation of intrapartum fetal well-being measurements are made within the context of the entire obstetric situation, including maternal and fetal factors and the course and anticipated duration and outcome of labor. The number of variables to consider and the often imprecise nature of the information make these among the most difficult of medical decisions. In-depth training and experience in obstetrics are required to adequately perform these complex tasks.

Sometimes, the fetal heart rate pattern will demonstrate a single pattern. If it is reassuring, no intervention is needed; if it is not reassuring, the appropriate intervention is often clear. More often, however, the observed FHR pattern is a mixture of two more patterns and variations of baseline values. In these cases, it is generally prudent to manage the obstetric situation based on the most ominous of the patterns present.

In general, if there is evidence of progressive fetal hypoxia and acidosis in a situation where the time of vaginal delivery is remote, operative delivery by cesarean section is indicated for fetal reasons. Awaiting vaginal delivery is appropriate if, in the judgment of the obstetric team, vaginal delivery will occur within a time wherein the progression of fetal distress will not result in permanent fetal injury and/or death, or where effective interventions to ameliorate the fetal distress may be taken. In general, a scalp pH greater than 7.24 is reassuring; certainly, good variability

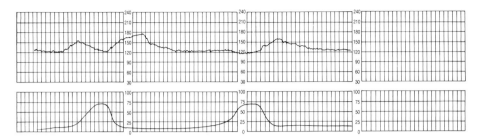

Figure 17-A-1.

on EFM is a reassuring factor. If meconium is present in the amniotic fluid, perinatal morbidity is increased by 5–10%, a condition that tends to dissuade continued labor with other evidence of fetal compromise also present. Certainly, in the face of historical evidence suggestive of fetal distress or a propensity for fetal distress, nonreassuring EFM tracings, and the inability to sample for scalp pH, expedited delivery is appropriate.

If the situation is appropriate to temporize while awaiting vaginal delivery, or while awaiting preparations for cesarean delivery, one or more of the following steps are appropriate: (*a*) discontinue oxytocin infusion that had been started for the purpose of induction or augmentation; (*b*) administer oxygen to the mother, usually 5–6 L/min by face mask; (*c*) check the maternal blood pressure, treating any hypotension discovered with intravenous fluids and, if needed, pressors such as ephedrine; (*d*) change the maternal position to left lateral position to decrease uterine pressure on the great vessels and thereby increase blood return to the heart, cardiac output, and uteroplacental blood flow; and (*e*) consider "intrauterine resuscitation," using an intravenous tocolytic (such as the β_2-sympathomimetic terbutaline) to relax the uterine tone and slow the contraction rate, thereby increasing uteroplacental blood flow. Umbilical arterial and venous blood gases should be drawn immediately after the delivery from the cord attached to the placenta prior to placental separation. The data will help the management of the newborn and shed light on the results of intrapartum interventions.

FURTHER READINGS

Depp R. Clinical evaluation of fetal status. In: Danforth D, Scott J, eds. Obstetrics and gynecology. Philadelphia: JB Lippincott, 1989:315–329.

Petrie RG. Intrapartum fetal evaluation. In: Gabbe S, Niebly JR, Simpson JL, eds. Obstetrics, normal and problem pregnancies. New York: Churchill Livingstone, 1991:457–492.

Quilligan EJ, Fitzsimmons J. Fetal monitoring. In: Pauerstein CJ, ed. Obstetrics. New York: John Wiley & Sons, 1987:249–266.

SELF-EVALUATION

Case 17-A

Your patient is a 24-year-old G3P2002 with an unremarkable antepartum course who presents at 41 weeks gestational age having uterine contractions of increasing severity for 8 hours before being seen. Her initial examination shows 3–4 cm, 80% effaced, −2 station, in cephalic presentation with intact membranes. She is admitted, an intravenous line and appropriate laboratory studies are initiated, and external electronic fetal monitoring is begun. After 30 minutes, the sample of EFM tracing seen in Figure 17-A-1 is representative of her tracing.

Question 17-A-1

Which statement best describes the patient's intrapartum clinical situation?

A. FHR bradycardia and poor variability

B. FHR tachycardia and good variability

C. normal FHR and good variability

D. normal FHR and intermittent late decelerations

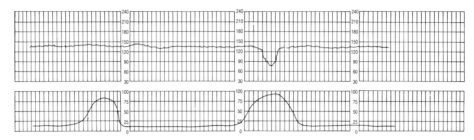

Figure 17-A-2.

Answer 17-A-1

Answer: C

The baseline FHR is 120–125 bpm, within the normal range, and there is short- and long-term variability. There are no decelerations. This is a completely reassuring FHR tracing.

Labor continues for 4 hours and the patient's pelvic examination then shows 6–7 cm, 100%, 0 station. Membranes are artificially ruptured, a FSE and an intrauterine pressure catheter (IUPC) are placed, and after 15 minutes the patient is given 25 mg of meperidine intravenously for pain. Thirty minutes thereafter, the sample of EFM tracing seen in Figure 17-A-2 is representative of her tracing.

Question 17-A-2

Which statement best describes the patient's intrapartum clinical situation?

A. FHR bradycardia and poor variability
B. normal FHR and poor variability
C. normal FHR, poor variability, and occasional variable decelerations
D. normal FHR, poor variability, and occasional late decelerations

Answer 17-A-2

Answer: B

Apart from being 41 weeks gestational age, there is no further historical information suggesting reasons for fetal distress. The patient's FHR tracing prior to the intravenous narcotic administration was normal, and the loss of variability after narcotic administration is consistent with narcotic effect. The single variable

deceleration may be explained by pressure on the fetal head, which is at 0 station.

Labor continues for 3 hours and the patient's pelvic examination then shows 9–10 cm, 100%, +1 station. A representative sample of her EFM tracing at this time is seen in Figure 17-A-3.

Question 17-A-3

Which statement best describes the patient's intrapartum clinical situation?

A. FHR tachycardia and poor variability
B. normal FHR and poor variability
C. normal FHR, poor variability, and occasional variable decelerations
D. normal FHR, poor variability, and occasional late decelerations

Answer 17-A-3

Answer: D

This is a mixed pattern, with reassuring return of variability now that the narcotic effect is gone, but occasional late decelerations are noted. There is no indication for operative delivery, as vaginal delivery may be expected in the near future in this multipara. Conservative interventions such as oxygen administration are indicated. Because she has had a previous cesarean section, and because of the intermittent late decelerations, close observation is indicated.

Case 17-B

Your patient is a 17-year-old G1 at 39 weeks who presents with premature spontaneous rupture of membranes (clear fluid) following an antepartum course remarkable only for an iron deficiency anemia, which responded to

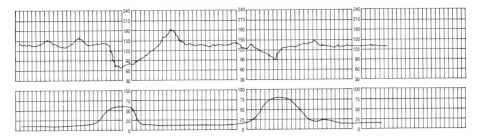

Figure 17-A-3.

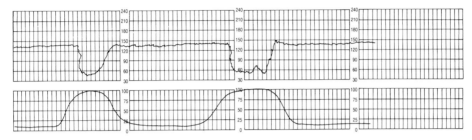

Figure 17-B-1.

hematemic therapy. After waiting 6 hours, you begin a Pitocin (oxytocin) induction of labor. The tracing seen in Figure 17-B-1 is representative of her EFM trace 3 hours later when pelvic examination shows 5 cm, 100%, 0/ + 1 station with a caput succedaneum, LOA, and the presence of the FSE and IUPC, which you placed prior to starting the induction.

Question 17-B-1

Which statement best describes the patient's intrapartum clinical situation?

A. normal FHR baseline and variability without decelerations

B. normal FHR baseline and variability with variable decelerations

C. normal FHR baseline and decreased variability without decelerations

D. normal FHR baseline and decreased variability with variable decelerations

E. normal FHR baseline and decreased variability with late decelerations

Answer 17-B-1

Answer: D

Although there is a normal FHR, there is poor variability and severe variable decelerations. In a primigravida delivery, this loss of variability is not reassuring and intervention is indicated.

For further consideration: What might be the causes for the FHR tracing seen in Figure 17-B-1? What interventions, if any, are appropriate and needed at this time? If this situation presents a risk, how much of a risk? Could it have been prevented by another management?

chapter 18

POSTPARTUM CARE

The *puerperium* is the 6-week period following birth during which the reproductive tract returns to its normal, nonpregnant state. Traditionally, the initial postpartum examination is scheduled at the end of this 6-week interval. However, many of the physiologic changes of pregnancy have returned to normal within 1–2 weeks after delivery, whereas others may take much longer. The initial postpartum examination is now often scheduled sooner than 6 weeks for these reasons as well as the fact that many patients return to full nonpregnant activity in a few weeks. This chapter focuses on the physiology of the puerperium, the immediate postpartum care of the puerpera, and the management of the patient at the first postpartum visit.

PHYSIOLOGY OF THE PUERPERIUM

UTERUS

The *uterus* weighs approximately 1000 g immediately after delivery compared with its nonpregnant weight of approximately 70 g. Immediately after delivery, the fundus of the uterus is easily palpable halfway between the pubic symphysis and the umbilicus. The *involution of the uterus* results in its return to the pelvis by 2 weeks postpartum and to its normal size by 6 weeks postpartum. Immediately after birth, uterine hemostasis is maintained as a result of the contraction of the smooth muscle of the arterial walls as well as compression of the vasculature by the uterine musculature. The uterus undergoes such a significant reduction in size because the uterus is no longer being stretched by the fetus and placenta and amniotic fluid as well as because of the loss of hormonal stimulation. There is also a marked reduction in the blood flow to the uterus. As the myometrial fibers contract, the blood clots from the uterus are expelled and the thrombi in the large vessels of the placental bed undergo organization. The *lochia* or uterine discharge contains blood as well as the remaining decidua and necrotic remnants of membranes. For the first 2–3 days, the lochia is red (lochia rubra). As hemostasis is established, the amount of blood in the lochia is reduced with a relative increase in serous secretion, resulting in a brownish color, ultimately becoming serous in appearance at the end of the first postpartum week (lochia serosa). At this time, the lochia contains more degenerated decidual material, as well as bacteria, resulting in a yellow appearance. This discharge is fairly heavy at first and rapidly decreases in amount over the first 2–3 days postpartum, although it may last for several weeks. In women who breast-feed, the lochia seems to resolve more rapidly when compared with those women who choose not to breast-feed. This may be due to a more rapid involution of the uterus due to uterine contractions associated with breast-feeding. In some patients, there is an increased amount of lochia 1–2 weeks after delivery because the eschar that developed over the site of placental attachment has been sloughed.

Within several hours of delivery, the *cervix* has reformed. The round shape of the nulliparous cervix is usually replaced by a transverse, fish-mouth-shaped external os, which is the result of laceration during delivery. This cervical change is permanent. *Vulvar* and *vaginal* tissues return to normal over the first several days, although the *vaginal mucosa* will reflect a hypoestrogenic state

195

should the woman choose to breast-feed, as ovarian suppression is continued during breast-feeding.

[Ovulation] can occur as early as 4 weeks postpartum if the woman chooses not to breast-feed. The mean time to ovulation in nonlactating women is approximately 10 weeks, with 50% of nonlacting women ovulating by 90 days postpartum (Fig. 18.1). Among breast-feeding women, the time to first ovulation is dependent on how long the woman breast-feeds. Ovulation is suppressed in the lactating woman in association with elevated prolactin levels. In these patients, prolactin remains elevated for 6 weeks, whereas in nonlactating women, prolactin levels return to normal by 3 weeks postpartum. Estrogen levels fall immediately after delivery in all patients, but begin to rise approximately 2 weeks after delivery if breast-feeding is not undertaken.

The changes seen in the cardiovascular system during pregnancy return to normal within 2–3 weeks after delivery. Immediately following delivery, plasma volume is reduced by approximately 1000 ml due primarily to blood loss at the time of delivery. During the immediate postpartum period, there is also a significant shift of extracellular fluid into the intravascular space. The elevated pulse rate seen during pregnancy persists for approximately 1 hour after delivery but then decreases. The increased cardiac output seen during pregnancy also persists into the first several hours of the postpartum period. This increased cardiac output at this time is felt to be the same result of increased venous return. This may contribute to decompensation seen in the early postpartum period in patients with heart disease. Immediately after delivery, approximately 5 kg of weight are lost as a result of diuresis and the loss of extravascular fluid. Further weight loss varies in rate and amount from patient to patient. The leukocytosis seen during labor persists into the early puerperium, thus minimizing the usefulness of identifying early postpartum infection by elevated white cell count. Renal function as evidenced by glomerular filtra-

↑ WBC

tion rate (GFR) returns to normal within a few weeks postpartum although the GFR remains elevated in the first few days postpartum.

MANAGEMENT OF THE IMMEDIATE POSTPARTUM PERIOD
Hospital Stay

The amount of time a patient remains in the hospital after delivery continues to decrease. In the past, patients were kept in the hospital for 3 days after the birth of their first child, and 2 days after subsequent deliveries. Postpartum hospital stays for cesarean section patients were routinely 4–5 days. The period of hospitalization for all patients has been significantly reduced. Many patients are now routinely discharged 24 hours after vaginal delivery and 72 hours after cesarean section. Figures 18.2 and 18.3 are examples of routine postpartum orders.

Maternal-Infant Bonding

It is recognized that shortly after delivery, the parents become totally engrossed in the events surrounding the newborn infant. Any significant separation of the mother from her infant, which reduces activity such as cuddling, fondling, kissing, or gazing at the infant, may have a negative impact on the involvement of maternal behaviors on a long-term basis. Modern labor and delivery suites have attempted to enhance these interactions by minimizing medical interventions, unless necessary, while increasing visitation by the father and other family members as well as rooming-in in the mother's room. A supportive environment to encourage breast-feeding also contributes to this atmosphere. Interaction between the infant and the new parents can also be observed by the nursing staff with the resultant ability to identify early in the postpartum course any problems such as negative or even abusive actions toward the newborn.

The likelihood of serious *postpartum complications* is greatest immediately after delivery. Significant hemorrhage occurs in ap-

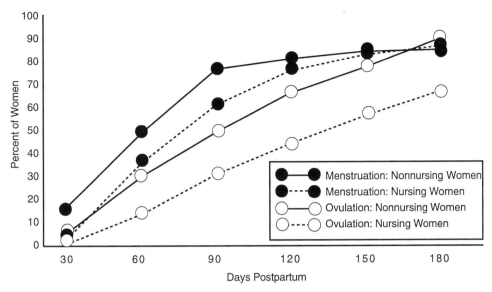

Figure 18.1. Menstruation and ovulation after delivery.

proximately 1% of patients; infection is seen in approximately 5% of patients. Immediately after the delivery of the placenta, the uterus is palpated bimanually to ascertain that it is firm. Uterine palpation through the abdominal wall is repeated at frequent intervals during the immediate postpartum period in order to ascertain uterine atony. Perineal pads are applied and the amount of blood on these pads, as well as pulse and pressure, are monitored closely for the first several hours after delivery in order to identify excessive blood loss.

Postpartum analgesia is primarily indicated for perineal discomfort resulting from lacerations, episiotomy, or hemorrhoids or for postoperative pain from cesarean section or postpartum tubal ligation. Patients may also require pain medication for "afterbirth pains," the painful uterine contractions following delivery. These are seen more prominently in breast-feeding women due to the release of oxytocin during suckling. Common medications for this include acetaminophen, aspirin, or nonsteroidal antiinflammatory drugs.

Breast engorgement in women who are not breast-feeding is commonly treated with the

prolactin inhibitor, bromocriptine (Parlodel). *Bromocriptine (Parlodel) Inhib. Prolactin and Breast Engorgment.* In addition to pharmacologic suppression, techniques such as breast binders and avoidance of nipple stimulation are now the most common ones used to suppress the breast engorgement typically seen at approximately 3 days postpartum. Oral analgesics, as well as ice packs applied locally, are also useful adjuncts. Occasionally, the breast-feeding mother may develop a *postpartum mastitis* manifest by fever and localized erythema and firmness of the breast as well as pain. Postpartum mastitis is usually caused by *Staphylococcus aureus* arising from the nursing infant's throat and nose and transmitted during nursing. Treatment includes penicillin G or a penicillinase-resistant drug such as dicloxacillin for penicillinase-reducing strains. For patients who are allergic to penicillin, erythromycin would be an appropriate alternative. Nursing from the affected size may be continued without danger to the infant. If an abscess develops, drainage of the abscess in addition to antibiotic therapy is necessary.

Women who do not have antirubella antibody should be immunized for *rubella* during the immediate postpartum period. Breast-feeding is not a contraindication to this im-

RUBELLA Immun

mastitis - Pen G or diclox.
S. Aureus   or erythrom if P:N allergy

NAME AND UNIT NUMBER   ADMISSION NUMBER   NURSING STATION

WOMEN'S HOSPITAL/PERINATAL CENTER

OBSTETRIC SERVICE

ROOM OR BED NUMBER

THE MED REGIONAL MEDICAL CENTER
AT MEMPHIS

DATE

DATE	HOUR	ROUTINE POSTPARTUM ORDERS
		These orders do NOT apply to postoperative, diabetic, hypertensive or preeclamptic-eclamptic patients.
		1. Patients with caudal, spinal or epidural must be able to move legs before leaving recovery room.
		2. BP, P fundal check and blood loss assessment q 15 min x 4, 1 h x 2; oral temperature qid for 48 hours,
		then 6 A.M. only (unless febrile > 100.4); notify physician if pulse > 110; systolic BP > 150 or
		< 90 distolic BP > 100; temp. > 100.4.
		3. Continue IV at 125-150 ml q h until discontinued.
		4. NPO until stable and normal observations for 1 h, then discontinue IV and place on regular diet.
		5. UP ad lib, unless spinal, epidural or saddle block must be able to move extremities and regain sensation
		in legs before getting out of bed.
		6. Encourage daily shower.
		7. If unable to void within 4-6 hours and bladder distended, catherize with #18 Foley; if volume > 500
		ml or necessary to catherize second time, leave Foley in place 24 hours; specimen to lab for C & S
		when catheter removed.
		8. Routine perineal and breast care daily; encourage use of supportive bra.
		9. Acetaminophen #3 p.o. q 3-4 h PRN pain; notify physician if pain relief inadequate.
		10 Promethazine 25 mg IM q 4 PRN nausea; notify physician if second dose is required.
		11. Dalmane 30 mg p.o. HS PRN
		12. Dioctyl sodium sulfosuccinate 100 mg p.o. tid.
		13. Bisacodyl USP suppository PRN the p.m. of the second postpartum day if no bowel movement since
		delivery.
		14. Hct in A.M. day after delivery. Notify physician if < 30%, UA.
		15. If mother D neg., Du neg.; check ABO, Rh and Coombs of baby and record on maternal chart.
		16. Type and crossmatch for anti-D immune globulin if appropriate after laboratory evaluation.
		17. Rooming in if desired.

Form #6091.011(Rev. 7/84)   PHYSICIAN'S ORDERS

Figure 18.2. Routine postpartum orders.

POST CESAREAN SECTION
PHYSICIAN'S ORDERS

DATE	HOUR	These orders do not apply to other postoperative, diabetic, hypertensive or preeclamptic-eclamptic patients.
		1. Patients with caudal, spinal or epidural must be able to move legs before leaving recovery room.
		2. BP, P, fundal check and blood loss assessment q 15 min x 4, q 1 h x 4, then per shift; notify physician if pulse >110; systolic BP > 150 or <90, diastolic BP >100.
		3. NPO, bedrest.
		4. Turn, cough and deep breath q 2 h x 6.
		5. Temp qid; notify if <100.4.
		6. #18 Foley catheter to dependent drainage.
		7. I&O q 4 h until Foley catheter removed; notify physician if output <100 ml in any 4 h interval.
		8. Each IV to run at 125-150 ml/h; do not exceed 250 ml in any hour.
		#1 1000 cc D5LR with 10 IU oxytocin added.
		#2 1000 cc D5 1/4NS with 10 IU oxytocin added.
		#3 1000 cc D5 1/4NS with 10 IU oxytocin added.
		#4 1000 cc D5 1/4NS at 50 cc/h to keep vein open until physician discontinues.
		9. Morphine sulfate 10 mg IM q3-4h, PRN pain, notify physician if pain relief inadequate; acetaminophen #3 p.o. 3-4 h PRN for mild discomfort after oral intake resumed or acetaminophen 600 mgm p.o. q 3-4 h PRN for pain.
		10. Promethazine 25 mg. IM q 4-6 h PRN nausea, notify physician if second dose is required.
		11. Encourage use of supportive bra.
		12. Bisacodyl USP suppository PRN in p.m. of the second postpartum day if no bowel movement since delivery; PRN Fleet's enema if no results from suppository.
		13. Dioctyl Sodium Sulfocuccinate 100 mgm p.o. tid when oral intake resumes.
		14. Antacid 30 cc p.o. PRN.
		15. Witchazel wipes PRN for Pericare.
		16. Dalmane 30 mg. p.o. HS PRN.
		17. Hct in a.m. and third postoperative day.
		18. If mother D Neg., check ABO, RH and Coombs' on baby and record on maternal chart.
		19. Type and crossmatch for anti-D immune globulin if appropriate after laboratory evaluation.
		20. Rooming-in if desired.

Signature _____

Form No. 6091.001 (Rev. 7/84)

Figure 18.3. Postcesarean section physician's orders.

munization. In some locations, a *tetanus tox-oid booster* injection is also given at this time if needed. If the woman is D-negative, is not isoimmunized, and has given birth to a D-positive infant, *anti-D immune globulin* (RhoGAM) should be administered shortly after delivery.

It is common for a patient not to have a bowel movement for the first 1–2 days after delivery, as patients have often not eaten for a long period of time. Stool softener is routinely prescribed in many institutions, especially if the patient has had a fourth degree episiotomy repair or a laceration involving the rectal mucosa. *Perineal pain* is minimized using oral analgesics, the application of an ice bag to minimize swelling, and/or a local anesthetic spray. Severe perineal pain unresponsive to usual analgesics may signify the development of a hematoma in that area.

Postpartum care in the hospital should always include discussion of contraception. As Figure 18.1 demonstrates, approximately 15% of nonnursing women are fertile at 6 weeks postpartum. All forms of contraception should be considered, with oral contraceptives no longer being considered contraindicated by breast-feeding. Once lactation is established, neither the volume nor composition of breast milk is adversely affected by the oral contraceptive.

Coitus may be resumed when the patient is comfortable. She should be counseled, especially if breast-feeding, that coitus may initially be uncomfortable because of a lack of lubrication and that the use of exogenous, water-soluble lubrication is helpful. The female superior position may be recommended, as the woman is thereby able to control the depth of penile penetration. The lactating patient may also be counseled to use topical estrogen to the vaginal mucosa to minimize the dyspareunia caused by coital trauma to the hypoestrogenic tissue. Signs and symptoms of other postpartum complications such as hemorrhage and fever should be reviewed with the patient.

Patient education at the time of discharge should not be solely focused on postpartum and contraceptive issues. This is a good opportunity to reinforce the value and need for preventive health care and health care maintenance for both mother and infant. This should include a review of follow-up that has been arranged for the newborn infant and frequency and scope of health care for the new mother. Previously identified high risk behaviors such as alcohol, tobacco, or drug abuse should once again be discussed with the patient. Any preexisting medical conditions should also be discussed as to the follow-up plans during the postpartum period.

Lactation and Breast-Feeding

An increasing belief in advantages of breast-feeding has led many physicians to recommend this form of infant nutrition and more patients to breast-feed and to breast-feed for a longer period of time than in previous years. The benefits of breast-feeding include increased convenience for some mothers, decreased cost, improved infant nutrition for a variable period of time, and some protection against infection and allergic reaction. Successful breast-feeding depends on several factors, most especially the motivation of the mother and her ability to include breast-feeding in her daily activities. For some women, breast-feeding may be impossible, even if desired, due to restrictions on time caused by work. Support by family and health care providers for the decision that best fits the total needs of the mother and baby is very important. If breast-feeding is chosen, rooming-in during the hospital stay allows the mother to begin the process in a less pressured setting while allowing the hospital staff to provide helpful recommendations and support. The decision to breast- or bottle-feed is best made prior to delivery and is facilitated by balanced discussion during the antepartum visits.

Suckling by the infant stimulates release of oxytocin from the neurohypophysis. The increased levels of oxytocin in the blood result in contraction of the myoepithelial cells and

hypoestrogenic tissues —poor lubrication.

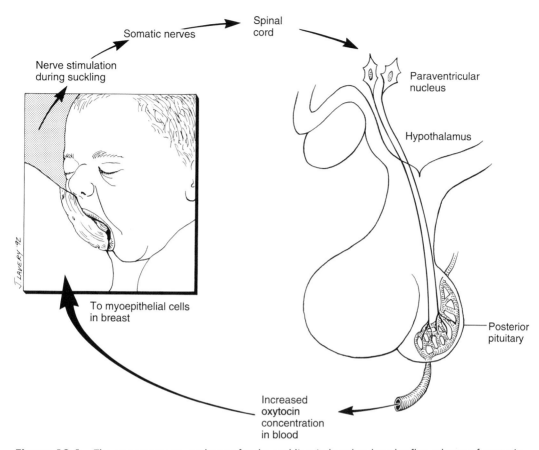

Figure 18.4. The somatosensory pathways for the suckling-induced reduced reflex release of oxytocin.

emptying of the alveolar lumen of the breast. Prolactin release is also stimulated by suckling with resultant secretion of fatty acids, lactose, and casein. In order for milk to be produced on an ongoing basis, there must be adequate insulin, cortisol, thyroid hormone, and adequate nutrients and fluids in the diet. In addition, the alveolar lumen must be emptied on a regular basis (Fig. 18.4).

Drugs in the breast milk is a common concern for the breast-feeding mother. Less than 1% of the total dosage of any medication is seen in breast milk. This should be considered when any medication is prescribed by a physician or when any over-the-counter medications are contemplated by the patient. Specific medications that would contraindicate breast-feeding include lithium carbonate, tetracycline, and any radioactive substance.

ANXIETY, DEPRESSION, AND THE POSTPARTUM PERIOD

Although pregnancy and childbirth is usually a joyous time, for some patients the experience is followed by significant emotional distress. Identification of specific risk factors for postpartum as well as antepartum anxiety and depression is an important first step in identifying and dealing with these problems. Of patients with previous postpartum mental disease, approximately 25% will have a recurrence after their next pregnancy. One third of patients with psychiatric illness during the postpartum period have a history of psychiatric disease. The exact cause of most of the postpartum emotional changes is unknown, although suggested etiologies include changing hormone levels (as is seen with premenstrual changes) and difficulty adjusting to a new life-style and the stresses of parenthood.

There is a wide spectrum of response to pregnancy and delivery, ranging from mild depression ("postpartum blues," which occurs in over 50% of the deliveries, typically occurring on postpartum day 2–3 and subsiding within 1–2 weeks) to postpartum depression (approximately 10% of women) to the extreme response of intense depression with suicidal ideation (occurring in approximately 1 in 2000 deliveries). Early symptoms of depression include sleeplessness, loss of self-esteem, irritability, and mood swings. More serious symptoms include anorexia, obsessive behavior, panic, and delusions. A most disturbing symptom is the patient's estrangement from the newborn.

Both internal and external forces may result in postpartum psychiatric illness. A patient who does not cope well with stress is particularly susceptible to such potentially traumatic stimuli as previous infertility, complications of the ante-, intra-, or postpartum course, or conflicts in the roles of mother and wife. A supportive spouse and family can minimize the severity of any symptom complex.

Anxiety is very common during the antepartum and intrapartum periods, but can be minimized by having the patient as an active participant in the planning of and carrying out of the birthing process plan. Prepared childbirth and the rational use of minimal anesthesia at the patient's discretion may help the patient feel a sense of control. Active involvement of nursing personnel in the identification of significant anxiety and depression is also critical, as they observe the patient on a more ongoing basis than do physicians during hospitalization.

Treatment must be tailored to the patient's individual situation with the vast majority of mild postpartum depression being managed by the attending physician in conjunction with the support of hospital staff such as nursing personnel and social workers. The mother who is fearful of, or is adverse to, contact with the newborn should not be forced into contact. Both psychotherapy and medication such as antidepressants or lithium carbonate may be provided, usually in consultation with a clinical psychologist or psychiatrist. If conditions worsen despite outpatient efforts, inpatient therapy is warranted.

Whether during the antepartum, intrapartum, or postpartum period, depression and anxiety should be viewed as significant problems. It should be noted, however, that they are not necessarily solely related to pregnancy or its complications. Specifically, women are clinically depressed twice as frequently as men. Anxiety accompanies depression in three fourths of cases. The earliest clinical clue to the diagnosis of depression may be in inability to experience pleasure or happiness. Women particularly susceptible to depression are those with young children, those who are living in poverty, those who are abused, and those who have professional careers.

There appears to be some evidence that there is a hereditary factor that predisposes some patients to developing anxiety disorders. This may occur in as high as 10–15% of the population. As all patients are subjected to some degree of stress, anxiety is generally seen in all patients, resulting in some shifts in mood as part of the normal life experience. As with depression, however, anxiety can become dysfunctional, with the patient seeing the world as a hostile or unsafe environment. Nonspecific nervousness, panic, irritability, and fear of losing control suggest significant anxiety disorder requiring treatment.

THE POSTPARTUM VISIT

At the time of the first postpartum visit, inquiries should be made into the following: status of breast-feeding, return of menstruation, resumption of coital activity, use of contraception, interaction of the newborn with the family, and resumption of other physical activities such as return to work. Involutional changes should have occurred in most instances. A full physical examination should be performed, including breast examination. It should be noted that inflammatory changes due to the healing of the cervix may result in minor atypia. Unless there is a past history of significant cervical dysplasia, repeating the Pap smear in three months is appropriate.

FURTHER READING

Zlatnik FJ. The puerperium: normal and abnormal. In: Scott JR, DiSaia PJ, Hammond CB, Spellacy WN, eds. Danforth's obstetrics and gynecology. 6th ed. Philadelphia: JB Lippincott, 1990:189–194.

SELF-EVALUATION

Case 18-A

A 24-year-old married woman has just delivered her first child, a healthy boy weighing 7 pounds. Her antepartum and intrapartum courses were unremarkable. On the first postpartum day, she is noted to cry easily and to have slept poorly.

Question 18-A-1

Which of the following are appropriate management steps at this time?

A. Reassure the patient that everything is O.K. and that feeling sad after a delivery is normal.
B. Ask the patient why she is crying.
C. Ask the nursing staff to ask the patient why she is crying.
D. Ask a psychiatrist to evaluate the patient's apparent sadness.
E. Ask a social worker to evaluate the patient's apparent sadness.

Answer 18-A-1

Answer: A, B, C

Discussion: Reassuring the patient is not inappropriate as a general measure, but it must be combined with some assessment of the apparent sadness. In general, this is best done at this level of distress by the physician or nursing staff; consultation to psychiatry or social services is generally not indicated.

chapter 19

POSTPARTUM HEMORRHAGE

Excessive bleeding in the minutes and hours following delivery is a serious and potentially fatal complication. Hemorrhage can be sudden and profuse or blood loss can occur more slowly but be prolonged and persistent. Traditionally, postpartum hemorrhage is defined as a blood loss in excess of 500 ml of blood associated with delivery. Many patients lose considerably more blood than this and the figure of 500 ml may actually represent the average amount of blood loss after vaginal delivery, with twice this amount lost at cesarean delivery. This chapter discusses the causes of postpartum hemorrhage followed by a general approach to the patient who bleeds excessively after giving birth.

MAJOR CAUSES OF POSTPARTUM HEMORRHAGE
Uterine Atony

Uterine atony is by far the most common cause of postpartum hemorrhage. The uterine corpus (or body) contracts promptly after delivery of the placenta constricting the spiral arteries in the newly created placental bed and preventing excessive bleeding from them. This muscular contraction, rather than coagulation, prevents excessive bleeding from the placental implantation site. When contraction does not occur as expected, the resulting uterine atony gives rise to postpartum hemorrhage.

A number of *factors predispose to uterine atony* as noted in Table 19.1. These include conditions in which there is extraordinary enlargement of the uterus, such as hydramnios or twins; abnormal labor (both precipitous, prolonged or augmented by oxytocin); and conditions that interfere with contrac-

Table 19.1.
Factors Predisposing to Uterine Atony

Precipitous labor
General anesthesia
Prolonged labor
Uterine leiomyomas
Macrosomia
Hydramnios
Twins
Amnionitis (sepsis)
Multiparity
Oxytocin use in labor
History of postpartum hemorrhage
Amniotic fluid embolus
Magnesium sulfate in laboring patient

tion of the uterus, such as uterine leiomyomas or use of magnesium sulfate. The clinical diagnosis of atony is based largely upon the tone of the uterine muscle on palpation. Instead of the normally firm, contracted uterine corpus, a softer, more pliable, often called "boggy" uterus is found. The cervix is usually open. Frequently the uterus will contract briefly when massaged, only to become more relaxed when the manipulation ceases.

Management of uterine atony is both preventive and therapeutic. In the management of a normal delivery, it is customary to infuse oxytocin diluted in intravenous fluids starting when the placenta has been delivered. Oxytocin promotes contraction of the uterine corpus and decreases the likelihood of uterine atony. It is given in dilute solution because the intravenous administration of undiluted oxytocin can cause significant hypotension. Once uterine atony is diagnosed, management can be categorized as manipulative, medical, and surgical. *Uterine massage* alone is often successful in causing uterine contraction and this should be done while preparations for other treatments are under way. Another manipulation, which is rarely used nowadays, is packing of the uterine cavity with gauze, which serves as a temporizing measure while awaiting definitive therapy. Medical treatments include oxytocin, Methergine (methylergonovine maleate), and several prostaglandin preparations, administered separately or in combination. *Methergine* is a potent constrictor that can cause uterine contractions within several minutes. It is always given intramuscularly since rapid intravenous administration can lead to dangerous hypertension. Prostaglandin $F_{2\alpha}$ may be given intramuscularly or directly into the myometrium, and prostaglandin E_2 may be given by vaginal suppository. Both result in very strong uterine contractions. Typically, oxytocin is given prophylactically as noted above; if uterine atony occurs, the infusion rate is increased and, in addition, Methergine, prostaglandin, or both are given.

Occasionally, uterine massage and oxytocics are unsuccessful in bringing about appropriate uterine contraction such that surgical measures must be utilized. Surgical management of uterine atony may include ligation of the uterine arteries or hypogastric arteries, selective arterial embolization, and hysterectomy. At times, these procedures may be lifesaving. Management must be individualized in cases of severe uterine atony, taking into account the degree of hemorrhage, the overall status of the patient, and her future childbearing desires (Table 19.2). When hemorrhage occurs, large-bore intravenous access should be obtained and blood typed and cross-matched for possible transfusion.

Lacerations of the Lower Genital Tract

Lacerations of the lower genital tract are far less common than uterine atony as a cause of postpartum hemorrhage, but can be serious and require prompt surgical repair. *Predisposing factors* include an instrumented delivery with forceps, a manipulative delivery such as a breech extraction, a precipitous labor, and a macrosomic infant.

Although minor lacerations to the cervix in the process of cervical dilation and delivery are routinely found, lacerations of greater than 2 cm in length and those that are actively bleeding generally require repair. In order to minimize blood loss due to significant cervical and vaginal lacerations, all patients with any predisposing factors or any patient in whom blood loss soon after delivery appears to be excessive despite a firm and contracted uterus, should have a careful repeat inspection of the lower genital tract. This examination may require assistance to allow adequate visualization. As a rule, repair of these lacerations is usually not difficult if adequate exposure is provided. Occasionally, however, extensive repair is required, necessitating general anesthesia.

Retained Placenta

Separation of the placenta from the uterus occurs because of cleavage between the *zona basalis* and the *zona spongiosa*. Once separation occurs, expulsion is caused by strong uterine contractions. Retained placenta can occur when either the process of separation or the process of expulsion is incomplete. Predisposing factors to retained placenta include a previous cesarean delivery, uterine leiomyomas, prior uterine curettage, and succenturiate placental lobe.

Placental tissue remaining within the uterus can prevent adequate contractions and predispose to excessive bleeding. After expulsion, every placenta should be inspected to detect missing cotyledons, which may remain in the uterus. If retained placenta is suspected, either because of apparent absent cotyledons or because of excessive bleeding, it can often be removed by inserting two fingers through the cervix into the uterus and manipulating the retained tissue downward into the vagina. If this is unsuccessful, or if there is uncertainty regarding the cause of hemorrhage, an ultrasound examination of the uterus is

Table 19.2.
Management of the Patient with Postpartum Hemorrhage

Evaluate promptly once excessive bleeding is detected.
Review clinical course for probable cause.
  Any difficulty removing placenta?
  Were forceps used?
  Other predisposing factors?
Perform bimanual examination in recovery area/delivery room.
  Uterus boggy? Massage. Initiate or increase oxytocin; give Methergine, 0.2 mg intramuscularly.
  Placental fragments within uterus on exploration or on ultrasound examination? If so, return to delivery
    room for curettage.
  Laceration or hematoma? Repair in delivery room.
Monitor and maintain circulation.
  Large-bore intravenous catheters: 1 or 2 well-functioning lines.
  Type and cross-match blood.
  Check hematocrit and coagulation profile with platelet count for baseline.
Notify obstetric physicians, nurses, and anesthesia and operating room personnel of potential need for
    surgical intervention.
Visualize cervix and vagina in search of lacerations. Repair if present.
Remember that postpartum hemorrhage may be from multiple causes, e.g., atony plus lacerations.
Observe patient constantly. Repeated bimanual examination. If bleeding persists, is the blood clotting?
Inform patient of the problem and what measures are being taken to correct it. Get an appreciation of her
    desires regarding further childbearing and hysterectomy.
Preoperative management options
  Uterine packing
  Prostaglandin (PG) administration
Operative measures
  Ligation of vessels
    Hypogastric artery ligation
    Uterine artery ligation
  Selective arterial embolization
  Hysterectomy is treatment of last resort in patient who wants to retain her uterus
Intensive care measures
  Hemodynamic, renal, and coagulation surveillance measures

very helpful. A firmly contracted uterus exhibits a characteristic "stripe" on ultrasound imaging representing the newly contracted endometrial cavity. Absence of such a stripe implies placental tissue and/or blood clots remaining within the uterine cavity. Curettage with a suction apparatus and/or a large sharp curet may remove the retained tissue. Care must be exercised to avoid perforation through the uterine fundus.

Placental tissue may also remain in the uterus because separation of the placenta from the uterus may not occur normally. At times, placental villi penetrate the uterine wall to form what is generally called *placenta accreta*. More specifically, abnormal adher-

ence of the placenta to the superficial lining of the uterus is termed *placenta accreta*, penetration into the uterine muscle itself is called *placenta increta*, and complete invasion through the thickness of the uterine muscle is termed *placenta percreta*. If this abnormal attachment involves the entire placenta, no part of the placenta separates. Much more commonly, however, attachment is not complete and a portion of the placenta separates while the remainder remains attached. Major, life-threatening hemorrhage can ensue. Hysterectomy is often required although in a woman who desires more children, an attempt to separate the placenta by curettage is usually appropriate in order to salvage the uterus.

OTHER CAUSES OF POSTPARTUM HEMORRHAGE

Hematomas

Hematomas can occur anywhere from the vulva to the upper vagina as a result of delivery trauma. The frequency of hematoma formation is higher for the vulva and lower vagina than the upper vagina, while, conversely, the morbidity is higher with hematomas in the less accessible upper vagina. Hematomas may also develop at the site of episiotomy or perineal laceration. Hematomas may occur without disruption of the vaginal mucosa, when the fetus or forceps cause shearing of the submucosal tissues without mucosal tearing.

Vulvar or vaginal hematomas are characterized by exquisite pain with or without signs of shock. Hematomas that are less than 5 cm in diameter and are not enlarging can usually be managed expectantly by frequent evaluation of the size of the hematoma and close monitoring of vital signs and urinary output. Application of ice packs can also be helpful. Larger and enlarging hematomas must be managed surgically. If the hematoma is at the site of episiotomy, the sutures should be removed and a search made for the actual bleeding site, which is then ligated. If not at the episiotomy site, the hematoma should be opened at its most dependent portion, the hematoma drained, the bleeding site identified, if possible, and the site closed with interlocking-hemostatic sutures. Drains and vaginal packs are often used to prevent reaccumulation of blood.

Coagulation Defects

Virtually any congenital or acquired abnormality in blood clotting can lead to postpartum hemorrhage. Abruptio placentae, amniotic fluid embolism, and severe preeclampsia are obstetric conditions commonly associated with coagulopathies. The treatment of coagulation defects is aimed at correcting the coagulation defect and eliminating the cause of the clotting abnormality. When assessing a patient with postpartum hemorrhage, it should always be noted whether or not the blood that is passing from the genital tract is clotting. It also should be recalled that profuse hemorrhage itself can lead to coagulopathy.

Amniotic Fluid Embolism

Amniotic fluid embolism is a rare, sudden, and often fatal obstetric complication caused by entry of amniotic fluid into the maternal circulation. The condition results in severe cardiorespiratory collapse and usually a coagulopathy. Treatment is directed toward total support of the cardiovascular and coagulation systems.

Uterine Inversion

Uterine inversion is a rare condition when the uterus literally turns inside out with the top of the uterine fundus extending through the cervix into the vagina, at times even past the introitus. Hemorrhage with uterine inversion is characteristically severe and sudden. Treatment includes administration of an anesthetic, which is a uterine relaxant (such as halothane), and replacement of the uterine corpus. If this fails, surgical treatment, possibly including hysterectomy, may be needed.

GENERAL MANAGEMENT OF PATIENTS WITH POSTPARTUM HEMORRHAGE

Once excessive blood loss occurs, prompt assessment is mandatory. A general approach to management is offered in Table 19.2. Because the vast majority of cases of postpartum hemorrhage are due to uterine atony, the uterus should be palpated abdominally seeking the soft, boggy consistency of the relaxed uterus. If found, oxytocin infusion should be increased and either Methergine or prostaglandins given if the excessive bleeding continues.

Other questions will help direct assessment:

Was expulsion of the placenta spontaneous and apparently complete?

Table 19.3.
Precautionary Measures to Prevent or Minimize Postpartum Hemorrhage

Before delivery
  Identify any predisposing factors
  Determine baseline hematocrit
  Send blood specimen to blood bank for group and screen
  Establish well-functioning intravenous line with large-bore catheter
  Obtain baseline coagulation studies and platelet count if indicated
In delivery room
  Avoid excessive traction on umbilical cord
  Inspect placenta for complete removal
  Perform digital exploration of uterus
  Massage uterus
  Visualize cervix and vagina
  Remove all clots in uterus and vagina before transfer to recovery area
In recovery area
  Closely observe patient for excessive bleeding
  Frequently palpate uterus with massage
  Determine vital signs frequently

Were forceps or other instrumentation used in delivery?

Was the baby large or the delivery difficult or precipitous?

Were the cervix and vagina inspected for lacerations?

Is the blood clotting?

As the cause of the hemorrhage is being identified, general supportive measures for patients with hemorrhage of any cause are initiated. Large-bore intravenous access; crystalloid infusions; type, cross-match, and administration of blood or blood components as needed; periodic assessment of hematocrit and coagulation profile; and monitoring of urinary output are all important.

The management of postpartum hemorrhage is greatly facilitated if patients at high risk are identified and preliminary preparations made. Table 19.3 reviews such precautionary measures.

FURTHER READINGS

Bowes WA. Postpartum care. In: Gabbe SG, Niebyl JR, Simpson JL, eds. Obstetrics: normal and problem pregnancies. 2nd ed. New York: Churchill Livingstone, 1991:753–779.

Cunningham FG, MacDonald PC, Gant NF. Williams obstetrics. 18th ed. East Norwalk, CN: Appleton & Lange, 1989:415–424, 695–701.

Herbert WNP, Cefalo RC. Management of postpartum hemorrhage. Clin Obstet Gynecol 1984;27:139–147.

SELF-EVALUATION

Case 19-A

A 25-year-old G1 has labor induced at 42 week's gestational age. Her induction is prolonged but finally results in a forceps-assisted delivery of a healthy 9½-pound infant. The placenta is expelled 9 minutes after delivery and appears intact. Intravenous oxytocin is begun in dilute solution at the time of placental delivery. During repair of the episiotomy, excessive bleeding from the uterus is noted. The patient is becoming tachycardic but her blood pressure is consistent with her intrapartum blood pressures.

Question 19-A-1

Which of the following causes of postpartum hemorrhage may be *excluded* from consideration based on the information provided so far?

A. coagulation defect
B. uterine atony
C. retained placental tissue
D. vaginal laceration
E. none may be excluded

Answer 19-A-1

Answer: E

At this time, none of these may be excluded. For example, the placenta may have *appeared* to be intact when in fact a placental fragment has remained in the uterus.

Question 19-A-2

Based on the information provided, which of the following seems *most likely* as the cause of this patient's postpartum hemorrhage?

A. coagulation defect
B. uterine atony
C. retained placental tissue
D. vaginal laceration

Answer 19-A-2

Answer: B

Given a prolonged labor induction with oxytocin and a large baby, uterine atony is most likely in this case. It is important to remember, however, that the forceps delivery of this large baby places this patient at risk for lacerations and, as noted, placental tissue may still be retained.

Case 19-B

A 32-year-old G2P001 undergoes a spontaneous vaginal delivery of a healthy 8-pound infant after an unremarkable spontaneous labor. After 10 minutes without spontaneous placental delivery, traction is applied to the umbilical cord. Placental tissue is expelled with the umbilical cord but vaginal hemorrhage ensues immediately thereafter. The placenta is clearly not intact.

Question 19-B-1

What are appropriate immediate interventions?

A. fluid resuscitation and cardiovascular support
B. oxytocin administration
C. manual exploration of the uterine cavity
D. uterine massage
E. notification of the operating room (OR) and anesthesia staff of a possible surgical emergency

Answer 19-B-1

Answer: A, B, C, D

All of these maneuvers are important for diagnostic and/or therapeutic reasons. Retained placental tissue can be assumed and treatment of an associated uterine atony should be undertaken immediately while attempts to remove the placental tissue proceed. The careful clinician should remember that lacerations are still a possible additional cause of this hemorrhage, albeit unlikely. The need for possible surgical intervention is still remote so that notifying the operating room is not necessary.

Question 19-B-2

Oxytocin administration, prostaglandin and Methergine administration, and uterine massage slow but do not stop the vaginal hemorrhage. Vaginal examination reveals placental tissue in the uterus, but repeated attempts to dislodge it are not successful. Indeed, careful examination cannot discover a "cleavage plane" between the retained placental tissue and the wall of the uterus. Placenta accreta is suspected.

For further consideration: What are your options in this situation? This young woman and her husband plan for a family of three. What implications does management of this condition have for their family plans? Are there other surgical procedures you may try before hysterectomy?

INFECTIONS IN THE POSTPARTUM PERIOD

fever after first 24°

Infections occurring during the puerperium represent a serious cause of morbidity, and rarely even mortality, in obstetric practice. This chapter addresses common causes of infections in the days following delivery, as well as mastitis, an infection that can occur in the weeks or months following childbirth.

The rising cesarean delivery rate carries with it an increase in the incidence of infection. Infection rates can vary from 10 to over 50%, depending upon a number of factors as seen in Table 20.1. Following vaginal delivery, infection occurs very infrequently. The most important determinant for the development of postpartum infection is whether or not the patient had a cesarean delivery.

PUERPERAL FEBRILE MORBIDITY

The definition of puerperal *febrile morbidity*, as determined many years ago by the Joint Committee on Maternal Welfare, is a "temperature of 38.0°C (100.4°F) or higher, the temperature to occur on any 2 of the first 10 days postpartum, exclusive of the first 24 hours, and to be taken by mouth by a standard technique at least four times daily." This guideline was proposed to help distinguish true infection from minor temperature elevations commonly seen in the early puerperium and presumed to be the result of breast engorgement. Practically speaking, significant elevations in maternal temperature even within the first 24 hours postpartum, especially when accompanied by other evidence of infection, is generally thought to represent frank infection and treatment is often instituted. However, this "official" definition of puerperal morbidity does serve as a reminder that not every temperature elevation reflects infection and that, in borderline cases, expectant management is warranted. A number of factors predispose to infection following delivery (Table 20.1). After a discussion of several common types of infections, an overview of the evaluation of the patient with fever in the early puerperium is provided.

METRITIS   *insidious – difficult to dx. – dur. labor/Rom. – amnionitis*

The most common infection following cesarean delivery is infection of the uterus. Often such infection is termed *endometritis* but, in fact, these infections usually extend well beyond the thin endometrial lining; hence the *preferred term is metritis*. Among the predisposing factors, the duration of labor, duration of rupture of membranes, and the presence of amnionitis during labor are signifi-

**Table 20.1
Factors That Predispose to Postpartum Infections**   *most imp is c/s*

Rupture of fetal membranes
Intraamniotic infection
Prolonged labor
Multiple pelvic examinations
Obesity
Anemia
Prolonged operating time
Low socioeconomic status
Internal electronic fetal monitoring
Use of prophylactic antibiotic

↑ risk in traumatic/surgical deliveries – presents early – can get metritis cultures.

211

Table 20.2
Common Organisms Associated with Pelvic Infections

Aerobes		Anaerobes	
Gram-positive	Gram-negative	Gram-positive	Gram-negative
Staphylococcus	Escherichia coli	Peptococcus	Bacteroides
Streptococcus (A, B, D)	Proteus	Peptostreptococcus	
Enterococcus	Klebsiella	Clostridium	

cant factors leading to the development of metritis.

Fever is the characteristic feature in the diagnosis of metritis, and it may be accompanied by *uterine tenderness.* If the infection has spread to the adnexa, tenderness may be present there as well. Signs of peritoneal irritation and diminished or absent bowel sounds, especially associated with ileus, indicate more serious infection.

As with virtually all pelvic infections, metritis is polymicrobial in origin. Both aerobic and anaerobic organisms are commonly isolated, with anaerobic organisms predominating. The most common of these organisms are listed in Table 20.2. Because bacteria are normally found in the vagina and endocervix, it is difficult to properly culture the endometrial cavity. On a practical basis, broad antibiotic coverage against a variety of common microorganisms is generally prescribed.

Various choices of *antibiotics* are utilized, most of which are successful. Single agent therapy has the benefit of ease of administration and is often cost saving; cephalosporins such as cefotetan and cefoxitin are commonly used. A combination of ampicillin and an aminoglycoside is also popular, as is the combination of clindamycin with gentamicin. Many such initial therapies have "gaps" in their total coverage, that is, one or more major pathogens are not sensitive to the antibiotic treatment. Therefore, it is customary to provide additional coverage if there has been no response within 48–72 hours. Intravenous antibiotic administration while the patient is hospitalized is preferred for initial treatment. Antibiotic therapy is continued until the patient is asymptomatic, has normal bowel

Some ampicillin

may need inpatient care.

function, and has been afebrile for at least 24 hours. Subsequent outpatient oral antibiotic treatment is usually unnecessary.

Occasionally a *pelvic abscess* will further complicate the patient's recovery. Evidence suggesting abscess formation includes persistent fever despite antibiotic therapy, protracted malaise, and delayed return of gastrointestinal function, localization of pain and/or tenderness in the abdominal cavity, and detection of a mass on pelvic/abdominal examination. Ultrasonography or other imaging scans (CT, MRI) may be helpful in diagnosing a pelvic abscess. Management of a persistent pelvic abscess includes drainage either by percutaneous techniques or laparotomy. Intraabdominal rupture of a pelvic abscess is a surgical emergency. Sepsis may occur in association with pelvic infection, with or without frank abscess formation.

Prophylactic antibiotic therapy at the time of cesarean delivery has been shown to significantly reduce the likelihood of postpartum infection. A single dose of a broad-spectrum antibiotic is generally given at the time of clamping of the umbilical cord, a practice designed to avoid interference with subsequent bacterial cultures of the infant should they be necessary. Additional doses of antibiotics given after surgery do not seem to provide added protection against infection.

2° cath.

URINARY TRACT INFECTIONS

Urinary tract infections are also commonly seen following cesarean delivery and may also occur after vaginal delivery. Bladder catheterization, a practice common with both cesarean deliveries and epidural anesthesia,

no breastfeeding complications

UTI - don't see dysuria / 1 freq. in PP.
as signs induc. intec.

CHAPTER 20 : INFECTIONS IN THE POSTPARTUM PERIOD   213

introduces bacteria into the lower urinary tract, which can lead to infection.

Dysuria (painful urination) is not as common in the puerperium as at other times because of a relative insensitivity of the bladder following delivery. *Frequency* of urination is also a normal occurrence postpartum, minimizing the value of this symptom during the postpartum period. *Costovertebral tenderness* may suggest an upper urinary tract infection. When a urinary tract infection is suspected, a "clean-catch" or catheterized urine sample should be obtained for urinalysis and for culture. Antibiotic treatment is begun with one of a variety of agents, most often ampicillin or a related drug. The antibiotic can be changed if the culture results obtained 24–48 hours later indicate insensitivity of the bacteria to the initial antibiotic, especially if symptoms persist.

✴ WOUND INFECTIONS   vag or staph aureus abd.

Infection of the *incision site* following cesarean delivery can occur but is uncommon. Fever accompanied by pain, tenderness, and erythema around the incision are seen most frequently on the third and fourth days after delivery. As with any wound infection, the incision must be probed for the extent of infection and to permit adequate drainage of purulent or serosanguineous material. A culture of the site should be obtained, after which broad-spectrum antibiotic treatment is often initiated. Drainage alone may be adequate, but given the likelihood of *Staphylococcus aureus* as a potential pathogen, antibiotic therapy is often initiated. Standard care of the open wound is also vital.

Infections of the episiotomy site are very uncommon, which is somewhat surprising given the bacteriologic milieu in that area. Infected episiotomy sites are tender and swollen. Poor tissue turgor often leads to breakdown of the sutures used in the initial repair. The sutures should be removed and drainage permitted both to limit further spread of infection and to promote healing. Sitz baths also help in healing. Subsequent repair of the episiotomy

site, if necessary, can be accomplished soon after the infection has cleared.

Necrotizing fasciitis is a rare infection that may be seen on the perineum or with abdominal incisions. This especially virulent and frequently fatal infective process involves the fascia, muscle, and subcutaneous tissue. It may spread downward along the thighs or upward onto the abdomen and chest. This necrotic tissue must be immediately debrided until healthy tissue is reached. Antibiotics, major cardiovascular system support, and subsequent skin grafting comprise the overall treatment. Without such vigorous care, fatality is virtually assured; even with treatment, approximately half the patients with necrotizing fasciitis do not survive. The important key is early recognition of the possibility that a wound infection, whether perineal or abdominal, may represent this overwhelming infection.

SEPTIC PELVIC THROMBOPHLEBITIS

This uncommon infection is a sequela of pelvic infection. The venous drainage of the pelvic organs tends to flow in a left-to-right fashion through the right ovarian vein. *Venous stasis* in these widely dilated veins, along with the presence of multiple bacteria if infection is present, can lead to thrombosis in these vessels; subsequent *microembolization* of the lungs or other organs via the inferior vena cava is possible.

Clinically, this infection is manifest as *residual fever* and *tachycardia* following several days of antibiotic treatment for presumed metritis. Usually the patient is asymptomatic with respect to uterine tenderness and bowel function. Although it is possible to diagnose this condition with CT scanning or other such imaging, it is customary to begin empiric treatment with *heparin*. Prompt resolution of the fever and tachycardia, usually within 24 hours, corroborates the diagnosis. The recommended duration of therapy with anticoagulation varies from 7 to more than 30 days.

Handwritten annotations in top margin: *dont get it in first week!* *very painful unilateral indurated tender* *fever* *staph aureus* *tx: diclox erythromycin keep nursing*

Handwritten annotation in left margin: *aware this out if fever in first week*

✳ MASTITIS

In the lactating woman, breast infection occurs most commonly from 1 to 3 months postpartum, but it can occur months later. Initially, symptoms can be misleading. Patients often complain of significant *fever* (often 103°F or more), *malaise*, and *general body aching*. Breast symptoms may be somewhat vague, although breast tenderness is described if patients are asked specifically about this. Commonly, patients think they have a generalized viral infection and call their physician seeking information regarding medications to take for the "flu" while lactating.

After the onset of these signs and symptoms, evidence of infection becomes more localized to the breasts over the following days. Erythema and tenderness are present, often with a brawny and indurated area to palpation, which may be segmented in orientation. The infection is virtually always unilateral. *S. aureus* is cultured from the breast milk in about half the cases; no single predominant organism is identified in other cases. The *origin* of the infection is, in fact, the infant's pharynx; accordingly, there should be no concern on the part of the mother with respect to transmitting the infection to the infant.

It is no longer common practice to culture the breast milk. However, because of the prevalence of the *S. aureus* as the offender, an antibiotic that is penicillinase-resistant, such as *dicloxacillin* is recommended. Resolution of symptoms is generally prompt, with marked improvement within 24–36 hours. Patients should be cautioned to complete the full antibiotic course to prevent recurrence. It *is not necessary to withhold nursing* on the infected breast, although some patients benefit greatly from uninterrupted rest for the first day or two of therapy.

Mastitis is generally distinguished from a blocked (inspissated) duct on the basis of fever. At times, however, it may be difficult to distinguish these two entities, and antibiotic treatment is generally begun empirically.

EVALUATION OF THE FEBRILE PATIENT

The *"sequence"* of infection sites is somewhat predictable *after surgery*. On the first day postoperatively, the lungs are the common cause of fever; on the second day, the urinary tract; on the third, the wound; on the fourth, the extremities. Metritis is usually associated with the development of fever on the first and second days postpartum.

When evaluating a febrile patient, a *history* of the labor and delivery can be helpful. If, for example, the patient had amnionitis and was febrile through labor, one would suspect metritis as the cause of fever. A careful history regarding pulmonary symptoms, urinary tract disturbance, and abdominopelvic pain and tenderness are of paramount importance. *Examination* should include the lungs, the back (for costovertebral tenderness), palpation of the abdomen, careful inspection of the incision site, a check for the presence of bowel sounds, examination of the perineum (if an episiotomy was performed or if a laceration occurred), a pelvic examination, and assessment for calf tenderness. Although a pelvic examination may not elicit any findings other than uterine tenderness, one can confirm that lochia drainage is, in fact, occurring and baseline information can be obtained concerning adnexal masses that may be important if the fever persists and an abscess develops. Blood cultures are not usually obtained unless the infection appears severe, if sepsis is suspected, if fever is especially high, or if response to limited therapy is delayed.

FURTHER READINGS

Bowes WA. Postpartum Care. In: Gabbe SG, Niebyl JR, Simpson JL. Obstetrics: normal and problem pregnancies. 2nd ed. New York: Churchill Livingstone, 1991:753–779.

Cunningham FG, MacDonald PC, Gant NF. *Williams Obstetrics*. 18th ed. East Norwalk, CN: Appleton & Lange, 1989:461–476.

SELF-EVALUATION

Case 20-A

Nine days postpartum, a new mother complains tha she feels awful, is running a fever of 99 to 100°F, and just aches all over. She is breast-feeding but the baby has been fretful the last 48 hours. She has no complaints of sore throat, dysuria, pelvic pain (except the uterine cramps she has come to expect with breast-feeding), or especially tender breasts.

On examination, the left breast is slightly warmer to touch and slightly more tender than the right.

Question 20-A-1

Appropriate management includes:

A. surgical drainage of the infected breast
B. cannulation of the breast ducts over the affected lobules
C. administation of an oral penicillinase-resistant antibiotic
D. instructions to cease breast-feeding until the infection clears

Answer 20-A-1

Answer: C

The presumptive diagnosis is early mastitis. Mastitis usually responds readily to oral antibiotic therapy. Surgical intervention for mastitis is not indicated, although drainage of an abscess may be. There is no risk to the baby or mother from continuing breast-feeding.

Case 20-B

When evaluating a patient, the timing of the onset of fever is often helpful in identifying the site of the infection.

Question 20-B-1

Match the site of infection with the days after surgery to create the class sequence of postoperative infection sites.

1. 1 day
2. 2 days
3. 3 days
4. 4 days

A. urinary tract
B. wound
C. extremities
D. lungs

Answer 20-B-1

1. D
2. A
3. B
4. C

Although the "wind-water-wound-walk" sequence is easy to remember, each patient should be thoroughly evaluated to rule out all causes of fever irrespective of when she presents.

FEVER

DAY 1 — Lungs
2 — UTI
3 — Wound
4 — EXT.

} METRITIS

wind water wound walk —

chapter 21

DISORDERS OF THE BREAST

Disorders of the female breast pose unique problems for patient and physician. Our society places special significance on the female breast, especially in matters of femininity and sexuality. In addition, there are appropriate fears of breast cancer, which are confounded by normal monthly changes that may be both uncomfortable and disconcerting. Consideration of both the medical disorder and its emotional sequelae is a challenge in the management of breast disorders.

The adult female breast is actually a large, modified sebaceous gland, located within the superficial fascia of the chest wall (Fig. 21.1). It weighs between 200 and 300 g and is made up primarily of fatty tissue, fibrous septa, and glandular structures. Breast tissue is organized into 12–20 triangular lobes with a central duct, collecting ducts, and secretory cells arranged in alveoli. Each of these lobes drains at the nipple. The breast has a rich blood supply and lymphatic system, which facilitate metastases of malignancies. Breast tissue may be located anywhere along "milk lines" that run from the axilla to the groin. Extra nipples (polythelia) are more common than true accessory breasts (polymastia).

Breast tissue is very sensitive to hormonal changes. The development of adult breast shape during puberty is a result of hormonal changes. The sensitivity to hormones is also responsible for cyclic changes that occur during the menstrual cycle and for the symptoms often reported by patients during therapeutic hormonal manipulations.

Each of the tissues of the breast may be the source of pathologic change. Fibrocystic changes and fibroadenomas may arise in the connective tissues of the breast. Fatty tissues may undergo necrosis in response to trauma or may harbor lipomas. The duct system of the breast may become dilated (duct ectasia or galactocele), contain papillary neoplasms, or undergo malignant change. Although more common to nursing mothers, infection of the breast (mastitis) also occurs in other women.

Breast cancer is the most common malignancy in women, accounting for roughly one quarter of all women's malignancies. With approximately 130,000 new cases and 40,000 breast cancer deaths per year in the United States, breast cancer is the most common cause of death in women in their 40's. Roughly *one woman in 10 will develop breast cancer in her lifetime.* Although there has been little change in the overall mortality from breast cancer over the past 40 years, newer diagnostic technologies and increased awareness promise earlier diagnosis and more successful treatment.

BENIGN BREAST DISEASE
Fibrocystic Change

The term "fibrocystic change" encompasses over 35 different processes including the misnomer "fibrocystic disease." Fibrocystic changes are *the most common of all benign breast conditions*. They may be present in one third to one half of premenopausal women and are a source of symptoms for roughly half of these women. The alterations associated with fibrocystic change may arise from an exaggerated response to hormones. Consequently, fibrocystic changes are most common during the reproductive years or occasionally during hormone replacement after

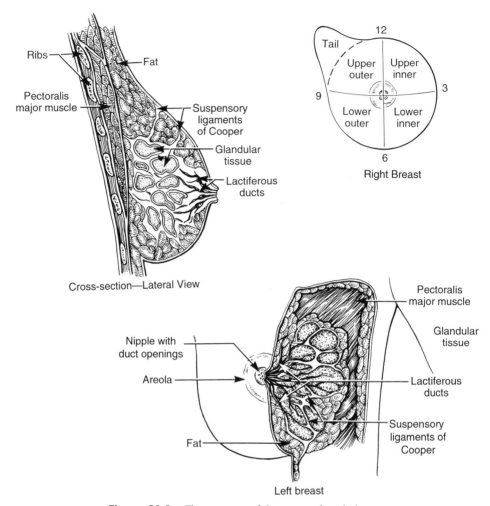

Figure 21.1. The structure of the mature female breast.

menopause. Disturbed ratios of estrogen and progesterone or an increased rate of prolactin secretion have both been suggested as causes for these changes. Neither of these theories has been conclusively proved, and there also is no evidence that fibrocystic changes are caused by oral contraceptives.

Histologically, fibrocystic changes occur in three stages. Initially there is a *proliferation of stroma*, especially in the upper outer quadrants of the breast, that leads to the induration and tenderness experienced by the patient. In the second phase, *adenosis* occurs, leading to cyst formation. During this phase,

cysts range from microscopic to 1 cm in diameter. Marked proliferation of the ducts and alveolar cells occur in this stage. In the late stages of fibrocystic change, *larger cysts* are present and *less pain* occurs (unless there is rapid change in a cyst). Proliferative changes may be marked in any of the involved tissues. When atypia is found in hyperplastic ducts or apocrine cells, there is a fivefold increase in the risk of future carcinoma.

Fibrocystic changes most commonly present as cyclic, bilateral pain (mastalgia) and engorgement. The pain associated with fibrocystic changes is diffuse, often with radiation to the shoulders or upper arms. Occasionally well-localized pain will occur when a cyst expands rapidly. On examination, diffuse bilateral nodularity is typical, with larger cysts taking on the character of a balloon filled with fluid. These changes are most prominent just prior to menstruation.

Fibroadenoma

Fibroadenomas are the second most common form of benign breast disease. They are most common in young women. These firm, painless, freely movable breast masses average 2–3 cm in diameter. Although generally solitary, multiple fibroadenomas develop in 15–20% of patients. These tumors do not change during the menstrual cycle and are generally slow growing. They are usually found during physical examination or during breast self-examination.

Lipomas and Fat Necrosis

The fatty tissue of the breast may be the source of benign tumors that are difficult to distinguish from malignancy. Both lipomas and fat necrosis may present as ill-defined tumors of the breast. Lipomas are generally nontender, but their diffuse character may raise suspicions of malignancy. Secondary signs suggestive of cancer (e.g., skin and nipple changes) are generally absent.

Fat necrosis is uncommon, and most often the result of trauma, although the causative event often cannot be identified. The patient usually presents with a solitary, tender, ill-defined mass. Skin retraction is present in some patients. Direct evidence of trauma is most often lacking. Even with a history of trauma, the commonality of findings between fat necrosis and cancer (on physical examination and mammography) generally require further evaluation and biopsy to establish the diagnosis.

Intraductal Papilloma

Intraductal papillomas are polypoid epithelial tumors arising in the ducts of the breast. These fibrovascular tumors are covered by benign ductal epithelium. Although these tumors may range from 2 to 5 mm in diameter, they are typically not palpable. The patient presents with a *spontaneous bloody, serous, or cloudy nipple discharge.* Although these polyps are *most often benign*, the similarity of symptoms to carcinoma mandates excisional biopsy for most patients.

Mammary Duct Ectasia and Galactocele

Mammary duct ectasia may arise from chronic intraductal and periductal inflammation, which causes *dilation of the ducts and inspissation of breast secretions.* Most common in the fifth decade of life, this condition presents with a thick gray-to-black nipple discharge, pain, and nipple tenderness. Palpation around the nipple will elicit discharge and may reveal thickening that may be difficult to distinguish from cancer. Nipple retraction is common. Biopsy will confirm the diagnosis, and once established, no further therapy is needed unless warranted by the patient's symptoms.

Ductal obstruction and inflammation during, or soon after, lactation may lead to the development of a *galactocele*. Galactoceles are cystic dilations of a duct or ducts. These ducts contain inspissated milky secretions that may become infected and lead to acute mastitis or abscess formation. When uncomplicated by infection, needle aspiration and decompression of the ducts is curative and excision is rarely required.

BREAST CANCER

Demographics

Much has been written about factors that increase a woman's risk of breast cancer (Table 21.1), but little is known about the actual cause. *Risk factors* themselves are of limited clinical value. Only 25% of patients with breast cancer are identified by risk factors. However, risk factors may be useful in planning detection strategies. For example, the incidence of breast cancer rises with age. Eighty-five percent of all breast cancer oc-

Table 21.1
Risk Factors for Breast Cancer

Factor	Relative risk
Family history of breast cancer	
First degree relative (sister or mother)	1.2–3.0
Menstrual history	
Menarche < age 12	1.3
More than 40 menstrual years	1.5–2.0
Pregnancy	
First delivery > age 35	2.0–3.0
Nulliparous	3.0
Other neoplasms	
Contralateral breast cancer	5.0
Carcinoma of uterus or ovary	2.0
Carcinoma of major salivary gland	4.0
Other conditions	
Atypical hyperplasia	4.0–6.0
Previous biopsy	1.9–2.1
North American (white or black)	5.0
Age 60 vs. age 40	2.0
"Moderate" alcohol use	1.5–2.0
Radiation exposure (>90 rads)	4.0
Obesity	Suggested but unknown
Large bowel cancer	Suggested but unknown
Increased dietary fat	Suggested but unknown

Table 21.2
Guidelines for Mammographic Screening

Baseline study between ages 35 and 40
Mammography every 1–2 years from age 40 to 49
Annual mammography from age 50 on
Screening mammography prior to age 35 may be appropriate in selected high risk patients

Table 21.3
Simplified Classification of Breast Cancer

Mammary duct cancers
  Infiltrating (80%)
    Papillary carcinoma
    Intraductal carcinoma
    Colloid carcinoma
    Medullary carcinoma
  Noninfiltrating (5%)
    Papillary carcinoma
    Intraductal carcinoma (comedocarcinoma)
    Intracystic carcinoma
Mammary lobule cancers
  In situ and infiltrating (12%)
Sarcomas
  Cystosarcoma phylloides
  Stromal sarcoma
  Liposarcoma
  Angiosarcoma
Lymphoma
Rare cancers
  Sweat gland carcinoma
  Tubular carcinoma
  Adenoid cystic carcinoma
  Metaplastic lesions
  Inflammatory carcinoma (2%)
  Paget's disease (1%)
  Metastatic cancers

many different cancer types can occur (Table 21.3). Breast cancer survival depends less on cell type than it does on the size of the tumor. Most breast tumors have a long latency from onset to clinically detectable size (Figure 21.2). For this reason, efforts to improve early detection are directed toward mammographic screening of those at high risk and increased public awareness, through programs such as breast self-examination.

Symptoms

In the early stages of cancer growth, the tumor is usually painless and may feel mobile. As the tumor grows, the borders become less distinct and fixation to the supporting ligaments or underlying fascia occurs. Nipple discharge and skin changes ("peau d'orange" or orange peel skin) are late occurrences and are associated with a poor prognosis. Eighty percent of breast cancers present as a mass.

curs after the age of 40 (66% over the age of 50). For this reason, current *recommendations for mammographic screening* for breast cancer depend on the patient's age (Table 21.2).

Types of Breast Cancer

Although 80% of breast cancers are of the nonspecific infiltrating intraductal type,

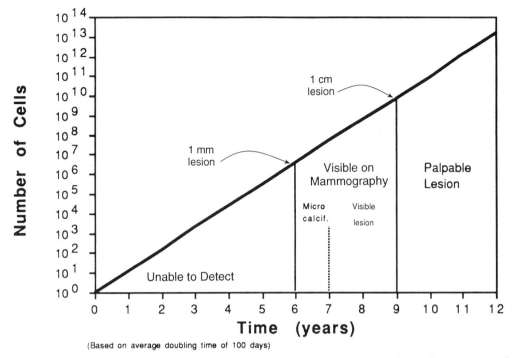

Figure 21.2. With a presumed doubling time of 100 days, breast cancer may be detected by mammography significantly before it becomes identifiable clinically. *Micro calcif.,* microcalcification.

Clinical Aspects

History and Physical Examination

With as many as one quarter of all breast cancers found during routine examination, the role of the careful history and physical examination cannot be overemphasized. All patients should be questioned on whether they practice *breast self-examination*. Breast self-examination should be done on a monthly basis. Since *90% of breast cancers are found by the patient*, this is an opportunity to both highlight an important screening test and obtain information that may be of help clinically. A general family, medical, menstrual, and obstetrical history should be obtained in all patients. Significant risk factors are also evaluated. Even though these risk factors will identify only 25% of cancer patients, they are helpful in planning screening and surveillance.

When obtaining the *history* of a patient with breast problems, information about the presenting complaint such as pain, tenderness, mass, or discharge may be obtained. The duration of symptoms as well as any changes in symptoms are also important. This is especially true of changes related to the menstrual cycle.

Physical examination of the breast should be performed by the physician annually and as a part of the evaluation of any breast complaint. The examination should begin with inspection of both breasts, looking for contour, symmetry, skin, or nipple changes. This should take place with the patient in both the upright and supine position, with arms both above the head and with the patient's hands on her hips contracting her pectoral muscles. Palpation of the breast tissue proceeds in a systematic way using the flat of the fingers, rolling the breast between the fingers and the underlying tissues. This may be carried out by quadrants or in a spiral fashion designed to insure that the entire breast is examined. Palpation of the axilla and supraclavicular area must be included.

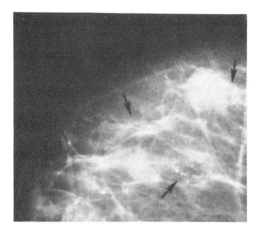

Figure 21.3. Multifocal duct carcinoma. Close-up shows multiple clusters of calcifications (*arrows*) and two masses. Only the larger mass was palpable.

Evaluation

The evaluation of any breast complaint is based on the history and physical examination, augmented by four additional modalities: imaging, fine needle aspiration, fine needle biopsy, and open biopsy.

Imaging

The only nonexperimental method of breast imaging and evaluation is *mammography.* Mammography provides the best mode currently available of screening for early lesions *and has been credited with reducing the mortality rate from breast cancer by up to 30%. Breast cancer mortality could be reduced by as much as one half if all women over the age of 40 were screened annually.* Mammography provides the opportunity to identify small lesions (1–2 mm) (Fig. 21.2), microcalcifications, or other changes suspicious for malignancy with a minimal radiation exposure (less than 1 rad) (Figs. 21.3 and 21.4). Mammography is approximately 85% accurate in diagnosing malignancy. For this reason, it provides an adjunct to clinical impressions and the definitive procedure of biopsy. *In large trials, mammographic screening has led to a 30% reduction in breast cancer mortality.*

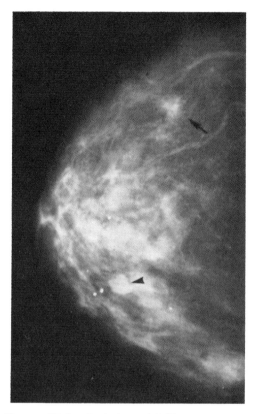

Figure 21.4. Cephalocaudal film-screen mammogram. Small scirrhous carcinoma (*arrow*) is contrasted with well-marginated fibroadenoma (*arrowhead*).

Ultrasonography has been proposed as useful in the evaluation of breast pathology. Although ultrasound is very good at differentiating between cystic and solid masses, it provides little additional information of help in the clinical management of the patient. Thermography and breast transillumination have not proven valuable as either screening or diagnostic tools. The role of magnetic resonance imaging is still under evaluation.

Breast Cyst Aspiration

A simple and very valuable diagnostic tool is simple *needle aspiration.* If the patient has a breast mass that feels cystic, aspiration with a 22- to 25-gauge needle may be both diagnostic and therapeutic. In women over the age of 35, mammography prior to aspiration should be considered because of the increased incidence of malignancy.

Fluid aspirated from patients with fibrocystic changes will customarily be straw colored. Fluid that is dark brown or green occurs in cysts that have been present for a long time. Cytologic evaluation of the fluid obtained is generally of little value.

Fine Needle Aspiration

Fine needle aspiration of cells from a breast mass is gaining acceptance in this country. In this procedure, a 16- to 22-gauge needle is inserted into the mass, negative pressure applied by a syringe, and cells or tissue is obtained. These are examined histologically or cytologically for signs of malignancy. This technique is 70–90% accurate, with a 20% false-negative rate. Therefore, if the aspiration is negative, open biopsy should still be performed.

Open Biopsy

The ultimate method of evaluation of any breast mass is open biopsy. This is often performed under local anesthesia through either radial or circumareolar incisions. For small lesions or those difficult to localize, preoperative identification and radiographically guided J-wire placement may be of value (so-called "needle-localized biopsy"). Post operative x-ray of the pathology specimen should confirm excision of the desired tissue.

Differential Diagnosis by Complaint or Finding

The most common presenting complaints are pain and the presence of a mass. Both of these complaints represent sources of great distress and emergency to the patient. Therefore, they deserve prompt and considerate attention.

Diffuse, bilateral breast pain occurring prior to menstruation is most often due to *fibrocystic changes. Dorsal radiculitis or inflammatory changes in the costal chondral junction* (Tietze's syndrome) may also present in this way. Well-localized breast pain may result from rapid expansion of a *cyst, obstruction of a duct*, or inflammation (such as *mastitis*). Breast pain is a presenting complaint in less than 10% of patients with breast cancer.

Masses in the breast, with the attendant fear of cancer, represent one of the most emotionally charged and difficult differential diagnoses the clinician must make. Masses that are firm, round and well demarcated are most likely to be *fibroadenomas*. Areas with a flattened, rubbery consistency, are suspicious for malignancy although other conditions such as fat necrosis may cause similar changes. With either mass, *further evaluation (such as tissue confirmation by open or needle biopsy) is mandatory*. One approach to this process is shown in Figure 21.5.

Although *bloody discharge* from the nipple is the hallmark of *intraductal papillomas*, any unilateral spontaneous nipple discharge requires a thorough evaluation. The color or clarity of the fluid does not rule out carcinoma. Cytologic evaluation of the nipple discharge is associated with a false-negative rate of almost 20%, significantly reducing its value. Mammography and biopsy are required to establish the diagnosis.

Nipple discharge associated with burning, itching, or nipple discomfort in older patients is suggestive of *ductal ectasia*. In these patients, the discharge is thick or sticky and gray to black in color. As with other sources of nipple discharge, excisional biopsy is often required.

GENERAL MANAGEMENT
Selection of Therapy

The treatment of *fibrocystic change* consists primarily of mechanical support. Diuretics and the reduction in the use of caffeine and tobacco are advocated. Oral contraceptives or supplemental progestins are successful for some patients. For patients with severe symptoms, danazol, bromocriptine, tamoxifen, or GnRH agonists may be useful. Rarely, patients with intractable pain that does not respond to medical management re-

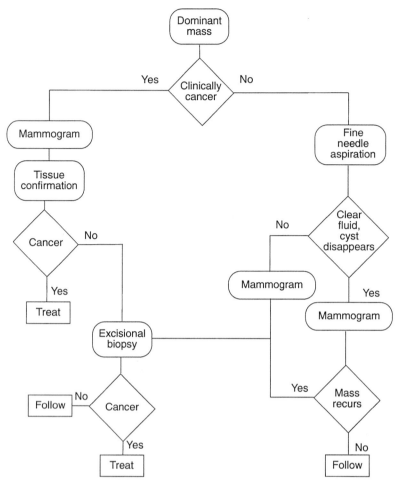

Figure 21.5. Management of a patient with a dominant breast mass.

quire subcutaneous mastectomy and subsequent or immediate breast implant.

Fibroadenomas are generally treated surgically by simple local excision, often under local anesthesia. Up to 20% of women with fibroadenomas will have recurrences.

The treatment of patients with breast cancer is directed toward three goals: control of local disease, treatment of distant disease, and improved quality of life. To this end, *most breast cancer is treated by surgical excision and adjunctive therapy. Breast cancer spreads by both vascular and lymphatic routes* with some direct infiltration. Recognition of this has led away from traditional radical surgical treatment, to therapy directed at both local and distant dis-

ease simultaneously. With local disease only, 5-year survival approaches 90%. This drops to 50–70% when there is regional involvement. Unfortunately, roughly one half of patients have axillary lymph node involvement at the time of diagnosis. Based on the stage of the disease (Table 21.4) and presence of hormone receptors, this adjunctive therapy may consist of radiation therapy, chemotherapy, hormonal manipulations, or a combination of these three. Like most conditions, the therapy of breast cancer must be individualized.

Follow-up of Therapy

Patients with diffuse tenderness and no dominant mass may be safely rechecked at a dif-

Table 21.4
Staging of Breast Cancer[a]

TNM Classification of Breast Cancer[b]

T	Primary tumors	
TIS	Paget's disease of the nipple with no demonstrable tumor	
TI	Tumor >2 cm	T1a, T2a, T3a with no fixation
T2	Tumor >2–5 cm	T1b, T2b, T3b with fixation to underlying pectoral fascia or muscle
T3	Tumor >5 cm	
T4	Tumor of any size with direct extension to chest wall or skin	
	T4a	With fixation to chest wall (including ribs, intercostal muscles, and serratus anterior muscle but not pectoral muscle)
	T4b	With edema (including peau d'orange), ulceration of skin of breast, or satellite skin nodules on same breast
	T4c	Both T4a and T4b
	T4d	Inflammatory cancer
	Dimpling of the skin, nipple retraction, or any other skin changes except those in T4b may occur in T1, T2, or T3 without changing the classification	
N	Regional lymp nodes	
NO	No palpable ipsilateral axillary nodes	
N1	Movable ipsilateral axillary nodes	
	N1a	Nodes not considered to contain growth
	N1b	Nodes considered to contain growth
N2	Ipsilateral nodes considered to contain growth and fixed to one another or to other structures	
N3	Ipsilateral supraclavicular or infraclavicular nodes considered to contain growth, or edema of the arm	
M	Distant metastasis	
MO	No known distant metastases	
M1	Distant metastases present	

Definitions of Clinical Stages I to IV Using TNM Classification				
Stage I	T1a	NO or N1a		MO
	T1b	NO or N1a		MO
Stage II	TO	N1b		MO
	T1a	N1b		MO
	T1b	N1b		MO
	T2a	NO, N1a, or N1b	MO	
	T2b	NO, N1a, or N1b	MO	
Stage III	T3	Any N		MO
	Any T	N2		MO
Stage IV	T4	Any N		Any M
	Any T	N3		Any M
	Any T	Any N		M1

[a]Staging system of International Union Against Cancer and American Joint Commission of Cancer Staging and End Results Reporting.
[b]TNM, tumor-node-metastasis.

ferent portion of the menstrual cycle. Patients who have undergone aspiration of a cyst (with clear fluid and disappearance of the palpable mass) should be rechecked in 2 weeks. Any reoccurrence of the cyst should prompt biopsy or additional evaluation. Some authors advocate a follow-up mammogram after cyst aspiration to delve for other lesions, although this is best individualized based on the needs and history of the patient.

Patients treated for breast cancer require frequent follow-up. Not only are these patients at higher risk for developing a new cancer on the opposite side, but two thirds of these patients will eventually develop distant metastasis. Any patient who has had breast cancer must be closely followed by physical examination and mammography (where appropriate). No biological markers yet exist to allow for either detection or monitoring of those with breast cancer.

FURTHER READINGS

Clarke-Pearson DL, Dawood MY. Breast disease. In Green's gynecology: essentials of clinical practice. 8th ed. Boston: Little, Brown & Co, 1990:473–489.

Droegemueller W. Breast disease. In: Herbst AL, Droegemueller W, Mishell DR, Stenchever MA. Comprehensive gynecology, 2nd ed. St. Louis, MO: CV Mosby, 1992.

Mitchell GW Jr, Bassett LW, eds. The female breast and its disorders. Baltimore: Williams & Wilkins, 1990.

SELF-EVALUATION

Case 21-A

A 24-year-old woman comes to your office with the complaint of a "breast lump" in her right breast. The patient has never been pregnant and currently is on triphasic oral contraception. She reluctantly admits that she did not find the mass and that she would not have known that it was there had it not been for her husband. She has not had any nipple discharge and does do breast self-examination "most months." She is very worried.

On your examination, you find no change in the contour of either breast. No skin changes or nipple discharge can be found. There is a 1-cm, firm, smooth, round, mobile, nontender mass located in the upper outer quadrant of the right breast, approximately 5 cm from the areola.

Question 21-A-1

Based on your history and physical examination, you tell the patient that the most likely diagnosis is:

A. fibrocystic change
B. fibroadenoma
C. hematoma
D. intraductal papilloma
E. fat necrosis

Answer 21-A-1

Answer: B

Even though this patient may have fat necrosis or a hematoma, they are less likely than fibroadenomas, based on the patient's age and findings. Fibrocystic change would be expected to demonstrate a longer history and cyclic changes. Intraductal papillomas are seldom felt as a mass, but rather present with bleeding from the nipple.

Question 21-A-2

The most appropriate next step would be:

A. reexamination in 3 weeks
B. mammography
C. needle aspiration or drainage
D. needle biopsy
E. excisional biopsy

Answer 21-A-2

Answer: A

Although it is likely that this mass will need to be removed by excisional biopsy, the low likelihood of malignancy and the possibility of cystic change is such that reexamination at a different part of the menstrual cycle is justified. Mammography is probably not needed for this patient and it exposes the breast to a small, but unneeded, amount of radiation. Because the mass is not cystic, needle aspiration is unlikely to be successful. Needle biopsy is best reserved for those patients in whom malignancy is suspected because a negative aspiration will not obviate the need for excisional biopsy.

Case 21-B

A 34-year-old G4P3 presents for her routine prenatal check at 26 weeks gestation. The pregnancy has been uneventful to date. At this visit, the patient tells you that she is experiencing occasional bloody discharge from her left nipple. The amount is small and she has had no other symptoms. She reminds you that her mother died of breast cancer and asks if she should be worried.

Your examination reveals only diffuse nodularity in both breasts and you are unable to express any nipple discharge.

Question 21-B-1

What is the most appropriate next step?

A. Reassure the patient that this may be colostrum.
B. Recheck the mass in 4 weeks at the next visit.
C. Have the patient obtain some of the discharge for cytologic evaluation.
D. Plan mammography for after delivery if the symptom persists.
E. Request a mammography now.

Answer 21-B-1

Answer: E

Although the appearance of colostrum in a multiparous patient may occur several weeks before delivery, the unilateral character, bloody appearance, and stage of gestation all make this option unlikely. Because of the nature of the complaint and the patient's family history, timely evaluation, including mammography (with uterine shielding) is required. Cytology of nipple discharges, even when obtained under ideal conditions, is generally of little value in ruling out malignancy.

For further consideration: If this patient's evaluation is normal, when should she have another mammogram? What can she do to minimize her risk of breast cancer?

chapter 22

CONTRACEPTION

The ability to control fertility has had more wide ranging impact than almost any other aspect of medical practice, past or present. Since the subject of contraception has personal, religious, and political overtones, it can often lead to conflict, emotionality, and confusion. Helping the patient and her partner sort through their options is both important and rewarding.

Before the physician can advise a couple on their contraceptive options, he or she must understand the physiologic or pharmacologic basis of action, the effectiveness, and the advantages and/or disadvantages of the contraceptive methods available. An awareness of the contraindications and complications associated with each method also is important.

Currently in the United States, there are many methods of contraception that might be considered "reliable," as well as numerous methods of dubious or no value arising from superstition or ignorance. Since no method is 100% reliable, failures are reflected in descriptive measures of "method failure" (the failure rate inherent in the method if applied correctly 100% of the time) or "failure" (the failure rate seen when patients use the method in actual clinic situations). Approximate pregnancy rates for various methods of contraception are shown in Table 22.1.

HOW CONTRACEPTIVES WORK

All contraceptive methods currently available act to prevent sperm and egg from uniting, or to prevent implantation and growth of the embryo. These goals are accomplished by: (*a*)

inhibiting the development and release of the egg (oral contraceptives); (*b*) imposing a mechanical, chemical, or temporal barrier between sperm and egg (condom, diaphragm, foam, rhythm); or (*c*) altering the ability of the fertilized egg to implant and grow (intrauterine devices, diethylstilbestrol, postcoital oral contraceptives, and inducing menstruation or abortion (RU 486)). Each method may be used successfully, individually or in combination, to prevent pregnancy, and each has its own unique advantages and disadvantages.

Table 22.1
Failure Rates for Various Contraceptive Methods

Method	Estimated pregnancy rates[a]
	%
Oral contraceptives	<1–2
Implantable rod	<1–3
Intrauterine device	2–4
Diaphragm (with spermicide)	10–20
Condom	5–15
Spermicide	
Foam	15–30
Jelly, cream	15–35
Rhythm	
Calendar	15–45
Temperature	1–20
Temperature + intercourse only after ovulation	1–10
Cervical mucus	1–25
Withdrawal	20–25
Postcoital douche	40
No method	90

[a]Rates are those during the first year of use, assuming variations in consistency of usage.

229

FACTORS AFFECTING CHOICE OF CONTRACEPTIVE METHOD

While efficacy is important in the choice of contraceptive methods, it is not the only factor upon which the final decision is based. Factors such as safety, availability, cost, degree to which method "interferes" with coitus (coital dependence), and personal acceptability all have a role to play in the decision. Although we tend to think of safety in terms of significant health risks, for many patients this also includes the possibilities of "side effects." For a couple to use a method, it must be accessible, that is, immediately available (especially in coitally dependent or "use oriented" methods) and of reasonable cost. The effects of a method on spontaneity or modes of sexual expression may be important in some cases. The ability of a contraceptive method to provide some protection against sexually transmitted diseases may also be relevant. Cultural, religious, or social considerations may also influence a couple's choice of contraceptive method. Finally, the couple's feelings about which partner should take responsibility for contraception may be important. The clinician must be sensitive to all these factors that might influence the decision and provide factual information that fits the needs of the patient and her partner. A "decision tree" based on this concept is presented in Figure 22.1.

HORMONAL CONTRACEPTIVES

For many women, "birth control" is synonymous with the oral contraceptive pill. Over 150 million women worldwide have used oral contraceptives and roughly one third of sexually active, fertile women in the United States currently use these agents. It is estimated that about one half of women in the United States 20–24 years old use oral contraceptives. Despite this widespread use, the "pill" is often mistrusted or misunderstood. In a 1985 Gallup pole, two thirds of the respondents said that they thought the pill was more dangerous than pregnancy, and up to one third thought that the pill caused cancer.

This lack of knowledge, combined with the high degree of use, make it important that the physician has an accurate understanding of this contraceptive method.

Oral contraceptive hormones are the *most effective method of reversible contraception* available approved by the Food and Drug Administration (FDA). *Failure rates* for oral contraceptives are in the range of *1%* or less. Failures are generally related to missed pills. In addition to oral administration, injectable or implantable long-acting hormones are available in many parts of the world, but have only recently been introduced into this country.

Biochemistry and Methods of Action

Most of the oral contraceptive formulations available are *combinations of an estrogen and a progestin*. Currently there are almost 30 estrogen-progesterone products on the market in the United States. The most frequently used synthetic estrogen is *ethinyl estradiol*, although a few products contain *mestranol*. The progestins are all androgens, which have the methyl group removed from the carbon 19 of the steroid molecule. Examples of these progestins include norethindrone and levonorgestrel. Most oral contraceptives contain a fixed ratio of estrogen and progestin. The newer "phasic" pills vary this ratio during the course of the month. This leads to a slight decrease in the total dose of hormone used per month but is also associated with a slightly higher rate of bleeding between periods. Progestin-only oral contraceptives have higher failure and complication rates and, as a result, are not widely used.

Oral contraceptive agents act to prevent pregnancy through several routes. These agents *block ovulation* by interfering with the pulsatile release of FSH and LH from the pituitary. This appears to be the main effect that confers protection from pregnancy. Oral contraceptives also *alter cervical mucus*, making it thicker and more difficult for sperm to penetrate. It has been postulated that they cause atrophic change in the en-

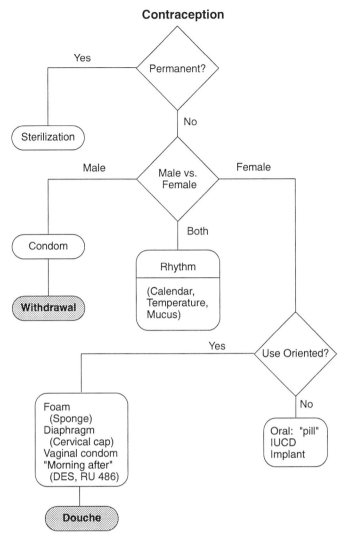

Figure 22.1. Contraception decision making. Methods shown in *gray* have a relatively higher failure rate and should not be used if pregnancy prevention is a high priority.

dometrium, but the role of this effect remains conjectural.

Effects of Oral Contraceptives

Oral contraceptives affect more than just the reproductive system. Estrogens cause alterations in glucose tolerance, affect lipid metabolism, potentiate sodium and water retention, increase renin substrate, and can reduce antithrombin III. Progestins increase sebum, facial and body hair, induce smooth muscle

relaxation, and increase the risk of cholestatic jaundice. However, newer progestational agents are being introduced that are anticipated to have less metabolic impact.

Oral contraceptives have many beneficial effects. Oral contraceptive users have a lower incidence of endometrial and ovarian cancer, benign breast and ovarian disease, and pelvic infection. Ectopic pregnancy is prevented along with the complications of intrauterine pregnancies. Menstrual periods are predictable, shorter, and less painful, and as a result

Table 22.2
Commonly Suggested Contraindications to Oral Contraceptive Use

Strongly suggested ("absolute") contraindications	Suggested ("relative") contraindications
Cardiovascular disease (severe)	Diabetes mellitus
Cerebrovascular disease (stroke)	Epilepsy
Hepatic disease with abnormal liver function	Gallbladder disease
Hepatic tumor	Sickle cell disease
Malignancy, current, of breast, endometrium, or ovary	Uterine fibroids
Pulmonary embolism	Vascular headache (migraine, cluster)
Age 35 with smoking	

the risk of iron deficiency anemia is reduced. There even appears to be a protective effect against rheumatoid arthritis.

High dose pills are associated with a greater risk of serious complications, whereas low dose products have a greater likelihood of *breakthrough bleeding and pregnancy*. Breakthrough bleeding is spotting that occurs in midcycle, most often alleviated by a few cycles on preparations with more estrogens. *Serious complications* such as venous thrombosis, pulmonary embolism, cholestasis and gallbladder disease, stroke, and myocardial infarction are more likely for women using oral contraceptives. Hepatic tumors have also been associated with the use of oral contraceptives. These tumors are rare and have been most closely associated with high dose, mestranol-containing drugs. Although all of these complications are from 2 to 10 times more likely in pill users, factors such as age, weight, and especially smoking also represent significant risk factors. These are important complications, but their infrequent occurrence must be balanced against the beneficial effects of oral contraceptive pill (OCP).

Less serious, but more common, side effects are also dependent on the dosage and type of hormones used. Estrogens may cause a feeling of bloating and weight gain, breast tenderness, nausea, fatigue, or headache.

Progestins are often blamed for symptoms such as acne or depression. Most of these minor side effects may be treated by altering the dose or composition of the agent used.

A better understanding of steroid biochemistry has led to a continuing decrease in the dosage of hormones needed to provide effective contraception, without the presence of complications or breakthrough bleeding. Every effort should be made to take advantage of lower dosage products, while balancing the need for reliability and freedom from menstrual disturbances.

Patient Evaluation for Oral Contraceptive Use

Before considering oral contraceptives for a patient, a careful evaluation is required. Not only is *the pill relatively or absolutely contraindicated in some patients (Table 22.2)*, but even factors such as previous menstrual history may have an impact on the choice of these agents. As an example, approximately 3% of patients may experience problems with resumption of their periods after prolonged oral contraceptive use ("postpill amenorrhea"). Young women and those with irregular periods in the past are much more likely to experience this problem. These patients deserve counseling about this potential complication, or a consideration of alternative methods.

Oral contraceptives may interact with other medications that the patient is taking. This interaction may reduce the efficacy of either the oral contraceptive or the other medications. Examples of drugs that decrease the effectiveness of oral contraceptives include penicillin-based antibiotics, tetracycline, barbiturates, ibuprofen, phenytoin, and the sulfonamides. Drugs that show retarded biotransformation when oral contraceptives are also used include anticoagulants, insulin, methyldopa, hypoglycemics, phenothiazides, and tricyclic antidepressants. With a woman using oral contraceptives, attention should be paid to possible drug interactions before prescribing medications.

"Long-acting" hormonal contraception is possible through the use of *injectable or implantable progestins* (Norplant). These methods offer *long-term reversible contraception* (about 5 years) without the adverse effects of estrogen. The preparation allows slow release of levonorgestrel, which acts to suppress ovulation and results in thickened cervical mucus and an unsuitable endometrium, all of which combine to prevent pregnancy. Norplant and other long-acting progestins are associated with a moderate incidence of random vaginal bleeding and progestin-related side effects. Although these methods may not be reversed as simply as merely discontinuing a daily tablet, they are a convenient and attractive alternative for many women.

BARRIER CONTRACEPTIVES

Among the oldest and most widely used contraceptive methods are those based on *providing a barrier between sperm and egg*. These include condoms (for one or both partners), diaphragms, and cervical caps. Each of these methods is *dependent on proper use before or at the time of intercourse and, as such, are subject to a higher failure rate than oral contraceptives, due to inconsistent or incorrect use*. Despite this, *these methods provide relatively good protection* from unwanted pregnancy, are inexpensive, may provide varying degrees of protection from sexually transmitted diseases, and in the case of condoms, do not require medical consultation.

Condoms

Condoms are sheaths worn over the erect penis or inside the vagina to prevent sperm from reaching the cervix and upper genital tract. Although almost half of all condoms are sold to women, the condom is the only reliable method available to males. Condoms are widely available and inexpensive. They may be made of latex or, less commonly, animal membrane (usually sheep cecum). They are available with or without lubricants or spermicides, plain or with reservoir tips, in colors, and with ridges. Although most of these choices are of personal preference only, lubrication and a reservoir tip both reduce the likelihood of breakage. The condom is well tolerated with only rare reports of skin irritation. Some men complain of reduced sensation with the use of condoms, but this may actually be an advantage for those with rapid or premature ejaculation.

The recent introduction of the female condom provides another option for some couples. This is a sheath, or vaginal "liner" that is inserted into the vagina prior to intercourse. Like the traditional male condom, this contraceptive relies on motivation to insure proper use with each episode of intercourse. Both male and female latex condoms are thought to provide *some protection against sexually transmitted diseases*. Neither method provides complete protection, and couples should still be cautioned about high risk behaviors.

Diaphragms

Diaphragms are a springy ring with a dome of rubber. When used properly, a contraceptive jelly or cream containing spermicide is applied to the rim of the diaphragm, which is then inserted into the vagina, over the cervix, and behind the pubic symphysis. In this position, the diaphragm covers the anterior vaginal wall and cervix. The diaphragm must be inserted before intercourse and be left in place for 6–8 hours after. It may then be removed, washed, and stored. Should additional intercourse be desired during the 6–8-hour waiting time, additional spermicide should be applied and the waiting time restarted.

Diaphragms must be fitted to the individual patient. Fit may change with significant weight change, vaginal birth, or pelvic surgery. The diaphragm should be the largest that can be comfortably inserted, worn, and removed. The patient must be initially instructed in the proper positioning of the diaphragm, with the correct position subsequently verified by the patient each time it is used. If the cervix can be felt through the dome of the diaphragm, the positioning is correct. Women who use diaphragms are slightly more susceptible to urinary tract infection.

The cervical cap is a smaller version of the diaphragm that is applied to the cervix itself. This method is associated with a relatively high degree of displacement, and therefore, of failure.

Spermicides

Although many "spermicidal" chemicals have been tried over the years, today's spermicides rely on one of two agents to immobilize or kill sperm: *nonoxynol 9* and *octoxynol 9.* Inserted into the vagina prior to intercourse, these compounds are delivered in a variety of ways: creams, jellies, foams, films, suppositories, and sponges. They should be applied from 15 to 60 minutes prior to each act of intercourse. Douching should be avoided for at least 8 hours after use. The spermicidal sponge was introduced to allow up to 24 hours of protection with a single application. However, a failure rate slightly higher than that of other spermicides, combined with reports of toxic shock, have tempered enthusiasm for this delivery system.

Spermicides are inexpensive, well tolerated, and provide good protection from pregnancy. *For a well-motivated couple who wish a greater degree of protection, spermicides are often combined with condoms to achieve failure rates that approach those of hormonal methods.*

INTRAUTERINE DEVICES

Intrauterine contraceptive devices (IUCDs) are inserted into the endometrial cavity and can remain for several years. This long-term contraception following a simple insertion is a main advantage of IUCDs. They act to *prevent implantation and growth* of the fertilized egg, although they are also thought to alter tubal transport and the chances of fertilization. These devices have been made of various materials, but are generally plastic. Some

IUCDs have increased efficiency through the addition of progesterone (Progestasert) or copper (Paragard).

Intrauterine devices have one or two filaments ("strings"), which protrude from the cervix. These serve to facilitate removal and allow confirmation of the IUCD's presence, minimizing the chance of undetected expulsion or migration. Should the IUCD become "lost," x-ray, ultrasound, laparoscopy, or hysteroscopy may be required to locate and retrieve the device.

Intrauterine contraceptive devices are associated with a *relatively low failure rate* but do suffer from a *higher rate of complications. Intermenstrual bleeding, menorrhagia, and menstrual pain* are more common in IUCD wearers. The prevalence of this may range as high as 20% for women who have not had children. *Ectopic pregnancies* are up to 10 times more common for women who wear IUCDs. This is thought to be due to the higher rate of *pelvic (tubal and ovarian) infections* also seen in IUCD users. Because of concerns about ectopic pregnancies and sepsis, any possible pregnancy should be aggressively investigated in women with an IUCD in place. Concerns about pelvic infections and subsequent fertility often limit the use of IUCDs to women who are at low risk for sexually transmitted disease and to those less likely to desire further children, i.e., monogamous, multigravid patients.

"NATURAL" FAMILY PLANNING

"Natural" family planning (also called rhythm) usually refers to methods that seek to *prevent pregnancy by either avoiding intercourse around the time of ovulation or using knowledge of the time of ovulation to augment other methods* such as barriers or spermicides. These methods are safe, cost little, and are more acceptable for religious reasons or for those couples who wish a more natural method. For couples who are highly motivated and where the woman has a regular menstrual cycle, these methods may provide acceptable contraception.

The *estimation of the woman's "fertile" period* is based on calendar calculations, variations in basal body temperature, changes in cervical mucus, or a combination of these methods. When the calendar is used, the fertile period would last from days 10 through 17 for a woman with absolutely regular 28-day cycles. Additional days are added to the fertile period based on the time of shortest and longest menstrual interval. Thus, a woman with periods every 28 ± 3 days would be considered to be fertile from days 7 (10 − 3) to 20 (17 + 3). Basal body temperatures (BBTs) and changes in cervical mucus are used to detect ovulation. A rise in BBT of ½–1°F or the presence of thin "stretchy" cervical mucus indicates ovulation. Couples using these methods avoid intercourse until a suitable period after ovulation (usually 2 or more days) has occurred.

These methods are less attractive to many couples because of the high level of motivation and cycle regularity required, along with the restrictions and loss of spontaneity placed on sexual relations.

POSTCOITAL INTERVENTION

Postcoital prevention of pregnancy is currently a poor substitute for planning and effective contraception. In instances of rape, unintended intercourse, IUCD expulsion, or barrier failure (such as condom breakage or diaphragm displacement), these methods have merit. The use of *high dose estrogen*, such as diethylstilbestrol (25–50 mg/day for 5 days) or oral contraceptives (Ovral, 2 tablets plus 2 tablets 12 hours later), *may be effective if begun within 72 hours of exposure*. After this time or with multiple episodes of intercourse, efficacy is markedly reduced. Insertion of an IUCD up to 5 days after unprotected intercourse is often successful. Each of these methods is associated with numerous side effects and the risk of failure. When failure occurs, exposure to intrauterine steroids or an IUCD can have significant effects on the developing embryo. For this reason, these approaches are often reserved for those who would undergo a pregnancy termination should failure ensue.

The use of the antiprogesterone RU 486 (mifepristone) holds promise as an effective menstrual induction agent and abortifacient. Studies of this new agent indicate that it is safe and effective in inducing "menstruation" either when taken at the time of anticipated bleeding or in the case of documented early pregnancy (induced abortion). Social and ethical considerations will affect the availability as well as the use of this or other postcoital agents.

INEFFECTIVE METHODS

Just as the clinician must provide information about effective contraception to those who request it, he or she must also counsel against routine use of less than effective techniques. Techniques such as postcoital douching, withdrawal prior to ejaculation, makeshift barriers (such as food wrap), and various coital positions should all be discouraged if pregnancy is to be avoided.

EXPERIMENTAL METHODS

Although there is very little new contraception research under way in this country, there are several options that may have a role in the future. Hormonal manipulations using gonadotropin-releasing hormone (GnRH) analogs to prevent ovulation or sperm formation may be possible. The use of implantable steroids to provide an effective male contraceptive may be perfected. Vaginal steroids in the form of vaginal rings or pessaries show some promise. Oral "antisperm" agents such as Gossypol may be perfected or point in new directions. Even such modalities as testicular heating hold possibilities. It is certain that the drive to control fertility will continue to demand much from our technology.

FURTHER READINGS

Mishell DR. Contraception, sterilization and pregnancy termination. In: Herbst AL, Mishell DR, Stenchever MA, Droegemueller W, eds. Comprehensive gynecology. St. Louis, MO: CV Mosby, 1992:295.
Oral contraception. ACOG technical bulletin. 1987;106.

The intrauterine device. ACOG technical bulletin. 1987; 104.

Wentz AC. Contraception and family planning. In: Novak's textbook of gynecology. 11th ed. Baltimore: Williams & Wilkins, 1988:204.

SELF-EVALUATION

Case 22-A

An 18-year-old nulligravid patient wants to know what is "the best method of birth control." She is not yet sexually active, although she and her boyfriend have been "close" on several occasions. The patient plans further education and correctly realizes that an unwanted pregnancy would spell disaster for her. She would not consider a pregnancy termination and the fear of pregnancy has become a problem for her and her boyfriend. Her history reveals that her periods are regular with cramping, for which she takes over-the-counter medications with some relief. She is currently taking no medications and knows of no allergies.

Question 22-A-1

In listing possible options, all of the following *might* be appropriate *except*:

A. oral contraceptives
B. vaginal spermicides
C. a diaphragm
D. an IUCD
E. rhythm

Answer 22-A-1

Answer: D

All of the methods listed might be possible for the couple to use. Given the patient's nulligravid status and history of dysmenorrhea, IUCDs are likely to be unsatisfactory.

Question 22-A-2

The patient tells you that because of her fear of pregnancy, oral stimulation has become an important part of her and her boyfriend's sexual expression. Because they may not always have control over when they might have the opportunity for intercourse, they would also like to avoid methods that interfere with spontaneity.

Based on this information, your best recommendation might be:

A. oral contraceptives
B. vaginal spermicides
C. a diaphragm
D. an IUCD
E. rhythm

Answer 22-A-2

Answer: A

Oral contraceptive pills do not interfere with spontaneity and are effective anytime the opportunity of intercourse presents itself. A diaphragm would not be a good method because it does interfere with spontaneity. The couple's preference for oral stimulation makes vaginal spermicides and diaphragms (which also use spermicides) less desirable. (These agents are not toxic, per se, but do provide an objectionable taste for most couples.) Oral contraceptives are also likely to provide relief from the patient's menstrual discomfort.

Case 22-B

A 38-year-old G3P2012 recently divorced business executive is taking a low dose monophasic oral contraceptive, which she has taken since the birth of her last child 6 years ago. She has had no particular problems and does not smoke. She is not currently dating but wishes to continue effective contraception. Her pelvic examination is normal with the exception of 10-week fibroids.

Question 22-B-1

Acceptable methods of contraception for this patient include:

A. tubal cautery
B. rhythm
C. oral contraceptives
D. condom/foam
E. IUCD

Answer 22-B-1

Answer: A, B, C, D, E

For a patient who is sexually active on a sporadic basis, a use-oriented method may provide excellent protection from pregnancy without the possible problems of an ongoing method. She is an educated, potentially motivated patient who could use foam/condom, a diaphragm, or even rhythm quite effectively. The patient's age and finding of fibroids make oral contraceptives less desirable, although not unreasonable as long as close follow-up is maintained. The decision to undergo sterilization is an option that can be discussed, but is a decision that only the patient can make. The history suggests that this option has not been chosen, although it may also not have received consideration. An IUCD is less desirable because of possible expulsion by the uterus with fibroids and the fact that she is not necessarily going to be monogamous. This case is a good example of how contraception choices must be individualized for each patient with relative risks of all alternatives discussed.

Question 22-B-2

For further consideration: What if this patient were sexually active on a regular basis? Could she continue to use the oral contraceptives? How would it affect your decision if she were a smoker? What if her partner refused to use a condom? How would you counsel her if she is "deathly afraid of AIDS?"

chapter 23

STERILIZATION

Sterilization offers highly effective birth control without continuing expense, effort, or motivation. *It is the most frequent method of controlling fertility used in the United States,* with close to a million procedures performed annually. About one in three married couples have chosen surgical sterilization as their method of contraception. Sterilization is the leading contraceptive method for couples where the wife is over 30 or for those who have been married more than 10 years.

Changes in operative techniques; anesthesia methods; and attitudes of the public, insurance providers, and physicians have all contributed to the rapid increase in the number of sterilization procedures performed each year. Modern methods of surgical sterilization are less invasive, less expensive, safer, and as effective, if not more effective, than those used 20 years ago. These factors have combined to decrease concern about the invasive nature of these procedures. *Counseling of patients must include the permanent nature of the procedures, the operative risks, and the chance of failure (pregnancy less than 1%). Despite careful counseling, approximately 1% of patients undergoing sterilization subsequently request reversal* of the procedure because of a change in marital status, loss of a child, or desire for more children. *Successful reversal occurs in only 40–60% of cases.*

All currently available surgical methods of sterilization prevent the union of sperm and egg, either by preventing the passage of sperm into the ejaculate (vasectomy), or by permanently occluding the fallopian tube (tubal ligation). The choice of which partner will undergo sterilization is generally a personal one. Although considerations of individual medical factors may affect this choice, the decision is most often based upon the motivation of the individuals involved.

STERILIZATION IN MEN

About one third of all surgical sterilization procedures are performed on men. Because the vas deferens is located outside the abdominal cavity, vasectomy is safer and generally less expensive than procedures done on women. Vasectomy is also more easily reversed than most female sterilization procedures. Vasectomy is routinely performed as an outpatient procedure, under local anesthesia. The procedure takes 15–20 minutes and consists of mobilizing the vas through a small incision in the scrotum, excision of a short segment of vas, and sealing the ends of the vas with suture, cautery, or clips. Postoperative complications include bleeding, hematomas, and local skin infections, but these occur in less than 3% of cases. Some authors report a greater incidence of depression and change in body image following vasectomy than after female sterilization. This risk may be minimized with preoperative counseling and education. Concern has been raised about the formation of sperm antibodies in approximately 50% of patients, but no adverse long-term effects of vasectomy have been identified.

Pregnancy after vasectomy occurs in about 1% of cases. Many of these pregnancies result from intercourse too soon after the procedure, rather than from recanalization. Vasectomy is not immediately effective. Multiple ejaculations are required before the proximal collecting system is emptied of sperm. For this reason, couples should use another method of contraception for 4–6 weeks or until azoospermia can be confirmed by semen analysis. Similar follow-up confirmation of efficacy is not routinely performed with female sterilization methods.

STERILIZATION IN WOMEN

Surgical sterilization techniques for women may be broadly divided into *postpartum* and *interval* (between pregnancies) *procedures*, although most techniques may be performed at either time. Factors such as parity, obesity, previous surgery or pelvic infections, and medical conditions, such as hypertension or respiratory diseases, may all affect the timing and method chosen.

Laparoscopy

The development of efficient light sources, fiberoptic light guides, and smaller instruments has led to a dramatic increase in the use of laparoscopy for female sterilization. Performed as an outpatient interval procedure, laparoscopic techniques may be carried out under either local, regional, or general anesthesia. Small incisions, a relatively low rate of complications, and a degree of flexibility in the procedures possible have led to high physician and patient acceptability.

In laparoscopic procedures, a small infraumbilical incision is made in the skin and a trocar and sheath placed into the abdominal cavity. Although most operators prefer to create a pneumoperitoneum prior to trocar placement, safe placement may also be accomplished without this step. The trocar is withdrawn and a laparoscope passed through the sheath into the abdominal cavity. For many procedures, a second, smaller trocar is passed (under direct vision) through the lower abdominal wall. A uterine manipulator is typically applied to the cervix to aid in visualizing pelvic structures and moving them into position for surgery. At the close of the procedure, the pneumoperitoneum is evacuated and the skin closed with one or two buried absorbable sutures and/or skin tapes.

Occlusion of the fallopian tubes may be accomplished through the use of electrocautery, the application of a plastic and spring clip (the Hulka clip), or Silastic band (Yoon or Falope ring) (Fig. 23.1). The choice among laparoscopic methods is often based on operator experience and training, even though there are some theoretical differences that could guide in the decision-making process. Electrocautery-based methods are fast and carry the lowest failure rates, but they carry a greater risk of inadvertent electrical damage to other structures, poorer reversibility, and a greater incidence of ectopic pregnancies when failure occurs (up to 25% of failures). The Hulka clip is the most readily reversed method because of its minimal tissue damage, but it also carries the greatest failure rate (up to 1%) for the same reason. The Falope ring falls between these two in both reversibility and failure rates, but may have a higher incidence of postoperative pain.

Laparotomy

The oldest methods of female sterilization have utilized laparotomy. Whether it is a small infraumbilical incision made in the postpartum period, or a small lower abdominal subrapubic incision (minilaparotomy) used as an interval procedure, laparotomy provides ready access to the uterine tubes. Permanent obstruction or interruption of the fallopian tubes may be then accomplished by a variety of means such as excision of all or part of the fallopian tube, or clips, rings, or cautery. Laparotomy techniques do not require the special tools or training needed for laparoscopy, which makes them attractive for many more physicians or smaller hospitals.

The most common method of tubal interruption done by laparotomy is the Pomeroy tubal ligation (Fig. 23.2). In this procedure, a segment of tube from the midportion is elevated and an absorbable ligature placed across the base, forming a loop, or knuckle, of tube.

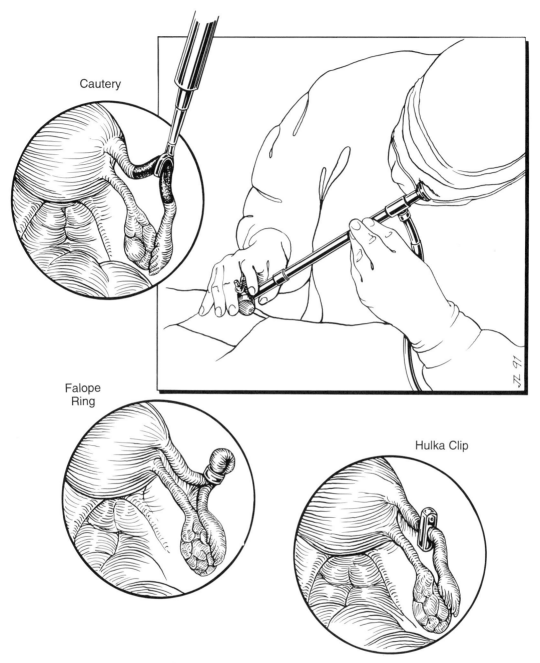

Cautery

Falope
Ring

Hulka Clip

Figure 23.1. Laparoscopic sterilization.

This is then excised and sent for histologic confirmation. When healing is complete, the ends of the tube will have sealed closed and there will be a 1–2-cm gap between the ends. *Failure* using this method is generally *in the range of one in 500 procedures*. Many modifica-

tions of this technique have been described. Burying of the proximal end of fallopian tube in the wall of the uterus (Irving method) or the broad ligament (Uchida method) have been proposed, as well as resection of the distal one third of the tube (fimbriectomy or

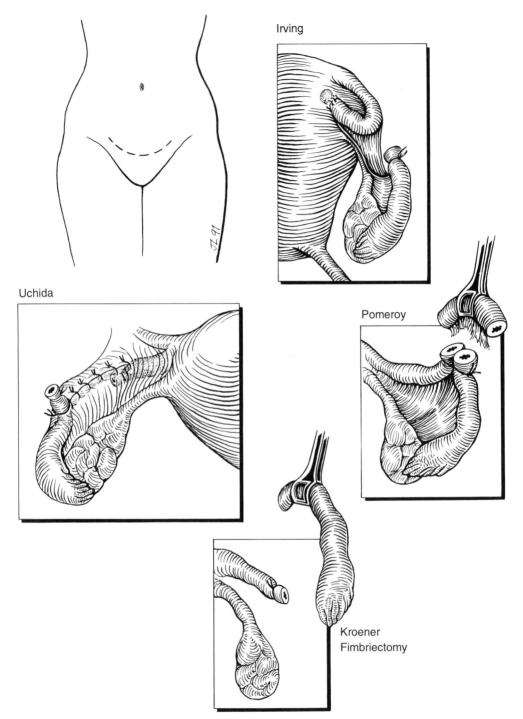

Figure 23.2. Sterilization at laparotomy.

Kroener method). These methods have acceptably low failure rates, but are not as popular as the Pomeroy technique. Electrocoagulation or the application of clips or bands may also be accomplished through a laparotomy incision, although these are more widely used via laparoscopy.

Colpotomy

The thin wall of tissue between the vaginal canal and the posterior cul-de-sac also offers a convenient port of entry into the peritoneal cavity for sterilization procedures. Although the occlusive techniques used in both laparoscopy and laparotomy may be applied to the fallopian tubes via this route, vaginal tubal procedures carry a high rate of cuff and ovarian infections if prophylactic antibiotics are not used. Vaginal tubal procedures require restrictions on intercourse and the use of tampons and douches for 2 weeks while healing takes place.

Hysteroscopy

The possibility of transcervical obstruction of the fallopian tube avoids the inherent risks in penetration of the peritoneal cavity. Methods that have been proposed include the development of formed-in-place silicon plugs, chemical cautery (e.g., phenol), or occlusive agents such as methyl cyanoacrylate. Endometrial ablation by cautery or laser has also been suggested. Although all of these procedures offer exciting possibilities, they remain in the developmental stage.

Nonsurgical Methods

A great deal of interest is currently focused on the development of permanent contraception based on nonsurgical methods. One such approach is the creation of an antipregnancy vaccine. Based on immunization to progesterone, this experimental technique appears promising. As more is learned about the biochemistry of reproduction, other alternatives may become available.

Side Effects and Complications

No surgically based technology is free of the possibility of complications or side effects. Infection, bleeding, injury to surrounding structures, or anesthetic complications may occur with any of the techniques for female sterilization listed above. Laparoscopic and hysteroscopic techniques carry risks that are unique to their special instrumentation, such as complications of trocar insertion or cervical damage, respectively. Failure of surgical sterilization occurs in 1% or less of all procedures and depends to some extent on the method chosen and operator experience.

Debate continues about the existence of a "posttubal ligation syndrome." It has been postulated that disruption of blood flow in the area of the fallopian tubes may influence ovarian function, leading to menstrual dysfunction and dysmenorrhea. Efforts to document or quantitate such an effect have not been successful and the existence of this syndrome remains conjectural.

FURTHER READINGS

Mishell DR. Contraception, sterilization and pregnancy termination. In: Herbst AL, Mishell DR, Stenchever MA, Droegemueller W, eds. Comprehensive gynecology. St. Louis, MO: CV Mosby, 1992:295.
Sterilization. ACOG technical bulletin. 1988;113.

SELF-EVALUATION

Case 23-A

A 26-year-old G3P2002 patient is in your office for a routine prenatal visit at 34 weeks gestation. She tells you that she and her husband of 8 years have decided that their family will be complete with the birth of this next child and they would like to know about sterilization options. Upon questioning, she says that she would like something done "right away, if the baby is O.K."

Question 23-A-1

Possible options for this couple include all of the following except:

A. Pomeroy tubal ligation

B. tubal electrocautery
C. Falope ring
D. vaginal tubal cautery
E. vasectomy

Answer 23-A-1

Answer: D

Because of uterine size and the rich vascular supply induced by pregnancy, vaginal tubal sterilization techniques are generally not employed within 3 months of a pregnancy. Any of the other methods, including vasectomy, would be reasonable to include in the counseling of this couple. Of the choices listed, Pomeroy tubal ligation through a small infraumbilical incision is most commonly used for the postpartum patient. Cautery or the Falope ring are usually used during interval laparoscopy procedures.

Case 23-B

A 23-year-old G2P2002 patient asks your advice in choosing a method of sterilization. She has read about the options and she presents you with a list of things she wants from her method: It should be reliable, safe, unlikely to cause future problems, quick and inexpensive, not affect libido, and "won't show."

Question 23-B-1

Which of the following should be included in your discussions with this patient? (Select all that apply.)

A. reversibility
B. operative techniques
C. anesthetic options
D. complications
E. reversible alternatives (temporary methods)

Answer 23-B-1

Answer: A, B, C, D, E

Even though a patient has "read all about" a topic, it is imperative that a full discussion be undertaken. The likelihood of disappointment, regret, hostility, and even lawsuits can be greatly reduced by insuring that the patient does, indeed, understand the ramifications of elective sterilization procedures. Each of the answers represents an important part of this counseling process, but by itself each is not sufficient to make an informed choice or provide an informed consent.

Question 23-B-2

For further consideration: How would you counsel the patient if she were 18 years old? What if she had recently undergone a difficult divorce? Would you be comfortable performing a sterilization if she had never had children?

chapter 24

DYSMENORRHEA AND CHRONIC PELVIC PAIN

Millions of hours each year are lost from school and work due to symptoms of dysmenorrhea and chronic pelvic pain. In today's society where many women work, the ability to diagnose and treat dysmenorrhea and chronic pelvic pain may be critical to a woman's economic status.

Painful menstruation (*dysmenorrhea*) may be due to clinically identifiable causes (*secondary dysmenorrhea*) or due to an excess of prostaglandins leading to painful uterine muscle activity (*primary dysmenorrhea*). The term *chronic pelvic pain* is generally applied to pelvic discomfort not solely associated with menstruation, of more than 6 months duration and of a severity sufficient to cause disability in some form.

Successful treatment of either dysmenorrhea or chronic pelvic pain requires a correct diagnosis. For most patients, this can be accomplished by a careful evaluation through history and physical examination. In some instances, evaluation using other modalities, including laparoscopy, may be needed. Once the diagnosis is established, specific and usually successful therapy may be instituted.

DYSMENORRHEA

Primary and secondary dysmenorrhea represent a source of *recurrent disability for about 10–15% of women* in their early reproductive years. It is uncommon for primary dysmenorrhea to occur during the first three to six menstrual cycles, when ovulation is not yet well established. The incidence of primary dysmenorrhea is greatest in women in their late teens to early twenties, and declines with age. Secondary dysmenorrhea becomes more common as a woman ages, as it accompanies rising prevalence of causal factors. The occurrence of either primary or secondary dysmenorrhea is not affected by childbearing.

The *causes of secondary dysmenorrhea* may be conveniently categorized into those processes that are outside the uterus, those within the wall of the uterus, and those that are internal or within the uterine cavity (see Table 24.1). The mechanism by which these processes bring about menstrual pain is generally apparent when one considers that pain anywhere in the body occurs when there is inflammation, ischemia, stretch or distention, hemorrhage, or perforation. Pain results when these processes alter pressure in or around the pelvic structures, change or restrict blood flow, or cause irritation of the pelvic peritoneum. This may occur in combination with the normal physiology of menstruation, creating discomfort, or it may arise independently with symptoms becoming more noticeable during menstruation. *When symptoms continue between menstrual periods, these processes may be the source of chronic pelvic pain.*

In patients with *primary dysmenorrhea*, no clinically identifiable cause of pain exists. Instead, there is an *excess of prostaglandin $F_{2\alpha}$* produced in the endometrium. This potent smooth muscle stimulant causes intense uterine contractions resulting in intrauterine pressures that can exceed 400 mm Hg. These prostaglandins also cause contraction in other smooth muscle, resulting in the nausea,

Table 24.1
Secondary Dysmenorrhea

Extrauterine causes
  Endometriosis
  Tumors (benign, malignant)
  Inflammation
  Adhesions
  Psychogenic (rare)
  Nongynecologic causes

Intramural causes
  Adenomyosis
  Leiomyomata

Intrauterine causes
  Leiomyomata
  Polyps
  Intrauterine contraceptive devices (IUCDs)
  Infection
  Cervical stenosis and cervical lesions

vomiting, and diarrhea reported by many women. Prostaglandin production in the uterus normally increases under the influence of progesterone, reaching a peak at, or soon after, the start of menstruation. With the onset of menstruation, formed prostaglandins are released from the shedding endometrium. In addition, the necrosis of endometrial cells provides increased substrate for prostaglandin synthesis. In addition to prostaglandin $F_{2\alpha}$, the potent smooth muscle stimulator and vasoconstrictor that is elevated in primary dysmenorrhea, prostaglandin E_2 is also produced in the uterus. Prostaglandin E_2, a potent vasodilator and inhibitor of platelet aggregation, has been implicated as a cause of primary menorrhagia.

Because of the prevalence of dysmenorrhea, every patient of reproductive age should be questioned about the presence of menstrual distress. By contrast, patients with chronic pelvic pain invariably exhibit this as their presenting complaint. The presence of one type of symptomatology (e.g., pelvic pain) does not preclude the possibility of other problems and, thus, a thorough evaluation is due each patient.

When *evaluating the patient with menstrual pain*, special attention should be paid to the patient's *history*. Patients with *primary dys-menorrhea* will present with recurrent, month-after-month, spasmodic lower abdominal pain, which occurs on the first 1–3 days of menstruation. The pain is often diffusely located in the lower abdomen and suprapubic area, with radiation around or through to the back. The pain is described as "coming and going," or labor-like. The patient will often illustrate their description with a fist opening and closing. This pain is frequently accompanied by moderate to severe nausea, vomiting and/or diarrhea. Fatigue, low backache, and headache are also common. Patients often assume a fetal position in an effort to gain relief and many will report having used a heating pad or hot water bottle in an effort to decrease their discomfort. Dyspareunia is generally not found in patients with primary dysmenorrhea, and, if present, should suggest a second cause.

In patients with *secondary dysmenorrhea*, symptoms may be slightly milder and are often more general in nature. The specific complaint that an individual patient may have will be determined by their underlying abnormality. Most frequently, a careful history will suggest the possibility of an ongoing problem and help direct further evaluations. Complaints of heavy menstrual flow, combined with pain, suggest uterine changes such as adenomyosis, myomas, or polyps. *Adenomyosis* is islands of endometrial tissue within the myometrium, resulting in a usually tender, symmetrically enlarged, "boggy" uterus. Menses are especially uncomfortable. The diagnosis is supported by exclusion of other causes of secondary dysmenorrhea, but can be definitely made only by histologic examination of a hysterectomy specimen. Pelvic heaviness or a change in abdominal contour should raise the possibility of large leiomyomata or intraabdominal neoplasia. Fever, chills, and malaise should suggest the presence of an inflammatory process. A coexisting complaint of infertility may suggest endometriosis or chronic inflammation disease. If the patient reports that her symptoms started only after placement of an intrauterine contraceptive device (IUCD), the IUCD must be regarded as the probable cause.

In patients with dysmenorrhea, the physical examination is always directed toward uncovering possible causes for secondary dysmenorrhea. The presence of asymmetry or irregular enlargement of the uterus should suggest myomas or other tumors. Symmetrical enlargement of the uterus is often found in patients with adenomyosis. Painful nodules in the posterior cul-de-sac and restricted motion of the uterus should suggest endometriosis. Restricted motion of the uterus is also found in cases of pelvic scarring from adhesions or inflammation. Thickening and tenderness of the adnexal structures due to inflammation may suggest this diagnosis as the cause of secondary dysmenorrhea. Cultures of the cervix for *N. gonorrhoeae* or *Chlamydia* may be obtained if infection is suspected.

Physical examination of patients with primary dysmenorrhea should be normal. There should be no palpable abnormalities of the uterus or adnexa, and no abnormalities should be found on speculum or abdominal examinations. Patients examined while experiencing symptoms will often appear pale and "shocky," but the abdomen will be soft and nontender, with a normal uterus.

In evaluating the patient with dysmenorrhea, the most important differential diagnosis to consider is that of secondary dysmenorrhea. Although the patient's history is often characteristic, a diagnosis of primary dysmenorrhea should not be made without a thorough evaluation to eliminate other possible causes. In patients with chronic pain, the clinician must always consider nongynecologic causes as a possibility. In some patients, a final diagnosis may not be established without invasive procedures, such as laparoscopy.

In patients with dysmenorrhea in whom no clinically identifiable cause is apparent, it is appropriate to presume a diagnosis of primary dysmenorrhea. Therapy with nonsteroidal antiinflammatory agents is generally so successful that, if some response is not evident, the diagnosis of primary dysmenorrhea should be reevaluated.

Patients with primary dysmenorrhea will generally experience exceptional pain relief through the use of nonsteroidal antiinflammatory drugs (NSAIDs). Treatments include 500 mg of mefenamic acid (Ponstel) followed by 250 mg every 4–6 hours; 1200–1600 mg of ibuprofen (Motrin) followed by 600–800 mg three times a day; or 150 mg of diclofenac (Voltaren) followed by 75 mg three times a day. Over-the-counter dosages of ibuprofen or other NSAIDs may be used in many patients with milder symptoms.

As in other areas of medicine, the best therapy is one directed toward the cause of the patient's problems. Hence, when a specific diagnosis is possible, therapy tailored to that process will be the most likely to succeed. Specific treatments for many of these processes are discussed in their respective chapters. When definitive therapy cannot be employed (e.g., in the case of a patient with adenomyosis in whom fertility is to be preserved, making hysterectomy inappropriate), symptomatic therapy in the form of analgesics and/or modification of the menstrual cycle may be effective. The dysmenorrhea may be improved with the use of low dose oral contraceptives in those patients who desire contraception and have no contraindications to their use.

CHRONIC PELVIC PAIN

The *prevalence* of chronic pelvic pain is less than that of dysmenorrhea, but still represents a source of significant disability. It is a problem that often demands a great deal of time and resources, from both physician and patient, in order to make a diagnosis and establish treatment. In these patients, the pathophysiology involved can be quite variable (Table 24.2). In some patients, the pain itself can become the disease. Indeed, in approximately one third of patients with chronic pelvic pain who undergo laparoscopic evaluation, no identifiable cause is found. However, two thirds of these patients will have potential causes identified where none was apparent prior to laparoscopy. A wide ranging, of-

Table 24.2
Chronic Pelvic Pain

Gynecologic causes	Mechanical *(continued)*
Adnexal	Obstruction (partial)
Adhesive disease	Torsion
Chronic infection	Intussusception
Chronic ectopic pregnancy	Other
Torsion of pelvic mass or organ (generally a	Neoplasia
cause of acute pain)	Parasites
Ovarian cyst (generally not painful without	
bleeding or growth)	Other causes
Uterine	Aneurysm
Fibroid tumors (uncommon cause of pain)	Musculoskeletal
Infection	Chronic back pain
Retrodisplacement (rare)	Radiculopathy
Urologic causes	Spondylolisthesis
Infection	Ankylosing spondylitis
Calculi	Strains
Tumors	Rectus hematoma
	Biochemical
Gastrointestinal causes	Sickle cell crisis/disease
Inflammatory	Acute intermittent porphyria
Chronic appendicitis	Heavy metal poisoning
Gastorenteritis	Black widow spider bites
Ulcerative colitis	Neurologic
Ulcer disease	Tabes
Irritable bowel syndrome	Herpes zoster (shingles)
Diverticulitis	Psychosocial
Mesenteric adenitis	Somatization
Biliary disease	Sleep disorders
Mechanical	Substance abuse
Constipation	Physical or sexual abuse
Herniation	Family or economic stress

ten multidisciplinary, approach to these patients will yield the best results.

The *history* reported in chronic pelvic pain can be varied. In general, it will relate to the underlying etiology. As with the evaluation of any pain, attention must be paid to the description and timing of the symptoms involved. The presence of gastrointestinal symptoms, urinary difficulties, or back problems should suggest the possibility of nongynecologic causes. The history must include a thorough medical, surgical, menstrual, and sexual history. Inquiries should be made into the patient's home and work status, social history, and family history (past and present). The patient should be questioned about sleep disturbances and other signs of depression.

As in patients with dysmenorrhea, the *physical examination* of patients with chronic pain is directed toward uncovering possible causative pathologies. The patient should be asked to indicate the location of the pain. This will act as a guide to further evaluation and provide some indication of the character of the pain by the way in which the patient points. For example, if the location of the pain is indicated with a single finger, you are probably dealing with a different process than when the patient uses a sweeping motion of the whole hand. Maneuvers that duplicate the patient's complaint should be noted, but undue discomfort avoided to minimize guarding, which would limit a thorough examination. Many of the same conditions that can cause secondary dysmenorrhea may cause chronic pain states. As in the evaluation of patients with dysmenorrhea, cervical cultures should be obtained if infection is suspected.

For most patients, a reasonably accurate differential diagnosis can be established through the history and physical examination. *At times, the wide range of differential di-*

agnoses possible in chronic pelvic pain lends itself to a multidisciplinary approach, which might include psychiatric evaluation and/or testing. Consultation with social workers, physical therapists, gastroenterologists, anesthesiologists, orthopedists, and others should be considered. The use of imaging technologies or laparoscopy may also be required to determine a diagnosis.

The evaluation should begin with the presumption that there is an organic cause for the pain. Even in patients with obvious psychosocial stress, organic pathology can and does occur. Only when other reasonable causes have been ruled out should psychiatric diagnoses such as somatization, depression, or sleep and personality disorders be entertained.

Patients with chronic pelvic pain offer a therapeutic challenge. In these patients, where pain can become the disease, care must be taken that the therapy offered does not potentiate the underlying problem. Analgesics may be used, but sparingly, and every effort must be made to reduce the risk of both emotional and physical dependence. Suppression of ovulation may be useful as either a therapeutic modality or as a diagnostic tool to assist in ruling out ovarian or cyclic processes. Surgical therapies are appropriate only when specific surgically treatable pathologies are present and thought to be the cause of the patient's complaints. Alternate treatment modalities such as transcutaneous electrical nerve stimulation (TENS), biofeedback, nerve blocks, laser ablation of the uterosacral ligaments, and presacral neurectomy may be used in selected patients. *In some cases, the physician and patient may come to the realization that the goal in treatment may not be a cure, i.e., elimination of chronic pain, but rather successful management of the symptoms.*

Patients begun on therapy for pelvic pain (dysmenorrhea or chronic pain states) should be carefully monitored for success and the possibility of complications from the therapy itself. Patients on oral contraceptives for the first time should be asked to return for follow-up after 2 months and again after 6 months. Once successful therapy is established, routine periodic health maintenance visits should continue. Patients with chronic pain should be encouraged to return for follow-up on a periodic basis, rather than only when pain is present, thus avoiding reinforcing pain behavior as a means to an end.

FURTHER READINGS

Dawood MY, McGuire JL, Demers LM, eds. Premenstrual syndrome and dysmenorrhea. Baltimore: Urban & Schwarzenberg, 1985.

Dysmenorrhea. ACOG technical bulletin. 1983;68.

Chronic pelvic pain. ACOG technical bulletin. 1989; 129.

SELF-EVALUATION

Case 24-A

An 18-year-old, virginal college student presents with the complaint of recurrent, severe menstrual distress, which begins a few hours after the onset of menstrual flow and lasts for the first 48 hours of menstruation. The pain is crampy, recurrent, and located in the lower abdomen, just above the symphysis. She occasionally experiences nausea with vomiting, but her pain is unchanged after she vomits. She has taken an over-the-counter pain reliever containing ibuprofen with only slight improvement. Her periods are regular and she is taking no other medications. Pelvic examination is difficult, but normal.

Question 24-A-1

The most likely diagnosis in this patient is:

A. leiomyomata
B. primary dysmenorrhea
C. endometriosis
D. irritable bowel syndrome
E. recurrent pelvic inflammatory disease

Answer 24-A-1

Answer: B

In a young virginal woman, the chance of leiomyomata, pelvic infection, or endometriosis is small. The patient's history offers no hint of symptoms that might be associated with irritable bowel disease and her physical examination does not offer evidence of other processes as a cause of secondary dysmenorrhea. This, combined with her typical history of crampy pain, makes primary dysmenorrhea the most likely diagnosis.

Question 24-A-2

The best therapy for this patient would be:

A. oral contraceptives
B. high bulk diet
C. Tylenol (acetaminophen) with codeine, 60 mg, q4h
D. ampicillin, 250 mg, qid. for 10 days
E. Ponstel, 250 mg, 2 at onset of pain and 1 q4–6h prn

Answer 24-A-2

Answer: E

Although the patient might get some relief from the use of oral contraceptives, unless she needs contraception, this may not be the best course of therapy. Treatment with high bulk diet or ampicillin does not appear to be supported by the patient's probable diagnosis. Even though the patient has tried NSAID therapy in the form of over-the-counter products, this is still the best option. It is likely that, in high prescription dosages, she will obtain relief. The lack of complete response is most likely due to the low dose in over-the-counter products and not necessarily to product selection. If higher dose NSAID therapy is unsuccessful, oral contraceptives should be considered, even though this patient is not sexually active.

Case 24-B

A 23-year-old, divorced mother of three, on government assistance, seeks help for symptoms of lower abdominal pain, which began 8 months ago. This coincided with her divorce and the loss of her job at a textile mill. Her pain is located in her left lower quadrant, but spreads to the right lower quadrant and to her back. The pain is worse with menstruation, bowel movements, and intercourse. She has tried multiple medications without benefit. Past history reveals an abusive marriage and two previous laparotomies for "ovarian cysts."

Question 24-B-1

Based on the most likely working diagnosis, the first examination or procedure that should be performed is:

A. laparoscopy
B. sigmoidoscopy
C. pelvic ultrasound
D. bimanual pelvic examination
E. psychological profile and depression index

Answer 24-B-1

Answer: D

Although it is very likely that this patient has some degree of depression and multiple psychosocial stresses, a physical cause must always be considered. Sigmoidoscopy and pelvic ultrasound are not indicated based on the symptoms presented. Laparoscopy is invasive and potentially carries more risk because of the patient's previous surgeries. Although it may be needed at some point in the future, it would be premature at this point. A pelvic examination offers the most information with the least risk as an initial step in evaluation of this patient with chronic pelvic pain.

Question 24-B-2

For further consideration: What if the second patient had been 45 years old with a history of repeated pelvic infections? What if she had had occasional bloody stools? Would your diagnosis be any different if she did not have any children, but had been infertile for 3 years? That is, how would your management approach change for different age patients with different histories?

chapter 25

PREMENSTRUAL SYNDROME

Premenstrual syndrome (PMS) is a group of physical, mood, and behavioral changes that occur in a regular, cyclical relationship to the luteal phase of the menstrual cycle. In affected women, these symptoms occur in most cycles, resolving near the onset of menses with a symptom-free interval of at least 1 week. They may be minimally to totally disruptive of the patient's normal daily activities and/or relationships. First described in 1931, premenstrual syndrome is still a poorly understood condition, as there is no consensus on critical issues such as its pathophysiology, its diagnostic criteria, and optimal therapies. In fact, it has been suggested that PMS is actually more than a single clinical entity. Despite these areas of confusion, it is clear that patients do present with symptoms that wax and wane in relationship to their menstrual cycles. Physicians must, therefore, be aware of potential causes for these changes, including the possibility of PMS.

INCIDENCE

Because of the wide variability in the signs and symptoms that are considered in making a diagnosis of PMS, the reported incidence of PMS is great, ranging between 10 and 90%. Severe, debilitating PMS is reported in less than 10% of patients, although 70% of all women have some physical or emotional premenstrual symptoms. PMS appears to be most prevalent in women in their thirties and forties, with a greater incidence in women with a past history of postpartum depression or other affective disorders. Accurate diagnosis is further confused by the similarity between some PMS symptoms and some psychiatric conditions.

SYMPTOMS

There have been well over 150 symptoms attributed to PMS. Each patient presents with her own constellation of symptoms, thus making specific symptomatology less important than the cyclic occurrence of the symptoms. Attempts have been made to classify PMS symptoms into subgroups, but none of these classification systems has been accepted universally. Somatic symptoms that are most common include breast swelling and pain, bloating, headache, constipation and/or diarrhea, and fatigue. The most common emotional symptoms include irritability, depression, anxiety, hostility, and changes in libido. Common behavioral symptoms include food cravings, poor concentration, sensitivity to noise, and loss of motor skills.

ETIOLOGY

Although the etiology of PMS has not yet been determined, there are many theories related to its pathogenesis. Each theory is supported by some scientific data and also explains a portion of the symptoms seen in patients. Unfortunately, *no single unified explanation accounts for the variations of PMS* seen in all patients. The theories of the basis of PMS include:

1. *Psychiatric Basis.* The high incidence of anxiety, depression, and other symptoms that simulate psychiatric disorders led to the theory that PMS is merely cyclic manifestations of underlying psychopathology.

2. *Endocrinologic Basis.* It was originally thought that PMS was related to abnormal luteal-phase steroid levels, predominantly higher estradiol levels relative to progesterone levels. Significant alterations in estradiol and/or progesterone levels have not been found. This theory remains viable, however, because of the cyclic nature of symptoms. It is known that progesterone does have a sedative effect on the central nervous system and that both estrogen and progesterone receptors exist in the brain.

3. *Endorphin Basis.* There is a relative decrease in the luteal-phase endorphin levels in some patients who suffer from PMS. Because these endogenous opiates are associated with a sense of well-being, a decline in their production is seen as a cause for some of the findings in these patients. In addition, PMS symptoms are mimicked by some symptoms of opiate withdrawal. A strong argument in favor of the endorphin basis of PMS comes from patients who describe alleviation of symptomatology when moderate exercise is undertaken, presumably because of an exercise-associated increase in endorphin production.

4. *Serotonin Basis.* Premenstrual serotonin levels in PMS patients have been reported to be lower than in control patients. Because lower serotonin levels have been associated with clinical depression, affective changes in PMS may be explained on this basis. In addition, anxiety has been described as a possible state of serotonin excess. Therefore, dysfunction in serotonin neurotransmission is an attractive explanation for many PMS symptoms.

5. *Prostaglandin Basis.* Because prostaglandins are produced in the breast, brain, gastrointestinal tract, kidney, and reproductive tract, and because these are areas that often present with physical symptoms in patients with PMS, a prostaglandin-associated basis for PMS remains attractive.

6. *Fluid Retention Basis.* Many women both with and without PMS report some premenstrual weight gain and edema. Although studies do not demonstrate an increased body weight in these patients, alterations of the renin-angiotensin-aldosterone axis as well as antidiuretic hormone have been suggested as a basis for PMS.

7. *Vitamin Basis.* Particular focus has also been placed on deficiency of vitamins A, B_6, and E as possible causes of PMS. Of note, vitamin B_6

Table 25.1
Differential Diagnosis of PMS

Psychiatric conditions	Medical conditions
Anxiety disorders	Dysmenorrhea
Major depression	Endometriosis
Bipolar disorders	Thyroid disorders
Personality disorders	Endocrinopathies
Life-circumstance disorders (marital discord, etc.)	Anemia
	Hypokalemia
Substance abuse	Lupus
Somatoform disorders (hypochondriasis, somatization disorders)	erythematosus
Eating disorders	

(pyridoxine) is a cofactor in the production of serotonin as well as prostaglandin.

8. *Others.* Other suggested bases for PMS include thyroid disorders, prolactin disorders, ovarian infection, and hypoglycemia.

DIFFERENTIAL DIAGNOSIS

Virtually any condition that results in mood or physical changes in any cyclic fashion may be included in the differential diagnosis of PMS. As a result, the physician must remain open-minded at the outset in order not to prematurely exclude the primary problem. Table 25.1 outlines the possible alternatives.

DIAGNOSIS

Because the etiology of PMS is unknown, there are no definitive historical, physical examination, or laboratory markers to aid in diagnosis. At present, the diagnosis of PMS is based upon documentation of the relationship of the patient's symptoms to the luteal phase. This is best done by *prospective documentation of symptoms using a menstrual diary* (Fig. 25.1). Since the patient's memory of daily symptoms cannot be depended upon for accuracy, she is asked to monitor and record key symptoms and their severity. To confirm the diagnosis of PMS, the patient must demonstrate a symptom-free follicular phase in contrast to the problems seen in the luteal phase.

A thorough *physical examination is necessary to rule out organic pathology* that might explain

NAME ______________________ AGE: ________ HEIGHT: ________ WEIGHT: ________

GRADING OF MENSES

0 - None
1 - Slight
2 - Moderate
3 - Heavy
4 - Heavy and clots

GRADING OF SYMPTOMS (COMPLAINTS)

0 - None
1 - Mild, present but does not interfere with activities
2 - Moderate, present and interferes with activities but not disabling
3 - Severe, disabling, unable to function

MONTH

DAY	1	2	3	4	5	6	7	8	9	10	11	12	13	14	15	16	17	18	19	20	21	22	23	24	25	26	27	28	29	30	31
Treatment Day																															
Menses																															

Nervous tension																															
Mood swings																															
Irritability																															
Anxiety																															

Weight gain																															
Swelling of extremities																															
Breast tenderness																															
Abdominal bloating																															

Headache																															
Fever, chills																															
Increased appetite																															
Heart pounding																															
Fatigue																															
Dizziness/faintness																															

Depression																															
Forgetfulness																															
Crying																															
Confusion																															
Insomnia																															

DYSMENORRHEA - PAIN

Cramps (low abdominal)																															
Muscle ache																															
Joint ache																															

Basal Weight in lbs.																															

Basal Body Temperature																															

NOTES:

SYMPTOM DIARY

Figure 25.1. Menstrual symptom diary.

some of the physical symptoms such as dysmenorrhea, cyclic pelvic pain, and breast tenderness. Otherwise, there are no specific physical findings helpful in diagnosing premenstrual syndrome.

TREATMENT

Because of the diverse symptoms of patients with PMS, a multidisciplinary team of providers including a gynecologist, psychiatrist, psychologist, endocrinologist, nutritionist, and social worker is often advocated. In addition, because the underlying pathophysiology is yet to be determined, a wide range of treatment protocols has been recommended. A major portion of any management scheme should include education of the patient as well her family in order to clarify what is known about PMS as well as what to expect from possible therapies that might be undertaken. Providing this patient education can, in and of itself, be therapeutic for patients who are otherwise lacking insight into the possible causes of their symptoms. As part of the educational process, prospective charting of symptoms not only documents the cyclic or noncyclic nature of the patient's symptoms, but also allows the patient to become a part of the diagnostic effort, thus helping her to take an active part in the diagnosis and management of her condition. Because the existence of cyclic patient symptom complexes cannot be disputed, it remains of critical importance for the physician to address the patient's specific concerns in a supportive fashion. In some cases, giving the symptoms a diagnostic label helps relieve the patient's concern that she may be "going crazy." Often a patient's symptoms will become less unbearable as she begins to understand her condition.

In addition to patient education, the following interventions have been shown to be helpful in selected groups of patients. Patients should be advised that no one therapy works for all patients and that a logical sequence of therapeutic manipulations may have to be done in order to achieve resolution of symptoms.

Diet recommendations emphasize fresh rather than processed foods. The patient is encouraged to eat more fresh fruits and vegetables and minimize refined sugars and fats. Some patients benefit by eating frequent small meals during the day rather than having three large meals, thereby minimizing hypoglycemia symptoms. Minimizing salt intake may help with bloating, and eliminating caffeine from the diet can reduce nervousness and anxiety.

Exercise has been found to be helpful in some patients, possibly by increasing endogenous production of β-endorphins.

Medications to induce anovulation have been reported to be of benefit in PMS. Since premenstrual symptoms are typically associated with ovulatory cycles, inducing an anovulatory state in women should be beneficial in many patients. This can be accomplished by using oral contraceptives, danazol, or gonadotropin-releasing hormone (GnRH) agonist. Oral contraceptives are a logical first choice for patients who also require contraception. Some patients, however, find a worsening of their symptoms when taking oral contraceptives. The use of danazol and GnRH agonist have been demonstrated to be beneficial in short-term studies, but long-term effects of either drug for PMS have not been fully evaluated. The use of either constitutes a "medical oophorectomy" and may be used as a trial before surgical therapy is undertaken.

Progesterone has been described to be effective delivered either as a vaginal or rectal suppository or as oral micronized progesterone. Although well-designed studies have not demonstrated its effectiveness, progesterone suppositories are widely used by patients who describe beneficial results.

Nonsteroidal and antiinflammatory agents have been found to be useful for symptoms other than dysmenorrhea. This is possibly related to prostaglandin production in various sites in the body.

Bromocriptine may be useful specifically for the treatment of mastodynia.

Diuretics such as spironolactone, an aldosterone antagonist, have been found helpful in controlling weight as well as some psychological symptoms. Bloating is also minimized in patients taking diuretics. Care should be taken to avoid using diuretics that might deplete the body of potassium.

Psychotropic and antidepressant medications have been widely studied and found to be useful in some patients. Alprazolam has been helpful for both physical and emotional symptoms. Serotonergic drugs such as buspirone, an anxiolytic, have been found useful, as have antidepressants such as fluoxetine.

Vitamin therapy, including administration of pyridoxine, a cofactor in the synthesis of serotonin, has been shown to be helpful in some patients. There are reported side effects including reversible peripheral neuropathy when large doses of pyridoxine are taken. Evening primrose oil, rich in vitamin E, has also been helpful in relieving both breast tenderness and depressive symptoms associated with PMS.

SELF-EVALUATION

Case 25-A

A 29-year-old G2P2 complains of periodic anxiety, depression, and irritability for 2 years. Her gynecologic history includes regular menses with mild cramps. Her breasts are also mildly tender before each period. She is presently using a diaphragm for contraception. Physical examination is normal.

Question 25-A-1

What initial evaluation(s) should be recommended?

A. pelvic ultrasound
B. psychiatric consult
C. monthly symptom calendar
D. mammogram
E. glucose tolerance test

Answer 25-A-1

Answer: C

Because of the periodic nature of these emotional symptoms, they may or may not be temporally related to the menstrual cycle. A prospective documentation of symptoms will aid in determining whether this is PMS or not. Pelvic ultrasound is unnecessary given the normal examination. A psychiatric consult may be needed if the patient's symptoms are severe, refractory to care, or causing significant emotional or interpersonal distress. A mammogram in this age group has little to offer in a patient with cyclic mastalgia. A glucose tolerance test is sometimes used to identify a patient with hypoglycemic episodes who might present with PMS-like symptoms, but would not be appropriate here.

Case 25-B

A 40-year-old G4P4 has struggled with documented PMS for several years. Despite treatments including vaginal progesterone, tranquilizers, vitamin B₆, and diuretics, she continues to have 10 days of premenstrual bloating, headaches, and mood swings. She requests a hysterectomy as definitive treatment.

Question 25-B-1

Which of the following medical therapies is most appropriate instead of hysterectomy?

A. fluoxetine
B. oral progesterone
C. bromocriptine
D. GnRH agonist
E. ibuprofen

Answer 25-B-1

Answer: D

GnRH agonist is the most appropriate of the drugs listed. The patient believes that removing the uterus will be a cure to her problems. Unfortunately, it is the ovaries, not the uterus, which may be linked with the symptoms. The uterus and monthly menses serve only as a reference point to which her symptoms are related. The GnRH can provide a temporary oophorectomy as a trial prior to any consideration for surgical oophorectomy. If the patient improves with GnRH agonist, then symptoms return when the medication is discontinued, bilateral oophorectomy with associated hysterectomy might be a consideration. All the other therapies have been utilized for patients with PMS, but will not affect the physiologic changes she is seeking. Each may have a role, however, in treatment of specific symptoms of PMS.

chapter 26

HUMAN SEXUALITY

An estimated 40% of couples have a sexual problem at some time during their relationship. Individuals not in a steady relationship experience sexual problems as well. Illness increases the frequency and often severity of these problems as well as engendering new ones. Physicians must be able to identify these problems and know whether to offer treatment or make referral to a specialist.

The first problem faced by the physician is to identify the sexual problem. By demonstrating a supportive and nonjudgmental attitude, the physician creates a sense that it is permissible to discuss sexual matters and problems. To create this kind of comfortable environment, each physician must explore his or her own attitudes about the range of sexual expressions that may be encountered, his or her own sexuality, and how to address both in a manner conducive to good patient care. In this chapter, we review some of the scientific information about sexuality and sexual dysfunction and how the primary physician may use this information to the benefit of patients.

DEVELOPMENT OF SEXUALITY

Human sexuality begins with the distribution of Y chromosomes, but thereafter the paths to an individual's present sexual status are complex. Various endocrinologic factors determine the development of the genetic sexual assignment of the individual. Overlaying this are the learned behaviors, first from parents, then siblings and peers, then by the individual's maturing evaluation of her own character. Most individuals are ultimately comfortable with a heterosexual identity, but others may choose gay/lesbian, bisexual, or asexual life-styles. Further, these sexual identities may change during the course of an adult's life. In addition, there are other sexual practices adding to the variety of situations encountered by the physician, including transvestism, sadomasochism, exhibitionism, voyeurism, and sexual experiences with animals. Whether any or all of these are considered "normal" is often as much a political/legal and theological question as it is a medical question.

HUMAN SEXUAL RESPONSE

The human sexual response, unlike the cycle-dependent estrus of lower animals, is *functionally volitional*. It is dependent on a complex interplay of emotional and physiological factors. As demonstrated in the work of William H. Masters and Virginia E. Johnson and that of Helen S. Kaplan, this variability allows considerable variety in the kinds of human sexual response (e.g., alternate sexual preferences, changes based on life-style or age, changes caused by physical or emotional disturbances, etc.) and opportunity for sexual dysfunction (e.g., vaginismus, changes associated with disease, etc.). Whatever the kind of sexual response possible for an individual, it is dependent upon two factors. First, an emotional and physical system that is sufficiently functional to allow a sexual response of some kind. Second, given a system with enough function for some response, a *sustained and sufficient sexual stimulation* to initiate the cascade of responses comprising the human sexual response. Sustained in this context means a stimulation that occurs over a long enough interval to effect arousal. Sufficient stimula-

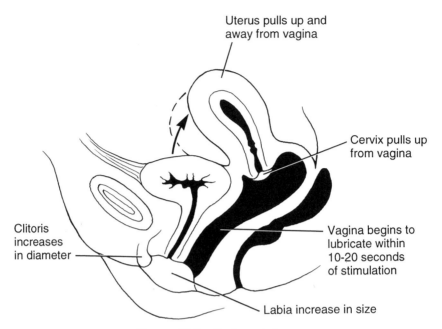

Uterus pulls up and away from vagina

Cervix pulls up from vagina

Clitoris increases in diameter

Vagina begins to lubricate within 10-20 seconds of stimulation

Labia increase in size

Figure 26.1. Excitement stage.

tion includes two parameters: physically correct and comfortable stimulation and stimulation effective enough to initiate and sustain the human sexual response. As we will see later, much of the sexual difficulties encountered in primary medical practice involve unsustained or insufficient stimulation.

With effective and sustained stimulation, the *human sexual response* may be initiated. Masters and Johnson, Kaplan, and others have demonstrated the value of considering the continuum of events comprising the human sexual response as consisting of "phases." Masters and Johnson have described four phases (excitement, plateau, orgasm, and resolution), whereas Kaplan has suggested a modification, combining the excitement and plateau phases and adding a desire phase at the start of the sexual response cycle. Both classifications are understood to be artificial in the sense that they describe highly variable components of a continuum of emotional and physiological events. The *physiological components of the human sexual response* are mediated primarily by two processes: (a) changes in muscle tone, myotonic activity, and (b) changes in blood flow, especially vasocongestion. Figures 26.1 through 26.4 demonstrate some of the physiological changes seen in these phases. The duration of each phase varies with each individual and for a given individual at different times in their life. The human sexual response is a continuum of events with no clear boundaries between the described "phases." The value of these classifications lies in their use to understand the events comprising the human sexual response and to assist in the clinical classification of sexual problems and dysfunctions.

EVALUATING SEXUAL CONCERNS
Sexual History and Physical Examination

Some patients will present with a complaint involving a sexual issue or of a specific sexual dysfunction. Relatively detailed and focused questions are appropriate early on in the history taking, as these patients, by raising their issues, have indicated a willingness to discuss them. Other patients will have a medical problem that is known to be associated with sexual issues or problems, such as concerns about ability to enjoy sex after hysterectomy.

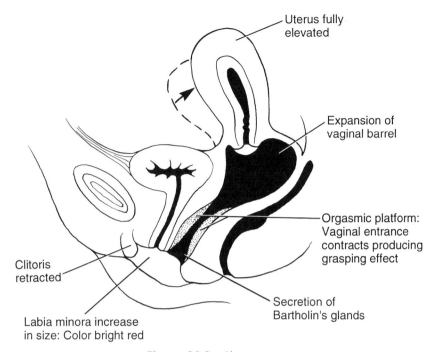

Figure 26.2. Plateau stage.

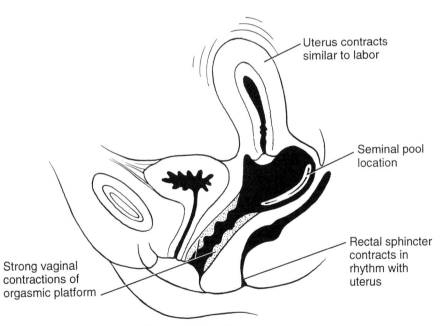

Figure 26.3. Orgasm stage.

Some of these patients will raise the related issues, whereas others will need to be carefully questioned, guiding them to a discussion of the associated sexual issue.

Many patients, however, will neither express a sexually related complaint nor have a medical problem with a commonly associated sexual issue. These patients, however, often

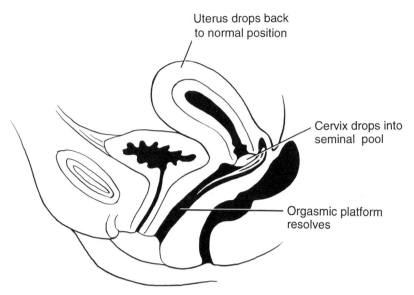

Figure 26.4. Resolution stage.

have sexually related problems, which need to be identified via the "sexual history" portion of the routine medical history. Introductory, nonobtrusive screening questions are useful. "How are things sexually?" "Do you have questions about sexual issues?" A question that gives much permission to discuss issues is: "Is there any way you would like your sex life to be different?"

The sexual history taken by the sex therapist is detailed and highly focused. For the primary care physician, its purposes are less ambitious and two in content. First, it should convey to the patient a sense of comfort and trust that the physician regards sexuality and related issues as a legitimate part of health care. This is facilitated by the physician's general behavior, but also more specifically by care to listen carefully for hints of sexually related issues followed by nonobtrusive questions that give the patient "permission" to discuss her problems. If a patient perceives the physician as harboring prejudice toward sexual values or issues, communication is doomed to failure. Second, the physician should obtain enough information to determine if a sexual problem exists and whether it is appropriate to treat the patient or to refer her for more specialized care.

Physical examination "for" sexually related issues is based on an excellent basic gynecologic examination. For example, dyspareunia in a young woman might be associated with extensive endometriosis or adhesions following PID and, in an older woman not on hormone replacement therapy (HRT), with atrophic vaginitis. Detailed "sexiological" examinations involving sexual evaluation, education, and counseling are appropriately reserved for sex therapists.

Barriers to Evaluating Sexual Problems

There are many barriers between the patient with a sexuality-related problem and effective care. One of the less discussed but potentially difficult barriers occurs *when the physician is uncomfortable with his or her own sexuality and/ or sexual issues*, conveying this discomfort to the patient so that she, in turn, is unable to discuss her problems. A task for each physician is to review his or her own attitudes and feelings about sexual issues, seeking help when needed to resolve them at least within the context of the professional relationship. A related barrier occurs *when the physician feels inadequately prepared in knowledge or skills or has insufficient* time to deal appropriately with a sexual problem. In this situation, the physician may directly or indirectly avoid identification of such problems. This barrier can be avoided by obtaining sufficient information and evaluation/management skills to identify a sexual problem, then treating the small number of problems amenable to limited care by a primary physician and referring the majority of problems to those with special training in sexual therapy.

Managing Sexual Problems

Some sexual problems/dysfunctions can be managed by the primary physician, whereas others are best referred immediately to a specialist in sex therapy. In general, single disorders of less than 1 year's duration in the context of a stable relationship are more likely to be amenable to simple interventions by a primary physician. Conversely, those patients whose dysfunction is comprised of multiple disorders, is of greater than a year's duration, and/or is in the context of a unstable relationship are usually best referred to a sex therapist. In addition, it is useful to determine whether a sexual complaint/dysfunction is primary (present throughout the patient's lifetime) or secondary (began after an interval of satisfactory sexuality) and whether it is constant (occurs in all situations, with all partners) or situational (occurs in some situations, with some partners). In general, dysfunctions that are secondary and/or situational are more easily and successfully treated than those that are primary and/or constant. The former often involve simple problems causing sexual stimulation to not be effective or sustained enough. Careful history taking to determine the problem and counseling will often relieve the barrier to effective, sustained stimulation and return the couple to satisfactory sexuality. Finally, it is also useful to determine where the dysfunction occurs in the human sexual response cycle. Sexual dysfunctions that occur in the later phases of the human sexual response cycle also tend to be easier to treat, with better outcomes expected,

whereas in general those occurring in the desire or early excitement phases are often composed of emotional and physical factors complexly interrelated. Patients with complex problems are best referred to a qualified sex therapist.

The *PLISSIT model for treatment of sexual problems* is useful for the primary care physician who chooses to treat a sexual problem along the guidelines noted and has sufficient although limited time for treatment. **P** *is permission*, giving the patient explicit or implicit permission to deal with sexual issues or problems. It also includes permission for normal behavior such as the normal exploration of sexuality via masturbation during the teen years. **LI** *is limited information*, providing the patient with pertinent limited amounts of useful information. In the former case, learning that limited masturbation is normal and not harmful facilitates the permission. **SS** *is specific suggestion*, giving the patient one or two specific suggestions for action. For example, following childbirth some couples have less satisfaction with coitus because the woman's vaginal walls are less elastic or the muscles looser than previously. Teaching the patient Kegel exercises to strengthen these muscles may alleviate this complaint. **IT** *is intensive therapy*, which in the context of the primary care physician means referral to a specialist in sexual therapy. Examples would be therapy for orgasmic dysfunction, male sexual dysfunction, dyspareunia, etc.

FURTHER READINGS

Annon J. Behavioral treatment of sexual problems: brief therapy. New York: Harper & Row, 1976.

Hammond DC. Screening for sexual dysfunction. Clin Obstet Gynecol 1984;27:732.

Reamy KJ. Sexual counseling for the nontherapist. Clin Obstet Gynecol 1984;27:781.

Reamy KJ, White SF. Sexuality in pregnancy and the puerperium: a review. Obstet Gynecol Surv 1985;40: 1–13.

Steege JF. Sexual function and dysfunction. In: Clarke-Pearson DL, Dawood MY, eds. Green's gynecology: essentials of clinical practice. 4th ed. Boston: Little, Brown & Co., 1990:Chapter 21.

SELF-EVALUATION

For each of the following situations, imagine yourself a primary care physician in a small town practice. You have been presented or discovered a sexual problem and taken a brief but reasonably complete history of the problem and a general sexual history. You must now decide whether to treat the patient yourself (A), perhaps using the PLISSIT model, or refer the patient to a specialist in the treatment of sexual problems (B).

Chose the possible answers:

A. Treat
B. Refer

Case 26-A

Your patient has been married for 6 months after a courtship of 2 years. At first, her marriage was fine, but now, with two new jobs and a first new home, she and her husband just aren't enjoying sex like they did before marriage. They are worried that something is wrong with them or that perhaps they made a mistake in getting married.

Answer 26-A

Answer: A

It is reasonable to treat this couple with the PLISSIT model. The most likely problems are inappropriate expectations of each other and of marriage, exhaustion, and coping with new and worrisome responsibilities. If permission, limited information, and perhaps specific suggestions are ineffective, referral would then be appropriate.

Case 26-B

After 6 years of marriage to her policeman husband, your patient is worried about her femininity, i.e., whether she is normal. Despite a vigorous and previously quite satisfactory sex life, she is unable to have multiple orgasms with her husband during intercourse. Both she and her husband are worried. Their relationship is strained; sex is now a feared chore.

Answer 26-B

Answer: A

Limited information from the PLISSIT model will help this couple understand that multiple orgasm is a possibility but not a requirement for all people for every sexual encounter. Permission to continue their previously satisfactory sex life should be helpful.

Case 26-C

Your patient has been at college for a year now, but has been unable to enjoy herself on a date, just as throughout high school. She "knows" that at her age she should enjoy sex, but it is simply repulsive to think about being touched by a man. She is afraid of her future, afraid she may actually be a lesbian, although she is aware of no more positive feelings about women then she has for men.

Answer 26-C

Answer: B

Whatever problems this young woman has, they are of long duration and by definition complex. The PLISSIT model helps in this case by allowing you to give her permission to be afraid, limited information that she can receive help, and referral for therapy.

chapter 27

VULVITIS AND VAGINITIS

Patients with vulvitis or vaginitis may present with acute, subacute, or indolent symptoms, which can range in intensity from minimal to incapacitating. Although generally nonspecific, the patient's history and symptoms may point to chemical, allergic, or other causes rather than infection. Irritation of the well-innervated tissues of the vulva often leads to intense pruritus. Edema, induration, and localized lesions, such as seen in herpes infection, may also be present (Table 27.1).

Vaginal secretions are always present to some extent, with the amount and character of these secretions dependent on the influence of chemical, mechanical, or pathologic conditions. Understanding the physiologic processes responsible for both normal and abnormal discharge will make the diagnosis of vulvitis and vaginitis more accurate.

The physician must be meticulous in the evaluation of these patients. There must be a careful history taken, including hygiene and sexual practices, and a thorough physical examination. The physician must also be familiar with office and laboratory methods for establishing the diagnosis. Inaccurate diagnosis or overtreatment of a physiologic condition is doomed to fail and may even make the patient worse.

The vulva and vagina are covered by stratified squamous epithelium. The vulva, but not the vagina, contains hair follicles and sebaceous, sweat, and apocrine glands. The epithelium of the vagina is nonkeratinized and lacks these specialized elements. The skin of the vulva is also vulnerable to secondary irritations such as from vaginal secretions, or contact with external irritants (such as soap residue, perfumes, fabric softeners, or infestation by pinworms).

Table 27.1
Clinical Aspects of Common Vaginal Infections

Characteristic	Physiologic	Gardnerella	Candidiasis	Trichomoniasis
Discharge				
Amount	Slight	Moderate	Variable	Moderate
Color	Yellow-white	Gray-white	White	Yellow-**green**[a]
Odor	−	+ + +	−	+
Character	Thin	Thin	**Thick, curdy**	**Frothy**
pH	**3.5–4.5**	**5–5.5**	**4–5**	**6–7**
Symptoms				
Itching	−	−	+ + + +	±
Burning	−	+	+ +	+
Findings				
Gross	Normal	Minimal erythema	Erythema, excoriation	**Petechiae**
Microscopic	**Few WBCs**	**"Clue Cells"**	**Mycelia on KOH**	***Trichomonas***

[a]Boldface items are of particular help in making a differential diagnosis.

VULVITIS

Vulvar irritation and itching are the reason for approximately 10% of all outpatient visits to gynecologists. Erythema, edema, and skin ulcers are all indications of possible *infection*. Ulcerative lesions should suggest the possibility of sexually transmitted disease such as *herpes or syphilis*. Other diseases, such as *Crohn's disease*, may also present in this manner. Papillary lesions suggest *condyloma acuminatum or Condyloma latum*. Screening should be done carefully for these and other sexually transmitted diseases. Excoriation caused by the patient's scratching, and fissuring of the skin of the vulva are often seen in vulvar irritation secondary to vaginal discharge. This must be investigated as a sign of vaginal infection.

Diffuse reddening of the vulvar skin accompanied by itching and/or burning, but without obvious cause, should suggest a *secondary allergic vulvitis*. The list of possible local irritants can be quite extensive, including feminine hygiene sprays, deodorants, tampons or pads (especially those with deodorants or perfumes), tight-fitting synthetic undergarments, colored or scented toilet paper, and laundry soap or fabric softener residues. Even locally used contraceptives or "sexual aides" may be the source of irritation. A careful history, combined with the removal of the suspected cause, will usually both confirm the diagnosis and constitute the needed therapy. In rare cases, the use of hydrocortisone cream may be needed to decrease the local inflammatory response. The possibility of a local *Candida infection*, which can mimic these symptoms, should be ruled out, especially in cases that do not respond or in patients with risk factors such as diabetes.

Allergic *causes of vulvitis* are also frequently found in the occasional pediatric patient who presents with vulvovaginal itching. However, the investigation in these cases must also include sources of irritations such as foreign bodies (especially with an accompanying vaginitis or discharge), sexual abuse, or pinworms.

In older patients, intense itching of the vulva may occur because of *atrophic changes* brought on by reduced estrogen levels. There will be a symmetrically reddened, smooth, and somewhat shiny look to the skin of the vulva and perineum. Biopsy will reflect the hypoplastic nature of this condition and will help to differentiate this from *lichen sclerosus*, which has a similar appearance. When atrophic change is the cause, estrogen replacement, either locally or systemically, is the treatment of choice. In the case of lichen sclerosus, local application of 2% testosterone cream is generally effective.

Vulvar itching may be caused by infestation with *Pthirus pubis* (*the crab louse*) or *Sarcoptes scabiei* (*the itch mite*). This is especially true when itching of the mons is part of the patient's complaint. The diagnosis is generally made by looking for small black specks (excreta) on the skin, or nits and eggs on hair shafts. Local treatment with two applications of a γ-benzene hexachloride lotion (Kwell) is generally successful.

VAGINITIS

The most common symptom associated with infections of the vagina is discharge. *Discharge from the vagina is normal physiologically; therefore, not all discharges from the vagina indicate infection*. This distinction is important to the diagnostic process, but occasionally difficult for the patient to understand or accept.

Vaginal secretions arise from several sources. The majority of the liquid portion consists of mucus from the cervix. A very small amount of moisture is contributed by endometrial fluid, exudates from accessory glands such as the Skene's and Bartholin's glands, and from vaginal transudate. Exfoliated squamous cells from the vaginal wall give the secretions a white to off-white color and provide some increase in consistency. The action of the indigenous vaginal flora also can contribute to the secretion. These components together constitute the normal vaginal secretions that provide the physiologic lubrication that prevents drying and irritation. The amount and character of this mixture vary under the influence of many factors, including hormonal and fluid status, pregnancy, immunosuppression, and inflammation. *Asymptomatic women produce, on the average, about 5 g of vaginal fluid per day. Normal vaginal secretions have no odor.*

After puberty, increased levels of glycogen in the vaginal tissues favor the growth of lactobacilli in the genital tract. These bacteria break down glycogen to lactic acid, lowering the pH from the 6–8 range, which is common before puberty (and after menopause), to the *normal menstrual vaginal pH range of 3.5–4.5.* In addition to the lactobacilli, a wide range of other aerobic and anaerobic bacteria may normally be found in the vagina at concentrations of 10^8 to 10^9 colonies per milliliter of vaginal fluid.

Increased vaginal discharge is associated with an identifiable microbiologic cause in 80–90% of cases. Hormonal or chemical causes account for most of the remaining cases. Most vaginal infections are caused by three infective agents: synergistic bacteria (bacteria vaginosis, nonspecific vaginitis), fungi (candidiasis), and protozoa, i.e., *Trichomonas* (trichomoniasis). Bacterial infections account for approximately 50% of infections, whereas fungi and *Trichomonas* account for roughly 25% each. Through gentle examination and simple microscopic investigation, the etiology of the patient's symptoms can be generally ascertained. *The value of microscopic examination of vaginal smears cannot be overstated. For this reason, any patient who complains of a vaginal discharge or irritation should be evaluated directly before therapy is suggested.*

Bacterial Vaginosis

Bacterial vaginosis is a diagnosis that has undergone a great deal of change and debate in the last few years. Once thought to be caused by the infection of *Gardnerella vaginalis* (formerly called *Haemophilus* or *Corynebacterium vaginale*), most now feel that bacterial vaginosis is actually *a symbiotic infection of anaerobic bacteria* (*Bacteroides* sp., *Peptococcus* sp., and *Mobiluncus* sp.) *and Gardnerella*, both of which contribute to the clinical findings.

Women with bacterial vaginosis generally complain of a *"musty" or "fishy" odor with an increased thin, gray-white to yellow, discharge.* The discharge may cause some mild vulvar irritation, but this is present in only about one fifth of the cases. On examination, the vaginal discharge will be found to be mildly adherent to the vaginal wall and have a pH of 5.0–5.5. Mixing some of these secretions with KOH (10%) will liberate amines that may be detected by their fishy odor (positive "whiff test"). Microscopic examination made under saline wet mount will show a slight increase in white blood cells, clumps of bacteria, and characteristic *"clue cells,"* which are epithelial cells with numerous bacilli attached to their surface, making them appear to have indistinct borders and a "ground glass" cytoplasm.

Bacterial vaginosis may be *treated* with oral metronidazole (500 mg twice a day for 7 days) or clindamycin (300 mg p.o. b.i.d. for 7 days). Because bacterial vaginosis may be transmitted sexually, treatment of the sexual partner(s) of patients with frequent recurrences should be considered.

Trichomonas Vaginitis

Trichomonas vaginalis is a flagellate protozoan that *lives only in the vagina, Skene's ducts, and male or female urethra* and may be freely transmitted by sexual intercourse. More than 60% of partners of women with *Trichomonas* infections will have a positive culture. Despite the large number of cases of symptomatic vaginitis caused by the organism, up to one half of women with *Trichomonas* in the vaginal canal are asymptomatic. *Symptoms* of *Trichomonas* infection vary from mild to severe and may include vulvar itching or burning, copious discharge with rancid odor, dysuria, and dyspareunia. Although not present in all women, the *discharge* associated with *Trichomonas* infections is generally "frothy," thin, and yellow-green to gray in color, with a pH of 6–6.5 or above. *Examination* may reveal edema or erythema of the vulva. Characteristic petechia, or strawberry patches, in the upper vagina or on the cervix, are found in about 10% of patients.

The *diagnosis* is confirmed by *microscopic examination* of vaginal secretions suspended in normal saline. This wet smear will show large numbers of mature epithelial cells, white blood cells, and the *Trichomonas* organism. *Trichomonas* is a fusiform protozoa just slightly larger than a white blood cell. The organism has three to five flagella extending from the narrow end. These flagella produce active movement that may facilitate identification of the organism.

Treatment of *Trichomonas* infections is by oral metronidazole. Because *Trichomonas* is very sensitive to *metronidazole*, 1-day therapy with 1 g in the morning and 1 g at bedtime will generally give a 90% cure rate. Treatment with 250 mg every 8 hours for 7 days or 2 g orally at one time will give comparable results. Many physicians prefer the single-day therapy because of its reduced cost and greater compliance. Debate continues with respect to treating asymptomatic partners of women with *Trichomonas* infections. If treatment is undertaken, the single-day therapy outlined above is usually adequate. Abstinence from alcohol use when taking metronidazole is necessary to avoid a possible disulfiram-like reaction. The use of metronidazole during pregnancy is not recommended because of reports of teratogenic effects. Many physicians, however, use the drug in the latter half of pregnancy for highly symptomatic patients.

Even though the pH generally associated with *Trichomonas* infections is different from that found with bacterial vaginosis, there are estimates of up to *a 25% prevalence of bacterial vaginosis in those patients with Trichomonas.* Because of the overlap in metronidazole therapy for these two conditions, this debate is not significant for most patients. It may, however, be worthy of consideration in patients who receive alternative therapies or those with frequent recurrences of "vaginal infections."

Although follow-up examination of patients with *Trichomonas* for test of care is often advocated, they are not cost-effective except in the rare patient with a history of frequent recurrences. In these patients, reinfection or poor compliance must be considered.

Candida (Monilial) Vaginitis

Monilial infections of the vagina are caused by *ubiquitous, airborne fungus.* Ninety percent of "yeast" infections are caused by *Candida albicans* with less than 10% caused by *C. glabrata, C. tropicalis,* or *Torulopsis glabrata.* *Candida* infections generally do not coexist with other infections and are not considered to be sexually transmitted even though 10% of male partners have concomitant penile infections. Candidiasis is more likely to occur in women who are pregnant, diabetic, obese, immunosuppressed, on oral contraceptives or corticosteroids, or have had broad-spectrum antibiotic therapy. Practices that keep the vaginal area warm and moist, such as wearing tight clothing or the habitual use of panty liners, may also increase the risk of *Candida* infections.

The most common presenting complaint for women with candidiasis *is itching*, although up to 20% of women may be asymptomatic. Burning, external dysuria, and dyspareunia are also common. The vulva and vaginal tissues will often be bright red in color and excoriation is not uncommon in severe cases. A thick, *adherent, "cottage cheese" discharge* with a *pH of 4–5* is generally found. *This discharge is odorless.*

The *diagnosis* of candidiasis is based on history and physical findings, and confirmed by the identification of hyphae and buds in wet mounts of vaginal secretions made with 10% KOH solution, which lyses most epithelial and white cells. There is no direct correlation between the degree of symptoms and the number of organisms present. Because false-negative wet preps are not uncommon, culture confirmation may be obtained using Nickerson's or Sabouraud's mediums.

Treatment of *Candida* infections is primarily with the topical application of one of the synthetic imidazoles: miconazole, clotrimazole, butoconazole, ketoconazole, or terconazole. These agents will give good cure rates after 3–7 days of treatment. Despite greater than 90% relief of symptoms with these therapies, 20–30% of patients will experience *recurrences* after 1 month. Treatments based on nystatin or povidone-iodine have proven to be less effective than the imidazoles. Resistant strains of *C. tropicalis* or *T. glabrata* may respond to therapy with terconazole or gentian violet. Treatment with oral agents or treatment of the male partner have not been effective in reducing the rate of recurrent infection. Patients with frequent recurrences should be carefully evaluated for possible risk factors such as diabetes or immune defects. For particularly susceptible patients, prophylactic local therapy with an antifungal agent should be considered when systemic antibiotics are prescribed.

"Chronic Vaginitis"

A problem for both physicians and patients is "chronic or recurrent vaginitis." Patients complain, often bitterly, of persistent vaginal discharge, odor, or both, without a readily identifiable cause or satisfactory response to treatment. These patients have frequently "tried everything," prescribed by several physicians, without success. A careful history must be obtained covering medical conditions and sexual and hygienic habits. A methodical physical examination and microscopic evaluations are also required.

In addition to the usual causes, one must evaluate alternative explanations for the patient's complaints. Victims of sexual assault (recent or past) may present in this manner. A frank explanation of the possibility of reinfection must be carried out in individuals with true recurrent infections. The existence of additional sexual contacts for the patient or her partner should be explored in an appropriately nonjudgmental way. Alternate sources of excessive vaginal moisture, such as

chronic cervical infections, must be evaluated. When the patient's complaints seem to exceed her physical and microscopic findings, the possibility of inappropriate expectations, inaccurate information, or psychologic dysfunction must be entertained.

FURTHER READINGS

Sweet RL, Gibbs RS. Infections of the female genital tract. 2nd ed. Baltimore: Williams & Wilkins, 1990.
Vulvovaginitis. ACOG technical bulletin, 1989;135.

SELF-EVALUATION

Case 27-A

A 36-year-old G3P2012 patient calls and states that she has one of her "yeast infections" again. She has just moved to the area, but her former physician would usually "just call something in" and she would like you to prescribe an antifungal agent. Upon further questioning, you find that the patient is experiencing vulvar itching, mild dysuria, a thick discharge, and a mild vaginal odor.

Question 27-A-1

The most appropriate initial action would be to:

A. prescribe miconazole suppositories for 3 days
B. prescribe metronidazole 1 g b.i.d. for 1 day
C. ask the patient to come in for an examination
D. refer the patient to the local STD clinic
E. prescribe oral nystatin therapy

Answer 27-A-1

Answer: C

Even though this patient may have a recurrent yeast infection, the symptoms of vaginal infections overlap to such a great extent that only a thorough evaluation (history, physical, and microscopic investigation) will reliably establish the diagnosis. Without a correct diagnosis, any therapy has the potential to either fail or make the patient worse. Especially in a patient whom you have never examined, treatment based on examination is appropriate rather than calling in a prescription.

Case 27-B

A 54-year-old patient comes to your office with the complaint of "vaginal itching." The patient is in good health and on no medications except for a mild diuretic for hypertension. Her last menstrual period was 3 years ago and she has recently begun experiencing mild hot flashes. On examination the patient's vulva is red but no edema is noted. The area of the Bartholin's glands appears to be normal. The vaginal canal is also slightly reddened and a small amount of slightly thickened discharge may be obtained from the vaginal apex.

Question 27-B-1

Which of the following tests performed on the vaginal secretions would *not* be of assistance in this case:

A. whiff test
B. 10% KOH wet prep
C. culture on Nickerson's medium
D. culture for bacteria
E. saline wet prep

Answer 27-B-1

Answer: D

The vagina is normally populated by many species of bacteria and, hence, culture of vaginal secretions for bacteria provides little useful information. Although it is likely that this patient is experiencing atrophic vulvitis and/or vaginitis, candidiasis or other infections are also possible and must be excluded by other means.

Case 27-C

A 22-year-old newlywed comes to your office with the complaint of vaginal "wetness" and excessive odor, which began 3 days ago. She notes that the vaginal "wetness" stains her underwear yellow. She notes some mild vulvar irritation, but no dysuria or dyspareunia. Physical examination shows diffuse redness of the vulva and vagina, with a copious amount of a yellow to gray discharge on the vaginal walls. Saline wet prep shows the following: 3+ epithelium, 2+ WBCs, 1+ motile sperm, moderate small rods, and occasional motile protozoa.

Question 27-C-1

The most likely diagnosis is:

A. mechanical vulvitis
B. contact dermatitis
C. bacterial vaginosis
D. trichomonas vaginitis
E. monilial vaginitis

Answer 27-C-1

Answer: D

The finding of motile protozoa is pathognomonic for a *Trichomonas* infection. Although each of the other options had to be considered initially, the microscopic findings establish the diagnosis in this case.

Question 27-C-2

For further consideration: What do you tell this patient about how she may have acquired this infection? Do you treat her husband? If so, should you examine him first? What do you tell him? What are her risks for other infections?

chapter 28

SEXUALLY TRANSMITTED DISEASES

Sexually transmitted diseases run the gamut from vaginitis to a life-threatening disease such as acquired immunodeficiency syndrome (AIDS). The increasing prevalence of sexually transmitted disease has resulted in increased awareness and, in some cases, even changes in attitudes about acceptable behaviors and standards. The impact of sexually transmitted diseases for the individual and for society cannot be overlooked or overemphasized. Although some of these diseases can be acquired though nonsexual means, sexual transmission represents the major route by which most are spread.

The impact of changing sexuality has had far-reaching implications, not the least of which has been the explosive increase in the number and types of sexually transmitted diseases. In recent years, there has been an increase of approximately 30% in the reported number of cases of syphilis. The physician must be alert to the possibility of sexually transmitted disease in all patients, perform diagnostic evaluations and institute appropriate treatments promptly, and attempt to educate patients regarding the risks involved in today's sexually open society (Table 28.1).

HISTORY AND PHYSICAL EXAMINATION

The sexual habits and modes of expression that individuals choose will affect their risk of infection, as well as the site and presentation by which infection is manifest. For this reason, a detailed sexual history is important for all patients, and invaluable for any in whom a sexually transmitted disease is either likely or suspected. Most of these infections require skin-to-skin contact or exchange of body fluids for transmission. Nonsexual activities that meet these criteria may also put the patient at risk.

All patients who are (or might be) sexually active should be examined with an awareness of the possibility of sexually transmitted disease. This is not a condemnation of the patient's life-style or personal choices, but rather a simple fact of life in today's society. The inguinal region should be inspected for rashes, lesions, and adenopathy. The vulva should be inspected for lesions, ulcerations, or abnormal discharge and palpated for thickening or swelling. The Bartholin's glands, Skene's ducts, and urethra cannot be overlooked. In patients with urinary symptoms, the urethra should be gently "milked" to express any discharge. The vagina and cervix must be inspected for lesions and abnormal discharge. When suspicion or risk is high, cultures of the urethra and cervix for gonorrhea, chlamydia, or other infections should be obtained. Lastly, the perineum and perianal areas must also be evaluated for signs of sexually transmitted diseases (Table 28.2). Cultures of the rectum for gonorrhea should be obtained in those patients who en-

Table 28.1
Most Common Sexually Transmitted Diseases (1987)

Herpes	20,000,000
Chlamydia	4,500,000
Gonorrhea	780,905
Human papilloma virus[a]	700,000
Syphilis	86,545
AIDS (women)[a]	7,523

[a]1989.

269

Table 28.2
Genital Lesions in Sexually Transmitted Diseases[a]

	Herpes	Genital warts	Syphilis	Chancroid	LGV[b]	Granuloma inguinale
Organism	Herpes simplex virus	Human papilloma virus	Treponema pallidum	Haemophilus ducreyi	Chlamydia trachomatis	Calymmato- bacterium granulo- matis
Incubation	3–7 days	1–8 months	10–60 days	2–6 days	1–4 weeks	8–12 weeks
Primary lesion	**Vesicle**	Papule/ polypoid	Papule (chancre)	Papule/ pustule	Papule/ pustule/ vesicle	Papule
Number	**Multiple coalesce**	Variable	1	1–3	Single	Single or multiple
Pain	**Yes**	No	**Rare**	**Often**	No	**Rare**
Shape	Regular	Irregular	Regular	Irregular	Regular	Regular
Margins	Flat	Raised	Raised	**Red, under- mined**	Flat	**Rolled, elevated**
Depth	Superficial	Raised	Superficial	**Excavated**	Superficial	Elevated
Base	Red, smooth	Normal, pink, white	Red, smooth	**Yellow, gray**	Variable	Red, **rough**
Induration	None	None	**Firm**	Rare, soft	None	**Firm**
Secretions	Serous	None	Serous	**Purulent, hemor- rhagic**	Variable	Rare, hemor- rhagic
Lymph nodes	Firm, tender	**Normal**	Firm, nontender	Tender, suppurative	Tender, suppurative	Pseudoade- nopathy
Duration	5–10 days, **recurrent**	Months	Weeks	Weeks	Days	Weeks

[a]Scabies, molluscum contagiosum, *Candida*, and other dermatologic conditions (e.g., hidradenitis suppurativa) may also cause genital lesions. Boldfaced items are of particular help in making a differential diagnosis.
[b]LGV, lymphogranuloma venereum.

gage in anal intercourse. For completeness, the oral cavity, as well as cervical and other lymph nodes, must be evaluated. The findings obtained by this process, combined with the patient's history, will generally make the establishment of the proper diagnosis much easier. Furthermore, the sexual partner(s) of patients diagnosed with or suspected of having a sexually transmitted disease (STD) should receive their own evaluation. It is vital to remember that *20–50% of patients with a sexually transmitted disease have one or more co-existing infections. When one venereal disease is found, others must be suspected.*

HERPES GENITALIS

Herpes simplex virus infection of the genital tract represents *one of the most common sexually acquired diseases.* Private patient office visits for this infection have increased tenfold in the past 10 years. It is estimated that there are approximately 500,000 new cases each year. Herpes simplex infections are *highly contagious.* Roughly 75% of sexual partners of infected individuals will themselves contract the disease.

The development of the *classic vesicular lesions is often preceded by a prodromal phase* of mild paresthesia and burning beginning approximately 2–5 days after infection in symptomatic patients. This will progress to very *painful vesicular and ulcerated lesions 3–7 days after exposure.* Dysuria due to vulvar lesions, or urethral and bladder involvement, may lead to urinary retention. Roughly 10% of patients with initial lesions will require hospitalization for pain control or management of urinary complications. Primary infections are also characterized by malaise, low grade fever, and inguinal adenopathy in 40% of patients. Aseptic meningitis with fever, headache, and meningismus can be found in some patients 5–7 days after the appearance of the genital lesions. This generally resolves over the period of a week.

Physical findings consist of clear vesicles, which lyse and progress to shallow, painful ulcers with a red border. These may coalesce and frequently become secondarily infected and necrotic. These lesions may be found on the vulva, vagina, cervix, or perineal and perianal skin, often extending onto the buttocks. There are recurrent lesions in roughly 30% of patients, which are similar in character, but milder in severity and shorter in duration than primary lesions.

The *diagnosis* of herpetic infections is made based on the characteristic history and physical findings. The diagnosis may be confirmed through the use of *viral cultures* taken by swab from the lesions. This is the most sensitive method of diagnosis and allows confirmation in as little as 48 hours. Scrapings from the base of vesicles may be stained by immunofluorescence techniques for the presence of viral particles. This technique is faster and carries approximately 80% agreement with culture results. *Smears* may also be stained with Wright's stain to visualize the characteristic giant multinucleated cells with eosinophilic intranuclear inclusions. The lesions of herpes simplex infections should be easily distinguished from the ulcers found in chancroid, syphilis, or granuloma inguinale by their appearance and extreme tenderness.

The *management of genital herpes* infections is generally directed toward the management of local lesions and symptoms. When treating initial infections, the lesions should be kept clean and dry. Sitz baths, followed by drying with a heat lamp or hair dryer, work well for this purpose. Occasionally, the use of a topical anesthetic, such as 2% Xylocaine jelly, may be required. If secondary infections occur, therapy with a local antibacterial cream such as Neosporin may be of help. Acyclovir 5% ointment may be applied to the lesions every 3 hours and is recommended to decrease the duration of symptoms and viral shedding. Unfortunately, this therapy does not decrease the likelihood of recurrence, and the decrease in symptom duration is often minimal. For patients who have frequent recurrences, oral acyclovir (200 mg t.i.d. increased to 5 times/day with lesions) is effective in decreasing both frequency and severity of flare-ups, but it should be limited to no more than 6 months of use. Hospitalization for intravenous acyclovir therapy may be required in cases of severe outbreak or in immunosuppressed or otherwise compromised patients. Until the vesicles are crusted over, the lesions are infectious and intercourse should be avoided.

In *pregnant patients* with active herpes infections, cesarean delivery should be considered. Vaginal delivery, when herpetic lesions are present, is associated with about a 50% chance that the baby will acquire the infection. In infants, this infection is associated with significant morbidity and an almost 80% mortality rate.

CHLAMYDIA TRACHOMATIS

The *second most common sexually transmitted disease* is infection by *Chlamydia trachomatis.* Infection by this *obligate intracellular parasite* may manifest as cervicitis, pelvic inflammatory disease, or as the much less common lymphogranuloma venereum. *More common than Neisseria gonorrhoeae by as much as 10:1 in some studies*, infections by *Chlamydia trachomatis* can be the source of significant complications and infertility. Infection rates are five times higher in women with three or more sexual partners, and four times higher in women using no contraception or nonbarrier methods.

Mild cases of cervicitis or pelvic infection by *Chlamydia* may be virtually asymptomatic yet culminate in infertility or ectopic pregnancy. Infection of the fallopian tubes causes a mild form of salpingitis with insidious symptoms. Once the infection is established, it may remain active for many months with increasing tubal damage. *Chlamydia* is also frequently found coexisting with or mimicking *N. Gonorrhoeae* infection. Chlamydial infections are also responsible for nongonococcal urethritis and inclusion conjunctivitis.

Physical findings in infections caused by *Chlamydia* are *often subtle and nonspecific*. Eversion of the cervix with mucopurulent cervicitis may suggest the diagnosis. Any patient with acute pelvic inflammatory disease (PID) or suspected of having gonorrhea should also be evaluated for *Chlamydia*.

The *diagnosis* of *Chlamydia* infection is suspected on clinical grounds. Cultures are generally used only to confirm the diagnosis. Two screening tests have recently gained clinical popularity: an enzyme immunoassay performed on cervical secretions and a monoclonal antibody test carried out on dried specimens. The immunoassay technique is easy to do and has a 95% specificity, but cannot be carried out rapidly. The monoclonal technique is faster, but requires precision in making the slide and the use of a fluorescent microscope for interpretation.

Treatment of suspected or confirmed infections with *Chlamydia* is with tetracycline (500 mg p.o., q.i.d. for 7 days) or doxycycline (100 mg p.o., b.i.d. for 7 days). Erythromycin (500 mg p.o., q.i.d. for 7 days) may be substituted for tetracycline in individuals unable to tolerate these medications or in pregnant patients. These treatments carry roughly 95% cure rates. Follow-up evaluation with culture or other tests as well as screening for other sexually transmitted diseases should be performed.

NEISSERIA GONORRHOEAE (GONORRHEA)

Infections with this *Gram-negative intracellular diplococcus* continue to be common. The emergence of penicillin-resistant strains, an increased frequency of asymptomatic infections, and changing patterns of sexual behavior have all contributed to the problem. The damage caused by *N. gonorrhoeae* infections can lead to recurrent infection, chronic pelvic pain, or infertility due to tubal damage or hydrosalpinx formation. *Infertility* occurs in approximately 15% of patients after a single episode of salpingitis and rises to 75% after three or more episodes. The risk of *ectopic pregnancy* is increased 7–10 times in women with a history of salpingitis.

Infections with N. gonorrhoeae can affect almost any part or organ of the body. Most commonly, the first signs or symptoms of infection occur 3–5 days after exposure, but are often mild enough to be overlooked. Infection in the *lower genital tract* is characterized by a malodorous, purulent discharge from the urethra, Skene's duct, cervix, vagina, or anus. Anal intercourse is not always a prerequisite to anal infection. The presence of greenish or yellow discharge from the cervix should alert the physician to the possibility of either *N. gonorrhoeae* or *C. trachomatis* infections. Infection of the Bartholin's glands is frequently encountered and can lead to secondary infections, abscesses, or cyst formation. Infection of the *pharynx* is found in 10–20% of heterosexual women with gonorrhea, and this site should not be overlooked when cultures are taken.

Fifteen percent of women with *N. gonorrhoeae infections of the cervix* will develop *acute pelvic infections*. *N. gonorrhoeae* infection of the fallopian tubes, adnexa, or pelvic peritoneum generally causes symptoms of pain and tenderness, fever or chills, and an elevated white blood count. Peritoneal involvement can include perihepatitis (Fitz-Hugh and Curtis

Table 28.3
Factors Suggesting Hospitalization for Patients with Pelvic Inflammatory Disease

Nulliparity
Paralytic ileus
Peritonitis or toxicity
Pregnancy
Intrauterine contraceptive device use
Previous treatment failure
Significant gastrointestinal symptoms
Significant pain
Temperature >39°C
Tubo-ovarian abscess
Uncertain or complicated differential diagnosis
Unreliable patient
White blood count >20,000 or <4,000

syndrome). *N. gonorrhoeae* is the causative agent in roughly 50% of patients with salpingitis. Many patients require hospitalization for adequate care (Table 28.3). In severe cases, or in patients with one or more prior episodes of PID, tubo-ovarian abscess formation may occur. These patients are acutely ill, with fevers of up to 39.5°C, tachycardia, severe pelvic and abdominal pain, and nausea and vomiting. Patients presenting with these symptoms must be differentiated from those with septic incomplete abortions, acute appendicitis, diverticular abscesses, and adnexal torsion.

On examination, patients with PID may exhibit muscular guarding, and/or rebound tenderness. A purulent discharge is often seen at the cervix and should be sampled for Gram staining and culture. On palpation, the adnexa will be exquisitely tender and a mass may be felt.

The *laboratory diagnosis* of *N. gonorrhoeae* infection is made by culture on Thayer-Martin agar plates kept in a CO_2-rich environment. Cultures should be obtained from the cervix, urethra, anus, and pharynx when appropriate. Cultures provide 80–95% diagnostic sensitivity. A solid phase enzyme immunoassay for the detection of *N. gonorrhoeae* antigen is also available. Gram stain of any cervical discharge for the presence of this Gram-negative intracellular diplococcus may support the presumptive diagnosis.

Aggressive *therapy* for patients with either suspected or confirmed *N. gonorrhoeae* infections should be tailored to the site of infection and the individual patient. Initial treatment should not be predicated on the results of cultures, but rather on clinical suspicion. General guidelines for treatment are shown in Table 28.4 and for the treatment of pelvic inflammatory disease in Table 28.5. Hospitalized patients require high dose intravenous antibiotic therapy with an antimicrobial spectrum that covers aerobic and anaerobic organisms and may also require surgical drainage of an abscess or even (rarely) hysterectomy. Rupture of a tubo-ovarian abscess, with septic shock, is a life-threatening complication. Follow-up cultures and examination of the patient should be performed 3–5 days after completion of therapy.

HUMAN PAPILLOMA VIRUS

Infection by the *human papilloma virus (HPV) is responsible for almost as many cases of sexually transmitted disease as N. gonorrhoeae*. This DNA virus is found in 2.5–4% of women. Over the past 15 years, the number of infected individuals has increased over fivefold. Unlike other sexually transmitted diseases, sequelae of HPV infection may take years to develop. At least three subtypes (16, 18, and 31 primarily) have been *associated with the development of cervical neoplasia*.

Infection by HPV causes soft, fleshy growths on the vulva, vagina, cervix, urethral meatus, perineum, and anus. They may occasionally also be found on the tongue or oral cavity. These growths are termed *condylomata acuminata or venereal warts*. These distinctive lesions may be single or multiple and generally cause few symptoms. They are often accompanied by *Trichomonas* or *Gardnerella* vaginal infections. Since human papilloma virus is spread by direct skin-to-skin contact, symmetrical lesions across the midline are common (often called "kissing lesions"). The diagnosis of condyloma acuminata is made based on physical examination, but may be confirmed through biopsy of the warts.

Table 28.4
Treatment of Gonorrhea

	Preferred treatment[a]	Alternative treatment[a]
Urethral/cervical	Ampicillin, 3.5 g, **or** amoxicillin, 3 g, + probenecid, 1 g p.o.	Aqueous penicillin G procaine, 4.8 MU i.m., + probenecid, 1 g p.o. **or** tetracycline, 500 mg p.o. q.i.d., × 7 days
Rectal	Ampicillin, 3.5 g, **or** amoxicillin, 3 g, + probenecid, 1 g p.o., **or** spectinomycin, 2 g i.m.	Aqueous penicillin G procaine, 4.8 MU i.m., + probenecid, 1 g p.o., **or** tetracycline, 500 mg p.o. q.i.d., × 7 days
Pharyngeal	Aqueous penicillin G, Aqueous, 4.8 MU i.m., + probenecid, 1 g p.o.	Tetracycline, 500 mg p.o. q.i.d., × 7 days
Arthritis	Crystalline penicillin G, 12–16 MU/day i.v. until improved, then ampicillin 500 mg p.o. q.i.d. to 7–10 days total, **or** ampicillin, 3.5 g, **or** amoxicillin, 3 g, + probenecid 1 g p.o., + ampicillin, 500 mg p.o. q.i.d. × 10–14 days	Cefoxitin, 2 g i.v. q8h until improved, then tetracycline, 500 mg p.o. q.i.d. to 7–10 days total
Penicillinase +	Spectinomycin, 2 g i.m.	Cefoxitin 2 g i.m. + probenecid, 1 g p.o.
Pharyngeal	Sulfamethoxazole, 400 mg/trimethoprim, 80 mg, 9 tab/day × 5 days in single daily dose	Aqueous penicillin G procaine, 4.8 MU i.m. + probenecid, 1 g p.o. **or** tetracycline, 500 mg p.o. q.i.d., × 7 days

[a]MU, milliunits.

Table 28.5
Treatment of PID

	Preferred treatment	Alternative treatment
PID (outpatient)	Cefoxitin, 2 g 9 i.v. every 6 h, or cefotetan, I.V. 2 g every 12 h, plus doxycycline, 100 mg every 12 h, orally, or i.v. The above regimen is given for at least 48 h after the patient clinically improves.	Clindamycin 900 mg I.V. every 8 hours plus gentamicin loading dose i.v. or (2 mg/kg) followed by a maintenance dose (1.5 mg/kg) every 8 h. The above regimen is given for at least 48 h after the patient improves.

While cytologic changes typical of HPV can be found on Pap smears, *Pap smears of the cervix will diagnose only about 5% of patients with the virus*. Because the condyloma lata of syphilis may be confused with venereal warts, some care must be taken in making the diagnosis in patients at high risk for both infections. Venereal warts are usually characterized by their narrower base and more "heaped-up" appearance, while condyloma lata lesions have a flattened top.

Small, uncomplicated venereal warts are treated medically with either an application of a 25% solution of podophyllin in tincture of benzoin or trichloroacetic acid. One of these solutions is carefully applied to the warts and allowed to remain for 30–60 minutes. Vaseline or other protective medium may be applied to the surrounding skin so that a chemical burn does not occur. Treatment may be repeated every 7–10 days as needed. Podophyllin should not be used during pregnancy because of potential fetal toxicity. If lesions persist or recur, cryosurgery, electrodesiccation, surgical excision, or laser vaporization may be required. Treatment with 5-fluorouracil cream is often used as an adjunct for cervical or vaginal lesions. Lesions will be more resistant to therapy during pregnancy, in diabetic patients, or in patients who are immunosuppressed. In patients with extensive vaginal or vulvar lesions, delivery via cesarean section may be required to avoid extensive vaginal lacerations and problems suturing tissues with these lesions. Cesarean delivery also decreases the possibility of transmission to the infant, which can cause subsequent development of laryngeal papillomata, although the risk is small and in and of itself not an indication for cesarean section.

Any patient with a history of condyloma should have at least yearly Pap smear evaluations of the cervix. The sexual partners of patients with HPV should also be screened for the development of genital warts.

SYPHILIS

Since antiquity, syphilis has been *the prototypic venereal disease*. The incidence of syphilis has been rising in the past several years. Contributing to this rise is today's increased use of nonpenicillin antibiotics to treat resistant gonorrhea, whereas in the past, penicillin treatment of gonorrhea provided treatment for coexisting syphilis.

Treponema pallidum, the causative organism of syphilis, is one of a very small group of *spirochetes* that are virulent for humans. Since this motile anaerobic spirochete can rapidly invade intact moist mucosa, the most common sites of entry for women are the vulva, vagina, and cervix. *Chancres* may also be found in or near the anus, rectum, pharynx, tongue, lips, fingers, or other areas. *Transplacental spread* occurs at any time during pregnancy and can result in *congenital syphilis*.

About 10–60 days after infection with *T. pallidum*, a painless ulcer will appear. This is the chancre of *primary syphilis*. The chancre has a firm, punched out appearance and has rolled edges. Even though it is often accompanied by adenopathy, the chancre is often missed. Serologic testing at this stage of syphilis will generally be negative. Healing of the chancre occurs spontaneously in 3–9 weeks.

Four to eight weeks after the primary chancre appears, manifestations of *secondary syphilis* develop. This stage is typically characterized by low grade fever, headache, malaise, sore throat, anorexia, generalized lymphadenopathy, and a diffuse, symmetric, asymptomatic maculopapular rash. This rash often is seen over the palm and soles and is sometimes referred to as "money spots." Highly infective secondary eruptions, called mucous patches, occur in 30% of patients during this stage. In moist areas of the body, flat-topped papules may coalesce, forming *condylomata lata*. These may be distinguished from venereal warts by their broad base and flatter appearance. In untreated individuals, this stage, too, will pass spontaneously in 2–6 weeks as the disease enters into the *latent phase*. In the late stages of the disease, transmission of the infection is unlikely, except via blood transfusion or placental transfer. However, crippling damage to the central nervous system, heart, or great vessels often develops. Destructive, necrotic, granulomatous lesions called *gummas* may develop 1–10 years after infection.

The *diagnosis* of syphilis may be made by *identifying motile spirochetes* on darkfield microscopic examination of material from primary or secondary lesions or lymph node aspirates. For most patients, the diagnosis will be established on the basis of serologic testing. The *VDRL or RPR* are nonspecific tests that are rapid, inexpensive, and useful for screening. The *FTA-ABS or MHA-TP* tests are specific treponemal antibody tests that are confirmatory or diagnostic, but are not used for routine screening. These latter tests are useful when assessing "false-positive" screening tests caused by such diverse conditions as atypical pneumonia, malaria, connective tissue disease, systemic lupus erythematosus, or some vaccinations. When neurosyphilis is suspected, a lumbar puncture with a VDRL performed on the spinal fluid is required.

The treatment of choice for syphilis is penicillin G benzathine as outlined in Table 28.6. The patient should be followed by quantitative VDRL titers and examinations at 3, 6, and 12 months.

Table 28.6
Treatment of Syphilis

	Preferred treatment	Alternative treatment
Syphilis 1°/2°/latent	Penicillin G benzathine, 2.4 MU i.m., **or** aqueous penicillin G procaine, 600,000 U i.m. every other day ×8 days. For latent: penicillin G benzathine, 2.4 MU i.m. weekly for 3 weeks	Tetracycline, 500 mg p.o. q.i.d. ×15 days Erythromycin 500 mg p.o. q.i.d. ×15 days in pregnant patients
Cardiovascular	Penicillin G benzathine, 2.4 MU i.m. weekly ×3 weeks **or** aqueous penicillin G procaine, 600,000 U i.m. every other day ×15 days	Tetracycline, 500 mg p.o. q.i.d. ×30 days Erythromycin 500 mg p.o. q.i.d. ×15 days in pregnant patients
Neurosyphilis	Crystalline penicillin G, 3–4 MU i.m. q4h for at least 10 days	

ACQUIRED IMMUNODEFICIENCY SYNDROME

Although transmission of the *human immunodeficiency virus (HIV)* may be accomplished via blood transfusion, pregnancy, or the use of contaminated drug equipment such as needles, the exchange of body fluids during sexual activity represents a major mode of spread, making AIDS a sexually transmitted disease. This virtually uniformly fatal disease is generally diagnosed either through screening of individuals at high risk, or suspicion when secondary infections or rare tumors, such as Kaposi's sarcoma, appear. Although women in heterosexual relationships are considered to be at somewhat lower risk than homosexual males and IV drug abusers, anyone with multiple sexual contacts risks exposure and infection. Women currently represent approximately 11% of AIDS cases (roughly 4000 cases to date), and this rate is rising. Because the risk of transmission of AIDS to a fetus is approximately 50% and the fact that maternal AIDS often worsens during pregnancy, pregnancy should be postponed until more is known or effective therapies become available.

The *diagnosis* of AIDS is made on the basis of serum screening tests (immunoassay) and confirmed through the use of western blot testing. Therapy with antimetabolities such as zidovudine (Retrovir) has been successful in delaying the progress of the disease for some patients. The results of long-term ther-apy and the development of improved treatment options have yet to become available.

MINOR SEXUALLY TRANSMITTED DISEASES

Chancroid, granuloma inguinale, lymphogranuloma venereum (LGV), molluscum contagiosum, parasite infections (such as pediculosis pubis or scabies), enteric infections, and some types of vaginitis (e.g., trichomoniasis) are all types of infections that are spread through sexual activities. Pertinent information about these infections, some of which are seldom seen, is summarized in Table 28.7.

FURTHER READINGS

Homes K, Mardh P, Sparling P, Wiesner P. Sexually transmitted diseases. New York: McGraw-Hill 1984.
Genital human papillomavirus infections. ACOG technical bulletin. 1988:105.
Gonorrhea and chlamydial infections. ACOG technical bulletin. 1985:89.
Gynecologic herpes simplex virus infections. ACOG technical bulletin. 1988:119.
Human immune deficiency virus infections. ACOG technical bulletin. 1988:123.

SELF-EVALUATION

Case 28-A

A 20-year-old college student comes to your office with the complaint of severe vulvar pain and itching, which has been present for 3 days. The patient first noted some "tingling" and irri-

Table 28.7
"Minor" sexually transmitted diseases

Disease	Causative agent	Main symptom[a]	Diagnosis	Treatment
Chancroid	*Haemophilus ducreyi*	Painful "soft chancres", adenopathy	Clinical, smears, culture	Erythromycin, 500 mg. q.i.d. for 10 days
Granuloma inguinale	*Calymmatobacterium granulomatis*	Raised, red lesions	Clinical, smears	Tetracycline, 500 mg q6h for 3 weeks
Lymphogranuloma venereum (LGV)	*Chlamydia trachomatis*	Vesicle, progressing to bubo	Clinical, complement fixation test	Tetracycline, 500 mg q6h for 3 weeks
Molluscum contagiosum	*Poxviridae*	Raised papule with waxy core	Clinical, inclusion bodies	Desiccation, cryotherapy, curettage
Parasites	*Pediculus Sarcoptes scabiei*	Itching	Inspection	Lindane 1%
Enteric infections	*Neisseria gonorrhoeae, Chlamydia trachomatis, Shigella, Salmonella, Protozoa*	Diarrhea	Culture	Based on agent
Vaginitis	*Trichomonas*	Odor, irritation	Microscopic examination of secretions	Metronidazole, 500 mg b.i.d. for 7 days

[a]See also Table 28.2.

tation, followed by the development of open sores that are extremely painful. The patient also complains of extreme pain on urination. She reports a low grade fever, but admits that she has not taken her temperature. When questioned, she concedes having broken up with her previous boyfriend and having become intimate with a new partner on one occasion about a week prior to the onset of symptoms. On examination, you find red, swollen labia with open ulcers that are painful to touch.

Question 28-A-1

To confirm your diagnostic suspicions, which of the following is most likely to be of help?

A. microscopic examination of vaginal secretions mixed with 10% KOH
B. a "whiff" of vaginal secretions mixed with 10% KOH
C. microscopic examination of material from the ulcerated lesions for giant cells
D. a cervical culture for gonorrhea

E. a serum test for syphilis (e.g., RPR)

Answer 28-A-1

Answer: C

The patient's history and physical findings suggest that this patient has a herpes vulvitis. If this is the case, screening for coexistent gonorrhea or syphilis is appropriate (answers D and E), but secondary to the diagnosis of the patient's complaint. Similarly, vaginal infections often occur as sexually transmitted diseases. Although *Trichomonas* infections are common in this group, they would not be tested for with the methods given in answers A and B. Screening for a vaginal infection is appropriate if history or physical findings suggest their presence.

Question 28-A-2

The most reasonable therapy for this patient would be:

A. soap and water cleansing, air drying

B. amoxicillin, 3 g, with probenicid, 1 g
C. podophyllin 25% in benzoin
D. metronidazade, 500 mg twice a day
E. local steroid cream therapy

Answer 28-A-2

Answer: A

For initial infections with herpes, local cleansing to decrease the risk of secondary infection is the best therapy. Amoxicillin would be an option for treating gonorrhea, whereas podophyllin is useful in treating condyloma, neither of which are likely in this patient. Similarly, metronidazole is indicated for *Trichomonas*. Because of the viral nature of herpes, local steroids should be avoided. Acyclovir therapy for herpes is best started within 48 hours of the onset of lesions and is best carried out by either local cream or a oral dose of 200 mg 5 times per day. A 3-times-a-day dosage is used for suppression of recurrences.

Case 28-B

A 24-year-old married mother of three comes to the clinic with the complaint of "something growing down there." The patient first noted small growths on her labia 3 weeks previously, at the end of her menstrual period. These growths have persisted and enlarged. Several small growths have now appeared on the other side. The growths do not cause symptoms, but the patient had an aunt with breast cancer and so was concerned about what these might be. Past medical and surgical history are unremarkable. On physical examination, several small raised, shaggy lesions, ranging in size from 1 to 7 mm are noted on both labia and the perineum.

Question 28-B-1

The most likely diagnosis in this patient is:

A. molluscum contagiosum
B. genital herpes
C. condyloma lata
D. condyloma acuminata
E. chancroid

Answer 28-B-1

Answer: D

The differential diagnosis of raised lesions must include Molluscum contagiosum and condyloma lata, in addition to the more common condyloma acuminata. The lesions of molluscum contagiosum are more common over the lower abdomen and are distinguished by their central umbilication and yellowish, cheesy appearance. Condyloma lata, found in syphilis, is usually flatter in appearance and has a broader base than is found in venereal warts.

Case 28-C

A 28-year-old unmarried nulligravid patient presents to you in the emergency room with a 6-hour history of diffuse lower abdominal pain. The pain was periumbilical, but has now moved into the lower abdomen. She complains of a fever, but has not taken her temperature. She notes mild nausea over the past hour. Past history reveals regular menstrual periods, with her last period occurring on schedule 1 week ago. She has had no previous surgeries or significant medical problems. She does note a similar episode 8 months previously for which she did not seek care. She is sexually active an has never used any contraception. On physical examination she has a pulse of 100, temperature of 38.1°C and a BP of 110/65. Examination of the abdomen finds diffuse tenderness in both lower quadrants. Pelvic examination is normal except for a yellowish discharge at the cervix, diffuse tenderness on motion of the uterus, and a tender fullness in both adenexa. You order a pregnancy test, CBC, and perform cervical cultures.

Question 28-C-1

While you await the results of your laboratory tests, what is the most reasonable working diagnosis?

A. ectopic pregnancy
B. salpingitis (PID)
C. appendicitis
D. gastroenteritis
E. threatened abortion

Question 28-C-2

The results of the CBC return and you find a WBC of 14,000 with 82% segmented polys. The pregnancy test is negative and the culture will not be available for 48 hours. Based on this additional information, what is the most reasonable diagnosis?

A. ectopic pregnancy
B. salpingitis (PID)
C. appendicitis
D. gastroenteritis
E. threatened abortion

Answers 28-C-1 and -2

Answer: B is correct for both.

Fever, lower abdominal pain, tachycardia, cervical and bilateral adnexal tenderness all point to an inflammatory process in the pelvis. In a patient with infertility and a similar previous episode recurrent salpingitis (PID) is more likely than appendicitis. This is supported by the elevated white blood count and differential. Broad-spectrum therapy should be implemented based on clinical suspicion, even if the cultures should eventually return as "negative."

Questions 28-C-3

For further consideration: What if the patient described in Case 28-B had been pregnant? How would that affect your therapy? What if the patient had been 65 years old? How would that affect your differential diagnosis? How do you answer the patient's question of "how did I get these?"

chapter 29

ABORTION

80% within first 12wks

< 20wks
< 500gm.

Abortion is the termination of a pregnancy prior to viability, typically defined as 20 weeks from the first day of the last normal menstrual period or a fetus of less than 500 g weight. Whether spontaneous or induced, there are profound medical as well as emotional implications associated with abortion. Because the lay expression for spontaneous abortion is "miscarriage," care should be taken to explain the terminology to the patient.

SPONTANEOUS ABORTION

The *incidence of spontaneous abortion* is estimated at *50%* of all pregnancies, an estimate based upon the assumption that many pregnancies spontaneously terminate without clinical recognition. An incidence of recognized spontaneous abortion of approximately 20–25% is commonly cited with approximately 80% occurring during the first 12 weeks of pregnancy.

Approximately 50% of early spontaneous abortions are attributed to chromosomal abnormalities. Risk factors associated with spontaneous abortion include increasing parity, increasing maternal age, increasing paternal age, and conception within 3 months of a live birth. Abnormal development of the early pregnancy (including the zygote, embryo, fetus, or placenta) is a common pathologic finding in spontaneous abortion. Expulsion of the pregnancy is typically preceded by death of the embryo or fetus.

As pregnancy progresses beyond the first trimester, the fetus may not have undergone fetal death before the pregnancy ends spontaneously. The etiologies of *second trimester abortions* are much less likely to be chromosomal and much more likely to be due to maternal systemic disease, abnormal placentation, or other anatomic considerations. This difference is of great clinical significance because there can be treatment for these conditions and, therefore, the possibility of preventing recurrent spontaneous abortion.

Maternal systemic conditions that have been associated with spontaneous abortion include infections such as *Listeria monocytogenes*, *Mycoplasma hominis*, *Ureaplasma urealyticum*, and *toxoplasmosis*. Insufficient secretion of progesterone by the corpus luteum or the placenta has also been associated with spontaneous abortion. Although uncommon, uncorrected medical conditions such as hyperthyroidism and diabetes are associated with an increased incidence of spontaneous abortion. Spontaneous abortion has also been related to environmental toxins, radiation, and immunologic factors. Both *smoking and alcohol consumption* have been linked to miscarriages. Women who smoke more than one pack of cigarettes per day have an almost twofold increase in their rate of spontaneous abortion. Women who drink more than 2 days per week experience twice the abortion rate of those who do not.

Leiomyomata uteri, especially when located in a submucous position, have been associated with spontaneous abortion. It is uncommon for subserous or intramural leiomyomata of the uterus to be a causative factor of spontaneous abortion. Removal of the leiomyomata (myomectomy) is recommended only if it is determined that pregnancy wastage has been caused by this anatomic distortion.

Table 29.1
Causes of Spontaneous Abortion

Genetic factors (10–50%)
    Nondisjunction
    Balanced translocation/carrier state
Endocrine abnormalities (25–50%)
    Luteal phase defect
    Thyroid disease
    Hyperandrogenism
    In utero DES exposure
Reproductive tract abnormalities (6–12%)
    Leiomyomata uteri (submucous)
    Septate uterus
    Bicornuate or unicornuate uterus
    Incompetent cervix
    Intrauterine adhesions
    Abnormality of placentation
Infection
    Listeria monocytogenes
    Mycoplasma hominis
    Ureaplasma urealyticum
    Toxoplasmosis
    Syphilis
    ?Chlamydia
    ?Herpes
Systemic disease
    Diabetes mellitus
    Chronic renal disease
    Chronic cardiovascular disease
    Systemic lupus/lupus anticoagulant
Environmental factors
    Toxins
    Radiation
    Smoking
    Alcohol
    Anesthetic gases

Spontaneous abortion can also be caused by a *unicornuate* or *septate uterus*, with 20–30% of women with a unicornuate or septate uterus having reproductive difficulties, most frequently recurrent pregnancy loss. In utero exposure to *diethylstilbestrol (DES)* has been associated with abnormally shaped uteri as well as cervical incompetence. *Intrauterine adhesions* synechiae (Asherman's syndrome) has been linked to spontaneous abortion due to an inadequate amount of endometrium to support implantation. This condition is typically a sequela of uterine curettage with subsequent destruction and scarring of the endometrium (Table 29.1).

DIFFERENTIAL DIAGNOSIS OF ABORTION

Because the differential diagnosis of bleeding in the first trimester of pregnancy includes such things as ectopic pregnancy, hydatidiform mole, cervical polyps, and cervicitis, the patient should be examined whenever bleeding occurs. Any vaginal bleeding in the first half of an intrauterine pregnancy is presumptively called a *threatened abortion* unless another specific diagnosis can be made. This threatened abortion occurs in up to 25% of pregnancies with approximately one half of these patients proceeding to spontaneous abortion. Those who carry a pregnancy complicated by threatened abortion to viability are at greater risk for preterm delivery, low birth weight, and a higher incidence of perinatal mortality. There does not, however, appear to be a higher incidence of congenital malformations in these newborns. Some patients describe bleeding at the time of their expected menses, sometimes referred to as the *placental sign* or *implantation bleeding*, which may be due to ruptured blood vessels in the endometrium.

Ultrasonography is especially useful to determine if an early pregnancy is intact. Lack of a gestational sac does not, however, rule out a very early viable pregnancy. Ultrasonography, in conjunction with quantitative human chorionic gonadotropin, has been used to identify viable pregnancies at various stages of gestation. Transabdominal ultrasonography can identify an intact gestation if the quantitative β-hCG exceeds 5000–6000 mIU/ml, whereas transvaginal ultrasonography can typically identify an early intact pregnancy when the β-hCG level exceeds 2000 mIU/ml.

An *inevitable abortion* is defined as rupture of the membranes and/or cervical dilation during the first half of pregnancy such that pregnancy loss is unavoidable. It is unusual for pregnancy to successfully reach viability in this circumstance. Uterine contractions typically follow and the products of conception are expelled. Conservative management of these patients significantly increases the risk of infection.

Completed abortion refers to the situation when a documented pregnancy spontaneously aborts and all of the products of conception are expelled. Early in pregnancy, the fetus and placenta are generally expelled in toto, but in those cases where some tissue is retained (*incomplete abortion*), bleeding and pain result. Suction curettage of the uterus is usually necessary to remove the remaining products of conception and prevent further bleeding and infection.

A *missed abortion* is the retention of a failed intrauterine pregnancy for an extended period, usually defined as more than two menstrual cycles. These patients present with an absence of uterine growth and may have lost some of the early symptoms of pregnancy. Although unusual, disseminated intravascular coagulopathy (DIC) can occur when an intrauterine fetal demise in the second trimester has been retained beyond 6 weeks after the death of the fetus. Evacuation of the uterus can be accomplished either through dilation and evacuation (D&E) or with the use of prostaglandin suppositories.

Recurrent abortion is a term used when a patient has had more than two consecutive or a total of three spontaneous abortions. In early abortions, there is a great likelihood of a chromosomal abnormality, whereas in later abortions, a maternal cause is more likely. Karyotyping is recommended for both parents when recurrent early abortion occurs. The possibility of immunologic factors should also be explored. Correction of maternal medical conditions and/or anatomic deformities should be pursued for those patients with recurrent late abortions. These include surgical correction of uterine abnormalities, cerclage of the incompetent cervix, or lysis of intrauterine synechiae. *adhesions*

TREATMENT OF SPONTANEOUS ABORTION

Intervention for patients with threatened abortion should be minimal, even if the bleeding is accompanied by low abdominal pain and cramping. If there is no evidence of significant pathology, the patient can be reassured and allowed to continue normal activities. Intercourse is usually proscribed for 2–3 weeks, or longer, depending on the etiology of bleeding. Although commonly recommended, a short period of bed rest has no documented benefit. ✱

If pain and bleeding persist, especially with significant hemodynamic alterations, or if ultrasound and hormonal evaluation identify a nonviable pregnancy, evacuation of the uterus should be carried out. Immediate considerations include control of bleeding, prevention of infection, pain relief (if needed), and emotional support. Bleeding is controlled by insuring that all the products of the conception have been expelled or removed from the uterus. This may be presumed in cases of complete abortion, or may be accomplished through curettage in cases of incomplete, inevitable, missed, or septic abortions. Hemostasis is enhanced through uterine contraction stimulated by intravenous oxytocin or intramuscular Methergine (methylergonavine maleate). Removal of the products of conception also decreases the risk of infection and this, combined with vaginal rest (no tampons, douches, or intercourse), provides adequate infection protection in most cases. A mild analgesic may be required and should be offered. Rh-negative mothers should receive Rh immune globulin (RhoGAM). Chromosomal evaluation of spontaneous abortions is not recommended unless there is a history of recurrent abortion. *if Rh– give RhoGAM*

Emotional support is important for both the short- and long-term well-being of the patient, as well as her partner. No matter how well prepared for the possibility of pregnancy loss a couple is, the event is a significant disappointment and stress. When appropriate, the couple should be reassured that the loss was not precipitated by anything that they did or did not do and that there was nothing that they could have done to prevent the loss. Although a potentially sensitive issue, there is a natural tendency to try to find "a reason" for this type of let down. This can lead to thoughts of "if we hadn't made love 2 weeks ago," or "if I hadn't let her pick up the grocery bag." These are clearly unrelated to the cause of most abortions and can easily lead to further stress in a relationship at a time when both partners need support the most. Couples are often reluctant to raise these issues in this situation, further increasing the risk of friction. These issues are best raised directly by the physician.

A follow-up office visit is generally scheduled for 2–6 weeks after the loss of a pregnancy. This is an appropriate time to evaluate uterine involution, assess the return of menses, and discuss reproductive plans. The causes (or lack of causes) of the pregnancy loss should also be reiterated. The impact of this loss on future childbearing should be discussed. A single pregnancy loss does not significantly increase the risk of future losses. Multiple pregnancy losses carry an increased risk for future pregnancies based, in part, on the higher likelihood of a continuing causative condition such as fibroids, immune diseases, or genetic disorders.

INDUCED ABORTION

Termination of an intact pregnancy prior to the time of viability can be done to safeguard the health of the mother or on a purely elective, i.e., voluntary, basis. Elective abortion has been legal since the Supreme Court decision of *Roe v. Wade*. Since that time, various local and state laws have been proposed to significantly limit access to elective abortion. These laws will continue to undergo many court challenges as our society struggles to define a consistent national policy.

Prior to embarking upon an elective abortion, patients must be aware that choices are available. These include: continuation of pregnancy with subsequent adoption, continuation of pregnancy and keeping the child, and elective abortion during either the first or second trimester. Medical complications are associated with all choices, with the least complications related to elective abortion in the first trimester. Although there are complications associated with pregnancy termination, they are significantly less than those associated with carrying a pregnancy. First trimester pregnancies are typically terminated by means of suction curettage, i.e., vacuum aspiration performed through the cervix. Second trimester abortions are most commonly performed through the cervix, using suction or destructive forceps, or by the use of prostaglandins, as in the form of intraamniotic injections or vaginal suppositories.

Risk of death from abortion during the first 2 months of pregnancy is less than 1 per 100,000 procedures, with increasing rates as pregnancy progresses. There is no apparent risk to future pregnancies if the first or second trimester abortion has been free of complications. There appears to be a slight increased risk of premature delivery if more than three first trimester pregnancies are terminated by elective abortion.

Other techniques used to perform abortions include hysterectomy, intrauterine infusion of hypertonic solutions such as saline and urea, and the as-yet unapproved antiprogesterone medication RU 486 (mifepristone).

SEPTIC ABORTION

Occasionally, patients may present with a *septic abortion*, an infected complete or incomplete abortion. It rarely occurs as a complication of a legal abortion, and it is most commonly associated with "criminal abortions." A criminal abortion is one done illegally, under unsterile conditions, by persons who may have little or no knowledge of medicine or anatomy. The patient can present with severe hemorrhage, bacteremia and septic shock with renal failure. Broad spectrum parenteral antibiotics, fluid therapy, and prompt evacuation of the uterus are indicated. A careful evaluation for trauma, including perforation of the uterus or vagina, should also be carried out.

FURTHER READINGS

Grief related to perinatal death. ACOG technical bulletin. 1985;86.

Methods of midtrimester abortion. ACOG technical bulletin. 1987;109.

Wentz AC, Cartwright PS. Recurrent and spontaneous abortion, In: Jones HW III, Wentz AC, Burnett LS, eds. Novak's textbook of gynecology. 11th ed. Baltimore: Williams & Wilkins, 1988:328–350.

SELF-EVALUATION

Case 29-A

A 20-year-old college student (G1P1) presents with the complaint of 2 days of vaginal bleeding, 6 weeks after her last menstrual period. She has had a positive home pregnancy test. The bleeding has been dark in color, painless, and began after intercourse.

Examination shows a small amount of dark blood in the vagina and at the cervical os. The cervix is closed and no tissue is visible. Bimanual examination reveals a slightly softened, normal size uterus and normal adnexa without masses or tenderness.

Question 29-A-1

Based on your assessment, your best course of management is:

A. Perform a culdocentesis.

B. Order a transvaginal ultrasound examination.

C. Prescribe medroxyprogesterone (Provera) 10 mg/day.

D. Recommend pelvic rest and light activity.

E. Advise evacuation of the uterus by suction curettage.

Answer 29-A-1

Answer: B, D

Assuming that the home pregnancy test is correct, the most likely diagnosis is a threatened abortion, and, as such, expectant management without other intervention is indicated. Roughly 30–40% of pregnancies experience early bleeding of this type, but less than one half end in pregnancy loss. A culdocentesis is valuable only in patients in whom intraperitoneal bleeding (such as with an ectopic pregnancy) is suspected. An ultrasound evaluation at 6 weeks of amenorrhea may help establish the viability of the pregnancy. A transvaginal ultrasound is more sensitive than a transabdominal scan, and in conjunction with a quantitative hCG may be helpful in an extremely early gestation. There is no evidence that synthetic progestin therapy benefits the pregnancy, and will only expose the fetus to unnecessary medication should the pregnancy continue. Evacuation of the uterus would be indicated only if nonviability were documented.

For further consideration: Would your management be any different if this patient had had a previous spontaneous abortion? Would your management be any different if this patient had had a previous elective abortion? What if she had passed some tissue? When do you advise this patient that she may safely resume sexual relations?

ECTOPIC PREGNANCY

Implantation outside of the uterine cavity is termed "ectopic pregnancy," an event that significantly jeopardizes both the pregnancy and the mother. Catastrophic bleeding may occur when the implanting pregnancy erodes into blood vessels or ruptures structures not suited to accommodate the growing conceptus. Primarily because of an increasing prevalence of pelvic inflammatory disease, the incidence of ectopic pregnancy has been increasing over the past few years. One ectopic pregnancy now occurs for every 66 intrauterine pregnancies. Despite this increase in the number of cases of ectopic pregnancy, maternal mortality has decreased markedly. In 1970, there were 3.5 maternal deaths per 1000 cases of ectopic pregnancy; now the rate is less than 1 per 1000. This improvement is primarily due to better detection, allowing early intervention.

Pregnancies may implant in many locations in the genital tract and pelvis (Fig. 30.1). The vast majority of ectopic gestations (95%) occur in the fallopian tube (tubal pregnancy). Four of five tubal pregnancies occur in the ampullary portion of the fallopian tube. Infrequent locations include the cervix, ovary, and peritoneal cavity (respectively, cervical, ovarian, and abdominal pregnancy). Patients with ectopic pregnancy are not only at risk for immediate morbidity and mortality from acute blood loss and risk of anatomic damage, but have a significantly reduced fertility rate, with fewer than one half of patients subsequently having a live birth. *As the second leading cause of maternal mortality in the United States, ectopic pregnancy should be high in the differential diagnosis for any woman of reproductive age with acute pelvic or lower abdominal pain, with or without abnormal vaginal bleeding.* Pain early in pregnancy should also raise the possibility of ectopic pregnancy.

CAUSES OF ECTOPIC PREGNANCY

Knowing which patients are at higher risk can aid the physician in making an early diagnosis. The primary risk factor for ectopic pregnancy is a prior history of *salpingitis.* Damage from such infection may retard the passage of the fertilized ovum through the tube to the endometrial cavity, facilitating extrauterine implantation. Women with a history of salpingitis have a sixfold increase in their risk of ectopic pregnancy. A previous ectopic pregnancy also increases the risk of future ectopic implantations by approximately 10-fold. *Age* is an important risk factor. Women 35–44 years old have a threefold increase in the rate of ectopic pregnancy, as compared with women 15–24 years old. Over half of all ectopic pregnancies occur in women who have had *three or more pregnancies.* Finally, *Black and Hispanic women* also have a significantly higher risk of ectopic pregnancy.

Contrary to some reports, *sterilization, contraception, and abortion do not increase ectopic pregnancy frequency.* Oral contraceptives prevent ovulation, thereby significantly reducing pregnancies in all locations. IUCDs prevent all types of pregnancies, although ectopic pregnancies may be reduced relatively less than intrauterine pregnancies, thereby giving the false impression that they are a risk factor. The higher prevalence of pelvic inflammatory disease in IUCD users, however, may increase the patient's risk even after the re-

287

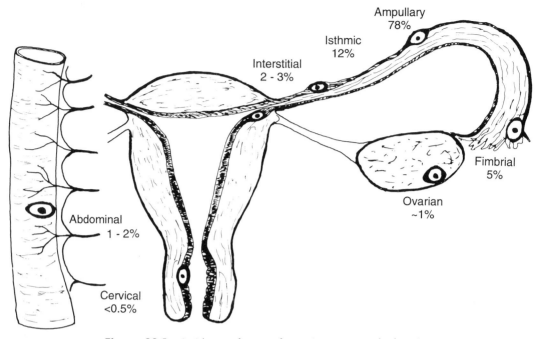

Figure 30.1. Incidence of types of ectopic pregnancy by location.

moval of the IUCD. In patients with previous sterilization, the chance of ectopic pregnancy is increased but because sterilization failures are so uncommon, the net effect of sterilization is to protect against ectopic pregnancies. Although 85% of sterilization failures are associated with intrauterine pregnancies, the possibility of an ectopic pregnancy should always be considered in patients with sterilization failures. Abortion itself does not predispose to ectopic pregnancy, although associated infection may do so. There has been a reported effect of ovulation induction in increasing the risk of ectopic pregnancy. This has been difficult to determine, because there is the potential for subclinical tubal disease in some infertile patients, which may itself be the primary cause of the ectopic pregnancy.

CLINICAL EVALUATION OF POSSIBLE ECTOPIC PREGNANCY

The classic presentation of a patient with an ectopic pregnancy includes *abdominal pain,* *amenorrhea,* and *vaginal bleeding,* although all of these symptoms are not always present.

The mechanism of *implantation* in ectopic pregnancies is similar to that of an intrauterine gestation. Symptoms arise from the development of hemoperitoneum, or the distention of a hollow viscus, such as the fallopian tube, or both. Early ectopic pregnancies are asymptomatic. As the pregnancy grows, the most common symptom is abdominal or pelvic pain, which is present in nearly all patients. The pain is generally described as colicky in character and may be unilateral (not necessarily on the same side as the ectopic) or bilateral, intermittent or constant, located in the lower or even upper abdomen. The proximal portions of the fallopian tube are not as able to adapt to the growing pregnancy, so an ectopic pregnancy in this area is likely to become symptomatic earlier in gestation. In up to one fourth of patients with extensive intraabdominal bleeding, irritation of the diaphragm causes referred pain to the shoulder. Irritation of the posterior cul-de-sac may cause an urge to defecate. These patients may present with a history of feeling faint or passing out while straining to have a bowel movement. Syncope occurs in approximately one third of patients with ruptured tubal pregnancies.

Although patients with ectopic pregnancy typically have missed their normal menses, this history is often not given. By the time symptoms have developed, it has usually been 6 weeks since the last normal menstrual period. At this early stage, symptoms of pregnancy are not always present and cannot be used to rule in or rule out ectopic pregnancy.

As long as placental hormones are produced, there is usually no vaginal bleeding. Irregular vaginal bleeding results from the sloughing of the decidua from the endometrial lining. Vaginal bleeding in patients with an ectopic gestation may range from little or none to heavy, menstrual-like flow. In some patients, the entire "decidual cast" is passed intact, simulating a spontaneous abortion. Histologic evaluation of this tissue will confirm whether placental villi are present. Whenever evaluation of tissue passed spontaneously or obtained by curettage does not demonstrate villi, an ectopic implantation should be assumed to be present until proven otherwise.

Physical examination findings range from a totally normal examination in early unruptured ectopic pregnancy to hypovolemic shock and an acute abdomen in cases of ruptured ectopic pregnancy. Most healthy reproductive age women are able to compensate for mild to moderate degrees of blood loss so that extensive blood loss is usually required to cause a fall in blood pressure and a rise in pulse. Only about 5% of patients present in hypovolemic shock, although blood loss is the major factor in 85% of ectopic pregnancy deaths.

Fever is not expected, although a mild elevation in temperature in response to intraperitoneal blood may occur. A temperature of greater than 38°C may suggest an infectious etiology to a patient's symptoms. Abdominal distention and tenderness, with or without rebound, rigidity, or decreased bowel sounds, may be seen in cases of intraabdominal bleeding, but tenderness is present in only about half of all patients with ectopic pregnancies. Cervical motion tenderness due to intraperitoneal irritation as well as adnexal tenderness are commonly found. An adnexal mass is present in roughly one third of cases but its absence does not rule out the possibility of an ectopic implantation. The uterus may enlarge and soften throughout the first trimester, thus simulating an intrauterine pregnancy. A slightly open cervix with blood or decidual tissue may be found and mistaken for a threatened abortion.

Ectopic implantations outside of the fallopian tube may present in a variety of ways related to the site of implantation. Pregnancies that implant on the surface of the bowel, mesentery, omentum (abdominal pregnancies), or on the surface of the ovary (ovarian pregnancies), may not be diagnosed until late in pregnancy. These pregnancies are rare and are effectively the only type of ectopic pregnancy in which fetal survival is possible although very uncommon. Also rare is implantation in the endocervical canal. *Cervical pregnancies* may present as catastrophic vaginal bleeding, frequently requiring emergency hysterectomy to save the mother's life.

The rapid and accurate diagnosis of ectopic pregnancy is imperative to reduce the risk of serious complications or death. Up to one half of ectopic pregnancy-related maternal deaths have had a lag in treatment due to delayed or inaccurate diagnoses. *Any sexually active woman in the reproductive age group who presents with pain, irregular bleeding, and/or amenorrhea should have ectopic pregnancy as a part of the initial differential diagnosis.* Other elements of the differential diagnosis include complications of an intrauterine pregnancy (threatened, missed, complete, or incomplete abortion), nonpregnancy-related gynecologic conditions (such as acute and chronic salpingitis, follicullar or corpus luteum cyst rupture, endometriosis, adnexal torsion) and nongynecologic conditions such as gastroenteritis and appendicitis.

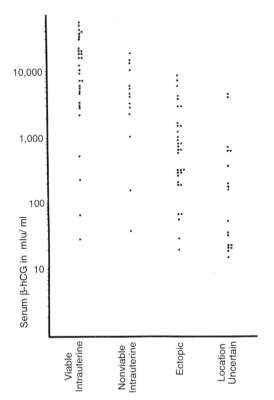

Figure 30.2. Serum β-hCG concentrations in relation to pregnancy outcome.

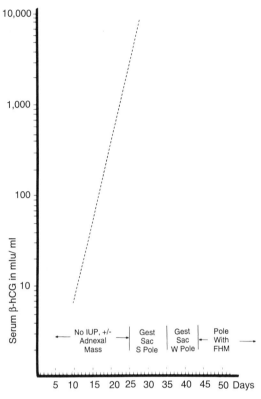

Figure 30.3. Serum β-hCG concentrations with corresponding ultrasound findings. *IUP*, intrauterine pregnancy; *Gest sac*, gestational sac; *pole*, fetal pole; *FHM*, fetal heart motion.

DIAGNOSTIC PROCEDURES

The initial assessment in the otherwise hemodynamically stable patient must include a *pregnancy* test. With the sensitive assays available today, a negative pregnancy test excludes the possibility of ectopic pregnancy. If positive, the remainder of the workup will focus on complications of pregnancy. *Quantitative* β-*hCG* levels can be followed at 2-day intervals. Early in pregnancy, these levels should increase by at least 66% in 48 hours. Failure to meet this criterion indicates a pregnancy not growing appropriately, thus increasing the suspicion of ectopic pregnancy (Fig. 30.2 and Fig. 30.3).

Although a low *hematocrit* is unusual, a complete blood count can document possible blood loss anemia and identify leukocytosis. If the *white blood count* is greater than 20,000

(WBC/dl), infection may be more likely than an ectopic pregnancy.

A useful adjunct to serial quantitative levels of hCG is *pelvic ultrasonography* (Fig. 30.4). Ultrasonography cannot be relied upon to image a pregnancy outside the uterine cavity but it can identify an intrauterine pregnancy, thus effectively ruling out a coexistent ectopic pregnancy (a very rare possibility). Transabdominal ultrasonography should be able to identify an intrauterine gestation by the time the hCG level reaches 6000 mlU/ml. The more sensitive transvaginal ultrasonography should show the pregnancy by the time the hCG level is 2000 mlU/ml. Failure to do so should further increase the suspicion that an ectopic pregnancy exists.

Serum progesterone concentration has also been used to identify an abnormal preg-

WBC ≥ 20,000 = Infection ? ectopic

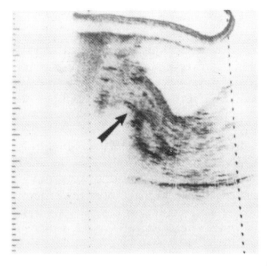

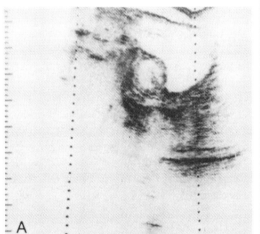

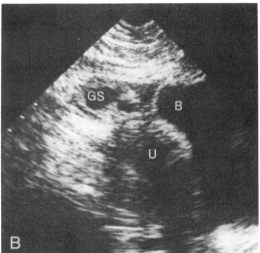

Figure 30.4. Sonogram findings in tubal ectopic pregnancy ultrasound findings. *GS,* gestational sac; *B,* bladder; *U,* uterus.

nancy. A progesterone less than 5.0 ng/ml indicates a nonviable pregnancy. Although it does not identify location, it helps raise the suspicion of an ectopic pregnancy.

In cases when the patient does not desire to continue a pregnancy, *curettage of the uterine cavity* can help rule out ectopic pregnancy. Although intrauterine and ectopic pregnancy can exist simultaneously in rare cases (approximately 1 in 8,000 to 1 in 30,000), identification of chorionic villi in curettings essentially rules out ectopic pregnancy. The Arias-Stella reaction of preg-

nancy seen on histologic examination is not useful in identifying the location of the pregnancy.

Culdocentesis can identify a hemoperitoneum. This involves insertion of an 18-gauge needle posterior to the cervix, between the uterosacral ligaments, and through the cul-de-sac, into the peritoneal cavity. Aspiration of clear peritoneal fluid (negative culdocentesis) indicates no hemorrhage into the abdominal cavity, but does not rule out an unruptured ectopic pregnancy. Aspiration of blood that clots can indicate either penetration of a vessel or rapid blood loss into the peritoneal cavity. Nonclotting blood is evidence of hemoperitoneum (positive culdocentesis) in which the blood has undergone fibrinolysis. If nothing is aspirated (equivocal or nondiagnostic culdocentesis), no information is obtained. Unfortunately, no finding on culdocentesis can definitively rule in or rule out ectopic pregnancy, although the findings may confirm the need for surgical evaluation or intervention.

The most accurate technique of identifying an ectopic pregnancy is by direct visualization, done most commonly via laparoscopy or laparotomy. Even laparoscopy carries a 2–5% misdiagnosis rate.

MANAGEMENT OF ECTOPIC PREGNANCY

The traditional management of a tubal pregnancy is surgical removal. Conservative surgical techniques have been developed that maximize preservation of reproductive organs. If done through the laparoscope, definitive diagnosis and treatment can be accomplished at the same operation with minimal morbidity, cost, and hospitalization. In a linear salpingostomy, the surgeon makes an incision of the fallopian tube over the site of implantation, removes the pregnancy, and allows the incision to heal by secondary intention. A "segmental resection" is the removal of a portion of the affected tube with the potential of reanastomosing the tube at a later time. Salpingectomy is removal of the entire tube, a procedure reserved for those cases in which little or no normal tube remains.

In selected cases, nonsurgical therapy may be advocated for the small, unruptured ectopic pregnancy. Expectant management involves no surgery and no medical therapy but allows the pregnancy to spontaneously regress as documented by serial hCG levels. Methotrexate, a folinic acid antagonist, has been successfully used to treat ectopic pregnancy via the oral or intramuscular routes, as well as by direct injection into the ectopic gestational sac.

When conservative surgery or nonsurgical treatment is utilized, the patient must be followed with serial quantitative β-hCG levels to monitor regression of the pregnancy. Surgery or methotrexate therapy may then be considered if trophoblastic function persists.

In the rare cases of abdominal pregnancy, survival of the fetus occurs in only 10–20% with up to one half having significant deformity. The patient is given the option of continuing the pregnancy to fetal viability and operative delivery, or operative termination of the pregnancy at the time of diagnosis. In either case, removal of the placenta is usually not attempted because of the risk of uncontrollable hemorrhage. Treatment with methotrexate is commonly used to deal with the retained placenta. Ovarian pregnancy very rarely proceeds to significant fetal age and is usually treated surgically at the time of diagnosis. Cervical pregnancy may be confused with an incomplete abortion and associated with uncontrollable hemorrhage from the lower uterine segment/endocervix once the placenta has been removed; hysterectomy is often required as a lifesaving measure.

Rh-negative mothers should receive *Rh immune globulin* (Rho-GAM) to prevent Rh sensitization.

FURTHER READINGS

Ectopic pregnancy. ACOG technical bulletin. 1990;150.
Cartwright PS. Ectopic pregnancy. In: Jones HW III, Wentz AC, Burnett LS, eds. Novak's textbook of gynecology. 11th ed. Baltimore: Williams & Wilkins, 1988:479–506.

SELF-EVALUATION

Case 30-A

A 20-year-old college student (G1P1) presents with the complaint of 2 days of vaginal bleeding, 6 weeks after her last menstrual period. She has had a positive pregnancy test. The bleeding has been dark in color, painless, and began after intercourse. She has had no prior surgeries. She has had one episode of "a pelvic infection" in the past.

Methotrexate · po/IM

Examination shows a small amount of dark blood in the vagina and at the cervical os. The cervix is closed and no tissue is visible. Bimanual examination reveals a slightly softened uterus and normal adnexae.

Question 30-A-1

Your best course of management is:

A. Advise an immediate culdocentesis.
B. Request a transvaginal ultrasound examination.
C. Prescribe medroxyprogesterone (Provera), 10 mg/day.
D. Recommend pelvic rest and light activity.
E. Advise evacuation of the uterus by suction curettage.

Answer 30-A-1

Answer: B, D

A likely diagnosis in this situation is a threatened abortion, but a history of a "pelvic infection" is present in up to 70% of patients with ectopic pregnancies and should increase the clinician's suspicion that an unruptured ectopic pregnancy may be present. A transvaginal ultrasound examination may help to identify the presence of an intrauterine pregnancy, making the diagnosis of threatened abortion more probable. Culdocentesis is a useful test to identify intraabdominal bleeding, but the patient's history is not suggestive of rupture or leakage from an ectopic implantation site. Because culdocentesis is invasive, it should be reserved for those cases where the possibility of intraabdominal bleeding is greater and the need for diagnostic information is more acute. Recommendations of therapy must be reserved until the possibility of an ectopic pregnancy has been addressed. If there is a delay prior to obtaining the ultrasound, treating the condition as a presumed threatened abortion is appropriate.

For further consideration: With this patient's history of a pelvic infection, how would you advise this patient regarding future fertility? What if she had had more than one "infection?" If this patient is treated for an ectopic pregnancy, how would you advise this patient regarding future fertility?

Case 30-B

A 25-year-old G1P0 patient begins to cramp and passes a clump of spongy tissue, which she brings to the office. A transvaginal ultrasound examination 1 week ago revealed an intrauterine gestational sac. On examination, her uterus is small and firm and her cervical os is closed with minimal bleeding.

Question 30-B-1

The best course of management is:

A. observe only
B. observe and send specimen for pathologic evaluation
C. D & C
D. diagnostic laparoscopy
E. methotrexate therapy

Answer 30-B-1

Answer: B

The specimen may represent a completed abortion, or it may be a decidual cast associated with an ectopic pregnancy. The latter is much less likely in this case because of the ultrasound documented intrauterine pregnancy 1 week ago. In general, any tissue must be sent for histologic evaluation. A D&C would be appropriate if bleeding is persistent and incomplete abortion was suspected. Diagnostic laparoscopy would be utilized only if ectopic pregnancy were more likely, and treatment such as methotrexate is inappropriate until ectopic pregnancy is diagnosed.

Case 30-C

A 32-year-old G2P2002 status post tubal ligation presents with 7 weeks of amenorrhea and vaginal spotting. Pelvic examination reveals a 6-week size anteverted uterus, a closed cervical os with minimal dark blood in the vaginal vault, and no palpable findings on adnexal examination. A urine pregnancy test is positive.

Question 30-C-1

Appropriate next steps in this patient's management include:

A. quantitative serum β-hCG
B. quantitative serum progesterone

C. transvaginal pelvic ultrasound
D. D&C
E. diagnostic laparoscopy

Answer 30-C-1

Answer: C

At 6 weeks gestational age with a positive urinary pregnancy test, transvaginal ultrasound will be able to differentiate an intrauterine pregnancy in virtually all cases. Invasive procedures are not indicated absent a diagnosis requiring them.

Question 30-C-2

Transvaginal ultrasound reveals an intrauterine gestational sac and fetal pole with fetal activity and a cystic adnexal mass with complex echoes.

For further consideration: Is the diagnosis of an intrauterine pregnancy secure? What is the possibility of a combined pregnancy, one in the uterus and another in the adnexae? How would you follow the patient for this possibility? What are likely causes of the adnexal mass? With this patient's history of a pelvic infection, how would you advise the patient regarding future fertility? What if she had had more than one "infection?" If this patient is treated for an ectopic pregnancy, how would you advise this patient regarding future fertility?

chapter 31

PELVIC RELAXATION, URINARY INCONTINENCE, AND INFECTION

Patients with pelvic relaxation present in many different and often subtle ways. In order to identify patients who would benefit from therapy, the physician should be familiar with the types of pelvic relaxation and the approach to the patient with symptoms suggestive of this problem. The physician must also be aware of common urinary tract conditions that frequently involve the female urinary system. Although pelvic relaxation or urinary tract disorders are frequently symptomatic, patients are often reluctant to voice their complaints. The physician must be sensitive to these complaints as well as to the physical findings that suggest a problem. Once a problem is identified, a logical and complete approach to evaluation and treatment will return the patient to normal health.

PELVIC RELAXATION AND URINARY INCONTINENCE

Our population is "aging." Although not exclusively the province of "old age," pelvic relaxation is more common as tissues become less resilient and the accumulated stresses of life have their effects. As a greater proportion of our patients move into their later years, more and more women will be at risk for pelvic relaxation and its attendant problems. Pelvic pressure and pain, dyspareunia, bowel and bladder dysfunction, and urinary incontinence may all result from loss of support for the pelvic organs. Almost half of all women have had the involuntary loss of a few drops of urine at some time in their life; 10–15% of

women suffer significant, recurrent loss. Loss of pelvic support can have both medical and social implications that necessitate evaluation and intervention.

CAUSES OF PELVIC RELAXATION

The pelvic organs are supported by a complex interaction of muscles (e.g., levator muscles), fasciae (urogenital diaphragm, endopelvic fascia), and ligaments (such as the uterosacral and cardinal ligaments). Each of these structures can lose its ability to provide support through birth trauma, chronic elevations of intraabdominal pressure (because of such problems as obesity, chronic cough, or heavy lifting), intrinsic weaknesses, or atrophic changes due to aging or estrogen loss. Loss of adequate support for the pelvic organs may be manifest by descent or prolapse of the urethra (*urethrocele*), bladder (*cystocele*), or rectum (*rectocele*). True herniation at the top of the vagina (*enterocele*) can also occur. These anatomic defects are illustrated in Figure 31.1. Loss of support for the uterus can lead to varying degrees of descent of the uterus (*uterine prolapse*). When the uterus descends beyond the vulva it is termed *procidentia*. In addition, prolapse of the vaginal vault can occur in patients who have had a hysterectomy. Although loss of support (*pelvic relaxation*) may affect any of the pelvic organs individually, multiple organ involvement is most common.

A common complaint of patients with a cystocele or urethrocele is *urinary incontinence*. This does not occur in all patients and

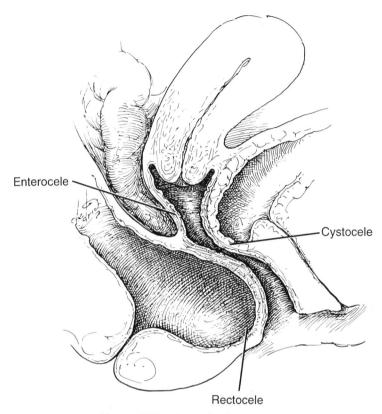

Figure 31.1. Loss of pelvic support.

the degree of incontinence is often not commensurate with the degree of pelvic relaxation. There is urine flow *anytime the pressure inside the bladder exceeds the pressure in the urethra.* This happens primarily during voluntary voiding when the muscles surrounding the urethra relax and the bladder contracts. It may also take place involuntarily when there is unequal transmission of intraabdominal pressure to the bladder and urethra, as seen with the loss of pelvic support. As the urethral support has been lost, it descends outside the influence of abdominal pressure. As a result, the bladder pressure exceeds urethral pressure briefly at times of strain or stress, thus the term stress incontinence. Also, if there is loss of normal innervation and control of bladder function, involuntary bladder contraction or bladder atony may result, leading to urgency and overflow incontinence, respectively. Loss of urine may ensue anytime there is a breakdown of the social or emotional competence of the patient (e.g., psychosis, neurosis, etc.) or when the normal continence mechanism is bypassed, such as with fistulous openings.

CLINICAL PRESENTATION

The *symptoms* caused by loss of pelvic support *will vary based on the structure or structures involved and the degree of prolapse.* The most common symptoms are those characterized as "pressure" or "heaviness." These symptoms are diffuse, low in the abdomen or pelvis, and are often worse late in the day, after lifting, or when standing for long periods. Backache and dyspareunia are also common complaints. When support for the bladder and urethra fails, urinary (stress) incontinence, frequency, hesitancy, incomplete voiding, or recurrent infections may result. A careful history that notes the associated

Table 31.1
Characteristics of Urinary Incontinence

	Stress	Urge	Overflow
Associated symptoms	None (occasional pelvic pressure)	Urgency, nocturia	Fullness, pressure, frequency
Amount of loss	Small, spurt	Large, complete emptying	Small, dribbling
Duration of loss	Brief, corresponds to stress	Moderate, several seconds	Often continuous
Associated event	Cough, laugh, sneeze, physical activity	None, change in position, running water	None
Position	Upright, sitting; rare supine or asleep	Any	Any
Cause	Structural (cystocele, urethrocele)	Loss of bladder inhibition	Obstruction, loss of neurologic control

symptoms and events, amount and duration of urine loss, and the position in which urine losses occur is important in establishing the correct diagnosis (Table 31.1).

Loss of rectal support may lead to problems such as constipation and painful or incomplete defecation. The patient may need to provide support to the posterior vagina with her fingers to promote bowel movements. When there is complete descent, the patient may be paradoxically asymptomatic and only note the protrusion of tissue from the vagina. Vaginal ulceration, bleeding, infection, or pain frequently accompany complete descent.

Pelvic relaxation is best demonstrated by observing the vaginal area while having the patient strain. This may be done in either, or both, the supine and standing positions. A urethrocele or cystocele may be demonstrated by separating the labia and asking the patient to "strain down" or cough. When a urethrocele or cystocele is present, a downward movement and rotation of the anterior vaginal wall toward the introitus will be seen. To more fully evaluate the presence of a cystocele, rectocele, or enterocele, inspection should be carried out using a Sims or the lower half of a Graves speculum. This facilitates the separate inspection of the anterior and posterior vaginal walls and allows differentiation of the structures involved. Descent of the uterus may be demonstrated either in this way or through palpation.

The *degree of pelvic relaxation* is often rated on a one to three scale based on the descent of the structure involved (Fig. 31.2). When descent is limited to the upper two thirds of the vagina, it is said to be first degree. Second-degree prolapse is present when the structure reaches the vaginal introitus. Descent of the structure to outside the vaginal opening (such as the body of the uterus in the case of *procidentia*) is classified as a third-degree defect. Cystourethroceles may be quantitated using the "*Q-tip test.*" This is done by placing a cotton swab in the urethra and measuring the angle of upward motion caused by the patient straining. Upward rotation of greater than 30° from the starting point is generally associated with urinary stress incontinence due to loss of support of the critical *urethrovesical junction.*

EVALUATION

The evaluation of patients with pelvic relaxation rests primarily on the history and physical examination. Additional evaluations should be dictated by the patient's symptoms and the anatomic defects found. Further evaluation is warranted anytime the patient's symptoms exceed or do not match the physical findings.

When a significant cystocele or urethrocele is found, *evaluation of urinary function* is advisable. Compromise of ureteral drainage may occur in cases of significant downward displacement of the trigone as is seen in some

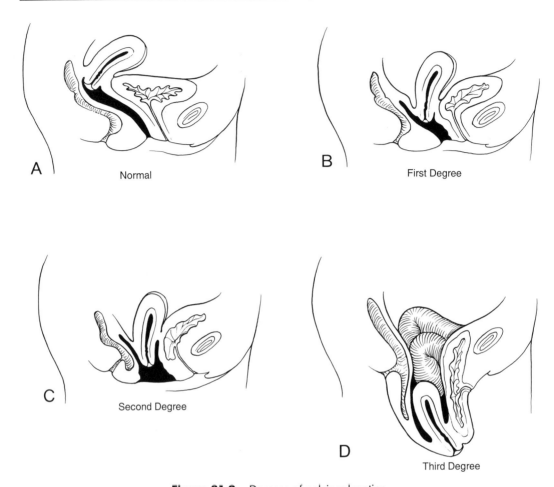

Figure 31.2. Degrees of pelvic relaxation.

cases of prodicentia. Urinary retention and subsequent infection may also occur and should be evaluated. Because of the frequent association of more than one cause of urinary incontinence, patients with incontinence should be considered for *urodynamics testing*.

Urodynamics testing refers to a group of procedures that evaluate bladder structure and functions. Although these procedures vary based upon the needs of the patient and the preferences of the physician, they generally include cystometrics, cystoscopy, and provocative tests such as coughing or straining. Most centers include sophisticated evaluation of bladder compliance and contractility, as well as evaluation of the voiding process itself. Pressure profiles of the bladder and urethra as well as fluoroscopic examina-

tions may also be included. This battery of tests is very important in the objective reproducible evaluation of proposed therapies. Clinically, these tests are very useful in the evaluation of patients where "mixed" etiologies are suspected, or prior to invasive intervention.

The *Q-tip test* is useful in documenting the degree of cystourethrocele present. The functional significance of a cystourethrocele may be gauged by elevating the bladder neck (using fingers or an instrument) and asking the patient to strain (called a Bonney or Marshall-Marchetti test). If continence is achieved, these tests help to anticipate the effect of pessaries or surgery. Care must be taken that the test accurately reflects elevation of the structures and not merely obstruction of the urethra. Because of this uncertainty, these tests have been accorded less significance and should not provide the sole means of evaluation.

Chronic constipation and difficulty passing stool may be symptoms of a rectocele but are compatible with obstructive lesions as well. *Anoscopy* or sigmoidoscopy should be considered, based on the needs of the individual patient.

DIFFERENTIAL DIAGNOSIS

The presumptive diagnosis of pelvic relaxation is based on the evaluation of the structural integrity of pelvic support. Often the characteristics of the patient's complaint may suggest a diagnosis (Table 31.1). Even though the differential diagnosis of pelvic relaxation is generally simple, *other processes* must be considered. Urethral diverticulum or Skene's gland abscesses may mimic a cystourethrocele. These may be identified through symptoms, careful "milking" of the urethra, or cystoscopy. The complaint of urinary loss may stem from mechanical factors (such as a cystourethrocele), irritation (mechanical or inflammatory trigonitis), neurologic causes (such as diabetes or detrusor instability), the effects of medications, or mental and psychosocial conditions. A vesicovaginal or ureterovaginal fistula must also be considered in the differential diagnosis. It is occasionally difficult to differentiate between a high rectocele and an enterocele. This distinction may be facilitated through rectal examination or the identification of small bowel in the hernia sac. It is common for the presence of an enterocele not to be established until surgical repair is undertaken.

Most pelvic relaxation is the result of structural failure of the tissues involved, but *other contributing factors* should be considered in the complete care of the patient. Has there been a change in intraabdominal pressure and why? Why does the patient have a chronic cough that has precipitated her symptoms? Is a neurologic process (such as diabetic neuropathy) complicating the pa-

tient's presenting complaint? Each of these issues should be considered prior to the selection of a diagnostic or therapeutic plan.

In the evaluation of involuntary loss of urine, the physician must also consider the possibility of *fistulae*. Fistulae between the vagina and the bladder (vesicovaginal), urethra (urethrovaginal), or the ureter (ureterovaginal) are generally the result of surgical trauma, irradiation, or malignancy. A communication between the bladder and the uterus (vesicouterine) may also be found on rare occasions. In addition, fistulae may occur between the rectum and vagina (rectovaginal fistulae) resulting in the passage of flatus and sometimes feces from the vagina.

NONSURGICAL TREATMENT OPTIONS

Because pelvic relaxation is a structural problem, the ultimate solutions are structural as well. These range from mechanical support (through pessaries) and exercises to strengthen the pelvic muscles, to surgical repair of the tissue defects. Estrogen replacement is also an important adjunct to other therapies in the postmenopausal woman.

In patients with urgency incontinence, *bladder training, biofeedback, or medical therapy* may be effective. Bladder training programs are directed toward increasing the patient's bladder control and capacity by gradually increasing the amount of time between voidings. Often successful by itself, this may be augmented in difficult cases by biofeedback when available. Treatment with anticholinergic drugs (Pro-Banthine (propantheline bromide), Ditropan (oxybutynin chloride)), β-sympathomimetic agonists (Alupent (metaproterenol sulfate)), musculotrophic drugs (Urispas (flavoxate hydrochloride), Valium (diazepam)), antidepressants (Tofranil (imipramine hydrochloride)), or dopamine agonists (Parlodel (bromocriptine mesylate)) have all had some success based on the character of the patient's problem.

The pelvic musculature may be strengthened through the use of Kegel exercises. This exercise

Table 31.2
Surgical Therapy for Urinary Incontinence

Type	Intent	Approach
Anterior vaginal repair (colporrhaphy, Kelly plication)	Provide support to the bladder and urethra by reinforcing the endopelvic fascia and vaginal epithelium	Vaginal
Retropubic suspension (Marshall-Marchetti-Krantz, Burch, paravaginal repair)	Repair defects in the endopelvic fascia and its attachments	Abdominal
Sling procedure (Pereyra, Stamey)	Supplement or replace the support of the bladder neck and urethra using suture or fascial slings	Combined abdominal and vaginal
Obliteration (LeFort, colpocleisis)	Provide support by obliterating the vaginal space	Vaginal

program consists of the repetitive contraction of the pelvic floor muscles as if trying to stop bladder emptying. This is repeated multiple times throughout the day. These exercises may be helpful for some patients with mild incontinence. They may also help to provide better tissues should surgical repair be attempted.

A mechanical buttress for the pelvic organs may be provided through the use of *pessaries*. These are devices worn in the vagina to furnish support. Pessaries come in a variety of types and sizes, all designed to replace the missing structural integrity of the pelvis or to diffuse the forces of descent over a wide area. The most common forms of pessary are the Smith-Hodge, the ring (or donut), the ball, and the cube. They are placed in the vagina in much the same way as a diaphragm. They occlude the vagina and hold the pelvic organs in a relatively normal position. Pessary therapy requires the cooperation and involvement of the patient, but offers a good alternative to surgical repair for properly selected, motivated patients.

Patients who are fitted with a pessary for the control of pelvic relaxation need careful initial monitoring. Reexamination in 5–7 days to confirm proper placement, hygiene, and the absence of pressure-related problems (vaginal trauma or necrosis) is required. Evaluation in 24 hours may be advisable in patients who are debilitated or require additional assistance.

SURGICAL THERAPY

Surgical repair of pelvic relaxation takes many forms, depending on the specific defect, ranging from hysterectomy to the creation of supportive slings to occlusion of the vagina to plastic repairs (Table 31.2). These procedures may be carried out from either the vaginal or abdominal approach, and each has its own set of indications, advantages, disadvantages, complications, and failures. No one procedure is best, and each surgical approach must be individualized. Success is based not only on the procedure chosen, but also on the skill of the surgeon, the degree of pelvic relaxation, and patient risk factors such as quality of tissues, obesity, and life-style.

Failure of rectovaginal support may be treated by reconstructing or reinforcing the rectovaginal space (posterior colporrhaphy). Prolapse of the vagina may be treated by suspending the vaginal vault to either the sacrospinous ligament (vaginal or abdominal approach) or to the sacrum itself (abdominal approach). Obliteration of the rectovaginal space (Moskowitz procedure) is also used to treat or prevent vaginal prolapse and enterocele formation. Enteroceles are treated like other hernias with dissection and high ligation of the hernia sac.

Because of the frequent concurrence of defects in pelvic support and uterine descent (i.e., prolapse), vaginal hysterectomy is often performed simultaneously with the reconstruction procedure. This corrects any symptoms referable to the descensus, provides access to the uterine support mechanism to reinforce other repairs, and prevents the uterus from tearing down anterior and posterior repairs should further descent occur.

In patients who cannot endure long procedures and are not sexually active, partial or complete obliteration of the vaginal canal (LeFort procedure, colpocleisis) may be done to provide support to the pelvic structures.

Therapy for fistulae is surgical. Some fistulae that occur following surgery will spontaneously heal when adequate drainage or diversion of the urinary or fecal flow is provided. In all other cases, the only successful therapy consists of meticulous dissection of the fistulous tract and careful reapproximation of tissues. Recurrence is a common problem, especially in patients who have had radiation therapy for malignancies.

URINARY TRACT INFECTIONS

Women suffer a urinary tract infection roughly 10 times more often than men. Approximately 15% of women will experience at least one urinary tract infection in their lifetime. This necessitates a familiarity with the diagnosis and treatment of a number of urologic disorders more common to women.

Most urinary tract infections in women ascend from bacterial contamination of the urethra. Except in the case of tuberculosis or immunosuppressed patients, infections will rarely be acquired by hematogenous or lymphatic spread. The relatively short female urethra, exposure of the meatus to vestibular and rectal pathogens, and sexual activity that may induce trauma or introduce other organisms, all increase the potential for infection. With estrogen deficiency there is also a decrease in urethral resistance to infection that contributes to ascending contamination. This change in resistance explains the almost 10% prevalence of asymptomatic bacteriuria found in postmenopausal women.

CLINICAL ASPECTS OF URINARY TRACT INFECTIONS

Ninety-five percent of urinary tract infections are symptomatic, uncomplicated, do not ascend to the kidneys, and produce no permanent damage. Ninety percent of first infections are caused by *Escherichia coli*, and these respond readily to antibiotic therapy. Anaerobic bacteria and yeasts are rare causes of infections except in diabetic or immunosuppressed patients or those with chronic indwelling catheters.

Patients with urinary tract infections will typically present with symptoms of frequency, urgency, nocturia, or dysuria. The symptoms found will vary somewhat with the site of the infection. When there is irritation of the bladder or trigone, urgency, frequency, and nocturia develop. Irritation of the urethra leads to frequency and dysuria. The physical examination will generally be nonspecific, although some patients may report suprapubic tenderness.

EVALUATION

The evaluation of the patient suspected of having a urinary tract infection should include a urinalysis and a urine culture and sensitivity. These are generally obtained through a "clean catch midstream" urine sample obtained by cleansing the vulva, and obtaining a portion of urine passed during the middle of uninterrupted voiding. Urine obtained from catheters or suprapubic aspiration may also be used.

Laboratory analysis of the urine may be carried out or the sample examined microscopically by the clinician. This microscopic evaluation is carried out using a drop of urine or the precipitate from a centrifuged specimen. For uncentrifuged samples, the presence of more than one white blood cell per high power field carries a 90% accuracy in detecting infection. Centrifuged specimens may be scanned with low power for the presence of large numbers of white cells. Pyuria is defined as the presence of more than five white cells per high power field in the centrifuged specimen. Gram stain of urine samples or sediments may also be helpful in establishing the diagnosis of infection. "Dipstick" tests for infection based on the presence of leukocyte esterace are also useful.

Culture of urine samples that show colony counts of greater than 100,000 of a single organism generally indicate infection. Colony counts as low as 10,000 *E. coli* are associated with infection when symptoms are present. Contamination of the specimen is indicated when cultures report multiple organisms.

Recurrent urinary tract infections should prompt a reevaluation. Possible causes that must be considered include incorrect or incomplete (e.g., noncompliant) therapy, mechanical factors such as obstruction, or compromised host defenses.

THERAPY

The selection of therapy for patients with urinary tract infections is simple and generally successful. Hydration, urinary acidification (with ascorbic acid, ammonium chloride, or acidic fruit juices), and urinary analgesics (Pyridium (phenazopyridine hydrochloride)) are helpful in most cases. Once confirmation by urinalysis or culture has been obtained, antibiotic therapy should be instituted. Nitrofurantoin (Macrodantin) produces good urinary antibiosis without undue alteration of other flora, although it is not effective against *Proteus* infections. Antibiotics such as ampicillin, tetracycline, and trimethoprim-sulfamethoxazole (Septra, Bactrim) provide good coverage in the urinary tract, but risk more alteration of vaginal or intestinal flora. Vaginal yeast infections may result from these antibiotic treatments. When pyelonephritis is suspected, aggressive antibiotic therapy with cephalosporins such as Keflex (cephalexin) or Duricef (cefadroxil) is indicated.

Patients who have been treated for urinary tract infections should have *follow-up urinalysis and culture* done 10–14 days after the initial diagnosis. This will document cure in most patients and identify those at risk for recurrence due to incomplete or ineffective therapy.

FURTHER READINGS

Urinary incontinence. ACOG technical bulletin. 1987; 100.

Ostergard DR, Bent AE. Urogynecology and urodynamics: theory and practice. 3rd ed. Baltimore: Williams & Wilkins, 1991.

Prevention of hospital-acquired urinary tract infections in gynecology patients. ACOG technical bulletin. 1977;46.

Antimicrobial therapy for obstetric patients. ACOG technical bulletin. 1988;117.

SELF-EVALUATION

Case 31-A

An 18-year-old nulligravid patient presents to your office with the complaint of 3 days of urinary frequency, urgency, and dysuria. She was married 2 weeks ago and the symptoms first appeared following a weekend "getaway" with her husband. She is using condom and foam for contraception. She reports no fever or chills and she is aware of no vaginal discharge. Your physical examination reveals no abnormal findings. You obtain a "clean catch" urine and centrifuge the specimen. You examine the sediment under the microscope and find 20–30 white cells, a moderate number of epithelial cells, and some bacteria in each low power field.

Question 31-A-1

The best working diagnosis at this point is:

A. cystitis
B. pyuria
C. traumatic urethritis/trigonitis
D. pyelonephritis
E. vaginitis

Answer 31-A-1

Answer: C

The finding of large numbers of white blood cells in the centrifuged urine specimen would normally be diagnostic of pyuria. This, combined with the patient's symptoms, would support the diagnosis of cystitis. In this case, however, the microscopic examination also showed a large number of epithelial cells, which means the specimen had had moderate contamination from vaginal secretions. Without symptoms of vaginal discharge or irritation, we cannot make the diagnosis of vaginitis, but we also cannot rely on the urine sample we have to make the diagnosis of urinary tract infection. Trauma to the urethra and bladder trigone ("honeymoon cystitis") may imitate infection. The patient's recent marriage, and the use of spermicides, could support the possibility of mechanical or chemical irritation. Although we have not ruled out the possibility of infection, the circumstances suggest it may be less likely than traumatic urethritis.

Question 31-A-2

To confirm your suspicions you might:

A. obtain a catheterized urine for examination
B. request a culture and sensitivity on the specimen you have
C. obtain a wet prep of vaginal secretions
D. obtain a more detailed sexual history
E. perform an intravenous pyelogram

Answer 31-A-2

Answer: D

Both a further exploration of the patient's sexual history and a better evaluation of the possibility of infection are indicated, but the invasive nature of urinary catheterization makes the evaluation of history a better choice. Based on the history, the need for a catheterized specimen may be better determined. We know from the presence of epithelial cells in the centrifuged specimen we have that the sample is contaminated and thus culture is useless. Although a microscopic examination of vaginal secretions is easy to accomplish, there is no evidence for vaginitis in the patient's history or physical examination. Intravenous pyelography is invasive, expensive, and would not contribute to the diagnostic possibilities in this case. A culture on the existing

urine specimen might be useful and is no risk to the patient.

Case 31-B

A 64-year-old G5P4 widowed patient comes to your office for her annual physical examination. She had a total hysterectomy 20 years ago for tumors. She takes iron and an antihypertensive medication. When you take your gynecologic history, the patient somewhat shyly admits that she is not sexually active but that she has recently "met someone" whom she likes. She also admits that she has begun experiencing a loss of urine when she coughs, laughs, or sneezes. This has made her self-conscious and she is considering giving up her seniors' aerobics class.

Your physical examination shows her to be an 87-kg woman with a blood pressure of 138/92 and a pulse of 84. Her abdomen is protuberant, but no masses or tenderness are noted. Pelvic examination reveals atrophic changes in the vulva and vagina, a second-degree cystocele, slight descensus of the vaginal vault, and no palpable adnexa.

Question 31-B-1

Which of the following is probably *not* indicated at this time:

A. weight reduction
B. vaginal estrogen therapy
C. Kegel exercises
D. anterior colporrhaphy
E. low-impact exercise program

Answer 31-B-1

Answer: D

The history and physical examination presented are consistent with stress incontinence due to a cystourethrocele. The patient's symptoms are mild and do not warrant surgical intervention at this time. Should the symptoms become worse, urodynamic evaluation should also be considered prior to scheduling a surgical repair. Estrogen therapy (systemic or vaginal), and Kegel exercises may both help to improve the patient's symptoms. Weight reduction is a worthwhile goal for general health and to decrease the possibility of progression of her pelvic relaxation. The addition of a low-impact exercise program may help the weight reduction program and support the patient's self-esteem. Reassurance is always indicated.

Question 31-B-2

What would your thoughts be if the patient reported loss of urine while in bed at night? How might a history of insulin-dependent diabetes affect your evaluation? If the patient wished to be sexually active, how would you counsel her?

chapter 32

ENDOMETRIOSIS

The *clinical impact* of endometriosis relates to its association with complaints such as infertility, dysmenorrhea, dyspareunia, and chronic pelvic pain. Initially described by Sampson in 1921, *endometriosis* is characterized by the *presence of endometrial tissue in extrauterine locations*, especially the ovaries, uterosacral ligaments, rectovaginal septum, and pelvic peritoneum. The term *endometrioma* has been used to described an isolated collection of endometriosis involving an ovary that is large enough to be considered a tumor. An out-dated term, endometriosis externa, has been used to differentiate it from endometriosis interna (adenomyosis); both terms should be relegated to historical interest only.

INCIDENCE AND PREVALENCE

Because histologic confirmation of endometriosis is required to make a definitive diagnosis, the true incidence of endometriosis is difficult to establish. Since laparotomy and/or endoscopy is required to confirm the diagnosis, there will be patients who have endometriosis that will be undetected because of a lack of symptomatology, and there also will be patients who undergo surgery for unrelated reasons who are found to have incidental findings of endometriosis. It is estimated that 1–2% of women in the general population have endometriosis and that this rate increases 10-fold in infertile women. Endometriosis occurs primarily in women in their twenties and thirties, although this may be a function of the frequency of evaluation of women in this age range for infertility and pelvic pain. Endometriosis is less frequently described in postmenopausal women. In adolescents, congenital anomalies that promote retrograde menstruation may be a common associated finding.

It has previously been thought that certain patient groups are at higher risk for developing endometriosis. Middle-class white patients who are described as high achieving and perfectionist were considered at higher risk. These stereotypical descriptions have not been proven valid. There is evidence, however, that there is a genetic predisposition in women whose first-degree relatives have had endometriosis.

PATHOGENESIS

The exact mechanism by which endometriosis develops is unknown. *Three major theories* are commonly cited:

1. *Direct implantation* of endometrial cells has been postulated, typically by means of retrograde menstruation. This appears to adequately explain the occurrence of pelvic endometriosis and its predilection for the ovaries and pelvic peritoneum. This also explains why endometriosis is found in sites such as an abdominal incision or episiotomy scar. This is commonly referenced to as Sampson's theory.
2. *Vascular and lymphatic dissemination* of endometrial cells suggests that distant sites of endometriosis can be explained by this process, for example, the presence of endometriosis in locations such as lymph nodes, pleural cavity, and kidney.
3. *Celomic metaplasia* suggests that there are *multipotential cells* in the peritoneal cavity that, under certain conditions, can develop into functional endometrial tissue.

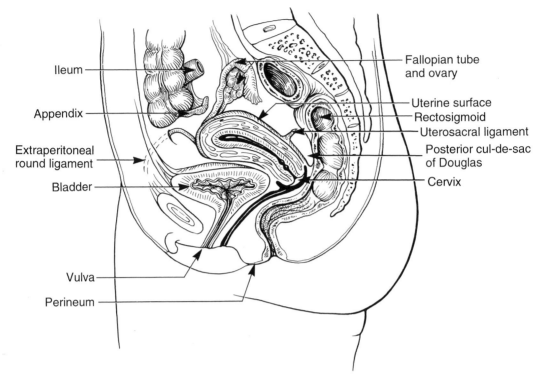

Figure 32.1. Sites of endometriosis.

Each of these major theories has its attractive aspects to explain the presence of endometriosis in its various locations. It is probable that more than one theory is necessary to explain the diverse nature of endometriosis. Underlying all of these possibilities is the yet-undiscovered immunologic factor which would be the "cause" why some women develop endometriosis while others with similar characteristics do not.

PATHOLOGY

Endometriosis is most commonly found on the ovary and is typically bilateral. Other common pelvic structures involved include the pouch of Douglas (particularly the uterosacral ligaments and rectovaginal septum), the round ligament, the fallopian tube, and the sigmoid colon (Fig. 32.1).

The gross appearance of endometriosis varies considerably. Subtle, minimal findings that have been biopsy-proven to be endome-

triosis can include 1-mm vascular hemorrhagic areas, white-opaque plaques on the peritoneal surfaces, and more classically, spots that have been described as "mulberry" or "raspberry" in appearance. These small areas may be rust-colored, dark brown, or like "powder burns" in appearance. There is reactive fibrosis surrounding these lesions, which give a puckered appearance. More advanced, disseminated disease causes further fibrosis and results in the typically dense adhesions seen in patients whose pelvic anatomy may be totally obscured by the disease.

The ovary itself can develop large collections of endometriosis, which form cysts on the ovary. These are filled with thick, chocolate appearing fluid, which is primarily old blood. These "chocolate cysts" are associated with endometriosis although hemorrhagic cysts of the ovary may also have this gross appearance.

The microscopic diagnosis of endometriosis is made when there are endometrial glands, stroma, and a presence of hemosiderin-laden macrophages. The glands and stroma do function histologically and physiologically like uterine mucosa in that cyclic changes are noted. It is not, however, as well ordered as that which occurs in the endometrial cavity. In as many as one third of cases, the microscopic diagnosis is not conclusive despite a "classic" clinical appearance.

CLINICAL FEATURES

Symptoms

Women with endometriosis demonstrate an exceptionally wide variation of symptomatology, the nature and severity of which depend on the both the location and gross severity of the disease. Women with extensive endometriosis may have few symptoms, whereas, paradoxically, those with minimal gross endometriosis may have severe pain. The *classic symptoms* of endometriosis include: (*a*) *dysmenorrhea*, (*b*) *dyspareunia*, (*c*) *infertility*, (*d*) *abnormal bleeding*, and (*e*) *pelvic pain*.

The *dysmenorrhea* associated with endometriosis is not directly related to the gross extent of the disease. Patients who present with dysmenorrhea that does not respond to oral contraceptives or nonsteroidal antiinflammatory agents should have endometriosis considered as a possible etiology. The *dyspareunia* is often associated with uterosacral or vaginal involvement with endometriosis. The dyspareunia is typically on deep penetration rather than entrance dyspareunia. The uterus may be retroverted and fixed in the cul-de-sac due to the extensive adhesions. There is, however, no correlation between dyspareunia and the extent of endometriosis.

Infertility is more frequent in women with endometriosis than in the general population. The exact mechanism for the infertility is unclear in patients with minimal endometriosis. Prostaglandins and autoantibodies have been implicated and with more extensive gross disease, adhesions and fibrosis of the pelvic distort normal anatomic relationships, thereby making the patient infertile. Infertility may, in some cases, be the only complaint. In these cases, endometriosis is discovered at the time of laparoscopic evaluation for the cause of infertility.

Abnormal bleeding occurs in approximately one third of women with endometriosis. In some cases, irregular menstrual periods are due to anovulation. In many cases, there is premenstrual spotting, possibly due to an associated luteal phase inadequacy.

Pelvic pain is a common finding in patients with endometriosis. In some cases, patients are unable to isolate their pelvic pain solely to the menstrual period or to coital activity, as suggested by the "classic" cases mentioned above. Chronic pelvic pain may be related to the adhesions and pelvic scarring found in association with endometriosis.

Other, *less common symptoms of endometriosis* include rectal bleeding and dyschezia in patients with bowel involvement with endometriosis. Occasionally, patients may present with an acute abdominal emergency, which may be associated with the rupture of an endometrioma.

Signs

The classic description of uterosacral nodularity on rectovaginal examination is consistent with significant disease. The uterus is often relatively fixed and retroflexed in the pelvis. Ovarian endometriomas may be tender, palpable, and freely mobile in the pelvis or adhered to the posterior leaf of the broad ligament or in the posterior cul-de-sac.

Physical findings in early endometriosis may be very subtle or even nonexistent. In cases of unexplained pelvic pain or infertility, the diagnosis of endometriosis should be entertained and diagnostic laparoscopy considered. It is recommended that visual and, ideally, histologic confirmation of endometriosis be obtained prior to institution of medical therapy for endometriosis. A summary of the clinical features of endometriosis is seen in Fig. 32.2.

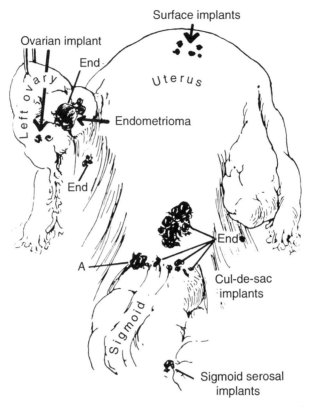

Figure 32.2. Clinical features of endometriosis (*End*). *A*, uterosacral implants.

DIFFERENTIAL DIAGNOSIS

Depending on how the patient presents, the primary differential diagnostic possibilities will vary. In patients who present with chronic abdominal pain, chronic pelvic inflammatory disease, pelvic adhesions, or other etiologies of chronic pelvic pain should be evaluated. In patients who present primarily with dysmenorrhea, both primary dysmenorrhea as well as other etiologies for secondary dysmenorrhea should be considered. In patients who present with dyspareunia, other considerations should include chronic pelvic inflammatory disease, ovarian cysts, and symptomatic uterine retroversion. If abnormal bleeding is the primary presentation, investigations focusing on anovulation (hypothyroidism, hyperprolactinemia) and premenstrual spotting (luteal phase defect) should be undertaken. If the patient presents with sudden abdominal pain, considerations other than a ruptured endometrioma would include ectopic pregnancy, acute pelvic inflammatory disease, adnexal torsion, and rupture of a corpus luetum cyst or other ovarian neoplasm.

DIAGNOSIS

Because of the diverse ways in which patients with endometriosis present, history taking and physical examination can be considered only preliminary in nature. Firm establishment of a diagnosis requires direct visualization at the time of diagnostic laparoscopy or laparotomy. Ideally, histologic confirmation of "endometriosis-appearing" lesions or implants should be obtained. Should rectal bleeding occur, barium enema and colonoscopy should be undertaken in order to exclude other primary gastrointestional disorders. Pelvic ultrasound cannot definitively

Table 32.1

THE AMERICAN FERTILITY SOCIETY
REVISED CLASSIFICATION OF ENDOMETRIOSIS

Patient's Name _____ Date_____

Stage I (Minimal) - 1-5
Stage II (Mild) - 6-15
Stage III (Moderate) - 16-40
Stage IV (Severe) - > 40
Total_____

Laparoscopy_____ Laparotomy_____ Photography_____
Recommended Treatment_____

Prognosis_____

			< 1cm	1-3cm	> 3cm
PERITONEUM	**ENDOMETRIOSIS**		< 1cm	1-3cm	> 3cm
		Superficial	1	2	4
		Deep	2	4	6
OVARY	R	Superficial	1	2	4
		Deep	4	16	20
	L	Superficial	1	2	4
		Deep	4	16	20

	POSTERIOR CULDESAC OBLITERATION	Partial	Complete
		4	40

			< 1/3 Enclosure	1/3-2/3 Enclosure	> 2/3 Enclosure
OVARY	**ADHESIONS**		< 1/3 Enclosure	1/3-2/3 Enclosure	> 2/3 Enclosure
	R	Filmy	1	2	4
		Dense	4	8	16
	L	Filmy	1	2	4
		Dense	4	8	16
TUBE	R	Filmy	1	2	4
		Dense	4*	8*	16
	L	Filmy	1	2	4
		Dense	4*	8*	16

*If the fimbriated end of the fallopian tube is completely enclosed, change the point assignment to 16.

make the diagnosis of endometriosis, nor are there any laboratory studies that are of specific value.

Once the diagnosis is made, the extent of the endometriosis should be properly documented. The most widely accepted classification system has been established by the American Fertility Society (Table 32.1). This standardizes the extent of the disease and aids in tracking progression or regression of endometriosis after therapy has been instituted.

PREVENTION

There is no known method to prevent endometriosis. Instead, the prevention of the spread of this disease should be the goal once the diagnosis has been established. Early diagnosis as a function of a high index of suspicion can allow for early treatment before the endometriosis has progressed extensively. As an example, conditions of the lower genital tract that may predispose to retrograde menstruation should be corrected as soon as they are found. As another example, diagnostic procedures that require retrograde insufflation of dye or gas through the fallopian tubes should not be done while the patient is menstruating. Because endometriosis appears to be suppressed by the hormonal effects of pregnancy, conception has traditionally been recommended as a way to prevent or minimize the effects of endometriosis. Unfortunately, there are no scientific data to support this latter recommendation.

TREATMENT

The diagnosis should be firmly established prior to instituting either medical or surgical therapy. The choice of therapy will depend on the patient's individual circumstances, which include: (*a*) presenting symptoms and their severity, (*b*) location and severity of endometriosis, and (*c*) desire for future childbearing. All of the medical treatments for endometriosis are temporizing measures to some extent. None can be expected to provide a permanent cure until extirpative surgery is undertaken.

Observation

There are selected cases in which patients can be treated expectantly, i.e., without either medical or surgical therapy. These include patients with very limited disease whose symptoms are minimal or nonexistent and/or those who are trying to get pregnant.

Medical Therapy

All forms of medical therapy are aimed at inducing relative inactivity of the endometrial tissue. Because the glands and stroma of endometriosis respond to both exogenous as well as endogenous hormones, suppression of endometriosis is based upon a medication's potential ability to induce atrophy of the endometrial tissue. This is optimal for the patients who are symptomatic, have documented endometriosis beyond minimal disease, and desire to conceive sometime in the future. The patient should be aware that recurrence after the completion of medical therapy is common and that medical therapy does not have an effect on adhesions and fibrosis caused by the endometriosis.

Beneficial effects have been obtained using *oral contraceptive* agents, i.e., combinations of estrogens and progestin. Commonly referred to as "pseudopregnancy," the use of oral contraceptives induces a decidual reaction in the functioning endometriotic tissue. Patients who are maintained on oral contraceptive agents without intermittent with-

drawal bleeding are rendered anovulatory as well as amenorrheic. They, thereby, avoid the ill effects of secondary dysmenorrhea. *Progestins* alone have also been administered by both the oral and parenteral routes.

A state of "pseudomenopause" can also be induced utilizing *danazol*, a 17α-ethinyl testosterone derivative. Danazol suppresses both LH and FSH midcycle surges so that the ovary no longer produces estrogen and progesterone, which stimulate endometriosis. The desired endometrial atrophy results, but the patient also experiences vasomotor symptoms and other hypoestrogenic symptoms. In spite of the term "pseudomenopause," FSH and LH levels are suppressed rather than elevated as they would be in the physiologic menopausal state. Side effects of danazol are also related to its androgenic properties, including acne, oily skin, growth of facial hair, and deepening of the voice. *GnRH agonists* have also been successfully used in treating endometriosis. Daily injections, monthly shots, and nasal spray have all been shown to be effective by "down-regulating" the pituitary. Efficacy appears to approximate that of danazol.

Surgical Therapy

The surgical management of endometriosis can be classified as either conservative or extirpative. *Conservative surgery* includes excision, cauterization or laser ablation of visible endometriotic lesions, and preservation of the uterus and other reproductive organs to allow for a possible future pregnancy. Conservative surgery is often undertaken at the time of the initial diagnosis. Whether the initial laparoscopy is performed for pain or infertility, attempts to remove the existent endometriosis are undertaken by the surgeon. If extensive disease is found, conservative surgery involves lysis of adhesions, removal of active endometriotic lesions, and possibly reconstruction of reproductive organs. Success rates of conservative surgery appear to correlate with the severity of the disease at the time of surgery. Medical therapy is often added either prior to surgery, in order to reduce the amount of endometriosis with which the surgeon has to contend, or post-operatively, to attempt to facilitate healing and avoid recurrence of the endometriosis.

Extirpative surgery for endometriosis is reserved only for cases where the disease is so extensive that conservative medical or surgical therapy is not feasible or when the patient has completed her family and wishes definitive final therapy. Definitive surgery includes *total abdominal hysterectomy, bilateral salpingo-oophorectomy, lysis of adhesions, and removal of endometriotic implants.* The ramifications of not being able to conceive in the future must be thoroughly explored with the patient. Assuming that all the ovarian tissue is removed at the time of surgery, it is anticipated that any residual endometriosis cannot be stimulated by further endogenous hormonal production. Occasionally in younger patients, ovarian tissue may be left in order to avoid the need for long-term estrogen replacement therapy. This should be done only with the understanding that further surgery may be necessary to remove the remaining ovary should endometriosis recur. Pregnancy is also possible after conservative surgical therapy, with 60% pregnancy rates seen in patients with moderate disease.

Estrogen replacement therapy after definitive surgery for endometriosis should not be avoided for fear of stimulating recurrent disease. Only rarely is reactivation of endometriosis noted, a far smaller risk than that associated with no estrogen therapy (e.g., bone loss, etc.).

FURTHER READINGS

Clarke-Pearson D, Dawood MY, eds. Green's gynecology: essentials of clinical practice, 8th ed. Boston: Little, Brown & Co, 1990.

Herbst AL, Mishell DR, Stenchever MA, Droegemueller W. Endometriosis and adenomyosis. In: Comprehensive gynecology, 2nd ed. St. Louis, MO: CV Mosby, 1992;545.

SELF-EVALUATION

Case 32-A

A 22-year-old woman seeks your help with her inability to become pregnant. She and her husband have been having intercourse without the use of birth control for the past 17 months. Her history includes an induced abortion at the age of 16 and two episodes of "pus tubes," which required hospitalization. She reports significant menstrual discomfort and pain "when he pushes deep" during intercourse. On your examination you find the uterus to be retroverted and somewhat fixed. The patient reports moderate discomfort to uterine and cervical motion. There is some enlargement of the adnexa bilaterally.

Question 32-A-1

The most likely diagnosis is:

A. acute pelvic inflammatory disease
B. ovarian endometriosis
C. primary dysmenorrhea
D. chronic pelvic inflammatory disease
E. pelvic scarring due to pelvic infections

Answer 32-A-1

Answer: E

By history, this patient is most likely to have inactive scarring due to pelvic inflammatory disease. The patient does not have any symptoms of an acute infection, decreasing the possibility of acute pelvic inflammatory disease. The history and physical examination provide enough suspicion of pelvic pathology to make secondary dysmenorrhea more likely than primary. Although endometriosis might explain the retroversion of the uterus and the patient's dyspareunia, endometriosis is not documented as yet.

Question 32-A-2

What is the best recommendation for this patient?

A. abdominal hysterectomy
B. in vitro fertilization
C. danazol treatment
D. diagnostic laparoscopy
E. observation

Answer 32-A-2

Answer: D

Although the patient's most likely diagnosis based on history and physical examination is pelvic adhesions, the diagnosis of that entity as well as endometriosis can be made only by direct observation. Only with a firm diagnosis can appropriate therapeutic options be presented to the patient for consideration.

Case 32-B

A 38-year-old woman presents for a premarital examination. She has never been pregnant and she uses a diaphragm for contraception. Over the past 3–4 years she has had increasing problems with cramps with her menstrual flow. The cramps use to improve with the use of an over-the-counter ibuprofen medication, but lately even this has not provided relief. Prior to her wedding she would also like you to check the fit of her diaphragm because "lately it has been causing some pelvic and rectal discomfort" when she uses it. On examination she has significant cervical motion tenderness and thickening of the uterosacral ligaments. Endometriosis is suspected.

Question 32-B-1

The patient should be advised that:

A. an immediate pregnancy is desirable.

B. switching to an oral contraceptive might be beneficial.

C. no therapy should be undertaken until exploratory surgery is performed.

D. therapy with a GnRh agonist should be started prior to her wedding.

E. no specific therapy is needed at this time.

Answer 32-B-1

Answer: B

Although this patient may experience problems conceiving, the decision to have a child is always up to the patient and her partner, not the physician. While the presumptive diagnosis of endometriosis may be correct, definitive diagnosis cannot be made unless endometriosis is visualized. Nevertheless, some suggestions based on this presumption are appropriate. Because the patient is symptomatic, suppression using oral contraceptives might be beneficial, although not without risk at this patient's age and, in fact, would be contraindicated if she were a smoker. Certainly aggressive therapy with GnRH agonist or danazol should be delayed until the diagnosis is established by laparoscopy.

For further consideration: What should you tell this patient about her future fertility? What factors would make you consider diagnostic laparoscopy? If the patient did not need contraception, would that affect your recommendation?

chapter 33

SEXUAL ASSAULT

Sexual assault is the nonconsensual performance of acts, which in a consensual setting would be sexual or which involve genital structures in such a manner that the victim perceives a sexual intrusion. An estimated one of every four women and children in the United States are sexual assault victims. Because of the stigmata associated with sexual assault, only one of 10 victims seeks help. Unfortunately, those victims who do seek help are often as traumatized by those from whom they seek help as by those who assaulted them. Because of the complex problems caused by sexual assault, treatment by a *multidisciplinary team* using prepared protocols is best. The health care team has three tasks: (*a*) *care for the victim's emotional needs,* (*b*) *evaluate and treat medically,* and (*c*) *collect forensic specimens.*

CARING FOR THE ADULT SEXUAL ASSAULT VICTIM
Rape Trauma Syndrome

During sexual assault, the victim realizes that she cannot escape the situation and has lost control. This *loss of control,* which is the most serious emotional problem faced by the victim, is based in fact, as *threatened or actual violence is always an integral part of sexual assault.* Victims of sexual assault may react to the experience in various ways. One recognized aftermath is the rape trauma syndrome. This syndrome has three phases. The *acute phase of rape trauma syndrome* begins with the assault, but may not be fully manifest until the time of initial disclosure when the victim first tells someone of the assault. In this emotionally volatile time, the victim may appear calm or may be tearful and agitated, or may move from one extreme to another. *An inability to think clearly or remember things such as her past medical history, termed "cognitive dysfunction," is a particularly distressing aspect of the syndrome.* The involuntary loss of cognition may raise fears of "being crazy" or of being perceived as "crazy" by others. It is also frustrating for the health team unless they realize that this is an involuntary reaction to the assault and not a willful action. After the assault and prior to seeking care, the victim may have performed routine tasks such as shopping or cleaning the house. This *retreat to routine activities* is an emotional attempt to regain control, the presence or absence of which is not related to the severity of the assault. *Safety and regaining control are the victim's main emotional needs during this time.* The patient should be reassured about her immediate safety and offered as much control over events as is reasonable for her clinical situation. Discussing the sexual assault within a supportive environmental facilitates a sense of control, even if the topics of discussion are themselves unpleasant.

During the *middle or "readjustment" phase* the patient appears to resolve most issues about the assault. This "resolution" involves a rationalization that she should or could have prevented the assault, coupled with unrealistic plans to avoid another assault. The plans of this phase ultimately break down in the *late or "reorganization" phase,* as the victim begins to deal with the reality of her victimization. The late phase, which may be quite lengthy, is a difficult and very painful time, often characterized by drastic changes in life-style, friends, and work. Ongoing counseling is important if the victim is to fully recover from the emotional traumas of the assault.

Initial Care of the Adult Victim

A team member should remain with the patient to help provide a sense of safety and security. The patient should be encouraged, in a supportive, nonjudgmental manner, to talk about the assault and her feelings. This starts the patient's emotional care, as well as providing historical data. Treatment for life-threatening trauma is, of course, begun immediately. Fortunately, such trauma is uncommon, although minor trauma is seen in one fourth of victims. Even in life-threatening situations, any sense of "control" that can be given the patient is helpful. Obtaining consents for treatment is not only a legal requirement but also an important aspect of the emotional care of the victim. Although patients are often reticent to do so, they should be gently encouraged to work with the police, as such cooperation is clearly associated with improved emotional outcomes for victims.

History taking about a sexual assault is uncomfortable for victims and health care providers alike. History taking is not, however, an additional trauma. Instead, it is both a necessary activity to gain medical and forensic information and an important therapeutic activity. Recalling the details of the assault in the supportive environment of the health care setting allows the victim to begin to gain an understanding of what has happened and to see that she and others can deal with the events. Victims of sexual assault characteristically perceive themselves as guilty of causing the assault, especially in situations where they have used poor judgment (e.g., hitchhiking). To say that any activity was acceptable when it involved poor judgment is a falsehood that destroys the patient's ultimate trust and the care provider's credibility. Reminding the patient that *"poor judgment is not a rapable offense"* helps the patient to start to place blame where it truly belongs: on the rapist.

Victims of sexual assault should be given a *complete general physical examination* including a pelvic examination. Forensic specimens should be collected and cultures for sexually transmitted diseases obtained. In collecting *forensic specimens*, it is critical to follow the directions on the forensic specimens kit. The forensic specimens are kept in a health professional's possession or control until turned over to an appropriate legal representative. This "protective custody" of the specimens assures that the correct specimen reaches the forensic laboratory and is called the "chain of evidence."

Initial *laboratory tests* should include cultures from vagina, anus, and usually also pharynx for gonorrhea and chlamydia, rapid plasma reagin (RPR, a test for syphilis), hepatitis antigens, HIV if indicated (usually), UA and C&S, and pregnancy test for menstrual age women regardless of contraceptive status.

Antibiotic prophylaxis should be offered to all adult victims. The risk of infection is unknown, but clearly higher than for a consensual sexual experience. Recommended regimens include oral *doxycycline* or oral *amoxicillin* plus *probenecid* followed by oral *erythromycin* base for pregnant victims or those allergic to tetracyclines. In areas with a prevalence rate greater than 1% for antibiotic resistant strains of *Neisseria gonorrhoeae*, ceftriaxone, 250 mg i.m., followed by oral doxycycline are recommended. Short courses of *Diethylstilbestrol (DES)* with *Compazine* (prochlorperazine) may be given as a *postcoital contraceptive medication*. If a postcoital contraception is chosen, the patient should be reminded that these medications may be teratogenic so that a therapeutic abortion is recommended if pregnancy does occur despite their use. *Tetanus toxoid* should be administered if indicated.

Within 24–48 hours, victims should be contacted by phone or seen for an *immediate posttreatment evaluation*. At this time, emotional or physical problems are managed and follow-up appointments arranged for 1 and 6 weeks. Potentially serious problems such as suicidal ideation, rectal bleeding, or evidence of pelvic infection may go unrecognized by the victim during this time because of fear or continued cognitive dysfunction. Gently stated but specific questions must be asked to ensure that such problems have not arisen.

Subsequent Care of Adult Victims

At the 1-week visit, a general review of the patient's progress is made and any specific new problems addressed. The next routine visit is at *6 weeks*, when a complete evaluation including physical examination, repeat cultures for sexually transmitted diseases, and a repeat RPR are performed. Another visit at 12–18 weeks may be indicated for repeat HIV virus titers, although the present understanding of HIV virus infection does not allow an estimate of the risk of exposure for sexual assault victims. Each victim should receive as much counseling and support as is necessary, with referral to a long-term counseling program if needed.

CARING FOR THE CHILD SEXUAL ASSAULT VICTIM

Ninety percent of child victimization is by parents, family members, or family friends; "stranger rape" is relatively uncommon in children. The assailants play upon the child's need for love and her dependency upon family. To get past this conflict, it is best to interview child victims apart from parents and other family members, if possible by interviewers skilled in child interview techniques. Although such interviewing and the interpretation of information gained is difficult, in general, a child who displays a knowledge of sexual matters, anatomy, or function beyond that expected for her years is very likely a victim of sexual abuse.

It is the responsibility of the care team to determine if the child may safely return home or if the risk of ongoing abuse requires foster home placement or hospitalization. Since *suspected child sexual abuse must be reported to police and child welfare authorities*, they officially may help in this decision, although responsibility rests with the care team at the time of the initial disclosure.

FURTHER READINGS

American Academy of Pediatrics, Committee on Child Abuse and Neglect. Guidelines for the evaluation of sexual abuse in children. Pediatrics 1991;B7:254–260.

Beckmann CRB. Sexual assault. In: Stovall TG, Summitt R, Beckmann CRB, Ling FW, eds. A clinical manual of Gynecology. 2nd ed. New York: Pergamon-Macmillan, 1991:Chapter 18.

Beckmann CRB. Sexual assault. In: Clarke-Pearson DL, Dawood MY, eds. Green's gynecology: essentials of clinical practice. 8th ed. Boston: Little, Brown & Co, 1990:Chapter 20.

Burgess A, Holstron G, Lytle L. Rape trauma syndrome. Am J Psychiatry 1974;131:981.

Sgroi S. Handbook of clinical intervention in child sexual abuse. Lexington, MA: DC Heath, 1985.

SELF-EVALUATION

Case 33-A

Your patient is a 15-year-old G2P2 who presents to your Emergency Room accompanied by police to whom she has reported a sexual assault. She is quiet but seems disoriented, dressed in a see-through blouse and tight stretch pants. She tells the nurses that she was raped by a "friend." The police ask that you speed your evaluation, as they have other calls and need to be on their way.

Question 33-A-1

Which of the following should guide your initial evaluation of this patient?

A. rapid conclusion of the evaluation to cooperate with the police

B. dismissing the claim of rape because it was a friend, hence clearly consensual sex rather than rape

C. concern that the historical information is incomplete, requiring a full evaluation regardless of pressure to proceed more rapidly

D. Since she is a minor, calling her parents to get permission to see the patient and obtaining further information

Answer 33-A-1

Answer: C

Your primary responsibilities are emotional and physical health care of the patient. Cooperation with police is important, especially in the initial phase to provide immediate information for pursuit of the assailant. Thereafter, police action is best left until after health care is completed. Knowing that sexual abuse in children is often performed by family members, you may contact parents but plan to pay special attention to the child's history. The patient's attire and anything it might imply about her life-style are irrelevant.

Question 33-A-2

Your sexual assault team completes its evaluation, and you discover that your patient lives with her mother and stepfather. She is afraid to tell your team about details of what has happened, but does indicate it has been going on for some time. She is frightened to return home.

Her physical examination is unremarkable except that her uterus is about 14 week size and soft. What laboratory tests are indicated?

A. UA
B. urine hCG
C. urine drug screen
D. Pap smear
E. hepatitis screen

Answer 33-A-2

Answer: B

By history and examination, pregnancy is likely and a pregnancy test is appropriate. The other tests listed may be useful in general, but do not address the specific issue: Who is abusing this child?

Question 33-A-3

When the pregnancy test is reported as positive, the police say the patient is just upset because she is pregnant and they insist on taking the patient home. She becomes tearful, but says she will go home if the police and her parents say she has to do so.

Answer 33-A-3

For further consideration: What do you do? What do you think really happened to this

young woman? Is it safe for her to go home? Does a report need to be made to welfare authorities? Do the police have the authority to make the decision about her?

Case 33-B

Your patient is a 35-year-old mother of three, the wife of a heavy equipment operator, who presents complaining that her husband raped her earlier in the day after she refused him "his sex." She says he threatened to beat her if she didn't "lie down and take it," so she did. Physical examination reveals only motile sperm in the vagina. The patient has had a postpartum tubal ligation. She says she wishes medical care but does not want the police notified, as they will "cause too much trouble." Her husband arrives, demands that you "get out of his business" and let his wife go so that she can fix dinner.

Question 33-B-1

Your appropriate response(s) to this situation include:

A. Tell the patient to go home, that how and when she and her husband have sex is their business and not yours.
B. Complete a sexual assault workup.
C. Notify the police.
D. Call psychiatry, as the patient is clearly not demonstrating an appropriate response to a sexual assault.

Answer 33-B-1

Answer: B, C.

In some states, a husband cannot by law rape his wife (in effect, she is in the eyes of the law his sexual property), whereas in other states, rape is defined as a nonconsensual experience. In either case, this legal decision is not properly made by you, but by the police, who should be notified. You may support the patient's decision not to talk to the police, although you should encourage her to do so, but you must call the police because a violent crime has been reported and because you do not know what the situation is at home, especially in relation to the safety of the children.

You, of course, complete a sexual assault workup, treating the patient emotionally and medically. You collect the forensic specimens. Whether or not they are used is up to the authorities. If you do not collect them now and they are needed later, it will be too late. You include a pregnancy test, as tubal ligations do fail on occasion. Psychiatry is rarely needed and in this case no demonstration of psychosis is evident. Referral to a "safe home" for battered and abused women may be helpful.

chapter 34

REPRODUCTIVE CYCLE

In the female reproductive cycle, ovulation is followed by menstrual bleeding in a recurring sequence if conception does not occur. This recurring sequence is established at puberty (around age 13) and continues until the time of menopause at around age 50. A regular, predictable reproductive cycle is usually established by age 15 and continues until age 45. Thus, a woman has approximately 30 years of optimal reproductive function. In healthy women, reproductive cycles occur at about 28-day intervals and most women ovulate 13–14 times per year unless ovulation is interrupted by pregnancy, lactation, or oral contraceptive use.

The reproductive cycle depends upon the cyclic interaction between hypothalamic gonadotropin-releasing hormone (GnRH), the pituitary gonadotropins follicle-stimulating hormone (FSH) and luteinizing hormone (LH), and the ovarian sex steroid hormones estradiol and progesterone. Through positive and negative feedback loops, these hormones stimulate ovulation, facilitate implantation of the fertilized ovum, and bring about menstruation. Feedback loops between the hypothalamus, pituitary gland, and ovaries are depicted in Figure 34.1. If any one (or more) of the above hormones becomes tonically elevated or suppressed, the reproductive cycle becomes disrupted; ovulation and menstruation cease. In the case of female reproductive dysfunction, it is essential to identify which hormones are either elevated or reduced.

HYPOTHALAMIC GnRH SECRETION

Hypothalamic GnRH (a decapeptide) is secreted in a pulsatile manner from the arcuate nucleus of the hypothalamus. The hypothalamus serves as the mainspring or pulse generator of the reproductive clock. Surgical ablation of the arcuate nucleus in animals disrupts ovarian function, as does continuous infusion of GnRH agonists. Ovarian function can be restored by the pulsatile infusion of GnRH at 70–90-minute intervals. The mechanism for stimulation of GnRH secretion is unknown; however, GnRH secretion is influenced by estradiol and by catecholamine neurotransmitters. The latter influence may help explain psychogenic influences on the reproductive cycle. GnRH reaches the anterior pituitary gland through the hypothalamic-pituitary portal plexus. Pituitary gonadotropin secretion is stimulated and modulated by the pulsatile secretion of GnRH.

PITUITARY GONADOTROPIN SECRETION

The pituitary gonadotropins *FSH* and *LH* are protein hormones secreted by the anterior pituitary gland. FSH and LH are also secreted in pulsatile fashion in concert with the pulsatile release of GnRH; the magnitude of secretion and the rates of secretion of FSH and/or LH are determined largely by the levels of ovarian steroid hormones and other ovarian factors. When a woman is in a state of relative estrogen deficiency, the principal gonadotropin secreted is FSH. As the ovary responds to FSH secretion with estradiol production, there is a negative feedback to the pituitary gland to inhibit FSH secretion and facilitate LH secretion. This is discussed in more detail in

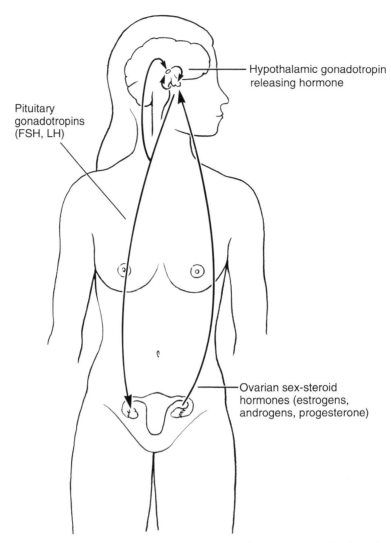

Figure 34.1. Cyclic interactions between the hypothalamus, pituitary gland, and ovaries.

association with the phases of the reproductive cycle.

OVARIAN SEX STEROID HORMONE SECRETION

Ovarian follicles respond to pituitary gonadotropin secretion by synthesizing the principal ovarian hormones, *estradiol* and *progesterone*. Increasing levels of estradiol on the pituitary gland via a negative feedback decreases secretion of FSH and increases secretion of LH. This results in a marked increase in LH secretion, known as the LH surge, which triggers ovulation. With ovulation, the ovarian follicle is converted into a corpus luteum and begins secreting progesterone.

At birth, the human ovary is filled with *primordial follicles*. Each follicle contains an oocyte that is arrested in the prophase stage of meiosis. The oocyte is surrounded by a single layer of pregranulosa cells, which will become the granulosa cells. The pregranulosa cells are surrounded by a matrix of cells that will become the theca cells. Some pri-

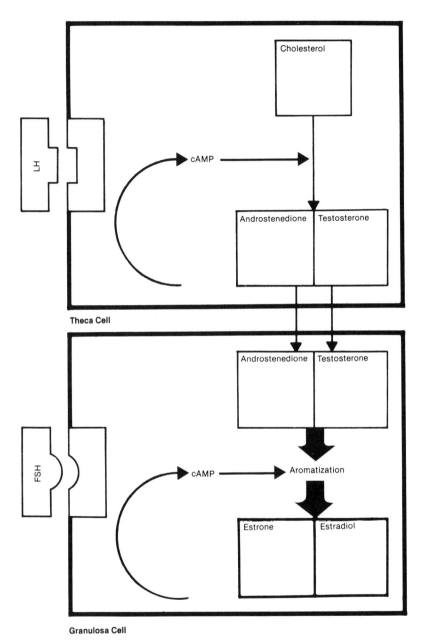

Figure 34.2. Two cell theories of estradiol production.

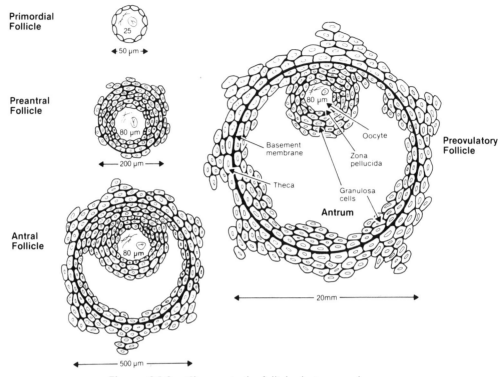

Figure 34.3. Changes in the follicle during a cycle.

mordial follicles respond to pituitary FSH during childhood, but ovulation does not occur until puberty, despite the stimulation and subsequent atresia of some follicles during childhood.

During a full reproductive cycle, one oocyte is brought to maturity prior to ovulation. In the process of bringing one oocyte to maturation, a number of oocytes are stimulated to partial maturation but subsequently undergo atresia before reaching ovulation. Why several oocytes are stimulated simultaneously, but only one is ovulated, is unknown.

During the process of follicular maturation, pregranulosa cells are stimulated by FSH to become *granulosa cells*, which begin secreting *estradiol*. Initially, there is a single layer of granulosa cells surrounding oocyte. Binding of FSH to receptors in the granulosa cells causes granulosa cell proliferation, increased binding of FSH, and increased pro-

duction of estradiol. The follicle with the greatest number of granulosa cells, FSH receptors, and the highest estradiol production becomes the dominant follicle from which ovulation will occur.

As a primordial follicle is stimulated, the pretheca cells surrounding the granulosa cells become *theca cells*. The theca cells secrete *androgens*, which serve as the precursors for estradiol production by the granulosa cells. Current scientific theory holds that estradiol is secreted through a two-cell mechanism (Fig. 34.2). Androgens are first secreted by the theca cells. These androgens enter the granulosa cells by diffusion, where they are aromatized to estradiol.

After ovulation, the dominant follicle becomes the *corpus luteum*, which secretes *progesterone* to prepare the endometrium for implantation of a fertilized oocyte. If pregnancy does not occur, menstruation begins and the cycle repeats. The changes in the follicle during the follicular phase of the cycle are presented in Figure 34.3.

For purposes of discussion, *the reproductive cycle is divided into three phases: menstruation and the follicular phase, ovulation*, and the *luteal phase*. These three phases refer to the status of the ovary during the reproductive cycle.

REPRODUCTIVE CYCLE

Phase I: Menstruation and the Follicular Phase

When the oocyte ovulated in the previous cycle fails to become fertilized, the cyclic interaction between the hypothalamus, pituitary gland, and ovaries is reset, initiating a new reproductive cycle. The first day of menstruation is considered day 1 of the menstrual cycle. During menstruation, the endometrium is sloughed in response to progesterone withdrawal. This is followed by the follicular phase where a new endometrial lining of the uterus is formed in preparation for implantation of an embryo.

Women usually menstruate for 3–5 days. A woman will shed approximately 30–50 ml of dark, nonclotting menstrual blood during menstruation. Occasionally, tissue elements of endometrium can be identified in the menstrual effluent.

There may be uterine cramps during the first day or two of menstrual bleeding. These occur due to the action of prostaglandins liberated from the endometrium at the beginning of menstruation. These prostaglandins stimulate uterine contractions that aid the expulsion of the menstrual effluent.

Menstruation also marks the beginning of the follicular phase of the cycle. With the beginning of menstruation, plasma concentrations of estradiol, progesterone, and LH reach their lowest point. Only FSH is increased at the beginning of menstruation. The increase in FSH begins about 2 days prior to onset of menstruation and is involved in the maturation of another group of ovarian follicles and the selection of a dominant follicle for ovulation in the next cycle.

FSH binds to receptors located in the granulosa cells of the primary oocyte. As FSH is bound to the granulosa cells, it stimulates their differentiation from a stratified squamous-type cell into a cuboidal cell. Moreover, FSH stimulates mitosis of the granulosa cells, thereby increasing the number of granulosa cells surrounding the oocyte. Under the influence of FSH, the granulosa cells begin to secrete estradiol.

Estradiol begins to rise in plasma by the fourth day of the cycle. Estradiol stimulates LH receptors on the theca cells, preparing them to increase secretion of androgen precursors to estradiol and preparing the granulosa and theca cells for progesterone production after ovulation.

With rising estradiol, there is negative feedback on the pituitary gland to decrease the release of FSH, and positive feedback on the pituitary gland to increase the release of LH. During the early follicular phase of the cycle, the FSH:LH ratio is greater than 1; as the cycle progresses, the FSH:LH ratio becomes less than 1, demonstrating both positive and negative feedback effects of estradiol on the pituitary gland.

As follicles enlarge, they secrete both androgens and estrogens; however, if the estradiol:androgen ratio within the follicular fluid becomes less than 1, that follicle will become atretic and never become a dominant follicle. The dominant follicle is the one that has a follicular fluid estradiol:androgen ratio of greater than 1.

As the dominant follicle secretes more and more estradiol, there is marked positive feedback to the pituitary gland to secrete LH. By day 11–13 of the normal cycle, an LH surge occurs, which triggers ovulation. Ovulation occurs within 30–36 hours of the LH surge, causing the oocyte to be expelled from the follicle and the follicle to be converted into a corpus luteum to facilitate progesterone production during the remainder of the cycle. At the time of the LH surge just prior to ovulation, there is a concomitant rise in FSH. The mechanism for this FSH rise and its effect on the follicle is unknown.

Phase II: Ovulation

The mechanism for ovulation is poorly understood. As the dominant follicle enlarges and accumulates follicular fluid, it is said to "ripen" and become ready for release. Through animal studies, it has been demonstrated that intrafollicular prostaglandins play an essential role in release of the oocyte and that the administration of prostaglandin synthetase inhibitors will cause the oocyte to be retained within the follicle during the luteal phase of the cycle.

Many women experience a twinge of pain ("mittelschmerz") at the time of ovulation and can distinguish the time of ovulation with precision. Others will not experience pain, but can appreciate the effects of changing hormone production that occur with ovulation.

The application of transvaginal ultrasound imaging has enabled physicians to follow the process of follicular growth and maturation and observe the collapse of the dominant follicle following ovulation. A condition of luteinized retained follicle has been recognized, in which the oocyte does not appear to be expelled from the follicle.

Phase III: Luteal Phase

The luteal phase of the cycle is characterized by a change in secretion of sex steroid hormones from estradiol predominance to progesterone predominance. As FSH rises early in the cycle and stimulates mitosis of granulosa cells and production of estradiol, additional LH receptors are created in the granulosa cells and theca cells. With the LH surge at the time of ovulation, these LH receptors bind LH and convert the enzymatic machinery of the granulosa and theca cells to facilitate production of progesterone.

Progesterone production depends upon the initial FSH and LH signals from the pituitary gland. Adequate progesterone production is necessary to facilitate implantation of the fertilized oocyte into the endometrium and to sustain pregnancy into the early first trimester. If the initial rise in FSH is inadequate, and if the LH surge does not achieve maximal amplitude, an "inadequate luteal phase," i.e., luteal phase defect, can occur. In the luteal phase defect, there is inadequate progesterone production to facilitate implantation of a fertilized oocyte or to sustain pregnancy.

The production of progesterone begins about 24 hours prior to ovulation and rises rapidly thereafter. A maximal production of progesterone occurs 3–4 days after ovulation and is maintained for approximately 11 days following ovulation. If fertilization and implantation do not occur, progesterone production diminishes rapidly, initiating events leading to the beginning of a new cycle.

The corpus luteum measures about 2.5 cm in diameter and has a characteristic deep yellow color. It can be seen on gross inspection of the ovary if laparoscopy or laparotomy are performed during the luteal phase of the cycle. As the corpus luteum fails, it decreases in volume and loses its yellow color. After a few months, the corpus luteum becomes a white fibrous streak within the ovary called the corpus albicans.

The corpus luteum has a fixed life span of 13–14 days unless pregnancy occurs. If the oocyte becomes fertilized and implants within the endometrium, the early pregnancy begins secreting human chorionic gonadotropin (hCG), which sustains the corpus luteum for another 6–7 weeks.

Progesterone has negative feedback on pituitary secretion of both FSH and LH. During the luteal phase of the cycle, both FSH and LH are suppressed to low levels. As the corpus luteum fails and progesterone secretion diminishes, FSH begins to rise to prepare a woman for the next reproductive cycle.

The cyclic changes in FSH, LH, estradiol, and progesterone along with the changes in the follicle, endometrium, vagina, and cervix are presented in Figure 34.4. Note the cyclic interaction between these four hormones during the course of a reproductive cycle.

Perimenopause

As a woman ages, the ovarian follicles diminish in number and become less sensitive to

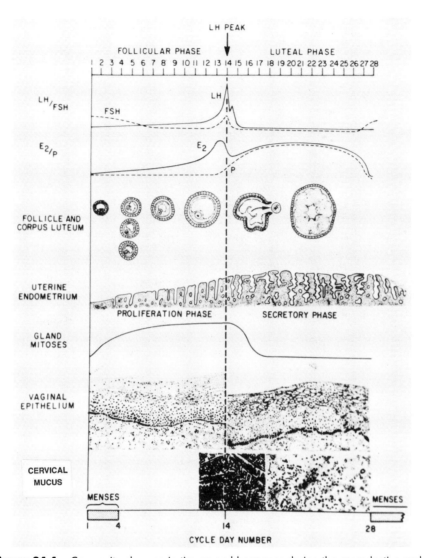

Figure 34.4. Composite changes in tissues and hormones during the reproductive cycle.

FSH. The process of ovulation becomes increasingly inefficient, less regular, and less predictable than in earlier years. A woman will begin to notice changes in her reproductive cycle at around age 38–42. Initially, she will notice a shortening of the cycle length. With increasing inefficiency of the reproductive cycle, the follicular phase shortens but the luteal phase is maintained at normal length. With the passing of time, some cycles become anovulatory so that the frequency of ovulation decreases.

As menopause approaches, the remaining follicles become almost totally resistant to FSH. The process of ovulation ceases entirely and cyclic hormone production ends with menopause.

CLINICAL MANIFESTATIONS OF HORMONAL CHANGES

The presence or absence of sex steroid hormones produce clinical manifestations that aid in establishing the phases of the reproductive cycle. The endometrium and endocervix, the breasts, the vagina, and the hypothalamic thermoregulating center all undergo cyclic changes in response to hormonal control. The changes in the endocervix and breasts can be directly observed and the changes in the hypothalamic thermoregulatory center can be measured by recording the basal body temperature. The changes in the vagina can be identified by cytologic examination of the vaginal epithelium, and the changes in the endometrium can be evaluated by endometrial biopsy followed by histologic examination of the biopsy sample. Other changes can be ascertained through a careful history. Some of these changes include alteration of libido, abdominal bloating, fluid retention, mood changes, and uterine cramps at the onset of menstruation.

Endometrium

The endometrial lining of the uterus undergoes dramatic histologic changes during the reproductive cycle. During menstruation, the endometrium is sloughed to a basal level consisting of compact stroma cells and short, narrow endometrial glands. Estrogen is a mitogenic hormone, which stimulates cell growth. With rising estradiol production during the follicular phase of the cycle, the endometrial stroma thickens and the endometrial glands become elongated; this is a proliferative endometrium. The endometrium reaches a maximal thickness at the time of ovulation. If ovulation does not occur, and a woman remains in an estrogenic state, the endometrium continues to thicken and the endometrial glands continue to elongate until the endometrium outgrows its blood supply and sloughs. This abnormal condition is the basis for dysfunctional uterine bleeding, which is discussed in Chapter 36, "Amenorrhea and Dysfunctional Uterine Bleeding."

When ovulation occurs the hormonal balance changes from an estrogenic state to a progestational state. Progesterone is not a mitogen, but causes differentiation of the tissues that contain progesterone receptors.

Progesterone converts the proliferative endometrium into a secretory endometrium. The endometrial stroma becomes loose and edematous, and blood vessels entering the endometrium become thickened. The endometrial glands, which were straight and tubular in the proliferative phase of the endometrium, become tortuous and contain secretory material within the lumina. Following ovulation, distinct, recognizable changes occur within the endometrium at almost daily intervals. Therefore, the quality of the corpus luteum and stage of the reproductive cycle can be evaluated by histologic examination of a small sample of endometrium.

Endocervix

The endocervix contains glands that secrete endocervical mucus in response to hormonal changes. Under the influence of estradiol, the endocervical glands secrete large quantities of thin, clear, watery, endocervical mucus. This mucus facilitates sperm capture, sperm storage, and sperm transport. Sperm can be stored in the crypts of the endocervical glands for up to 7 days and then released into the upper genital tract for fertilization of an oocyte. Endocervical mucus production is maximal at the time of ovulation. With ovulation and the shift in hormone production from estradiol to progesterone, the endocervical mucus becomes thick, opaque, and tenacious. This type of mucus is an impediment to sperm capture, storage, and transport.

Breasts

The ductal elements of the breasts, nipples, and areolae respond to estradiol secretion. The breasts have a relatively tubular shape during the follicular phase of the cycle. After ovulation, progesterone stimulates the acinar (milk producing) glands. Since the acinar glands are located in the tails of the breasts, this gives the breasts a more rounded configuration. Moreover, progesterone makes the venous pattern on the surface of the breasts appear more prominent and accentuates the small Montgomery glands contained within the areolae. These dynamic changes can be observed during the reproductive cycle and are seen in the development states of puberty.

Vagina

Estradiol stimulates vaginal thickening and maturation of the surface epithelial cells of the vaginal mucosa. Estradiol also stimulates vaginal transudation during sexual excitement, creating a moist, lubricated vagina for sexual intercourse. During the luteal phase of the cycle, the vaginal epithelium retains its thickness but the secretory changes are markedly diminished. Women report less sexual desire and sexual enjoyment during the luteal phase. This loss of sexual desire is even more marked during the early weeks of pregnancy.

Hypothalamic Thermoregulating Center

Progesterone shifts the basal body temperature upward by 0.6 to 1.0°F. This shift occurs abruptly with the beginning of the progesterone secretion and wanes abruptly with loss of progesterone secretion. The changes in the basal body temperature reflect the changing plasma progesterone concentration. The basal body temperature record is a useful tool for women and their physicians who want to evaluate the reproductive cycle in a dynamic and inexpensive way.

CLINICAL IMPLICATIONS OF THE REPRODUCTIVE CYCLE

Some women have exaggerated responses to the changing hormonal environment of the reproductive cycle and experience troublesome symptoms. The two conditions for which women seek medical attention as a result of the reproductive cycle are premenstrual syndrome (PMS) and primary dysmenorrhea.

The etiology and pathogenesis of premenstrual syndrome are poorly understood. There are many theories to explain this common condition and a number of treatments

devised for its correction; however, none has withstood scientific scrutiny. The emotional, physical, and behavioral symptoms of premenstrual syndrome occur during the luteal phase of the reproductive cycle and these symptoms do not occur in anovulatory women. Thus, premenstrual syndrome is directly associated with the reproductive cycle.

Primary dysmenorrhea is the occurrence of debilitating uterine cramps during the first 2 days of menstruation. Associated symptoms are diarrhea, nausea, vomiting and headache. These symptoms are self-limiting and abate as menstruation ceases. The etiology of primary dysmenorrhea is linked to the endometrial production and secretion of prostaglandins just prior to and during menstruation. Symptoms of primary dysmenorrhea can be directly alleviated by the administration of prostaglandin synthetase inhibitors and moderately by oral contraceptives to inhibit ovulation.

FURTHER READINGS

Speroff L, Glass RH, Kase NG. Regulation of the menstrual cycle. In: Clinical gynecologic endocrinology and infertility. 4th ed. Baltimore: Williams & Wilkins, 1989:91–119.

Rebar RW. Reproductive endocrinology. In: Berkow R, ed. The Merck manual. 15th ed. Rahway, NJ: Merck Sharp & Dohme Research Laboratories, 1987:1678–1687.

Ross GT. Disorders of the ovary and the female reproductive tract. In: Wilson JD, Foster DW, eds. Williams textbook of endocrinology. 7th ed. Philadelphia: WB Saunders, 1985:206–258.

SELF-EVALUATION

Case 34-A-1

A 24-year-old woman has regular, predictable menstrual cycles, which began at age 13.

Question 34-A-1

Which of the following statements about the follicular phase of her cycle are correct?

A. Follicle-stimulating hormone initiates the development of a cohort of follicles, one of which will become the dominant follicle.

B. Endometrial biopsy would reveal presence of a secretory endometrium.
C. Endocervical mucus would be thin, clear, and watery during the late follicular phase.
D. Estradiol is the predominant steroid hormone.

Answer 34-A-1

Answer: A, C, D

The only incorrect statement is regarding the state of the endometrium, which would be proliferative. Secretory endometrium reflects a state of progesterone dominance and occurs in the luteal phase.

Question 34-A-2

Which of the following statements about the luteal phase of the cycle are correct?

A. Progesterone is the predominant steroid hormone.
B. Endocervical mucus is thick, sticky, and tenacious.
C. Basal body temperature is elevated.
D. It is during this phase of the reproductive cycle that some women develop cyclic emotional, physical, and behavioral symptoms.

Answer 34-A-2

Answer: A, B, C, D

Each of the options are correct and each statement has clinical relevance in certain patients. A basic understanding of the underlying reproductive cycle physiology will facilitate diagnosis as well as treatment.

Case 34-B

A 45-year-old woman notices a lengthening of her cycle from the usual 29 days to 50–60 days. She also experiences occasional hot flushes.

Question 34-B-1

Which of the following statements are correct?

A. The number of ovarian follicles is still adequate for ovulation.
B. Her FSH concentration is tonically elevated.
C. Her FSH hormone has altered and the ovarian follicles are less responsive to the altered molecule.
D. Her plasma estradiol concentration is zero.

Answer 34-B-1

Answer: A

Although the total number of follicles continues to decrease with each cycle, the woman is apparently still having ovulatory cycles. The FSH concentration is not tonically elevated until the ovary no longer responds to FSH stimulation. Until then, it continues to fluctuate. The FSH molecule itself does not change in configuration during the perimenopausal period. The estradiol concentration is not zero, as the ovary continues to produce estradiol, albeit in less efficient fashion. The occasional vasomotor symptoms suggest waning of but not lack of ovarian function.

chapter 35

PUBERTY

Puberty is the physical, emotional, and sexual transition from childhood to adulthood. Although the transition occurs gradually, it contains a series of well-defined events and milestones. Few individuals have problems with this endocrine process. However, when puberty is delayed or advanced, an understanding of the hormonal events of puberty and the sequence of physical changes is essential for the physician to be able to evaluate the process and progress of sexual development. Moreover, an understanding of puberty is essential for an understanding of the process of reproduction.

The endocrine events that initiate the onset of secondary sexual maturation are unknown. The hypothalamic-pituitary-gonadal axis functions during fetal life and during the first few weeks following birth, after which the axis becomes quiescent. At about age 8 in boys and girls, the adrenal glands begin to secrete increasing quantities of dehydroepiandrosterone; approximately 2 years later, the gonads begin secreting gonadal sex steroid hormones. The process of secondary sexual maturation requires about 4 years from its beginning until full sexual maturation has been achieved; this process takes place in an orderly, predictable sequence. The events, age, and hormone(s) responsible for the sequence of *sexual maturation* in girls is presented in Table 35.1. The sequence of breast development (thelarche) is presented in Figure 35.1.

These events are predictable and reflect the secretion and action of hypothalamic peptide hormones and pituitary protein hormones, adrenal steroid hormones, and gonadal sex-steroid hormones. An alteration in the sequence of these events suggests that there is an alteration in normal hormone secretion and action.

Three known critical elements play a role in the timing of *secondary sexual maturation*. These are adequate body fat, adequate sleep, and vision (optic exposure to sunlight).

Girls must attain a *critical body weight* — irrespective of height — before breast development begins. Moreover, a body weight of *106 pounds* must be achieved before menses begins, and a proportion of *body fat of 24%* is required to sustain ovulatory cycles. This theory of critical body weight has been challenged by a number of investigators but has held up well in clinical observations and practice. Girls who engage in strenuous exercise programs prior to puberty have delayed sexual development; girls who are obese as children have early menarche. The role of body weight in male secondary sexual maturation and in sustaining male reproductive function is not defined.

Sleep has varying effects on the gonadotropin secretory pattern in prepubertal children, intrapubertal children, and sexually mature

Table 35.1
Sequence of Sexual Maturation in Girls

Event	Age	Hormone(s)
	years	
Breast budding	10–11	Estradiol
Sexual hair growth	10.5–11.5	Androgens
Growth spurt	11–12	Growth hormone
Menarche	11.5–13	Estradiol
Adult breast development	12.5–15	Progesterone
Adult sexual hair	13.5–16	Androgens

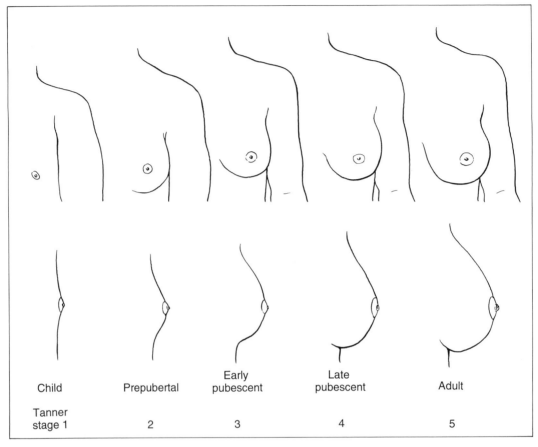

Child	Prepubertal	Early pubescent	Late pubescent	Adult
Tanner stage 1	2	3	4	5

Figure 35.1. Sequence of breast development in pubertal girls as described by Tanner.

adolescents. In prepubertal children, there is no correlation between sleep cycle and gonadotropin secretion. In intrapubertal adolescents — girls who have breast development and sexual hair growth but who have not menstruated, and males who have penile and testicular enlargement but who have not ejaculated — there is a sleep-entrained gonadotropin secretory cycle. That is, during sleep, there is a marked increased in the secretion of follicle-stimulating hormone (FSH) and luteinizing hormone (LH). In sexually mature adolescents, the release of gonadotropins bears no relationship to the sleep cycle. Instead, gonadotropins are released at 6- to 8-hour intervals. This pattern is maintained for the remainder of a person's reproductive life unless reproductive dysfunction occurs.

Optic exposure to sunlight is essential for timely secondary sexual development. Blind girls have delayed menarche and blind boys have delayed spermatogenesis and ejaculation. In hibernating animals who obviously have limited optic exposure, pituitary secretion of gonadotropins is suppressed during the period of hibernation. A similar mechanism is postulated for humans with decreased exposure to sunlight for any reason.

The relationships of *sleep* and body fat and the sequence of secondary sexual maturational events are particularly useful for understanding problems of puberty and for understanding problems of reproductive function during adult life.

Abrupt *mood changes* occur during the period of secondary sexual maturation in girls

Table 35.2
Causes of Delayed Puberty

Premature ovarian failure
  Turner syndrome
  Long-arm X chromosomal deletion
  Alkylating chemotherapy
Inadequate gonadotropin-releasing hormone
secretion
  Olfactory tract hypoplasia (Kallmann syndrome)
  Constitutional delayed puberty
  Craniopharyngioma
  Hypothalamic hamartoma
  Marijuana use
Inadequate gonadotropin secretion
  Isolated gonadotropin deficiency
  Prolactin-secreting pituitary adenoma
Inadequate body fat
  Anorexia nervosa
  Exercise-induced hypothalamic dysfunction
Genital tract abnormalities
  Imperforate hymen
  Vaginal and uterine agenesis (Rokitansky-
    Küster-Hauser syndrome)

and boys. Periods of depression, euphoria, and even violent behavior occur to some extent in many intrapubertal adolescents. Once full sexual maturation—with release of gametes—is completed, these mood changes disappear, so the physician can be reassuring to concerned, distraught parents that mood changes will abate with time.

ABNORMALITIES OF PUBERTAL DEVELOPMENT

The abnormalities of puberty are delayed sexual maturation, incomplete sexual maturation, primary amenorrhea, and precocious puberty. The presence of these disorders requires investigation of the hypothalamic-pituitary-gonadal axis and the reproductive outflow tract. The initial investigation must begin with measurement of pituitary gonadotropins (FSH and LH). These hormones distinguish a hypothalamic-pituitary etiology from a gonadal etiology.

Delayed Sexual Maturation

The first step in sexual maturation is breast budding, which usually begins between 10 and

11 years in most girls. Some girls will begin breast budding by 8 years, and this falls within the range of normal. However, if breast budding does not begin by 13 years, puberty may be delayed or may not begin spontaneously. *Failure to establish a breast bud by age 13* should cause the physician to initiate an endocrine evaluation to elucidate the cause of pubertal delay. Moreover, if *sexual hair growth precedes breast budding by more than 6 to 9 months* the physician should likewise initiate an endocrine evaluation. The most *common causes of delayed puberty* are presented in Table 35.2.

Premature Ovarian Failure

Ovarian failure can occur anytime prior to the expected time of menopause. *Ovarian failure is characterized by diminished or absent estrogen production in association with elevated gonadotropins.* The most common form of premature ovarian failure seen in prepubertal and pubertal girls is the *Turner syndrome.* The features of Turner syndrome are failure to establish secondary sexual development along with somatic changes such as short stature, a webbed neck (pterygium colli), a shield chest with widely spaced nipples, and an increased carrying angle of the elbow (cubitus valgus).

The fundamental genetic defect in girls with Turner syndrome is absence of an X chromosome. Genetic information that regulates the rate of ovarian follicular atresia is carried on the long arm of the X chromosome, whereas somatic information is carried on the short arm of the X chromosome. The absence of the entire X chromosome leads to loss of ovarian function and to the somatic features described above.

Partial deletions of the long arm of the X chromosome cause premature ovarian failure to occur at varying chronological ages. For example, complete loss of the long arm of the X chromosome results in premature ovarian failure prior to puberty, whereas a small fragmentary loss of the X-chromosome may not result in ovarian failure until many years after a normal puberty.

When breast development fails to occur at the expected age, or if breast development begins and then fails to be completed, the physician should consider premature ovarian failure. This diagnosis is established easily by the finding of elevated gonadotropins. The diagnosis must be established promptly and estrogen administration initiated as soon as possible. Estrogen is necessary to stimulate breast development, genital tract maturation, and the beginning of menstruation. A delay in estrogen administration can lead to the development of osteoporosis beginning during the teen years.

Hypothalamic Dysfunction

The arcuate nucleus of the hypothalamus secretes gonadotropin-releasing hormone (GnRH) in cyclic bursts, which stimulates release of gonadotropins from the anterior pituitary gland. Dysfunction of the arcuate nucleus disrupts the short hormonal loop between the hypothalamus and pituitary, resulting in no pituitary gland secretion of FSH or LH. In consequence, the ovaries are not stimulated to secrete estradiol, and secondary sexual maturation is delayed.

An unusual cause of hypothalamic dysfunction is the *Kallmann syndrome*. In this disorder, the olfactory tracts are hypoplastic and the arcuate nucleus does not secrete GnRH. Young women with Kallmann syndrome have no sense of smell and fail to have breast development and secondary sexual hair growth. The diagnosis of this condition can be made on initial physical examination by challenging olfactory function with known odors. Patients with this disorder will fail to recognize common odors such as coffee or rubbing alcohol. The prognosis for successful secondary sexual maturation and reproduction is excellent in Kallmann syndrome. Secondary sexual maturation can be stimulated by the administration of exogenous hormones, or by the administration of pulsatile GnRH. When pregnancy is desired, ovulation can be induced by exogenous gonadotropin administration or by administration of pulsatile GnRH. Once pregnancy is established, the lack of pituitary secretions has no adverse effects.

Less common causes of hypothalamic dysfunction are *neoplasms and inflammatory disorders of the hypothalamic-pituitary axis*. Examples are craniopharyngioma, hamartoma of the pituitary stalk, and sarcoidosis of the hypothalamus. Over 70% of cases will be associated with calcifications in the suprasellar region on plain skull x-ray. If a suprasellar neoplasm is strongly suspected, a magnetic resonance image of the hypothalamic-pituitary area is indicated.

Use of marijuana by prepubertal and intrapubertal boys and girls will delay the onset of puberty. Marijuana blocks the release of GnRH from the hypothalamus; thus, marijuana truncates gonadotropin secretion by the pituitary gland, which in turn delays gonadal function. With the increasing incidence of drug abuse by adolescents, this must be considered in the differential diagnosis of hypogonadotropic-hypogonadism.

Body Weight

Body weight seems to be a critical element for establishing full secondary sexual maturation, including the capacity for reproduction. Girls who are *underweight* have delayed puberty. Moreover, girls who participate in *strenuous athletics* such as gymnastics, ballet, and competitive running may experience pubertal delay. Young female athletes who have pubertal delay will have the normal onset and sequence of secondary sexual maturation when they decrease their level of training. No residual harm results from this pubertal delay. Full reproductive function will be attained. However, there is risk of osteoporosis if ovarian estrogen secretion is delayed for many years.

Genital Tract Anomalies

During fetal life, müllerian ducts develop and fuse in the female fetus to form the upper reproductive tract, that is, the fallopian tubes, uterus, and the upper vagina. The lower and midportion of the vagina develop from the canalization of the genital plate. One in 10,000 females has a birth defect of the reproductive tract that presents as primary amenorrhea at the time of puberty. The simplest genital tract anomaly is *imperforate hymen*. In this condition, the genital plate canalization is incomplete and the hymen is, therefore, closed. In this simple defect, menarche occurs at the appropriate time. Since there is obstruction to the passage of menstrual blood, menarche is not apparent. This condition presents with pain in the area of the uterus and a bulging vaginal introitus. Hymenotomy is the definitive therapy.

In *müllerian agenesis (Rokitansky-Küster-Hauser syndrome)*, the uterus is absent along with its cervical extremity and the vagina. All of the endocrine events of puberty occur at the proper time as the young woman establishes normal breast development, sexual hair growth, and ovulation. Yet, there is no menstruation. Physical examination leads to the diagnosis of müllerian agenesis. Renal anomalies such as reduplication of the ureters, horseshoe kidney, or unilateral renal agenesis occur in 25–35% of cases, and skeletal anomalies such as scoliosis occur in 15–25% of these women. There are several therapeutic approaches to this condition. An artificial vagina may be created by repetitive pressure to the perineum or by surgical construction followed by a split-thickness skin graft. After creation of a vagina, these women are able to enjoy sexual intercourse. With the advances in assisted reproductive technologies including in vitro fertilization (IVF) and surrogacy, it is possible for women with this condition to have their genetic child.

Precocious Puberty

If physical signs of *secondary sexual development* appear *before the age of 8 years*, the physician should consider the diagnosis of precocious puberty. Precocious puberty occurs in girls more frequently than in boys. Most precocious puberty is isosexual, that is, the sequence of pubertal events is appropriate for sexual development and leads to full sexual maturation. Idiopathic isosexual precocious puberty has no serious pathology. It only causes an advance in sexual maturation and carries the risk of short stature due to premature closure of the epiphyseal plates.

Occasionally, isosexual precocious puberty results from *tumors of the hypothalamic-pituitary stalk or transient inflammatory conditions of the hypothalamus*. In these situations, although sexual development begins early, the rate of sexual development is slowed compared with the usual rate. In the case of inflammatory conditions, sexual development may begin and end abruptly. Laboratory studies show an appropriate rise in either gonadotropins or gonadotropins in the prepubertal range.

Precocious puberty may be the result of *inappropriate secretion of androgens or estrogens*. The most common cause of inappropriate hormone secretion is *congenital adrenal hyperplasia 21-hydroxylase type*. In this disorder, the adrenal glands are unable to produce adequate cortisol as a result of a partial block in the conversion of progesterone to desoxycorticosterone. Since this step is mediated by the enzymatic action of 21-hydroxylase, deficiency of the enzyme leads to an accumulation of adrenal androgens, which results in precocious adrenarche. In girls, there is premature development of pubic hair followed by axillary hair. Breast development either does not occur or is incomplete for the stage of sexual development. Measurement of adrenal androgens—such as dehydroepiandrosterone, dehyderoepiandrosterone sulfate, and androstenedione—leads to the diagnosis.

In males with this condition, there is premature enlargement of the phallus and the appearance of axillary and pubic hair. However, the testicles remain small because the source of androgens is of adrenal rather than testicular origin. Again, adrenal hormones are elevated. Once the diagnosis is established, treatment should commence immediately. If not, short stature will result.

Rarely, there will be *inappropriate secretion of estrogens* in girls. This can result from ovarian neoplasms or from inappropriate secretion of chorionic gonadotropin by hepatic or gonadal neoplasms. In these conditions, there will be rapid breast development without sexual hair growth. Menarche may be established within a few months of thelarche. This deviation from the expected pattern of secondary sexual maturation suggests an abnormality.

Isosexual precocious puberty can be treated by the administration of an exogenous GnRH agonist. These agents block the periodic secretion of GnRH and suppress pituitary gonadotropin secretion. If precocious puberty is within a few months of the expected time of normal puberty, it is probably wise to allow puberty to progress. However, if puberty is advanced by several years, the process should be arrested. If the events of puberty do not progress in the expected way, an evaluation for hormonal abnormalities and/or hypothalamic-pituitary tumors is advised. If an abnormality is found, it should be treated specifically.

FURTHER READINGS

Cowell CA, ed. Pediatric and adolescent gynecology. Pediatr Clin Nor Am, 1981;28.

Kulin HE. Disorders of sexual maturation: delayed adolescence and precocious puberty. In: DeGroot LJ. Endocrinology. 2nd ed. Philadelphia: WB Saunders, 1989:1873–1899.

Styne DM, Grumbach MM. Puberty in the male and female. Its physiology and disorders. In: Yen SSC, Jaffe RB, eds. Reproductive endocrinology. 2nd ed. Philadelphia: WB Saunders, 1986:313–384.

SELF-EVALUATION

Case 35-A

A 15-year-old girl is brought by her mother for evaluation because she has never menstruated.

Question 35-A-1

Which of the following is the normal sequence in secondary sexual maturation?

A. hair growth, growth spurt, thelarche, menarche

B. growth spurt, hair growth, thelarche, menarche

C. thelarche, hair growth, growth spurt, menarche

D. thelarche, growth spurt, menarche, hair growth

Answer 35-A-1

Answer: C

Secondary sexual maturation should occur in an orderly sequence. Table 35.1 summarizes these events.

Question 35-A-2

Which of the following laboratory studies would be indicated on *initial* evaluation on this patient?

A. chromosomal karyotype

B. CAT scan of the pituitary gland

C. FSH and LH

D. progesterone

Answer 35-A-2

Answer: C

Although all the tests listed may be utilized as part of evaluation in different situations, for the initial evaluation of the patient described, gonadotropin measurement is the most cost effective.

Question 35-A-3

Initial laboratory studies suggest premature ovarian failure. Which of the following would be the most useful diagnostic test in establishing this diagnosis?

A. chromosomal karyotype

B. CAT scan of the pituitary gland

C. dehydroepiandrosterone, dehydroepiandrosterone sulfate

D. progesterone

Answer 35-A-3

Answer: A

Premature ovarian failure is diagnosed by finding elevated (i.e., menopausal) gonadotropin levels. The most common etiology of this in prepubertal girls is Turner syndrome in which an X chromosome is absent. Chromosomal karyotype is, therefore, the most appropriate test.

Case 35-B

A 16-year-old girl presents with primary amenorrhea. She has normal secondary sexual development including breast development, pubic and axillary hair growth, and adult height.

Question 35-B-1

The differential diagnosis would include all of the following *except*:

A. müllerian agenesis
B. pregnancy
C. premature ovarian failure
D. Kallmann syndrome

Answer 35-B-1

Answer: D

Patients with Kallmann syndrome do not have spontaneous breast development or sexual hair growth and, therefore, would not fit this clinical presentation.

Question 35-B-2

A physical examination reveals absence of the vagina. Based on this additional information, which management would you institute?

A. creation of an artificial vagina
B. administration of exogenous estrogen
C. administration of pulsatile GnRH
D. counseling to decrease strenuous physical activity

Answer 35-B-2

Answer: A

The patient described has müllerian agenesis (Rokitansky-Küster-Hauser syndrome). Because there is no uterus, the patient will never have periods. Once the vagina is developed, either by surgical construction or by a series of perineal pressure exercises, normal sexual activity can be anticipated.

chapter 36

AMENORRHEA AND DYSFUNCTIONAL UTERINE BLEEDING

Menstruation (cyclic uterine bleeding) is usually established by age 13 and continues until about age 45–50. Each menstrual cycle should follow ovulation. Once established at puberty, in most women menstrual cycles remain regular and predictable until menopause approaches.

Amenorrhea and dysfunctional uterine bleeding are the most common gynecologic disorders of reproductive age women. *Absence of menstruation is amenorrhea; irregular menstruation without anatomic lesions of the uterus is dysfunctional uterine bleeding.* Amenorrhea and dysfunctional uterine bleeding are discussed as separate topics in this chapter. However, the pathophysiology underlying amenorrhea and dysfunctional uterine bleeding may be the same.

AMENORRHEA

If a young woman has never menstruated, she is classified as having *primary amenorrhea*. If a woman has previously menstruated, but has failed to menstruate within 6 months, she is classified as having *secondary amenorrhea*. The designation of primary or secondary amenorrhea has no bearing on the severity of the underlying disorder or on the prognosis for restoring cyclic ovulation.

The physiology of ovulatory menstrual cycles is presented in Chapter 34, "Reproductive Cycle." When there is disruption of hypothalamic-pituitary-ovarian endocrine function or alteration of the genital outflow tract (obstruction of the uterus, cervix, or vagina, or scarring of the endometrium) menstrua-

tion will cease. Causes of amenorrhea will be divided into those arising from: (*a*) pregnancy, (*b*) hypothalamic-pituitary dysfunction, (*c*) ovarian dysfunction, and (*d*) alteration of the genital outflow tract.

Pregnancy

Since *the most common cause of amenorrhea is pregnancy*, it is essential to exclude pregnancy in the evaluation of amenorrhea. Often, a history of breast fullness, weight gain, nausea, and a "feeling of pregnancy" suggests the diagnosis of pregnancy. The diagnosis can be confirmed by a pregnancy test.

It is important to rule out pregnancy because a great deal of anxiety can be created for the patient if other causes of amenorrhea are presumed, and much money can be wasted to evaluate amenorrhea when a simple pregnancy test will establish the cause. Also, some of the treatments for amenorrhea can be harmful to a pregnancy.

Hypothalamic-Pituitary Dysfunction

Release of hypothalamic gonadotropin-releasing hormone (GnRH) occurs in a pulsatile fashion. When this pulsatile secretion of GnRH is disrupted or altered, the anterior pituitary gland is not stimulated to secrete follicle-stimulating hormone (FSH) and luteinizing hormone (LH). The result is cessation of ovulation and menstruation.

GnRH release is modulated by catecholamine secretion from the central nervous system and by feedback of sex steroids from

**Table 36.1
Causes of Hypothalamic-Pituitary
Amenorrhea**

Functional causes
  Weight loss
  Chronic anxiety
  Excessive exercise
Drug-induced causes
  Marijuana use
  Tranquilizer use
Neoplastic causes
  Prolactin-secreting pituitary adenomas
  Craniopharyngioma
  Hypothalamic hamartoma
Other causes
  Head injury
  Chronic medical illness

**Table 36.2
Signs and Symptoms of Ovarian-
Associated Estrogen Deficiency**

Symptoms	Signs
Hot flushes	Vaginal dryness
Mood changes	Thin vaginal epithelium
Sleep disturbances	Thinning of skin
Vaginal dryness	Hot flushes
Dyspareunia	

the ovaries. Alterations in catecholamine secretion and metabolism and in sex steroid hormone feedback disrupt ovulation and menstruation. In addition, alteration of bood flow from the hypothalamus to the pituitary gland through the hypothalamic-pituitary portal plexus can disrupt the signaling process that leads to ovulation. This alteration can be caused by tumors that alter blood flow.

The most common causes of hypothalamic-pituitary dysfunction are presented in Table 36.1. Most hypothalamic-pituitary amenorrhea is of functional origin and can be corrected by modifying causal behavior or by stimulating gonadotropin secretion.

In each of the disorders resulting in hypothalamic-pituitary amenorrhea, there is interference with the hypothalamic release of GnRH or interference with the pituitary secretion of FSH and LH. The physician cannot differentiate hypothalamic-pituitary causes of amenorrhea from ovarian or genital outflow causes by medical history or even physical examination alone. However, there are some clues in the medical history and physical examination that would suggest a hypothalamic-pituitary etiology for amenorrhea. A history of any condition listed in Table 36.1 should cause the physician to consider hypothalamic-pituitary dysfunction. Moreover, women with hypothalamic-pitui-

tary dysfunction usually do not complain of hot flushes and sleep problems as do women who have ovarian failure.

The way to definitively identify hypothalamic-pituitary dysfunction is to measure FSH, LH, and prolactin in blood. In these conditions, FSH and LH are in the low range. Prolactin will be normal in most conditions but will be elevated in prolactin-secreting pituitary adenomas.

Ovarian Failure

In the ovarian failure, the ovarian follicles are either exhausted or are resistant to stimulation by pituitary FSH and LH. As the ovaries fail, blood concentrations of FSH and LH increase. This is the basis for the chemical diagnosis of ovarian failure. Women with ovarian failure experience the symptoms and signs of estrogen deficiency that are listed in Table 36.2.

Women with estrogen deficiency due to ovarian failure usually experience hot flushes, whereas those with estrogen deficiency due to hypothalamic-pituitary dysfunction usually do not experience hot flushes. This is an important differential point in the medical history.

A summary of causes is presented in Table 36.3. A detailed description of these causes is presented in the chapter on menopause.

Obstruction of the Genital Outflow Tract

Obstruction of the genital outflow tract will prevent menstruation even if ovulation occurs. Most cases of outflow obstruction result

Table 36.3
Causes of Ovarian Failure

Chromosomal causes of ovarian failure
  Turner syndrome (45,X gonadal dysgenesis)
  X chromosome long-arm deletion (46,XX q−)
Unknown causes
  Gonadotropin-resistant ovary syndrome (Savage
    syndrome)
  Premature natural menopause
Immunologic cause
  Autoimmune ovarian failure (Blizzard syndrome)
Iatrogenic cause
  Ovarian failure due to effects of alkylating
    chemotherapy

from congenital *abnormalities in the development and canalization of the müllerian ducts.* Imperforate hymen, absence of uterus and vagina, or absence of the vagina are the most common anomalies that result in primary amenorrhea. Even with attempted surgical correction, menstruation and fertility may not be restored.

Scarring of the uterus (Asherman syndrome) is the most frequent cause of secondary amenorrhea of anatomic origin. Women who undergo dilation and curettage for retained products of pregnancy are at particular risk for developing scarring of the uterus. Moreover, scarring may occur as the result of infection of the uterine cavity. Cases of mild scarring can be corrected by surgical lysis of the adhesions performed by D&C or hysteroscopy. However, severe cases are often refractory to therapy. Estrogen therapy should be added to the surgical treatment to stimulate endometrial regeneration to "cover" the uterine lesions.

Treatment of Amenorrhea

It is essential to first establish a cause for the amenorrhea. In hypothalamic amenorrhea, ovulation can usually be restored by changing behavior in women who have functional amenorrhea. Women with central nervous system tumors should be considered on an individual basis for surgical therapy. Often, central nervous system tumors are benign and need not be removed. Ovulation can be induced by the administration of gonadotropins. Women with genital tract obstruction require surgery to create a vagina or to restore genital tract integrity. In some, menstruation will never be established if the uterus is absent. Women with premature ovarian failure require exogenous estrogen replacement. Hormone replacement regimens are discussed in Chapter 37, "Menopause."

DYSFUNCTIONAL UTERINE BLEEDING

Failure to ovulate results in either amenorrhea or irregular uterine bleeding. *Irregular bleeding, unrelated to anatomic lesions of the uterus, is dysfunctional uterine bleeding.*

Patients with amenorrhea do not ovulate at all and those with dysfunctional bleeding do not ovulate or do so only periodically. However, while women with amenorrhea do not menstruate, women with dysfunctional uterine bleeding have irregular, often heavy, uterine bleeding. How can these two disparate conditions result from the same cause? The answer relates to estrogen levels. Women with *amenorrhea* are in a state of estrogen deficiency. There is inadequate estrogen to stimulate growth and development of the endometrium. Therefore, there is inadequate endometrium for uterine bleeding to occur. Women with *dysfunctional uterine bleeding* are in a state of *chronic estrus.* They have constant, noncyclic blood estrogen concentrations that stimulate growth and development of the endometrium. Eventually, the endometrium outgrows its blood supply and support and sloughs from the uterus. When there is chronic stimulation of the endometrium from low plasma concentrations of estrogens, the episodes of dysfunctional uterine bleeding will be infrequent and light. Alternatively, when there is chronic stimulation of the endometrium from increased plasma concentrations of estrogens, the episodes of dysfunctional uterine bleeding can be frequent and heavy. In this situation, the dysfunctional uterine bleeding can result in hemorrhage so heavy that it requires hospitalization for intense medical treatment or even minor surgical therapy (dilation of the cervix and curettage of the uterine cavity) if medical therapy is not successful.

Dysfunctional uterine bleeding is most likely to occur in association with polycystic ovarian disease, exogenous obesity, and adrenal hyperplasia.

Women who develop secondary amenorrhea may first experience a phase of dysfunctional uterine bleeding. This can occur due to weight loss, prolactin-secreting pituitary adenomas, premature ovarian failure, and other causes of amenorrhea. Since amenorrhea and dysfunctional uterine bleeding result from anovulation, it is not surprising that they can occur in association.

Dysfunctional uterine bleeding can occur in association with ovulation. Although this may seem a contradiction, subtle alterations in the mechanisms of ovulation can produce abnormal cycles even when ovulation occurs. The luteal phase defect is such an example. In the *luteal phase defect*, ovulation does occur; however, the corpus luteum of the ovary is not fully developed to secrete adequate quantities of progesterone to support the endometrium for the usual 13–14 days and is not adequate to support a pregnancy if conception occurs. The menstrual cycle is shortened, and menstruation occurs earlier than expected. Although this is not classical dysfunctional uterine bleeding, it is considered to be in the same category.

Diagnosis of Dysfunctional Uterine Bleeding

Dysfunctional uterine bleeding should be suspected when menstrual cycles are not regular and predictable and when cycles are not associated with the premenstrual molimina associated with ovulatory cycles, breast fullness, abdominal bloating, mood changes, edema, weight gain, and menstrual cramps.

Before a diagnosis of dysfunctional uterine bleeding is made, anatomical causes of abnormal uterine bleeding must be excluded. These include uterine leiomyomata, carcinoma of the cervix, carcinoma of the endometrium, cervical erosions, cervical polyps, or lesions of the vagina. Women with these conditions have regular, ovulatory cycles with superimposed irregular bleeding.

If the diagnosis is uncertain from history and physical examination alone, a woman may keep a *basal body temperature chart* for 6–8 weeks to look for the shift in the basal temperature that occurs with ovulation. Occasionally, an *endometrial biopsy* is necessary to demonstrate endometrial hyperplasia, which may be associated with dysfunctional uterine bleeding. Since dysfunctional uterine bleeding results from chronic, unopposed estrogenic stimulation of the endometrium, the endometrium will be in a proliferative phase, or with prolonged estrogenic stimulation, in a hyperplastic phase.

Treatment of Dysfunctional Uterine Bleeding

The risks to a woman with dysfunctional uterine bleeding are incapacitating blood loss and/or hyperplasia or carcinoma of the endometrium. Uterine bleeding can become so severe as to require hospitalization. Hemorrhage as well as endometrial hyperplasia can be prevented by appropriate management.

The goal of treatment of dysfunctional uterine bleeding is to convert the proliferative endometrium into secretory endometrium, which results in predictable withdrawal uterine bleeding. This goal can be achieved by administration of a progestational agent for a minimum of 7–10 days. When the progestational agent is discontinued, uterine withdrawal bleeding will ensue, thereby mimicking physiologic withdrawal of progesterone.

Administration of oral contraceptives will suppress the endometrium and establish regular, predictable withdrawal cycles. Women who take oral contraceptives as treatment for dysfunctional uterine bleeding will often resume dysfunctional uterine bleeding after therapy is discontinued.

FURTHER READINGS

Baird DT, Amenorrhea, anovulation, and dysfunctional uterine bleeding. In: DeGroot LJ, ed. Endocrinology, 2nd ed. Philadelphia: WB Saunders, 1989:1950.

Ross GT. Disorders of the ovary and female reproductive tract. In: Wilson JD, Foster DW, eds. Williams textbook of endocrinology. 7th ed. Philadelphia: WB Saunders, 1985:206.

Speroff L, Glass RH, Kase NG. Clinical gynecologic endocrinology and infertility. 4th ed. Baltimore: Williams & Wilkins, 1989:165.

SELF-EVALUATION

Case 36-A

A 27-year-old woman complains of 6 months of amenorrhea.

Question 36-A-1

All of the following could affect her menstrual cycles except:

A. change in body weight
B. marijuana use
C. müllerian agenesis
D. pregnancy

Answer 36-A-1

Answer: C

Patients with müllerian agenesis would present with primary amenorrhea rather than secondary amenorrhea as this patient does. In all patients of reproductive age, pregnancy should be ruled out as the first stage of evaluation.

Question 36-A-2

If evaluation reveals elevated gonadotropins, which of the following statements are correct?

A. The patient may have a loss of chromosomal material on the long arm of the X chromosome.
B. Her ovaries may be depleted of ovarian follicles.
C. She may have numerous ovarian follicles that are resistant to FSH and LH.
D. She may have hypothalamic dysfunction.

Answer 36-A-2

Answer: A, B, C

A, B, and C are all clinical circumstances that can result in elevated gonodatropins. Each can be described as ovarian failure. The elevated gonadotropins are a result of the ovary not producing adequate amounts of hormones to feed back to the pituitary. Hypothalamus dysfunction would result in lower or normal gonadotropins.

Question 36-A-3

If evaluation reveals low gonadotropins, which of the following statements are correct?

A. The patient has decreased hypothalamic release of gonadotropin-releasing hormone.
B. Her ovaries are depleted of ovarian follicles.
C. Ovulation can be induced by administration of exogenous FSH and LH.
D. The examiner should inquire about changes in body weight, stress, and marijuana use.

Answer 36-A-3

Answer: C, D

A low level of gonadotropins does not usually suggest decreased GnRH release, as any aberration in the normally delicate pulsatile release can result in loss of physiologic mechanisms. The importance of low gonadotropin levels is that it is not ovarian failure that has caused amenorrhea.

Case 36-B

A 33-year-old woman gives a history of irregular menstrual cycles. She has basal body temperature records of 12 months duration that reveal ovulation occurring three times during that period.

Question 36-B-1

Which of the following statements are correct?

A. The patient has interruption of the cyclic interaction between gonadotropins and sex steroid hormones.
B. The endometrium varies between a proliferative endometrium and a secretory endometrium every month.

C. The patient is at high risk for endometrial hyperplasia.

D. She does not need to use contraception to prevent pregnancy.

Answer 36-B-1

Answer: A

This is a good example of intermittent ovulation resulting in dysfunctional bleeding. The patient's risk of endometrial hyperplasia is very low since the intermittent progestational effect of ovulatory cycles is protective. The endometium will become secretory only when ovulation has occurred in this patient three times in a year. Contraception is still needed, as there is no way to predict when she will ovulate.

Question 36-B-2

Further evaluation reveals tonic elevation of LH. Based on this additional data, which of the following statements are correct?

A. LH can be suppressed by administration of oral contraceptives.

B. Ovulation can probably be induced by administration of clomiphene citrate.

C. The patient may have elevated androgens.

D. Obesity frequently coexists with dysfunctional uterine bleeding.

Answer 36-B-2

Answer: A, B, C, D

This clinical picture is commonly seen in patients with oligo-ovulation and oligomenorrhea. If the patient desires to conceive, medical induction of ovulation can usually be accomplished. Otherwise, oral contraceptives are commonly used to regulate menstrual periods. Hyperandrogenism may be a contributory factor to the irregular ovulation (see Chapter 39, "Hirsutism and Virilization"). Obesity can also contribute, as peripheral fat stores convert androstenedione to estrone, thereby chemically increasing estrogen production and adversely affecting cyclic estrogen feedback.

chapter 37

MENOPAUSE

Ovarian function ceases by age 55 years in 95% of women. The cessation of menses is *menopause*. The *climacteric* is the transition from the reproductive to the nonreproductive years.

Unlike the male who is able to renew gametes on a daily basis, the female has a fixed number of gametes for her reproductive life. In the fetus, approximately 8 million primordial oocytes migrate into the ovarian stroma at about 20 weeks of gestation. The process of follicular atresia begins prior to birth. At the time of birth, the female infant has approximately 1–2 million oocytes; by puberty, she has about 400,000 oocytes remaining. By age 30–35, the number of oocytes has decreased to about 100,000. For the remaining reproductive years, the process of oocyte maturation and ovulation becomes increasingly inefficient.

A woman will ovulate approximately 400 oocytes during her reproductive years. The process of *oocyte selection* is poorly understood. During the reproductive cycle, a cohort of oocytes is stimulated to begin maturation, but only one or two complete the process and are eventually ovulated. It is unclear why one oocyte becomes atretic and degenerates while another oocyte achieves full maturation and ovulation.

Follicular maturation is induced and stimulated by pituitary release of follicle-stimulating hormone (FSH) and luteinizing hormone (LH). FSH binds to its receptors in the follicular membrane of the oocyte and stimulates follicular maturation. LH stimulates the theca luteal cells surrounding the oocyte to produce androgens as well as estrogens and serves as the triggering mechanism to induce ovulation. With advancing reproductive age, remaining oocytes become increasingly resistant to FSH. Thus, plasma concentrations of FSH begin to increase several years in advance of actual menopause.

Menopause marks the end of a woman's reproductive life. The mean age of menopause throughout the world today is 50 years. Twenty-five percent of women will experience menopause prior to age 45 years; 95% of women will be menopausal by age 55 years. Menopause is a physiologic process. However, the consequences of ovarian failure can diminish a woman's quality of life and can predispose her to osteoporosis and an increased risk of cardiovascular disease.

SYMPTOMS AND SIGNS OF OVARIAN FAILURE
Menstrual Cycle Alterations

Soon after an adolescent woman has her first menstrual cycle, regular, predictable menstrual cycles are established that continue until about 40 years of age. Around 40 years, the number of ovarian follicles becomes substantially depleted and subtle changes occur in the frequency and length of menstrual cycles. A woman may note shortening or lengthening of her cycles. The luteal phase of the cycle remains constant at 13–14 days, whereas the variation of cycle length is related to a change in the follicular phase. Women in their twenties and thirties will ovulate 13–14 times per year. Several years in advance of menopause, the frequency of ovulation decreases to 11–12 times per year, and with advancing reproductive age will decrease to 3–4 times per year.

Table 37.1
Relative Changes in FSH as a Function of Life Stages

Life stage	FSH
	mIU/ml
Childhood	<4
Prime reproductive years	6–10
Perimenopause	14–24
Menopause	>30

With the change in reproductive cycle length and frequency, there are concomitant changes in the plasma concentration of FSH and LH. More *FSH* is required to stimulate follicular maturation. Beginning in the late thirties and early forties, the concentration of FSH begins to increase. This is the first chemical evidence of ovarian failure. The 5–10-year period prior to menopause is termed *perimenopause*. During the perimenopausal years, women begin to experience symptoms and signs of estrogen deficiency as reproductive function becomes increasingly inefficient. Relative changes in FSH as a function of stage of life is presented in Table 37.1.

Hot Flushes and Vasomotor Instability

Coincident with the change in reproductive cycle length and frequency, the hot flush is the first physical manifestation of ovarian failure. Occasional hot flushes begin several years prior to actual menopause. The *hot flush is the most common symptom of impending ovarian failure*. Over 95% of perimenopausal and menopausal women experience hot flushes.

Hot flushes have rapid onset and resolution. When a hot flush occurs, a woman experiences a sudden sensation of warmth. The skin of the face and the anterior chest wall become flushed for approximately 90 seconds. With resolution of the hot flush, a woman feels cold and will break out into a cold sweat. The entire phenomenon lasts less than 3 minutes. The hot flush is the result of declining estradiol-17β secretion by the ovarian follicles. As a woman approaches menopause, the frequency and intensity of hot flushes increases. Hot flushes may be disabling by producing *diaphoresis*, especially at night. When perimenopausal and postmenopausal women receive estrogen replacement, hot flushes usually resolve in 3–6 weeks. If a menopausal woman does not receive estrogen replacement therapy, hot flushes will usually resolve spontaneously within 2–3 years.

Sleep Disturbances

Ovarian failure with consequent declining estradiol induces a change in a woman's sleep cycle so that restful sleep becomes difficult. The latent phase of sleep, i.e., the time required to fall asleep, is lengthened; the actual period of sleep is shortened. Therefore, perimenopausal and postmenopausal women complain of having difficulty falling asleep and waking up soon after going to sleep. The sleep cycle is restored to the premenopausal state by the administration of replacement estrogens.

Vaginal Dryness and Genital Tract Atrophy

The vaginal mucosa, cervix, endocervix, endometrium, and myometrium are estrogen-dependent tissues. With decreasing estrogen production, these tissues become atrophic. The vaginal epithelium becomes thin; vaginal and cervical secretions diminish. Women experience vaginal dryness while attempting or having sexual intercourse; as a result of vaginal dryness and hormonal changes, they have diminished sexual pleasure as well.

Also, the endometrium becomes atrophic and a woman ceases having menstruation. The paravaginal tissues that support the bladder and rectum become atrophic so that there is a loss of support of the pelvic viscera. Some women experience bladder and rectal prolapse with genital tract atrophy. Due to atrophy of the urinary tract, there may be symptoms of dysuria and urinary frequency.

Therapy with replacement estrogens restores the integrity of the vaginal epithelium and promotes natural secretions from the vagina and endocervix. Sexual pleasure is often restored. In addition, vaginal lubricants may be used by couples who are experiencing vaginal dryness to enhance sexual intercourse. Estrogen replacement therapy partially restores the integrity and support of the tissues surrounding the vagina. If a menopausal woman has symptomatic pelvic relaxation, estrogen replacement therapy should be administered for several months before surgical correction is considered.

Mood Changes

Perimenopausal and postmenopausal women often complain of volatility of affect. Some women experience depression, apathy, and "crying spells." Not only are these emotional symptoms disturbing to a woman, but her inability to control these feelings is equally concerning. The physician should provide counseling and emotional support as well as medical therapy. The role of estrogens in central nervous system function is unknown. However, it is well established that sex steroid hormone receptors are protean in the central nervous system. Estrogen replacement in perimenopausal and postmenopausal women often diminishes these mood swings.

Skin, Hair, and Nail Changes

Estrogen influences *skin* thickness. With declining estrogen production, skin tends to become thin and less elastic. Estrogen replacement helps restore the thickness and elasticity of skin.

Some women will notice changes in their hair and nails with the hormonal changes of menopause. Estrogen stimulates the production of sex hormone binding globulin, which binds androgens and estrogens. With declining estrogen production, there is less available sex hormone binding globulin, which results in more free testosterone. This may result in increased facial hair. Moreover, changes in estrogen production affect the rate of hair shedding. Hair from the scalp is normally lost and replaced in an asynchro-

nous way. With changes in estrogen production, hair is shed and replaced in a synchronous way resulting in the appearance of increased scalp hair loss. This is a self-limiting condition and requires no therapy, but patients do require reassurance. Nails become thin and brittle with estrogen deprivation, but are restored to normal with estrogen replacement.

Osteoporosis

Bone demineralization is a natural consequence of aging. Diminishing bone density occurs in both men and women. However, the onset of bone demineralization occurs 15–20 years earlier in women than in men and is accelerated after ovarian function ceases. Not only does bone demineralization occur with natural menopause but has been reported in association with decreased estrogen production in certain groups of young women.

The role of estrogen in stimulating and maintaining *bone density* is unclear. Estrogen receptors have been demonstrated in osteoblasts. This finding suggests a permissive and perhaps even essential role for estrogen in bone formation. Bone density diminishes at the rate of approximately 1–2% per year in postmenopausal women compared with approximately $\frac{1}{2}$% per year in perimenopausal women. Of all the therapies utilized for the prevention and treatment of osteoporosis, estrogen replacement seems to be best.

If a woman does not receive estrogen in the first 5 years following menopause, she will have a progressive, linear decrease in bone mineral mass. However, if estrogen replacement is initiated prior to or at the time of menopause, bone density is maintained at the premenopausal levels.

It remains controversial as to whether estrogen replacement in women 5 years or more menopausal has an effect on bone density. Some investigators report that administration of estrogens to elderly women will stabilize bone density and even partially restore bone mineral mass.

Calcium supplementation is not a substitute for estrogen replacement. In several studies comparing estrogen with calcium, patients who received calcium alone had continued loss of bone mineral mass, whereas those who received estrogens had a stabilization of bone mineral mass.

Cardiovascular Lipid Changes

With approaching ovarian failure, changes occur in the cardiovascular lipid profile. Total cholesterol increases, high density lipoprotein (HDL) cholesterol decreases, and low density lipoprotein (LDL) cholesterol increases.

The administration of exogenous estrogens to perimenopausal and postmenopausal women promotes normalization of the cardiovascular lipid profile. Women who receive estrogen replacement therapy have a lowered incidence of myocardial infarction and stroke than women who do not receive estrogen replacement therapy.

PREMATURE OVARIAN FAILURE

By definition, *premature ovarian failure is menopause that occurs prior to age 42 years.* Approximately 5% of women will experience premature menopause. For some, premature ovarian failure may be the cause of infertility and for others, the cause for the menopausal symptoms.

Genetic Factors

There are several factors that influence a woman's reproductive life span. Genetic information that determines the length of a woman's reproductive life is carried on the distal long arm of the X chromosome. Partial deletion of the long arm of one X chromosome results in premature ovarian failure. Total loss of the long arm of the X chromosome, as seen in Turner's syndrome, results in ovarian failure at birth or in early childhood. When suspected, these diagnoses can be established by careful mapping of the X chromosome.

Gonadotropin-Resistant Ovary Syndrome (Savage Syndrome)

Some women with premature ovarian menopause have an adequate number of ovarian follicles, yet these follicles are resistant to FSH and LH. A number of pregnancies have been reported in women with the gonadotropin-resistant ovary syndrome during the administration of exogenous estrogen. This fact suggests a role for estrogens in stimulating FSH receptors in the ovarian follicles.

Autoimmune Disorders

Some women develop autoantibodies against thyroid, adrenal, and ovarian endocrine tissues. These autoantibodies cause ovarian failure. Some women will respond to estrogen replacement therapy with resumption of ovulation.

Smoking

Women who smoke tobacco can undergo ovarian failure some 3–5 years earlier than the expected time of menopause. It is established that women who smoke tobacco metabolize estradiol primarily to 2-hydroxyestradiol. The 2-hydroxylated estrogens are termed catechol estrogens because of their structural similarity to catecholamines. The catechol estrogens act as antiestrogens and block estrogen action. The mechanism for premature ovarian failure in women smokers is unknown. However, smoking effect should be considered in women smokers who are experiencing symptoms of estrogen deficiency.

Alkylating Cancer Chemotherapy

Alkylating cancer chemotherapeutic agents affect the membrane of ovarian follicles and hasten follicular atresia. One of the consequences of cancer chemotherapy in reproductive age women is loss of ovarian function. Young women being treated for malignant neoplasms should be counseled of this possibility.

Hysterectomy

Surgical removal of the uterus (hysterectomy) in reproductive age women is associated with ovarian failure some 3–5 years earlier than the expected age. The mechanism for this occurrence is unknown. It is likely associated with alteration of ovarian blood flow resulting from the surgery.

Low Body Weight

Since adipocytes play a role in estrogen production and estrogen storage, slender women experience menopausal symptoms earlier than women of normal body habitus and obese women. Moreover, slender women tend to be more difficult to normalize with exogenous estrogen replacement during the menopausal years. Physicians should counsel women to gain to their ideal body weight by the time of menopause.

MANAGEMENT OF MENOPAUSE

All of the signs and symptoms of menopause result from declining estradiol-17β production by the ovarian follicles. *Exogenous estrogen administration* to the perimenopausal and postmenopausal woman will obviate most of these changes. In addition, estrone and estriol are metabolic by-products of estradiol-17β.

The *objective of estrogen replacement* therapy should be to diminish the signs and symptoms of ovarian failure and restore estrogen homeostasis. There are several different estrogen preparations available through various routes of administration. Estradiol-17β can be administered orally; however, it then is oxidized in the enterohepatic circulation to estrone. Estradiol-17β remains unaltered if it is administered transdermally, transbucally, transvaginally, intravenously, or intramuscularly. Unfortunately, intramuscular estradiol administration results in unpredictable fluctuations in plasma concentration. When estradiol is administered across the vaginal epithelium, absorption is poorly controlled and pharmacologic plasma concentrations of estradiol can result. The *transdermal administration of estradiol* results in steady, sustained estrogen blood levels because of controlled absorption.

Conjugated estrogens such as estrone sulfate have been used as an oral medication for decades as a primary hormone preparation for estrogen replacement. Conjugated estrogens are unconjugated in the gastrointestinal tract and delivered to the target tissues as estrone. Conjugated estrogens are effective in diminishing the symptoms of estrogen deficiency, in maintaining bone mass, and restoring plasma lipids to more normal levels.

The administration of continuous *unopposed estrogens* can produce endometrial hyperplasia and lead to endometrial adenocarcinoma. Therefore, it is essential to administer a progestin in conjunction with estrogens to prevent endometrial hyperplasia in women who have not undergone hysterectomy.

There are two principal *regimens for estrogen replacement* therapy. Continuous estrogen replacement with cyclic progestin administration results in excellent resolution of symptoms and cyclic withdrawal bleeding from the endometrium. One of the difficulties of this method of therapy is that many postmenopausal women do not want to continue having menstrual cycles. As a result, many physicians choose to avoid the problem of cyclic withdrawal bleeding by the daily administration of combined estrogen and progestins.

There is a wide *variety of estrogen preparations* available. The following are comparable dosages: conjugated equine estrogens, 0.625 mg; estrone sulfate, 0.625 mg; estradiol-17β, 1 mg; and transdermal estradiol-17β, 50 μg. Most perimenopausal and menopausal women will respond to one of these preparations, all of which are adequate to prevent osteoporosis and to provide protection from cardiovascular disease. Most women will experience relief from hot flushes, vaginal dryness, sleep disturbances, and mood changes. The administration of 5 mg of *medroxyprogesterone* acetate (Provera) given for 12 days each month will convert the proliferative endometrium into a secretory endometrium and bring about endometrial sloughing. If continuous progestin therapy is used to produce endometrial atrophy, 2.5 mg of medroxyprogesterone per day is utilized.

An annual pelvic examination with Pap smear and mammogram (after age 50) is advisable for all women given hormone replacement therapy.

CAUTIONS IN ESTROGEN REPLACEMENT

Patients with unexplained abnormal vaginal bleeding should not receive estrogen replacement until the cause of the bleeding is ascertained and treated appropriately. In addition, patients with active liver disease or chronically impaired liver function should generally not receive estrogen replacement.

Carcinoma of the Breast

Carcinoma of the breast is felt to be a relative contraindication for estrogen replacement. It may be reasonable, however, to administer estrogen replacement to women who have documented estrogen-receptor negative breast tumors and negative axillary lymph nodes. Nonetheless, *caution must be exercised when making the decision to administer estrogen to women with a history of breast cancer.*

Thromboembolic Disease

Oral estrogens stimulate the production of clotting factors, but estradiol administered by the transdermal route has no effect on clotting. Therefore, women with a history of thromboembolic disease can safely receive transdermal estradiol therapy.

Endometrial Carcinoma

There is little evidence to suggest that estrogens should be withheld from women with a history of carcinoma of the endometrium if the tumor was limited to the endometrium and myometrium. Women with metastatic endometrial carcinoma should not receive exogenous estrogens.

FURTHER READINGS

Buchsbaum HJ, ed. The menopause. New York: Springer-Verlag, 1983.

Byyny RL, Speroff L. A clinical guide for the care of older women. Baltimore: Williams & Wilkins, 1990.

Hormone replacement therapy. ACOG Technical Bulletin No. 166. April, 1992.

Jaffe RB. The menopause and perimenopausal period. In: Yen SSC, Jaffe RB. Reproductive endocrinology. 2nd ed. Philadelphia: WB Saunders, 1986:406.

Odell WD. The menopause. In: DeGroot LJ. 2nd ed. Endocrinology. Philadelphia: WB Saunders, 1989: 2009.

Speroff L, Glass RH, Kase NG. The ovary from conception to senescence. In: Clinical gynecological endocrinology and infertility. Baltimore: Williams & Wilkins, 1989:121.

SELF-EVALUATION

Case 37-A

A 46-year-old woman complains of increasing irritability, hot flushes, and an increasingly irregular menstrual cycle over the last 12 months. Her mother died of breast cancer. She had three uncomplicated pregnancies and has been well, with no other problems other than varicose veins.

Question 37-A-1

Which of the following signs and symptoms would be expected?

A. sleep disturbance
B. dry skin
C. loss of hair
D. vaginal irritation after coitus
E. oily skin

Answer 37-A-1

Answer: A, B, C, D

The loss of estrogen can result in many physiologic changes. Of those listed, only oily skin is not due to estrogen deprivation.

Question 37-A-2

Which of the following findings would be expected?

A. increased FSH
B. decreased FSH
C. increased LH

D. decreased LH
E. increased bone density
F. decreased bone density
G. increased total cholesterol
H. decreased total cholesterol

Answer 37-A-2

Answer: A, C, G

If this patient is experiencing early menopause, FSH and LH will be elevated and total cholesterol may be increased. Untreated, bone density will decline over several years, but the findings now would most likely be normal.

Question 37-A-3

Which are appropriate therapeutic steps?
A. oral progestin
B. oral estrogen
C. oral calcium
D. oral tranquilizers
E. parenteral progesterone
F. parenteral estrogen
G. parenteral calcium
H. parenteral tranquilizers

Answer 37-A-3

Answer: A, B, C

Oral estrogen replacement is appropriate for treatment of menopause symptoms. Progestin therapy is indicated in addition to estrogen whenever the patient still has a uterus. Calcium supplementation is also a good idea as additional therapy to prevent osteoporosis. Parenteral preparations of any of these drugs are rarely needed. Tranquilizers are not routinely indicated, as estrogen replacement therapy usually successfully treats the mood changes. Because of the first degree relative with breast carcinoma, yearly breast examination by a physician and yearly screening mammography are indicated.

Case 37-B

A 27-year-old woman presents with a history of amenorrhea and hot flushes for the last 6 months. Laboratory studies reveal elevated FSH and LH.

Question 37-B-1

The differential diagnosis would include all of the following except:
A. gonadotropin-resistant ovary syndrome
B. 46,XX q-ovarian dysgenesis
C. idiopathic ovarian failure
D. pituitary prolactinoma

Answer 37-B-1

Answer: D

A pituitary prolactinoma would present with amenorrhea, but the gonadotrophs would not be elevated as seen in this case. An elevated prolactin level would be expected if a prolactinoma were present.

Question 37-B-2

Which of the following is *not* a potential therapy for this patient?
A. estrogen and progestin replacement
B. securing a donor oocyte
C. biopsy of the ovaries
D. maintaining ideal body weight

Answer 37-B-2

Answer: D

The vasomotor symptoms of premature ovarian failure should respond to estrogen replacement. Progestin is a part of the therapeutic regimen to prevent endometrial hyperplasia. The use of donor oocytes could be utilized if assisted reproductive technology were to be utilized in the future. Biopsy of the ovary may be considered if ovarian dysgenesis is a possibility. Body weight is often associated with anovulation and amenorrhea, but is not a factor in premature ovarian failure.

chapter 38

EVALUATION OF THE INFERTILE COUPLE

Infertility affects 15% of reproductive age couples in the United States. During the 20-year period from 1970 to 1990, the incidence of infertility appeared to increase; however, the incidence now appears stable. *Infertility is defined as a couple's failure to conceive following 1 year of unprotected sexual intercourse.* The reasons for an increasing incidence of infertility may be related to life-style, e.g., such as maintaining low body weight, marijuana use, deferred childbearing, and increased incidence of pelvic inflammatory diseases.

Reproductive age is synonymous with a woman's reproductive years (ages 15–44 years). Since this is the healthiest segment of the population, it is surprising that 15% of this group experiences reproductive dysfunction. With such a high incidence in an otherwise healthy population, one must look for causes of infertility resulting from environment and life-style. During the 20-year period when incidence of infertility was rising, there was a corresponding increase in the knowledge of reproductive physiology and in the diagnosis and treatment of infertility. Formerly, there was little hope for the infertile couple; today, 85% of couples can expect to have a child with appropriate diagnosis and treatment for "infertility."

The inability to conceive a child or carry a pregnancy places a great emotional burden on infertile couples. The quest to have a child becomes the driving force in the infertile couple's life. Friends, family, and often occupation can be subordinated to this medical problem. Unlike dysfunction of other organ systems, dysfunction of the reproductive system does not directly produce physical or mental abnormalities. Yet, the mental anguish of infertility is nearly as incapacitating as the pain or life restrictions of other diseases. The emotional needs of infertile couples must be recognized.

CAUSES OF INFERTILITY

Infertility can be reduced to *three generic causes* that account for *95% of reproductive dysfunction.* These causes are: (*a*) *anovulation,* (*b*) *anatomical defects* of the female genital tract, and (*c*) *abnormal spermatogenesis.* The frequency of these causes is presented in Figure 38.1. In the initial investigation of the infertile couple, it is important for the physician to establish, as rapidly as possible, the major cause(s) of the infertility. Each of these categories can be investigated by a simple diagnostic procedure, which gives a high probability of establishing a cause.

The *initial evaluation of the infertile couple* should include the following studies:

1. Basal body temperature recording of the female partner
2. Semen analysis
3. Hysterosalpingogram

The *basal body temperature* recording is an excellent screening test for ovulation. The characteristic biphasic temperature shift occurs in over 90% of ovulating women (an example is shown in Figure 38.2). Note the rise in temperature that coincides with ovulation. Thirteen to fourteen days after ovulation, the basal temperature drops and menstruation begins within 24–36 hours. A temperature elevation of longer than 16-days suggests pregnancy.

Analysis of a semen specimen obtained by masturbation provides immediate informa-

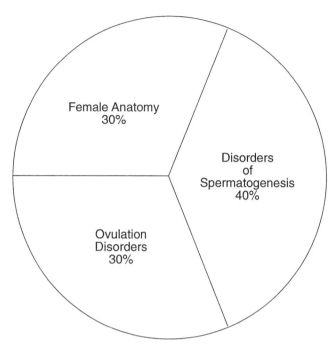

Figure 38.1. A pie graph presenting the distribution of common causes of infertility.

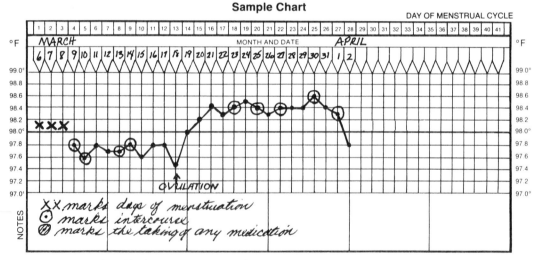

Figure 38.2. A basal body temperature record in an infertile woman receiving clomiphene citrate. Note the biphasic temperature shift on day 15. That a temperature remains elevated for more than 16 days may indicate pregnancy.

Table 38.1
Tests in the Infertility Workup

Possible cause	Test	Comments
Anovulation	Basal body temperature chart	Patient must do each morning
	Endometrial biopsy	Office procedure in late luteal phase
	Serum progesterone	Blood test
	Urinary ovulation detection kit	Home use at midcycle
Anatomic disorder	Hysterosalpingogram	X-ray in proliferative phase
	Diagnostic laparoscopy	View external surfaces of internal structures
	Hysteroscopy	Visualize endometrial cavity
Abnormal spermatogenesis	Semen analysis	Normal value 20 million/ml, 2 ml volume, 60% motility
	Postcoital test	Midcycle timing
Immunologic disorder	Antisperm antibodies	Male and female tested

tion about the quantity and quality of seminal fluid, the density of the sperm, the morphology of sperm, and the motility of sperm. A normal semen specimen should contain a concentration of motile sperm of >20 million/ml with at least 60% motile sperm. A normal semen analysis excludes a male cause for infertility in over 90% of couples.

The *hysterosalpingogram*, an x-ray study of the internal female genital tract, provides important information about the tract's architecture and integrity. A radiopaque dye is injected under pressure past the cervix and through the uterine cavity and fallopian tubes. The internal architure of these structures is then outlined on x-ray. The hysterosalpingogram has a diagnostic accuracy of approximately 70% for detecting anatomical abnormalities of the genital tract. A diagnostic laparoscopy is another diagnostic step to evaluate the genital tract, used in conjunction with the hysterosalpingogram for evaluating internal female anatomy (Table 38.1).

Anovulation

A healthy woman between ages 18 and 36 ovulates 13–14 times per year. The typical menstrual cycle is 28 days in length with ovulation occurring on the 14th day. Menstruation begins on the 28th day and lasts approximately 5 days. *The ovulatory menstrual cycle* is divided into two phases, the follicular phase and the luteal phase. During the *follicular phase* of the menstrual cycle, estradiol-17β is the predominant hormone. Its actions on its target tissues result in increased turgor of the ductal elements of the breasts, increased production of clear, watery endocervical mucous, and proliferation of the endometrium. The *luteal phase* of the menstrual cycle is dominated by the secretion of progesterone by the corpus luteum. Progesterone acts on the acinar elements of the breasts to produce rounding of the lateral quadrants, and upon the endocervix to convert the thin, clear endocervical mucous into a sticky mucoid material. Progesterone also converts the endometrium to a secretory one, which accepts the embryo for implantation and supports subsequent fetal growth and development.

Progesterone shifts the thermoregulatory center and increases the set point of the basal body temperature. Following ovulation, the basal body temperature increases by approximately 0.6°F and remains elevated until menstruation begins. With involution of the corpus luteum, progesterone production abruptly decreases and the basal body temperature shifts downward; menstruation ensues soon after.

The menstrual history helps the physician ascertain if a woman ovulates regularly. Ovulating women characteristically experience cyclic changes in the breasts, cervix and vagina, integument, and in mood and emotion. They may also experience the symptoms of the premenstrual syndrome. Characteristically, *following ovulation* and preceding menstruation, an ovulating woman will experience some fullness and heaviness of the breasts, decreased vaginal secretions, abdominal bloating, mild peripheral edema with slight increase in body weight, and occasional episodes of depression. These changes do not occur in anovulatory women. Therefore, *a history of these cyclic changes are presumptive evidence of ovulation.*

Diagnostic studies to confirm ovulation, in addition to recording the basal body temperature, include the endometrial biopsy, measurement of serum progesterone, and the urinary ovulation detection kit. The *endometrium* undergoes specific histologic changes on an almost daily basis following ovulation. These changes can be detected from an endometrial biopsy. This is a useful procedure for evaluating certain causes of infertility, but is expensive and provides only static information. *Progesterone* increases in plasma following ovulation and can be measured to confirm that ovulation has occurred. However, a single measurement provides little information that cannot be obtained by a basal body temperature chart. *Ovulation detection kits* are available that measure changes in urinary LH. As the LH surge begins, more LH will be excreted in urine and can be measured by qualitative detection kits. This is useful in helping to predict ovulation but does not confirm ovulation. Ovulation detection kits should not be used routinely, but can be useful where ovulation prediction is needed, such as in the timing of artificial insemination.

Symptoms such as irregular unpredictable menstrual cycles and episodes of amenorrhea, as well as signs of hirsutism, acne, galactorrhea, and increased or decreased vaginal secretions *suggest anovulation.* A woman with irregular menstrual cycles can be presumed to be anovulatory. In this case, maintaining a basal body temperature record is not necessary.

Given a history of irregular menstrual cycles the physician should look for signs of abnormal androgen, prolactin, and gonadotrophin secretion.

A woman who is anovulatory should have plasma concentrations of follicle-stimulating hormone (FSH), luteinizing hormone (LH), prolactin, androstenedione, total testosterone, and dehydroepiandrosterone (DHEA) measured. If thyroid dysfunction is suspected, thyroxin (T_4) and thyroid-stimulating hormone (TSH) should be measured as well. The results of these hormonal studies will help the physician understand the etiology of the chronic anovulation. Once the etiology of anovulation is established, a treatment regimen designed to induce ovulation can be developed for the patient. Any agent that will set in cyclical motion the secretion of gonadotrophins or estradiol will stimulate ovulation.

Anatomic Disorders of the Female Genital Tract

Sperm Transport, Fertilization, and Implantation

The female genital tract facilitates the migration of sperm from the posterior vaginal fornix toward the unfertilized egg. *Cervical mucus* secreted by the endocervix traps the coagulated ejaculate, where the sperm are stored and capacitated for immediate or later migration into the endometrial cavity and fallopian tubes.

At the time of ovulation, the oocyte is either picked up directly by the fimbriated extremity of the fallopian tube or retrieved from the pelvic cul-de-sac. The oocyte is then transported to the proximal portion of the fallopian tube, where fertilization occurs. The fertilized oocyte cleaves and forms a zygote and then an embryo. Three to five days following fertilization, the embryo enters the *endometrial cavity*, where it implants into the secretory endometrium for subsequent growth and development. The cells of the cervix, endometrium, and endosalpinx respond to progesterone secretion from the ovarian follicle. *The internal anatomic genital tract serves as more than a simple conduit for sperm and eggs. Indeed, these are dynamic structures that are essential for normal transportation, fertilization, and implantation.*

Disorders

The most *common disorders* of the female genital tract are acquired during the early reproductive years. The most common cause of fallopian tube disease is acute *salpingitis*. Organisms that infect the fallopian tubes include *Neisseria gonorrhoeae* and *Chlamydia trachomatis*. These organisms alter the functional integrity of the fallopian tubes and can lead to fallopian tube obstruction.

Hysterosalpingography

Less common congenital anatomical abnormalities of the female genital tract can range from a simple septum of the upper uterine cavity to a complete reduplication of the genital tract with a double vagina, double cervix, and double uterus. Endometriosis, scarring and adhesions from pelvic inflammation or surgery, tumors of the uterus (e.g., leiomyoma) and ovary (e.g. cystadenoma), and rarely sequelae of trauma may also distort the reproductive tract anatomy.

The hysterosalpingogram is an essential diagnostic tool for evaluation of the internal genital structures. The hysterosalpingogram should be performed between the 7th and 11th day of the menstrual cycle. If it were performed during menses, the risk of iatrogenic retrograde menstruation would be increased. If performed later, it could interfere with the possible ovum transport, fertilization, or implantation.

There are several important characteristics of the normal hysterosalpingogram (Fig. 38.3). The endometrial cavity should be smooth and symmetrical. Indentations and irregularities of the endometrial cavity suggest uterine leiomyomata or chronic scarring of the endometrium from previous surgery. The proximal two thirds of the fallopian tubes should be slender, approximating the diameter of a pencil lead. The distal one third of the fallopian tubes is the ampulla and should appear dilated compared with the proximal two thirds. The fimbrial folds should appear as linear radiolucencies along the longitudinal axis of the tube.

During the radiographic study, dye should *spill* promptly from the fallopian tubes into the peritoneal cavity. In a pelvis free of adhesions, dye will intersperse between loops of bowel, producing characteristic radiographic crescents throughout the pelvis. Moreover, dye should spill freely into the cul-de-sac and dispense throughout the pelvis. Failure to observe these late changes in the hysterosalpingogram suggests the possibility of peritubal adhesions or endometriosis, restricting normal fallopian tube mobility.

A hysterosalpingogram that shows an abnormality of the fallopian tubes should be followed with a *diagnostic laparoscopy*. *The hysterosalpingogram provides information about the surfaces of the genital tract organs, whereas diagnostic laparoscopy provides information about the external surfaces of these organs.* In addition, hysteroscopy can allow direct visualization of the endometrial cavity, as well as access to possible connections in patients with suggested lesions.

Abnormalities of Spermatogenesis

Problems of spermatogenesis account for over *40% of cases of infertility*. Unlike oocytes, which are ovulated periodically, sperm are being constantly produced by the germinal epithelium of the testicles. As sperm mature within the germinal epithelium, they are released into the epididymis where maturation occurs prior to ejaculation.

The *sperm generation time* is approximately 73 days. Thus, an abnormal sperm count is a reflection of events that occurred 73 days prior to the collection of a semen specimen. Alternatively, a minimum of 73 days is required to observe the change in sperm production following therapy for oligospermia.

Sperm production is thermoregulated. Intratesticular temperature is regulated by contraction and relaxation of the scrotum. Sperm production occurs at a temperature of approximately 1°F less than body temperature. External thermal shock to the testicles can result in reduced sperm production. Examples include spending time in a hot tub, sit-

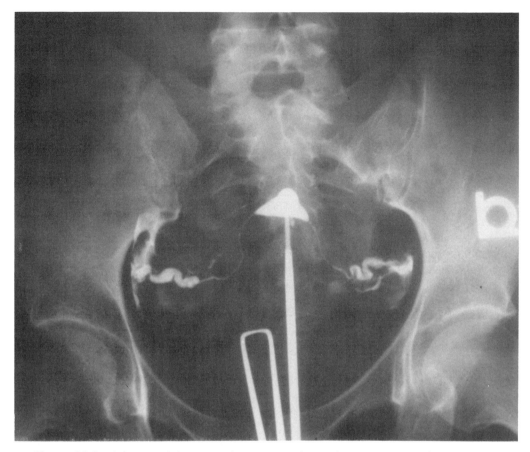

Figure 38.3. A hysterosalpingogram showing normal genital tract anatomy and architecture.

ting on the testicles for long periods of time with poor heat dispersion, or wearing tight clothing that pulls the testicles against the body for extended periods of time. In many cases, one of these causes can be discovered from a carefully obtained history or from observation.

As the follicle of the ovary responds to FSH and LH, the Leydig cells and germinal epithelium of the testicles also respond to gonadotropic stimulation. In some males, the germinal epithelium becomes fibrotic and sperm production is diminished. In others, testosterone production by Leydig cells is decreased. Men with oligospermia should have gonadotropin hormones measured to exclude testicular failure. Suspected testicular failure should be confirmed by testicular biopsy.

The man who has *poor sperm production* as a result of hormonal abnormalities does not respond well to induction of spermatogenesis. Some men with marginal testicular failure or poor gonadotropic production will respond to the administration of clomiphene citrate. This is appropriate therapy for a limited time.

Another method besides sperm analysis is to evaluate sperm density and sperm motility is the *postcoital test (Sims-Huhner test)*. The test should be timed to take place during the late follicular phase of the menstrual cycle just prior to ovulation. At this time of the cycle, cervical mucus is abundant and facilitates sperm survival and transport. The couple should have intercourse approximately 8 hours before the test is scheduled. The female partner undergoes a speculum examination to expose the cervix. With a tuberculin syringe, a small sample of endocervical mucus is aspirated from the endocervical canal. This is placed on a glass side and examined under a microscope. Normally 8–10 motile sperm are seen per high powered field in the cervical mucus. This simple test provides important information about coitus, ejaculation, sperm pickup, and sperm storage within the endocervical canal. Preferably, this test is done with both partners in attendance. The male then has the opportunity to better understand his partner's reproductive system and both can view the cervical mucus under the microscope.

Recently, *immunologic causes of infertility* have received attention. Both men and women can produce *antisperm antibodies*. If the woman produces antisperm antibodies, sperm will be immobilized in the cervical mucus. If the male produces antisperm antibodies, sperm will agglutinate and will be unable to penetrate the cervical mucus. The diagnosis of antisperm antibodies is made by performing immunologic studies on both partners. If antisperm antibodies exist in the woman, timed intrauterine insemination of washed sperm into the endometrial cavity may produce a pregnancy. There is no known effective treatment for men with antisperm antibodies.

For some couples, there will be no biological explanation for their infertility. Physicians must look for men and women with low body weight, individuals or couples who use marijuana, or something else in their lifestyle that may compromise reproduction.

TREATMENT OF THE INFERTILE COUPLE

Once a cause for infertility has been established, a treatment program can be developed. If *anovulation* is the cause of infertility, therapy should be directed to *restore ovulation by the administration of ovulation-inducing agents*. The most frequently used therapy is *clomiphene citrate*. Clomiphene citrate is an antiestrogen, which stimulates increased production of follicle-stimulating hormone, which acts to trigger ovulation. Ovulation can also be triggered by the exogenous administration of human chorionic gonadotropin, which serves as a surrogate luteinizing hormone. This is typically administered in conjunction with clomiphene. If a woman fails to respond to clomiphene citrate, *follicle-stimulating hormone* can be administered directly to stimulate follicular growth. A purified preparation of gonadotropins from the urine of postmenopausal women (Pergonal (menotropins)) is usually used. Pergonal contains about 75 IU of FSH or LH per dose and must be given parenterally, as it is inactivated if given orally. When clomiphene citrate is used, ovulation can be monitored simply by maintaining a basal body temperature record. On the other hand, if exogenous follicle-stimulating hormone is administered, monitoring requires frequent measurement of estradiol-17β and frequent imaging of the ovarian follicles.

Anatomic Abnormalities

In the event an anatomical abnormality of the genital tract is discovered, a *surgical treatment* is developed. Lysis of pelvic adhesions will result in freeing of entrapped internal genital structures. In case of fallopian tube obstruction, the obstruction can be corrected surgically. However, for these operations to be successful, the endosalpinx must be healthy. If the endosalpinx has been altered such that ovum pickup and transport cannot occur, one of the assisted reproductive technologies—primarily in vitro fertilization—must be considered as an option.

Inadequate Spermatogenesis

Problems of spermatogenesis should be addressed by trying to eliminate alterations of thermoregulation. Attempts at induction of spermatogenesis can be made by the administration of clomiphene citrate. However, the response to this therapy is usually less than 20%.

If spermatogenesis cannot be improved, couples may choose to utilize *artificial insemination using donor sperm* (AID), or one of the assisted reproductive technologies such as gamete intrafallopian tube transfer (GIFT) or in vitro fertilization (IVF) to facilitate fertilization using the infertile partner's sperm.

Assisted Reproductive Technologies

An explosion of assisted reproductive technologies has occurred in the last decade. These include in vitro fertilization, gamete intrafallopian tube transfer, and zygote intrafallopian tube transfer (ZIFT). These technologies provide infertility specialists with tools to bypass the normal mechanisms of gamete transportation and fertilization. However, IVF, GIFT, and ZIFT are expensive and place infertile couples on an emotional roller coaster. The expected successful outcome from IVF in properly selected couples is approximately 18–22% per cycle. The expected successful outcome for properly selected couples for GIFT and ZIFT is approximately 22–28% per cycle. Strict indications for the use of these procedures must be maintained to prevent misuse and exploitation of couples. The probability of pregnancy in a healthy couple is approximately 18–20% per cycle. Assisted reproductive technologies do not enhance the possibility of pregnancy in couples who do not have indications for their use.

With the array of imaging techniques, pharmacologic agents, and surgical procedures available to the physician, there are many treatment options for infertile couples. Thus, the physician can be optimistic in counseling infertile couples about the prognosis for having a child. At the same time, while offering encouragement, the physician must be aware of the psychological impact that infertility has on both partners and their family. Appropriate therapy must include psychological support.

FURTHER READINGS

Aiman EJ, ed. Infertility. New York: Springer-Verlag, 1984.

Damewood MD, ed. The Johns Hopkins handbook of in vitro fertilization and assisted reproductive technologies. Boston: Little, Brown & Co, 1990.

Seibel MM. Infertility. A comprehensive text. East Norwalk, CT: Appleton & Lange, 1990.

Speroff L, Glass RH, Kase NG. Clinical gynecologic endocrinology and infertility. 4th ed. Baltimore: Williams & Wilkins, 1989.

SELF-EVALUATION

Case 38-A

A couple in their late 20's presents for evaluation of infertility. The woman is G0 and has regular menses. The husband has never fathered a child. They have had unprotected sexual intercourse for 18 months. Neither has a history of sexually transmitted disease nor major illness. The male reports no difficulty with erection or ejaculation.

Question 38-A-1

Which of the following is the most likely cause of their infertility?

A. an ovulation disorder
B. an abnormality of spermatogenesis
C. an anatomic disorder of the female's reproductive tract
D. immunologic disorder

Answer 38-A-1

Answer: B

Problems with spermatogenesis are found in about 40% of couples with infertility, whereas abnormalities of ovulation and anatomical disorders of the female reproductive tract account for about 30% each of infertility cases. An ovulation disorder is unlikely, given her regular menstrual history. There is no reason to expect an anatomic abnormality, but this will need to be evaluated, as well as the possibility of infertility of immunologic etiology.

Question 38-A-2

Which of the following diagnostic studies *would not* be indicated as part of this couple's *initial* evaluation?

A. basal body temperature record
B. semen analysis

C. hysterosalpingogram
D. diagnostic laparoscopy

Answer 38-A-2

Answer: D

Basal body temperature records are an excellent method of confirmation of ovulation, and semen analysis, of confirmation of spermatogenesis. Hysterosalpingography should be a part of initial infertility evaluations to rule out possible endometrial or tubal pathology. Diagnostic laparoscopy is used to evaluate the external surfaces of the female reproductive tract but requires a hospital surgical procedure. It should, therefore, be reserved until other initial tests are completed. Hysteroscopy may also be used for detailed evaluation of the intrauterine cavity and is commonly performed in conjunction with laparoscopy.

Question 38-A-3

The female partner is found to have anovulation. The next step in the evaluation is to:
A. Induce ovulation with clomiphene citrate.
B. Perform artificial insemination.
C. Induce ovulation with exogenous gonadotropins.
D. Perform diagnostic laparoscopy to rule out other causes of infertility.

Answer 38-A-3

Answer: A

Initial treatment with clomiphene citrate will often be sufficient to induce ovulation. Occasionally, other agents such as hCG and Pergonal may be necessary. If ovulation does not occur, evaluation as to the etiology is indicated. Artificial insemination is not yet indicated since it does not address the identical dysfunction. Laparoscopy would be premature at this point also.

Case 38-B

A 37-year-old woman with a history of gonococcal salpingitis presents with her husband and expresses a complaint of infertility.

Question 38-B-1

Which of the following studies is indicated on initial evaluation?
A. basal body temperature record
B. semen analysis
C. hysterosalpingogram
D. endometrial biopsy

Answer 38-B-1

Answer: A, B, C

Without evidence of anovulation, the endometrial biopsy is not indicated, whereas evaluation of the male (semen analysis) is routine and the hysterosalpingogram is performed to rule out fallopian tube obstruction.

Question 38-B-2

The hysterosalpingogram reveals bilateral tubal obstruction. A consultant advises against corrective surgery because of a very poor prognosis for successful outcome. You recommend which of the following?
A. gamete intrafallopian tube transfer
B. homologous intrauterine insemination
C. in vitro fertilization
D. adoption

Answer 38-B-2

Answer: C

chapter 39

HIRSUTISM AND VIRILIZATION

A woman who complains of being too hairy or too masculine presents a diagnostic and therapeutic challenge for the physician. Hirsutism and virilization may be clinical clues to an underlying androgen excess disorder. The physician should consider the sites of androgen production and the mechanisms of androgen action when evaluating and treating hirsutism and virilization. The most common cause of hirsutism is polycystic ovarian disease, the second most common cause, adrenal hyperplasia. These conditions must be established by laboratory diagnosis. Treatment of androgen excess should be directed at suppressing the source of androgen excess or blocking androgen action at the receptor site.

Androgens play three essential roles in female reproductive function: (*a*) they are precursors for estrogen biosynthesis, (*b*) they stimulate and maintain sexual hair growth, and (*c*) they drive the female libido. However, exposure to excess androgens, through either excess production or increased action, results in increased body hair and acne.

Hirsutism is defined as excess body hair. It is manifested initially by the appearance of midline *terminal hair*. Terminal hair is dark, coarse, somewhat kinky hair as compared with vellus hair, which is soft, downy, fine hair. When a woman is exposed to excess androgens, terminal hair will first appear on the lower abdomen and around the nipples, next around the chin and upper lip, and finally between the breasts and on the lower back. Usually a woman with hirsutism will also have *acne*. In western cultures, terminal hair on the abdomen, breasts, and face is considered unsightly and presents a cosmetic prob-

lem for women. At the first sign of hirsutism, women often consult their physician to seek a cause for the excess hair growth and seek treatment to eliminate it.

Virilization is defined as masculinization of a woman. It is associated with marked increase in circulating *testosterone*. As a woman becomes virilized, she first notices enlargement of the clitoris followed by temporal balding, deepening of the voice, involution of the breasts, and a remodeling of the limb-shoulder girdle. Over time, she takes on a more masculine appearance as presented in Figure 39.1.

ANDROGEN PRODUCTION AND ANDROGEN ACTION

In women, *androgens are produced* in the adrenal glands, the ovaries, and adipose tissue where there is extraglandular production of testosterone from androstenedione. The following three androgens must be measured in evaluating a woman with hirsutism and virilization:

1. *Dehydroepiandrosterone (DHEA)*—a weak carbon 5 androgen secreted principally by the *adrenal glands*.
2. *Androstenedione (A)*—a weak carbon 4 androgen secreted in equal amounts by the *adrenal glands and ovaries*.
3. *Testosterone (T)*—a potent carbon 4 androgen secreted by the *adrenal glands and ovaries* and produced in *adipose* tissue from the conversion of androstenedione.

The sites of androgen production and proportions produced are presented in Table 39.1.

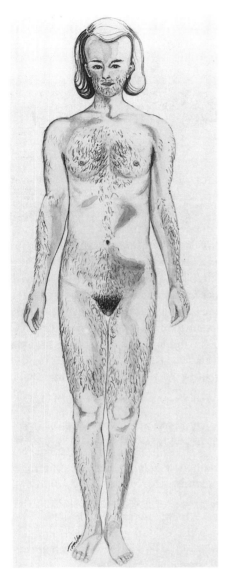

Figure 39.1. An illustration of a woman with virilization. Note the clitoral enlargement, temporal balding, masculine body habitus, and hirsutism.

Table 39.1
Sites of Androgen Production

	DHEA	Androstenedione	Testosterone
	%	%	%
Adrenal glands	90	50	25
Ovaries	10	50	25
Extraglandular	0	0	50

Adrenal androgen production is regulated by pituitary secretion of adrenocorticotropic hormone (ACTH). ACTH stimulates the adrenal cortical production of cortisol. In the metabolic sequence of cortisol production, DHEA is one precursor hormone. In enzymatic deficiencies of adrenal steroidogenesis (21-hydroxylase deficiency and 11β-hydroxylase deficiency), DHEA accumulates and is further metabolized to androstenedione and testosterone. The flow of adrenal hormone production is presented in Figure 39.2.

Ovarian androgen production is largely under the control of luteinizing hormone (LH) secretion from the pituitary gland. LH stimulates theca-lutein cells surrounding the ovarian follicles to secrete androstenedione, and to a lesser extent, testosterone. These androgens are precursors for estrogen production by granulosa cells of the ovarian follicles. In conditions of sustained or increased LH secretion, androstenedione and testosterone increase. The metabolic relationship between androgens and estrogens is presented in Figure 39.3.

Extraglandular testosterone production occurs in adipocytes (fat cells) and depends upon the magnitude of adrenal and ovarian androstenedione production. When androstenedione production increases, there is a dependent increase in extraglandular testosterone production. When a woman becomes obese, the conversion of androstenedione to testosterone in adipocytes increases.

Testosterone is the primary androgen that causes increased hair growth, acne, and the physical changes associated with virilization. After testosterone is secreted from its site of production, it is bound to a carrier protein — *sex hormone binding globulin (SHBG)* — and

In addition, testosterone is also converted within the hair follicle and within genital skin to *dihydrotestosterone (DHT)*, which is an androgen even more potent than testosterone. This metabolic conversion is the result of the local action of 5α-reductase on testosterone at these sites. This is the basis for constitutional hirsutism, which is discussed later.

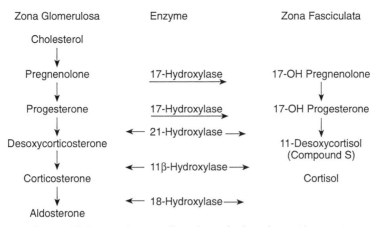

Figure 39.2. A schematic flow chart of adrenal steroidogenesis.

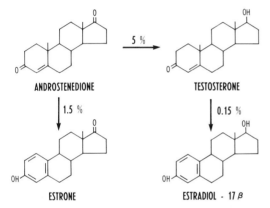

Figure 39.3. The metabolic interrelationships between androgens and estrogens. The percentages indicate the extent of metabolism in adipocytes.

circulates in plasma as a bound steroid hormone. Only a small fraction (1–3%) of testosterone is unbound (free). Bound testosterone is unable to attach to testosterone receptors and is, therefore, metabolically inactive. It is the small fraction of free hormone that exerts the effects. SHBG is produced by the liver. Estrogens stimulate hepatic production of SHBG. Greater estrogen production is associated with less free testosterone, whereas decreased estrogen production is associated with increased free testosterone. Therefore, measurement of total testosterone alone may not reflect the fraction of free testosterone.

Testosterone receptors are scattered throughout the body. For the purpose of this discussion, testosterone receptors will be considered only in hair follicles, sebaceous glands, and genital skin. Free testosterone enters the cytosol of testosterone-dependent cells. There it is bound to a testosterone receptor and carried into the nucleus of the cell to initiate its metabolic action. *When testosterone is excessive*, there is: increased hair growth, acne, increased libido, and rugation of the genital skin. Moreover, some individuals have increased 5α-reductase within hair follicles resulting in excessive production of DHT.

CONDITIONS DUE TO OVARIAN ANDROGEN EXCESS
Polycystic Ovarian Disease (PCOD)

Polycystic ovarian disease is the *most common cause of androgen excess and hirsutism*. The etiology of this disorder is unknown. Some cases appear to result from a genetic predisposition, whereas others seem to result from obesity or other causes of luteinizing hormone (LH) excess. One proposed mechanism for PCOD is presented in Figure 39.4.

The symptoms of polycystic ovarian disease include *oligomenorrhea*, *amenorrhea*, *anovulation*, *acne*, *hirsutism*, and *infertility*. The disorder is characterized by chronic anovulation or extended periods of anovulation.

PCOD is related to obesity by the following mechanism. LH stimulates the theca-

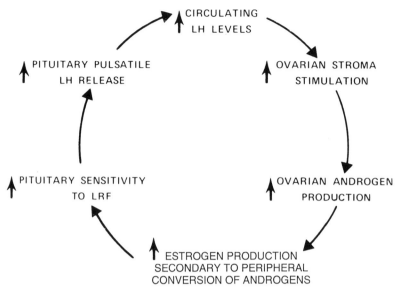

Figure 39.4. A mechanism for polycystic ovarian disease proposed by Yen. *LRF*, luteinizing releasing factor.

lutein cells to increase androstenedione production. Androstenedione undergoes aromatization to estrone within adipocytes. Although estrone is a weak estrogen, it has a positive feedback action or stimulating effect on the pituitary secretion of LH. LH secretion is, therefore, stimulated by increased estrogen. With increasing obesity, there is increased conversion of androstenedione to estrone. In many women with PCOD, obesity seems to be the common factor, and the acquisition of body fat coincides with the onset of PCOD. With the increased rise in androstenedione, there is coincident increased testosterone production, which causes acne and hirsutism.

PCOD is a functional disorder whose treatment should be targeted to interrupt the disorder's positive feedback cycle. Hormonal studies in women with PCOD show the following: (*a*) increased LH:FSH ratio, (*b*) estrone in greater concentration than estradiol, (*c*) androstenedione at the upper limits of normal or increased, and (*d*) testosterone at the upper limits of normal or slightly increased.

The most common therapy for PCOD is the *administration of oral contraceptives*, which will suppress pituitary LH production. Oral contraceptives have several beneficial effects. By suppressing LH, there is decreased production of androstenedione and testosterone. The ovarian contribution to the total androgen pool is thereby decreased. Acne clears, new hair growth is prevented, and there is decreased androgenic stimulation of existing hair follicles. By preventing estrogen excess, oral contraceptives also prevent endometrial hyperplasia. In addition, the women will have cyclic predictable withdrawal bleeding episodes.

If a woman with PCOD wishes to conceive, oral contraceptive therapy is not a suitable choice. If the patient is obese, a *weight reduction* diet designed to restore the patient to a normal weight should be instituted. With body weight reduction alone, many women resume regular ovulatory cycles and conceive spontaneously. With weight reduction, there is decreased aromatization, which interrupts PCOD at the level of the adipocyte. In some women desiring pregnancy, ovulation induction with clomiphene citrate is needed. Ovulation induction is facilitated by weight reduction in obese women.

In some women, a *variation of PCOD* occurs in which *the patient also has insulin-resistant diabetes mellitus*. A common physical sign of this condition is acanthosis nigricans in the skin folds. *Acanthosis nigricans* is characterized by thickening of the skin on the back of the neck, under the breasts, and in the intertriginous areas of the thighs. This is found most often in obese patients, and with weight loss, the skin changes resolve spontaneously.

Hyperthecosis

Hyperthecosis is a *more severe form of polycystic ovarian disease*. In cases of hyperthecosis, *androstenedione* production may be so great that testosterone reaches concentrations such that early signs of *virilization* appear. Women with this condition may exhibit some temporal balding, clitoral enlargement, deepening of the voice, and remodeling at the limb-shoulder girdle.

Hyperthecosis is refractory to oral contraceptive suppression. It is also more difficult to successfully induce ovulation in women with this condition.

Sertoli-Leydig Cell Tumors

Sertoli-Leydig cell tumors are *ovarian neoplasms that secrete testosterone*. These tumors usually occur in women between the ages of 20 and 40 years. The tumor is most often unilateral and may reach a size of 7–10 cm in diameter.

Women with a Sertoli-Leydig cell tumor will have a rapid onset of *acne, hirsutism, amenorrhea*, and *virilization*. In the short span of 6 months, a woman may cease having ovulatory menses and exhibit extensive body hair, temporal hair recession, clitoral enlargement, and deepening of the voice.

Laboratory studies of this disorder show suppression of FSH and LH, a low plasma androstenedione, and a marked elevation of testosterone. An *ovarian mass* is usually palpable on pelvic examination and confirmed by sonography. Once the diagnosis is suspected, there should be no delay in *surgical removal* of the involved ovary. The contralateral ovary

should be inspected, and if it is found to be enlarged should be bisected for gross inspection.

Following surgical removal of a Sertoli-Leydig cell tumor, ovulatory cycles return spontaneously and further progression of hirsutism is arrested. If the clitoris has become enlarged, it will not revert to its pretreatment size. However, temporal hair is restored and the body habitus will become feminine once again.

ADRENAL ANDROGEN EXCESS DISORDERS
Congenital Adrenal Hyperplasia

In the sequence of adrenal steroidogenesis, *dehydroepiandrosterone DHEA* is a key hormone. DHEA is a precursor for androstenedione and testosterone. The most common cause of increased adrenal androgen production is adrenal hyperplasia due to *21-hydroxylase deficiency*. 21-Hydroxylase catalyzes the conversion of progesterone and 17α-hydroxyprogesterone to desoxycorticosterone and compound S. When 21-hydroxylase is deficient, there is an accumulation of progesterone and 17α-hydroxyprogesterone, which are metabolized subsequently to dehydroepiandrosterone. This disorder affects approximately 2% of the population and is due to an alteration in the gene for 21-hydroxylase that is carried on chromosome 6. The genetic defect is autosomal recessive and has variable penetrance.

In the most severe form of 21-hydroxylase deficiency, the newly born female infant is virilized. However, milder forms are more common and can appear at puberty or even later in adult life. A mild deficiency of 21-hydroxylase is frequently associated wth terminal body hair, acne, subtle alterations in menstrual cycles, and infertility. *When 21-hydroxylase deficiency is manifested at puberty*, adrenarche may precede thelarche. The history of pubic hair growth occurring prior to the onset of breast development may be a clinical clue to this disorder. The *diagnosis* of 21-hydroxylase deficiency is made by measuring *increased dehydroepiandrosterone sulfate (DS) and androstenedione* in plasma.

The diagnosis of *late-onset adrenal hyperplasia* is suspected in a woman with hirsutism, acne, and menstrual irregularities. This diagnosis is established by measuring plasma concentrations of DS, androstenedione, and testosterone. In this condition, it is not unusual to find an increased plasma DS, increased androstenedione, and normal or slightly increased testosterone. When this hormone pattern is reported, the physician should follow up with an *ACTH stimulation test.*

A less common cause of adrenal hyperplasia is *11β-hydroxylase deficiency.* 11β-Hydroxylase catalyzes the conversion of desoxycorticosterone to cortisol. A deficiency in this enzyme also results in increased androgen production. The clinical features of 11β-hydroxylase deficiency are mild hypertension and mild hirsutism. The *diagnosis* of 11β-hydroxylase deficiency is made by demonstrating increased plasma desoxycorticosterone.

Treatment of Adrenal Hyperplasia

In adrenal hyperplasia, the adrenal glands require increased ACTH secretion to stimulate adequate cortisol production. To maintain normal cortisol production, the adrenal glands oversecrete androgens.

This condition can be managed easily by *supplementing glucocorticoids.* Usually, prednisone, 2.5 mg daily, will suppress adrenal androgen production to within the normal range. When this therapy is instituted, facial acne usually clears promptly, ovulation is restored, and there is no new terminal hair growth.

Medical therapy for adrenal and ovarian disorders cannot resolve hirsutism; it can only suppress new hair growth. Hair that is present must be controlled by shaving, by use of depilatory agents, or by electrolysis.

Adrenal Neoplasms

An adrenal adenoma is a rare causes of hirsutism. In androgen-secreting adrenal adenomas, there is a rapid increase in hair growth associated with severe acne, amenorrhea, and sometimes virilization. In androgen-secreting adenomas, DS is usually elevated above 6 μg/ml. The diagnosis is established by computed axial tomography or magnetic resonance imaging of the adrenal glands, which shows the adrenal adenoma. Adrenal adenomas must be removed surgically.

CONSTITUTIONAL HIRSUTISM

Occasionally after a diagnostic evaluation for hirsutism, there will be no explanation for the cause of the disorder. By exclusion, this condition is often called "constitutional hirsutism." Data support the hypothesis that women with constitutional hirsutism have *greater activity of 5α-reductase* than do unaffected women. These women ovulate regularly and have normal hormone concentrations. Women with constitutional hirsutism may respond to treatment with *spironolactone*, a mild diuretic designed to limit aldosterone production. This drug *binds androgen receptors*, thus blocking androgenic activity. A dosage of 50–100 mg/day will suffice for the treatment of constitutional hirsutism.

IATROGENIC ANDROGEN EXCESS
Danazol

Danazol is an *attenuated androgen designed for the suppression of pelvic endometriosis.* It has androgenic properties, and some women will develop hirsutism, acne, and deepening of the voice while taking the drug. If these symptoms develop, the value of the danazol should be weighed against the side effects before continuing therapy.

Pregnancy should be ruled out before initiating a course of danazol therapy, as it can produce virilization of the female fetus.

Oral Contraceptives

The progestins in oral contraceptives are impeded androgens. Rarely, a woman taking oral contraceptives will develop acne and even hirsutism. If this occurs, another product with a less androgenic progestin should be selected or the pill should be discontinued. Moreover, evaluation for the coincidental development of late-onset adrenal hyperplasia should be done.

FURTHER READINGS

Bondy PK. Disorders of the adrenal cortex. In: Wilson JD, Foster DW, eds. Williams textbook of endocrinology. 7th ed. Philadelphia: WB Saunders, 1985: 816–890.

Rebar RW. Hirsutism, hyperandrogenism, and polycystic ovarian disease. In: DeGroot LJ, ed. Endocrinology. 2nd ed. Philadelphia: WB Saunders, 1989:1982–1983.

Yen SSC. Chronic anovulation caused by peripheral endocrine disorders. In: Yen SSC, Jaffe RB. Reproductive endocrinology: physiology, pathophysiology, and clinical management. 2nd ed. Philadelphia: WB Saunders, 1986:441–499.

SELF-EVALUATION

Case 39-A

A 19-year-old unmarried woman presents with a complaint of being "too hairy." Her history includes severe irregular menstrual cycles, worsening acne, and hair growth on the face, breasts, and lower abdomen. She is on no medication, is sexually active, uses condoms for contraception, and otherwise feels well. She is depressed about the new hair growth.

Question 39-A-1

The most likely cause for this group of symptoms is:

A. congenital adrenal hyperplasia
B. Sertoli-Leydig cell tumor of the ovary
C. polycystic ovarian disease
D. constitutional hirsutism

Answer 39-A-1

Answer: C

PCOD is the most common cause of this patient's complaints. Although she was focused on the increase hair growth, further history revealed andogen excess, in general, with symptoms comparable with PCOD.

Question 39-A-2

Which of the following laboratory studies should be performed?

A. DHEA
B. progesterone
C. androstenedione
D. testosterone

Answer 39-A-2

Answer: A, C, D

LH stimulates androstenedione production, which is aromatized in the fat cells to estrone, which stimulates pituitary LH production: a positive feedback loop. Very high testosterone levels may suggest the need for a Gyn ultrasound examination of the ovaries, as such levels are associated with Sertoli-Leydig cell tumors. DHEA is the "key hormone" in adrenal hyperplasia. Progesterone levels are not helpful in the workup of hirsuitism.

Question 39-A-3

A diagnosis of polycystic ovarian disease is made. An initial treatment plan should include:

A. clomiphene citrate
B. oral contraceptives
C. prednisone
D. spironolactone

Answer 39-A-3

Answer: B

Because this patient does not desire to get pregnant, oral contraceptive therapy will be the best choice of therapy, as it provides effective contraception, as well as suppresses LH production.

Case 39-B

A 27-year-old G0 complains of the gradual appearance of terminal hair on the face and lower abdomen. She has noted subtle changes in her menstrual cycle length. She has tried to conceive for 1½ years but has been unsuccessful. Her blood pressure is normal.

Question 39-B-1

Of the following, which is the most likely cause for these symptoms?

A. hyperthecosis
B. constitutional hirsutism
C. late-onset adrenal hyperplasia (21-hydroxylase type)
D. late-onset adrenal hyperplasia (11α-hydroxylase type)

Answer 39-B-1

Answer: C

Late-onset adrenal hyperplasia should be suspected in women with hirsutism, acne, and menstrual irregularities. Infertility is also common.

Question 39-B-2

Initial laboratory studies show an elevated dehydroepiandrosterone sulfate (DS). Which of the following is the most appropriate next diagnostic study?

A. GnRH stimulation test
B. ACTH stimulation test
C. FSH and LH measurement
D. thyroid stimulation test

Answer 39-B-2

Answer: B

DS and androstenedione are elevated in 21-hydroxylase deficiency, the most common disorder causing adrenal hyperplasia. ACTH stimulation will confirm this diagnosis.

Question 39-B-3

A diagnosis of late-onset adrenal hyperplasia (21-hydroxylase type) is made. Which of the following therapies should be initiated?

A. clomiphene citrate
B. oral contraceptive suppression
C. prednisone
D. thyroid replacement therapy

Answer 39-B-3

Answer: C

Glucocorticoid supplementation will suppress adrenal androgen production. Facial acne usually clears and ovulation resumes.

chapter 40

CELL BIOLOGY AND PRINCIPLES OF CANCER THERAPY

Treatment of cancers involving the breast and genital organs can involve surgery, chemotherapy, radiation therapy, and hormone therapy, used alone or in combination. The specific treatment plan will depend on the type of cancer, the stage of the cancer, and the characteristics of the individual patient. Individualizing treatment is an important characteristic of cancer therapy.

THE CELL CYCLE AND CANCER THERAPY

Knowledge of the cell cycle is important in understanding cancer therapies. Many treatments are based on the fact that cancer cells are constantly dividing, making them more vulnerable to agents that interfere with the cell division process.

The cell cycle consists of four phases (as shown in Figure 40.1). During the G_1 phase, there is synthesis of RNA and protein that prepares the cell for DNA synthesis, which occurs in the S phase. The G_2 phase is a period of additional RNA, protein, and specialized DNA synthesis. This leads to mitosis (M phase), where cell division occurs. After mitosis, cells can again enter the G_1 phase or can "drop out" of the cell cycle and enter a resting phase (G_0). Cells in G_0 do not engage in the synthetic activities characteristic of the cell cycle. The *growth fraction* is the number of cells in a tumor that are actively involved in cell division (that is, not in the G_0 phase). The growth fraction of tumors decreases as they enlarge, since vascular supply and oxygen levels are decreased. *Surgical removal of tumor tissue* (cytoreductive debulking surgery) *can result in G_0 cells reentering the cell cycle, thus making them more vulnerable to chemotherapy and radiation therapy.*

The *generation time* is the length of the cell cycle, from M phase to M phase. For a given cell type, the lengths of the S and M phases are relatively constant, whereas G_2 and, especially, G_1 vary. The variable length of G_1 can be explained by cells entering G_0 for a period and then reentering the cycle.

Chemotherapeutic agents and radiation kill cancer cells by first-order kinetics. This means that they kill a constant fraction of tumor cells, instead of a constant number. The implication of this is that a number of intermittent doses are more likely to be curative than a single large dose.

CHEMOTHERAPY

Chemotherapeutic agents can be (a) cell cycle (phase) nonspecific, which means that they can kill in all phases of the cell cycle and are useful in tumors where the growth index is low, *or (b) cell cycle (phase) specific,* which kill in a specific phase of the cell cycle and are most useful in tumors where a large proportion of cells are actively dividing. Figure 40.1 contains examples of common drugs and their sites of action within the cycle.

There are several *classes of antineoplastic drugs* (Table 40.1). *Alkylating agents* primarily interact with DNA molecules to interfere with base pairing, produce cross-links, and cause single- and double-strand breaks. This interferes with DNA, RNA, and protein syn-

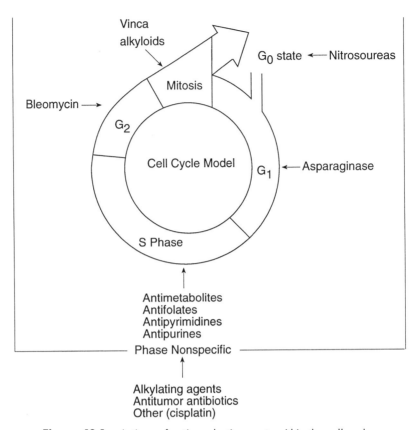

Figure 40.1. Actions of antineoplastic agents within the cell cycle.

thesis. Most alkylating agents are active in both resting (G_0) and dividing cells. Alkylating-like agents probably act, in part, through the formation of interstrand and intrastrand linkages in DNA.

The *antitumor antibiotics* intercalate between DNA base pairs to inhibit DNA-directed RNA synthesis and also are involved in the formation of free radicals, causing strand breakage. They probably are effective in all phases of the cell cycle.

The *antimetabolites* are structural analogs of normal molecules necessary for cell function. They competitively interfere with the normal synthesis of nucleic acids, and, therefore, are most active during the S phase of cell division.

Plant (vinca) alkaloids primarily prevent the assembly of microtubules, thus interfering with the M phase of cell division.

Antineoplastic drugs are toxic because they act on normal as well as cancer cells. Rapidly dividing cell types are most sensitive. For example, the cells of the erythroid, myeloid, and megakaryocytic series are damaged by common neoplastic drugs. Granulocytopenia and thrombocytopenia are predictable side effects. Patients with low granulocyte counts are at high risk for fatal sepsis, and those with sustained thrombocytopenia are at risk for spontaneous gastrointestinal or acute intracranial hemorrhage. Prophylactic antibiotics are usually administered to febrile patients to prevent serious infection, and platelet transfusions are employed to decrease the risk of hemorrhage. Table 40.2 describes the major side effects of antineoplastic agents.

There are limitations in the use of single agents. These include the development of drug resistance and the limitations on dura-

Table 40.1
Examples of Antineoplastic Drugs

Alkylating agents
    Nitrogen mustard (Mustargen, HN_2)
    Busulfan (Myleran)
    Melphalan (Alkeran, L-PAM)
    Chlorambucil (Leukeran)
Antitumor antibiotics
    Doxorubicin (Adriamycin)
    Daunorubicin (Daunomycin)
    Bleomycin (Blenoxane)
    Actinomycin D (dactinomycin, Cosmegen)
    Mitomycin C (Mutamycin)
Antimetabolites
    Methotrexate (MTX, amethopterin)
    6-Mercaptopurine (6-MP, Purinethol)
    5-Fluorouracil (fluorouracil, 5-FU)
    Hydroxyurea (Hydrea)
Plant alkaloids
    Vinblastine (Velban)
    Vincristine (Oncovin)
Other
    cis-Diamminedichloroplatinum (cisplatin)

Table 40.2
Major Side Effects of Antineoplastic Drugs

Hematologic
    Granulocytopenia
    Thrombocytopenia
Gastrointestinal
    Mucositis
    Necrotizing entercolitis
Immunosuppression
Dermatologic
    Alopecia
Hepatic
Pulmonary
    Interstitial pneumonitis
Cardiac
    Cardiomyopathy
Urinary
    Chronic azotemia
    Acute renal failure
Neurological
    Peripheral neuropathies
    Ototoxicity
    Paresthesias
Reproductive
    Amenorrhea

tion of treatment and dosage caused by toxicity. As a consequence, combination chemotherapy has come into use.

The *interactions between drugs used in combination* are defined as *synergistic* (result in improved antitumor activity or decreased toxicity than with each agent alone), *additive* (result in enhanced antitumor activity equal to the sum of each individual agent), or *antagonistic* (result in less antitumor activity than each individual agent). Drugs used in combinations should: (*a*) be effective when used singly, (*b*) have different mechanisms of action, and (*c*) be additive or, preferably, synergistic in action.

RADIATION THERAPY

Ionizing radiation causes the production of free hydrogen ions and hydroxyl (OH^-) radicals. In the presence of sufficient oxygen, H_2O_2 is formed, which affects DNA and, eventually, the cell's ability to divide. As with chemotherapy, killing is by first order kinetics. Since dividing cells are more sensitive to radiation damage, and since not all cells in a given tumor are dividing at any one time,

fractionated doses of radiation are more likely to be effective than a single dose. Providing multiple lower doses of radiation also reduces the deleterious effects on normal tissues.

The basis of fractionated dosage comes from the *"four R's" of radiobiology.*

1. *Repair of Sublethal Injury.* When a dose is divided, the number of cells that survive is greater than if the dose were given at one time (higher total amounts of radiation can be tolerated in fractionated as opposed to single doses).
2. *Repopulation.* Reactivation of stem cells occurs when radiation is stopped; thus, regenerative capacity depends on the number of available stem cells.
3. *Reoxygenation.* Cells are more vulnerable to radiation damage in the presence of oxygen; as tumor cells are killed, surviving cells will be brought into contact with capillaries, making them radiosensitive.
4. *Redistribution in the Cell Cycle.* Since tumor cells are in various phases of the cell cycle, fractionated doses make it more likely that a given cell will be irradiated when it is most vulnerable.

The *rad* has been used as a measure of the amount of energy absorbed per unit mass of tissue. A new standard measure of absorbed dose is the *Gray*, which is defined as 1 joule per kilogram. *One Gray is equal to 100 rad.* Radiation is delivered in two general ways: external irradiation (teletherapy) and local irradiation (brachytherapy). *Teletherapy* now depends on the use of high energy (over 1 million eV) beams, as this spares the skin and delivers less toxic radiation to bone. Tolerance for external radiation is dependent on the vulnerability of surrounding normal tissues. Teletherapy usually is used to shrink tumors prior to localized radiation. *Brachytherapy* depends on the inverse square law: the dose of radiation at a given point is inversely proportional to the square of the distance from the radiation source. To put the radioactive material at the closest possible distance, brachytherapy uses intracavity devices containing radioactive materials and interstitial (intratumor) implants. *Intracavity devices* can be placed within the uterus or vagina and then afterloaded with radioactive sources (radium or cesium). This method protects health personnel from radiation exposure. *Interstitial implants* use isotopes (iridium-192, iodine-125) formulated as wires or seeds. These implants are usually temporary.

Complications associated with radiation therapy can be acute or late (chronic). *Acute reactions* affect rapidly dividing tissues, such as epithelia (skin, gastrointestinal mucosa, bone marrow, reproductive cells). Manifestations are cessation of mitotic activity, cellular swelling, tissue edema, and tissue necrosis. Early problems associated with irradiation of gynecologic cancers include enteritis, acute cystitis, vulvitis, proctosigmoiditis, and occasionally, bone marrow depression. *Chronic complications* occur months to years after completion of radiation therapy. These include obliteration of small blood vessels or thickening of the vessel wall, fibrosis, and reductions in epithelial and parenchymal cell populations. This results in chronic proctitis, hemorrhagic cystitis, formation of uterovaginal or vesicovaginal fistula, and rectal or sigmoid stenosis as well as gastrointestinal fistulae.

HORMONAL THERAPY

The therapeutic importance of the presence of cellular *estrogen receptors* (ER) has been well established in breast cancers. There is a good relationship between the presence of ER and the response of patients to endocrine therapy. Normally, estrogen enters cells and binds to ER in the cytoplasm. The complex is translocated to the nucleus, where it binds to acceptor sites on chromosomes, resulting in activation of RNA and protein synthesis. The drug tamoxifen acts as a competitive inhibitor of estrogen binding. The tamoxifen-ER complex also binds to chromosomes, but does not activate cell metabolism. This decreases cellular activity and cell division, thus reducing tumor growth.

There also are *progestin receptors* (PR), which appear to be located in the nucleus of progestin-sensitive cells. Binding of the progestin-PR complex to DNA results in a decrease in the synthesis of both ER and PR and other antiestrogenic effects.

FURTHER READINGS

Berek J, Hacker N. Practical gynecologic oncology. Baltimore: Williams & Wilkins, 1989:Chapters 1 and 2.

Chabner BA, Collins JM. Cancer chemotherapy: principles and practice. Philadelphia: JB Lippincott, 1990.

SELF-EVALUATION

Case 40-A

A patient with a large ovarian tumor undergoes total abdominal hysterectomy with bilateral salpingo-oophorectomy for widespread disease. Most of the tumor mass is removed.

Question 40-A-1

Which of the following is a likely result of this operation?

A. The proportion of tumor cells in G_0 will increase.

B. The growth fraction of the remaining tumor will decrease.

C. The proportion of tumor cells that are sensitive to antineoplastic agents will increase.

D. A single dose of chemotherapy will be able to kill the remaining tumor cells.

Answer 40-A-1

Answer: C

Removal of part of a tumor mass increases the growth fraction (the number of cells that are actively dividing). Therefore, the proportion of cells in G_0 (the nondividing phase) will decrease, and the proportion of cells sensitive to antineoplastic agents will increase (since dividing cells are more sensitive). A single dose of chemotherapy will probably not be sufficient to kill the remaining tumor cells, since cells still will be killed by first-order kinetics.

For further consideration: What do you tell the patient about chemotherapy? Side effects? Value of repeated courses of treatment?

chapter 41

VULVAR DISEASE AND NEOPLASIA

Appreciation of vulvar symptoms and examination for vulvar dermatologic pathology constitute a significant part of primary health care for women. Noninflammatory vulvar pathology is found in women of all ages, but is particularly significant in peri- and postmenopausal women because of concern regarding the possibility of vulvar neoplasia. The major symptoms of vulvar disease include pruritis, burning, nonspecific irritation, and/or appreciation of a mass. Diagnostic aids for the assessment of noninflammatory conditions are likewise relatively limited in number and include, in addition to careful history, inspection and biopsy. Because vulvar lesions are often difficult to diagnose, liberal use of vulvar biopsy is central to good care.

This chapter discusses a range of vulvar pathologic conditions: nonneoplastic dermatoses, white lesions including both atrophic and hyperkeratotic lesions, vulvar intraepithelial neoplasia (VIN), and vulvar cancer. Inflammatory conditions of the vulva are included in Chapter 27, "Vulvitis and Vaginitis." Table 41.1 outlines common vulvar diseases.

COMMON VULVAR DERMATOSES
Lichen Simplex Chronicus (LSC)

In contrast to many dermatologic conditions that may be described as "rashes that itch," lichen simplex chronicus can be described as *"an itch that rashes."* Although oversimplified, this dermatologic maxim adequately describes the condition. It is thought that the majority of patients develop this disorder secondary *to an irritant dermatitis, which pro-gresses to lichen simplex chronicus as a result of the effects of chronic mechanical irritation* from scratching and rubbing an already irritated area. The mechanical irritation contributes to epidermal hyperplasia, which, in turn, leads to heightened sensitivity which triggers more mechanical irritation.

Accordingly, the history of these patients is one of *progressive vulvar pruritis and/or burning*, which is temporarily relieved by scratching or rubbing with a washcloth or some similar material. *Etiologic factors* for the original pruritic symptoms often are unknown, but may include sources of skin irritation such as laundry detergents, fabric softeners, scented hygienic preparations, and the use of colored or scented tissue. These potential sources of symptoms must be investigated. Any domestic or hygienic irritants must be removed, in combination with treatment, in order to break the cycle described above.

Table 41.1
Common Vulvar Diseases

Common vulvar dermatoses
  Lichen simplex chronicus (LSC)
  Lichen planus
  Psoriasis
  Seborrheic dermatitis
White lesions
  Hyperplastic vulvar dystrophy
  Lichen sclerosis
Vulvar intraepithelial neoplasia (VIN)
  Without atypia
  With atypia including carcinoma in situ
Vulvar carcinoma
  Paget's disease
  Squamous cell carcinoma

On *clinical inspection*, the skin of the labia majora, labia minora, and perineal body often shows diffusely reddened areas with occasional hyperplastic or hyperpigmented plaques of red to reddish brown. One may also find occasional areas of linear hyperplasia, which show the effect of grossly hyperkeratotic ridges of epidermis. Biopsy of patients who have these characteristics findings is usually not warranted.

Empiric *treatment* to include antipruritic *medications* such as Benadryl (diphenhydramine hydrocloride) or Atarax (hydroxyzine hydrochloride) that inhibit nighttime, unconscious scratching, combined with a mild to moderate topical *steroid cream* applied to the vulva, will usually provide relief. A steroid cream such as hydrocortisone (1 or 2%) or, for patients with significant areas of obvious hyperkeratosis, triamcinolone acetonide (0.1%) (Kenalog) or betamethasone valerate (0.1%) (Valisone) may be used. *If significant relief is not obtained within 3 months, diagnostic vulvar biopsy is warranted.*

Lichen Planus

Although lichen planus is usually a desquamative lesion of the vagina, occasional patients will develop lesions on the vulva near the inner aspects of the labia minora. Patients may have areas of whitish, lacy bands of keratosis near the reddish ulcerated-like lesions characteristic of the disease. Typically, complaints including *chronic vulvar burning and/or pruritis* and insertional, i.e., entrance, dyspareunia. Because of the patchiness of this lesion and the concern raised by atypical hyperplastic lesions, *biopsy is warranted* to confirm the diagnosis. In lichen planus, biopsy shows an absence of atypia in the hyperplastic area.

Treatment for lichen planus is topical *steroid perparations* similar to those described above. In patients with marked degrees of hyperkeratosis, a stronger steroid preparation such as fluocinonide 0.05% (Lidex cream) or triamcinolone acetonide (0.5%) (Aristocort) may be used. Length of treatment for these patients is often shorter than that required to treat lichen simplex chronicus, although lichen planus is more likely to reoccur.

Psoriasis

Psoriasis may involve the vulvar skin as part of a generalized dermatologic process. With approximately 2% of the general population suffering from psoriasis, the physician should be alert to its prevalence and likelihood of vulvar manifestation. Moreover, because it may appear at menarche, pregnancy, and menopause, the physician may be consulted by the patient for what she perceives to be a gynecologic disorder.

The *lesions* are typically slightly raised round or ovoid patches with a silver scale appearance atop an erythematous base. These lesions most often measure approximately 1×1 to 1×2 cm. Most patients are concerned by the appearance of this lesion, as pruritis is usually not marked. *The diagnosis is generally known because of psoriasis found elsewhere on the body, obviating the need for vulvar biopsy* to confirm the diagnosis.

Treatment often occurs in conjunction with consultation by a dermatologist. Like lesions elsewhere, vulvar lesions usually respond to topical cold tar preparations, followed by exposure to ultraviolet light, as well as corticosteroid medications, either topically or by intralesional injection. Since vulvar application of some of the photoactivated preparations can be somewhat awkward, topical steroids are most effective, using compounds such as betamethasone valerate (Valisone) 0.1%.

Seborrheic Dermatitis

Isolated vulvar seborrheic dermatitis is rare. The diagnosis is usually made in patients complaining of vulvar pruritis who are known to have seborrheic dermatitis in the scalp or other hair-bearing areas of the body. The lesion my mimic other entities such as psoriasis, tinea cruris (jock itch), or lichen simplex chronicus. The *lesions are pale red to a yellowish pink and may be covered by an oily-appearing, scaly crust.* Because this area of the body remains continually moist, occasional exudative lesions include raw "weeping" patches, due to skin maceration, which are exacerbated by the patient's scratching. As with psoriasis, *vulvar biopsy is usually not needed* when the diagnosis is made in conjunction with known seborrheic dermatitis in other hair-bearing areas.

For patients with acute exudative variations of seborrheic dermatitis, initial perineal hygiene includes the use of *Burow's solution soaks.* After remediation of the exudative phase, standard treatment includes *topical corticosteroid lotions or creams* containing a mixture of an agent that penetrates well such as betamethasone valerate in conjunction with Eurax (crotamiton) to control the intense pruritus. As with lichen simplex chronicus, the use of antipruritus agents such as Atarax or Benadryl as a bedtime dose in the first 10 days to 2 weeks of treatment will frequently help break the sleep/scratch cycle and allow the lesions to heal.

VULVAR NEOPLASIA

Historically, the classification of vulvar disease has used descriptive terminology based on gross morphologic appearance. Accordingly, such terms as leukoplakia, kraurosis vulvae, and vulvar dystrophy have been used. Standardization of nomenclature and classification by symptoms, gross appearance, and histology were lacking. In order to improve standardization and thus treatment of these disorders, the International Society for the Study of Vulvar Disease (ISSVD) established a modified classification in 1987. This classification has generally been accepted by different medical disciplines including gynecology, dermatology, and pathology. The rationale for the new description is based on both gross and microscopic morphology (Table 41.2).

Vulvar dermatoses have been described previously. The following discussion includes a description of squamous cell hyperplasia

Table 41.2
ISSVD Classification

I.	Squamous cell hyperplasia
II.	Lichen sclerosis
III.	Other dermatoses

(formerly hyperplastic dystrophy) and lichen sclerosis.

Squamous Cell Hyperplasia (Hyperplastic Dystrophy)

In considering the various types of vulvar neoplasia, the clinician should be aware that gross appearance may not be consistent with underlying cellular architecture and that often atrophic lesions, such as lichen sclerosis, may appear grossly to be hyperplastic. Further, within the group of true hyperplasia lesions, there is a need to confirm whether the hyperplasia is accompanied by atypia. As a result, classification of intraepithelial vulvar disease becomes a matter of close cooperation between the clinician, who must first appreciate the need for thorough investigation, and the pathologist, who is called upon to confirm the presence of lesions that may have premalignant or malignant potential. Because these distinctions cannot always be made on physical examination alone and because many of these lesions present with similar symptoms, *liberal use of vulvar biopsy is encouraged to provide definitive diagnosis and assure rational treatment.*

Many hyperplastic lesions without atypia evolve from chronic irritation and secondary thickening of the vulvar skin and are classified under the LSC group. These have been discussed previously. As with many of the other lesions, vulvar pruritus is the main presenting symptom. On gross inspection of the vulva, areas may be isolated and include obviously hyperkeratotic skin with secondary excoriation. These changes may diffusely involve the vulva or may occur as isolated ridges or patches. In the presence of gross abnormalities of the vulvar skin, directed biopsies of the lesions are warranted.

The microscopic appearance confirms the diagnosis. *Squamous cell hyperplasia without atypia* characteristically shows hyperkeratosis as well as acanthosis with an absence of mitotic figures. These lesions are usually treated as described in the previous discussion of lichen simplex chronicus, using various types of *topical, highly penetrating corticosteroid creams.* The patient can be reassured that these lesions usually respond to treatment with complete resolution and do not predispose to further premalignant or malignant vulvar disease.

Lichen Sclerosis

Lichen sclerosis, previously called lichen sclerosis et atrophicus, has confused both clinicians and pathologists because of inconsistent terminology and because it is associated with other types of vulvar pathology, including those of the hyperplastic variety. As with the other disorders, *chronic vulvar pruritus* occurs in most patients. Typically, *the vulva is diffusely involved with very thin, whitish epithelial areas* termed "onion skin" epithelium. Most patients have involvement on both sides of the vulva, with the most common sites being the labia majora, labia minora, the clitoral and periclitoral epithelium, and the perineal body. The lesion may extend to include a perianal "halo" of atrophic, whitish epithelium. In severe cases, there is loss of many normal anatomic landmarks, including obliteration of labial and periclitoral architecture, as well as severe stenosis of the vaginal introitus. Some patients will have areas of cracked skin, which are prone to bleeding with minimal trauma. Patients with these severe anatomic changes complain of difficulty in having normal coital function.

Microscopic confirmation of lichen sclerosis is mandatory. The histologic features are pathognomonic and include areas of hyperkeratosis despite epithelial thinning, a zone of homogenous, pink-staining collagenous-like material directly under the epithelial layer, and a band of chronic inflammatory cells consisting mostly of lymphocytes.

It is important to remember that there may be associated areas of hyperplasia mixed throughout or adjacent to these typically atrophic-appearing areas. In patients with this so-called *"mixed dystrophy,"* there is a need to treat both components to effect resolution of symptoms. Patients with histologic confirmation of a large hyperplastic component should initially be treated with well-penetrating corticosteroid creams. With improvement of these areas (usually 2–3 weeks), therapy can then be directed to the lichen sclerosis component.

The *treatment of choice for lichen sclerosis is topical testosterone appropionate (2%) in white petrolatum.* This is applied twice daily for 3 months and, with improvement in symptoms, may be used on a chronic basis once or twice a week depending on the need. Patients need to be reassured that this disorder is not premalignant, but that the lesion is unlikely to totally resolve. Intermittent treatment may be needed indefinitely. This is in marked contrast to the hyperplastic lesions without atypia, which usually totally resolve within 6 months.

Neither lichen sclerosis nor hyperplastic dystrophy without atypia significantly increase the patient's risk of developing cancer. It has been estimated that this risk is in the 2–3% range when there is no preexisting atypical hyperplasia. However, since patients who have had these disorders are more likely to eventually develop atypical hyperplasia, they need to be followed carefully and rebiopsied liberally if there is a return of vulvar symptoms or new lesions.

VULVAR INTRAEPITHELIAL NEOPLASIA (VIN)

Vulvar intraepithelial neoplasia may be classified as: VIN-I, mild dysplasia; VIN-II, moderate dysplasia; or VIN-III, severe dysplasia, carcinoma in situ.

Also included in the category of intraepithelial neoplasia lesions are vulvar condylomata. Other lesions represented include Paget's disease and level 1 melanomas. Condylomata are discussed in the section on inflammatory vulvar lesions, and Paget's disease and level I melanomas are mentioned briefly later in this chapter.

VIN-I and VIN-II

Early vulvar intraepithelial neoplasia (VIN-I and VIN-II) represents *true neoplastic lesions* that, as with their counterparts in the cervix, are thought to have a *high predilection for progression* to severe intraepithelial lesions and eventually carcinoma.

Presenting complaints include *vulvar pruritus, chronic irritation*, and *a development of raised mass lesions*. Usually, the lesions are localized and fairly well-isolated and are raised above the normal epithelial surface to include a slightly rough texture. These lesions are usually found along the posterior vulva and in the perineal body, although they may occur anywhere on the vulva. They typically have a whitish cast or hue. As with other vulvar lesions, diagnosis by biopsy is mandatory.

Microscopically, these lesions mimic intraepithelial neoplasia elsewhere, including mitotic figures and nuclear pleomorphism, with loss of normal differentiation in the lower one third to one half of the epithelial layer. As with the cervix, the degree of dysplasia increases to a point where full thickness change indicates severe intraepithelial neoplasia and/or carcinoma in situ. Changes consistent with human papilloma virus (HPV) infection are occasionally seen with these lesions and suggest an association between various types of HPV and the occurrence of vulvar intraepithelial neoplasia. Lesions that are typically condyloma in origin will not have features of attenuated maturation and have an absence of pleomorphism and atypical mitotic figures.

VIN-III (Carcinoma in Situ)

Full thickness loss of maturation indicates lesions that are at least severely dysplastic, including areas that may represent true carcinoma in situ. Common presenting complaints include *intractable pruritus* and *nonspecific vulvar irritation* with *gross lesions that are similar to earlier grades of VIN* occurring in patchy, fairly well-isolated areas. Occasional patients may have extensive vulvar involvement. The color changes in these lesions range from white, hyperplastic areas to reddened or dusky patch-like involvement, depending on whether there is associated hyperkeratosis.

Diagnosis

As with the other vulvar disorders, *diagnosis of vulvar intraepithelial neoplasia is made by biopsy*. In patients without obvious raised or isolated lesions, careful inspection of the vulva is warranted using a magnifying device such as a hand lens or visor. Washing the vulvar skin with a dilute solution of 3% acetic acid often accentuates the white lesions and may also help in revealing abnormal vascular patterns. When present, these areas should be selectively biopsied in multiple sites to thoroughly investigate the grade of vulvar intraepithelial neoplasia and reliably exclude the presence of invasive carcinoma.

Treatment

The goal in treating VIN is to quickly and completely remove all involved areas of skin. A variety of treatments are available, depending on the extent of the lesion and the severity of the dysplasia. Most *isolated and limited VIN-I or VIN-II lesions* may be removed by local excision in the office or by *cryocautery, electrodesiccation*, or *laser cautery* with local anesthetic. Extended lesions showing VIN-I or VIN-II are usually treated with *laser ablation* in an ambulatory surgery area using a general anesthetic.

VIN-III, including carcinoma in situ, is best treated by wide *local excision with or without combination laser ablation*, depending on the area of involvement. This usually requires a general or regional anesthetic and often requires inpatient hospitalization, depending on the extent of the vulvar surgery. Occasionally, for diffuse or recurrent disease, simple vulvectomy is warranted.

Paget's Disease

Paget's disease is characterized by extensive intraepithelial disease including characteristic intraepithelial pathologic findings. It is identical histologically to Paget's disease of the breast. Although not common, Paget's disease of the vulva may be associated with carcinoma of the skin. Similarly, patients with Paget's disease of the vulva have a higher incidence of underlying internal carcinoma, particularly of the colon and breast.

The treatment for vulvar Paget's disease is wide local excision or simple vulvectomy, depending on the amount of involvement. Recurrences are more common with this disorder than with vulvar intraepithelial neoplasia, necessitating wider margins when local excision or vulvectomy is performed.

Melanoma

Vulvar melanoma usually presents with a *raised, irritated, pruritic, pigmented lesion*. Melanoma accounts for only 5% of all vulvar malignancies, and when suspected, *wide local excision* is necessary for diagnosis and staging. For level I melanoma, wide local excision is usually adequate. An in-depth discussion of this entity is beyond the scope of this book; however, the clinician should be aware that irritated, pigmented, vulvar lesions mandate excisional biopsy for definitive diagnosis.

VULVAR CANCER

Vulvar carcinoma accounts for approximately 4% of all gynecologic malignancies, with 90% of these carcinomas being of the *squamous cell* variety. The typical clinical profile includes women in their *postmenopausal years*, most commonly between the ages of 65 and 70. *Vulvar pruritis* is the most common presenting complaint. In addition, patients may notice a red or white, ulcerative or exophytic lesion arising most commonly on the posterior two thirds of either labium majus. An exophytic ulcerative lesion need not be present, further underscoring the need for thorough biopsy in patients of the age group who complain of vulvar symptoms. There is *often a delay in treatment of these patients* because of reluctance of a patient in this age group to present to her physician and further reluctance on the physician's part to investigate the symptoms and findings thoroughly by utilizing vulvar biopsy.

Although a specific *etiology* for vulvar cancer is not known, it has been shown that there may be progression from prior intraepithelial lesions including those that are associated with certain types of human papilloma virus.

Natural History

Squamous cell carcinoma of the vulva generally *remains localized for long periods of time* and *then spreads in a predictable fashion to the regional lymph nodes*, including those of the inguinal and femoral chain. Lesions of greater than 2 cm in diameter and $\frac{1}{2}$ cm in depth have an increased chance of nodal metastases. Lesions arising in the anterior one third of the vulva may spread to the deep pelvic nodes, bypassing regional inguinal and femoral lymphatics.

Evaluation

After suspicious lesions are biopsied and the diagnosis of invasive squamous cell carcinoma of the vulva confirmed, other studies that may be obtained include *chest x-ray and intravenous pyelogram*. For patients with lesions near the urethra and/or patients with lesions involving the anus or perineal area, preoperative *cystoscopy and proctoscopy*, respectively, are indicated.

The *staging classification* was altered by the Federation of Gynecology and Obstetrics (FIGO) in 1988 (Table 41.3). The new staging convention uses the analysis of the removed vulvar tumor and microscopic assessment of the regional lymph nodes as its basis. The change from clinical staging to this surgical staging convention was necessitated by the observation that clinical assessment of this disease contained many errors, in particular, the assessment of inguinal and femoral adenopathy.

Table 41.3
FIGO Staging for Carcinoma of the Vulva[*]

Stage 0		
Tis	Carcinoma in situ; intraepithelial carcinoma	
Stage I		
T1 N0 M0	Tumor confined to the vulva and/or perineum—2 cm or less in greatest dimension, nodes are not palpable	
Stage II		
T2 N0 M0	Tumor confined to the vulva and/or perineum—more than 2 cm in greatest dimension, nodes are not palpable	
Stage III		
T3 N0 M0	Tumor of any size with. . .	
T3 N1 M0	1) Adjacent spread to the lower urethra and/or the vagina, or the anus, and/or. . .	
T1 N1 M0	2) Unilateral regional lymph node metastasis	
T2 N1 M0		
Stage IVA		
T1 N2 M0	Tumor invades any of the following:	
T2 N2 M0	Upper urethra, bladder mucosa, rectal mucosa, pelvic bone, and/or bilateral regional node metastasis	
T3 N2 M0		
T4 any N M0		

Stage IVB		
Any T	Any distant metastasis including	
Any N, M1	pelvic lymph nodes	

Rules for Clinical Staging

The rules for staging are similar to those for carcinoma of the cervix.

TNM Classification of Carcinoma of the Vulva (FIGO)

T	Primary tumor	
Tis	Preinvasive carcinoma (carcinoma in situ)	
T1	Tumor confined to the vulva and/or perineum—$\leq$2 cm in greatest dimension	
T2	Tumor confined to the vulva and/or perineum—>2 cm in greatest dimension	
T3	Tumor of any size with adjacent spread to the urethra and/or vagina and/or to the anus	
T4	Tumor of any size infiltrating the bladder mucosa and/or the rectal mucosa, including the upper part of the urethral mucosa and/or fixed to the bone	
N	Regional lymph nodes	
N0	No lymph node metastasis	
N1	Unilateral regional lymph node metastasis	
N2	Bilateral regional lymph node metastasis	
M	Distant metastasis	
M0	No clinical metastasis	
M1	Distant metastasis (including pelvic lymph node metastasis)	

[*]FIGO, International Federation of Gynecology and Obstetrics.

Treatment

The mainstay of treatment for invasive squamous cell vulvar carcinoma is radical *vulvectomy with concomitant bilateral inguinal and femoral node dissection*. Adjunctive treatment for advanced disease such as radiation therapy and chemotherapy are only of selective value.

Prognosis

The corrected 5-year survival rate for all vulvar carcinoma is approximately 80% and is especially favorable if the patient has negative inguinal and femoral lymph nodes at the time of her first surgery. If metastatic disease is found in the regional nodes, survival falls off dramatically to as low as 20% if the deep pelvic nodes are involved.

FURTHER READINGS

Clarke-Pearson DL, Dawood MY, eds. Green's gynecology: essentials of clinical practice. 8th ed. Boston: Little, Brown & Co., 1990:503–506, 553–559.

Kaufman R, Friedrich E, Gardner H. Benign diseases of the vulva and vagina. 3rd ed. St. Louis, MO: Mosby-Year Book, 1989.

SELF-EVALUATION

Case 41-A

A 72-year-old woman comes in with a complaint of vulvar itching for the past 8 months. This has become progressively worse over the last 2 months to the point where it awakens her *two or three times* at night as she finds herself scratching unconsciously. Her past gyneco-logic history is unremarkable. She underwent normal menopause in her early fifties and is on no chronic medication. Her general health is excellent.

Examination reveals external genitalia that are somewhat atrophic as appropriate for her age. Circumferentially around the inner aspect of the labia majora, the lateral aspect of the labia minora, and the skin over the clitoral hood there is a diffuse whitish epithelial change. This coalesces in the perineal body and extends to within a centimeter of the anal verge. Scattered throughout this area are patches of what appear to be hyperkeratotic skin in the perineal body and some isolated excoriation presumably secondary to her scratching. The remainder of the Gyn exami-nation is normal.

Question 41-A-1

What is the next step in the management of this patient?

A. Administer topical testosterone propion-ate.
B. Administer topical corticosteroid cream.
C. Administer topical antifungal prepara-tions.
D. Administer Benadryl at bedtime.
E. Perform directed vulvar biopsy(ies).

Answer 41-A-1

Answer: E

This case illustrates a postmenopausal patient with inflammation of the vulva secondary to one of the so-called "vulvar dystrophies." Since it is unclear as to the histologic variation and since intraepithelial neoplasia cannot be ruled out by gross examination, it is manda-tory to perform a vulvar biopsy in this patient. If the entire lesion is homogenous and a single biopsy would be representative, this is proba-bly adequate. If on the other hand, as with this patient, there are areas of heterogeneity (hy-perkeratosis and/or ulceration or excoria-

tion), two or three biopsies may be warranted in order to make the diagnosis. Application of the appropriate medication and/or surgical treatment can then be offered after histologic verification of the problem.

Case 41-B

A 67-year-old-patient presents to the office having noticed a "sore" on her vulva. She has been aware of this for approximately 8 months but has not come in hoping it would go away. Currently, it is bleeding slightly and is irritated by her underclothing.

Vulvar examination reveals a 1 × 1 cm slightly raised but "cratered lesion" in the pos-terior left labium majus. There are no other apparent abnormalties. Examination of her groin reveals two "marble sized" lymph nodes in her left inguinal ligament area.

Question 41-B-1

The most likely diagnosis is:

A. epidermoid carcinoma of the vulva
B. chancroid
C. amelanotic melanoma
D. granuloma inguinale
E. lymphogranuloma venereum

Answer 41-B-1

Answer: A

Given the patient's age and physical findings, she most probably has squamous cell carci-noma of the vulva. This is suggested by an ex-ophytic but "cratered" lesion in the posterior two thirds of the vulva with a highly suspicious groin examination. It is mandatory in this pa-tient to obtain one or two vulvar biopsies at the margin of the "puckered" epithelium in or-der to confirm the diagnosis.

For further considerations: Vulvar biopsy shows squamous cell carcinoma. What further consideration is indicated? What treatment options are available? Do the inguinal nodes suggest anything about her prognosis?

chapter 42

CERVICAL NEOPLASIA AND CARCINOMA

Cervical carcinoma serves as the model of a "controllable" cancer, controllable in the sense that there is: (*a*) an identifiable precursor lesion (cervical intraepithelial neoplasia (CIN)) with a natural history of usually slow progression to frank cervical cancer, (*b*) a cheap and noninvasive screening test (the Pap smear) and a follow-up diagnostic procedure (colposcopy) for diagnosis, and (*c*) simple and effective treatments of the precursor lesion (cyrotherapy, laser ablation, cone biopsy) with high cure rates. Because it is usually possible to identify and treat the asymptomatic precursor lesion, cervical cancer is now the second rather than most common malignancy in women. Further, with improved treatment of cervical cancer when disease progression has gone beyond the precursor lesion, cure rates of up to 90% are seen in early stage disease (stage 1A and 1B), and increased life expectancy is seen in advanced stage disease. The salubrious effect of these interventions is graphically seen in the fall in the mortality rate for cervical cancer as compared to ovarian carcinoma, where no treatable precursor lesion can be easily identified (Fig. 42.1).

Of the means by which the "control" of CIN/cervical cancer has occurred, the annual Pap smear is most important. The recogni-

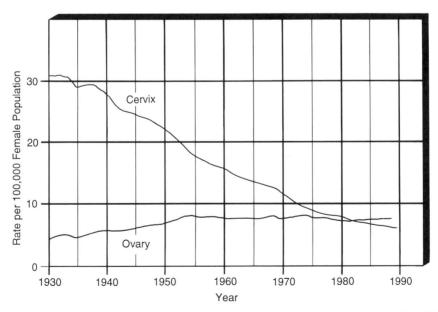

Figure 42.1. Age-adjusted death rate for cervical cancer in the United States, 1930–1987.

tion of the 1–10% of abnormal Pap smears and their appropriate evaluation and treatment before progression to cancer is one of the great success stories of modern medicine. In the years to come, it is hoped that similar progress will be made in further identification of the causes of CIN/cervical cancer and development of a preventive treatment.

In this chapter we review the natural history, evaluation, and treatment of CIN and cervical cancer, with special attention to the precursor lesion CIN and its early recognition, a responsibility of all physicians who see women for primary care.

CERVICAL INTRAEPITHELIAL NEOPLASIA

Pathology of Cervical Intraepithelial Neoplasia: The Squamocolumnar Junction

An understanding of the pathophysiology of CIN and its association with the *squamocolumnar junction* (transformation zone) of the cervix is necessary in order to understand the rationale behind cervical Pap smear screening, diagnostic colposcopy, and the treatment of CIN. The development of the transformation zone is a process that occurs through the development of squamous epithelium distal to the squamocolumnar junction. Proximal to the squamocolumnar junction (SCJ) is glandular epithelium of the endocervix, whereas distal to the SCJ is squamous epithelium of the portio. The border between these is the *transformation zone* (Fig. 42.2). With sexual maturation and eventual hormone influence produced from the maturing ovary, the transformation zone usually lies just outside the external cervical os and can be visualized by the naked eye. This slightly reddened or orange-red tissue proximal to the transformation zone surrounding the os is then glandular tissue of the exposed endocervical canal. Through repeated trauma and exposure to chronic irritants, there are usually some areas of squamous metaplasia at the transformation zone in most patients.

In certain patients, *carcinogen exposure* may cause an abnormal maturation process at the transformation zone and begin the process of intraepithelial neoplasia. *Ninty-five percent of squamous intraepithelial neoplasia occurs within the transformation zone.* Although the carcinogenicity of most suspected carcinogens remains unproven, certain agents are known to be associated with the development of dysplasia (abnormal growth, in this case CIN). These include *cigarette smoke* (secreted through the endocervical glandular mucus), undefined factors transmitted through intercourse at a young age when the transformation zone is immature, and the human papilloma virus (HPV). Although it is unclear if HPV is a direct cervical carcinogen, it is clear that *HPV of certain types (6, 11, 16, and 18) is closely associated with the development of dysplasia.* It is speculated that HPV may serve as a cofactor in the abnormal maturation and mitotic process of the epithelial cells. A distinct rise in the incidence of intraepithelial neoplasia in association with cytologic confirmation of HPV is well known.

Screening for Cervical Intraepithelial Neoplasia: The Pap Smear

During the early 1940s, George Papanicolaou developed a method to examine single cell morphology based on an exfoliative cell specimen scraped from the cervix at the time of routine pelvic examination. The accuracy of this cytologic assessment by *Pap smear* is dependent on a number of factors including: the degree of cervical inflammation and concomitant infection which may obscure early dysplastic changes, adequacy of the specimen obtained, and expeditious fixation of the specimen on the glass slide so as to avoid air-drying cytologic artifacts. Currently, the most accurate samples are obtained by using both the cervical spatula and the endocervical brush.

At the present time, the American College of Obstetricians and Gynecologists recommends obtaining the *first Pap smear at the time a woman becomes sexually active or by the*

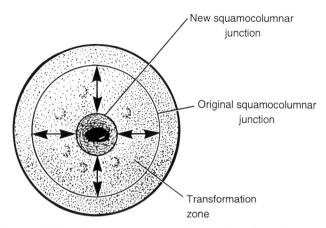

New squamocolumnar
junction

Original squamocolumnar
junction

Transformation
zone

Figure 42.2. Squamocolumnar junction and transformation zone.

age of 18, and yearly thereafter. Reasons cited for these recommendations include: the ease with which the Pap smear is obtained, the improvement in the morbidity and mortality from CIN and cervical cancer associated with Pap smear screening, and the health promotion benefits of the examination. However, the indications and frequency for obtaining a PAP smear have been questioned by other professional groups. They suggest that low risk patients (defined as women who have had three consecutive normal Pap smears, who have become sexually active after the age of 25, and who have only one sexual partner) may have intervals of Pap smear screening of up to 3 years. Those who advocate this delayed interval as more appropriately cost-effective cite the observation that cervical intraepithelial neoplasia is generally a slowly progressing process in its transformation to more severe degrees of CIN and to frank cervical cancer. However, in most office settings the performance of the Pap smear at the time of an annual examination remains the accepted standard of care.

Pap smear classification is confusing because of the use of different classification systems. The most common systems are: the *class system* (class I to V); the cervical intraepithelial neoplasia or *CIN system*, which provides a description of the degree of abnormality (CIN-I to CIN-III); and a more recently advocated convention describing squamous in-

traepithelial lesions, the *SIL system*. This most recent convention is also called the Bethesda system and purports to provide a more descriptive diagnosis of cellular architecture. Within this system, lesions are described as "low grade SIL and high grade SIL." In addition, when cellular architecture suggests the involvement of human papilloma virus (HPV), this description is added to either the low grade or high grade SIL description. Currently, the class and CIN systems are most widely used, although many advocate conversion to the Bethesda system. Table 42.1 compares and contrasts the three systems.

The basis for these classification systems is the likelihood of the progression of precursor lesions to more advanced degrees of cervical intraepithelial neoplasia and eventully to carcinoma. Generally, more severe intraepithelial lesions progress more quickly, whereas less severe intraepithelial lesions may take as long as 7–8 years to progress to carcinoma. The term *dysplasia* is used to describe these intraepithelial cellular abnormalities, including an altered nuclear-cytoplasmic ratio, an increased staining of chromatin material, and other cellular characteristics that suggest a less orderly maturation process. For example, considering all cases of mild dysplasia (CIN-I, class II–III, or low grade SIL), approximately 65% of these lesions will spontaneously regress, whereas approximately 20% will re-

Table 42.1
Comparisons of PAP Smear Descriptive Conventions

Descriptive Convention	Class System	CIN System	Bethesda System	Histology
	Class I (Normal)	Normal	Within Normal Limits	
	Class II Inflammation	Inflammatory	Inflammatory a) Without atypia b) With atypia	
	Class III Mild Dysplasia or Moderate Dysplasia	CIN I or CIN II	Low Grade SIL	
	Class IV Severe Dysplasia CIS	CIN III	High Grade SIL	
	Class V Suggestive of Cancer	Suggestive of Cancer	Squamous Cell Cancer	

Labels: Invasive Cervical Cancer; WBCs; Basal Cells; Basement Membrane

CIN = cervical intraepithelial neoplasia.
SIL = squamous intraepithelial lesion.

main the same, leaving 15% to progress to worsening disease. Because there is no way to predict which of these lesions is destined to progress and which is not, *further investigation is warranted for even mildly abnormal Pap smears*. Further investigation is also indicated to identify women with disease that is more severe than indicated by their screening Pap smear. *Specifically, this investigation involves histologic diagnosis of the nature and grade of dysplasia/carcinoma which is suggested by the screening cytologic evaluation obtained at Pap smear*. This is accomplished by means of colposcopy and directed biopsy or cone biopsy of the cervix.

Histologic Evaluation of the Abnormal Pap Smear

A colposcope is a sophisticated binocular stereomicroscope with variable magnification (usually $\times$ 1 to 14) and a variable intensity light source with green filters, which aid in the identification of blood vessels. With *colposcopy*, small, often subtle areas of dysplastic change on the cervix can be evaluated and appropriate sites for biopsy chosen. Colposcopic criteria such as white epithelium, abnormal vascular patterns, and punctate lesions help identify such areas. To facilitate the examination, the cervix is washed with dilute 3–4% acetic acid solution, which also acts as an epithelial desiccant, enhancing visualization of dysplastic lesions, which usually appear with relatively discrete borders at or near the squamocolumnar junction. *Visualization of the entire squamocolumnar junction is required for a satisfactory colposcopic examination* since approximately 95% of the CIN/cervical cancer will arise in the transformation zone. If the squamocolumnar junction is not visualized in its entirety, or if the margins of abnormal areas are not seen in their entirety, the colposcopic assessment is unsatisfactory and other evaluation is needed. This is the *first reason for cervical conization: unsatisfactory colposcopy*. Conization is described in the section on surgical excision.

The number of colposcopically directed biopsies obtained will vary, depending on the number of abnormal areas found and the severity of the involvement based on colposcopically defined criteria. After sampling the colposcopically identified lesions, an *endocervical curettage (ECC)* using a small curette is performed. This simple sampling procedure may be performed without cervical dilation, as in a dilation and curettage. This endocervical sample is obtained so that potential disease further inside the cervical canal, which is not visualized by the colposcope, may be detected. The cervical biopsies and endocervical curettage are then submitted separately for pathologic assessment. Endocervical curettage will be positive for dysplasia in 5–10% of women with a dysplastic Pap smear. Because of the absence of tissue orientation from endocervical curettings, the degree of dysplasia from endocervical curettings is difficult to assess. This is *the second reason for cervical conization: positive endocervical curettage*.

In approximately 10% of colposcopies with directed biopsies and endocervical curettage, there will be a discrepancy between the screening Pap smear and the histologic data from biopsy and ECC, e.g., if the Pap smear is read as severely dysplastic (CIN-III or high grade SIL) and the direct biopsies only show mild dysplasia (CIN-I or low grade SIL). Directed biopsy of the cervix should vary no more than one grade with the reference Pap smear. When a "two-step" discrepancy occurs, further tissue diagnosis by cervical conization is necessary so that the most severe abnormality can be explained histologically. By obtaining the cone-shaped biopsy of the entire squamocolumnar junction and identified lesions as well as a portion of the endocervical canal, the pathologist can determine the most severe lesions by histologic, hence diagnostic, criteria. Often, the cone biopsy may prove to be therapeutic as well as diagnostic since the entire lesion is removed. This is *the third indication for cervical conization: a "two-step" discrepancy between Pap smear and biopsy results*.

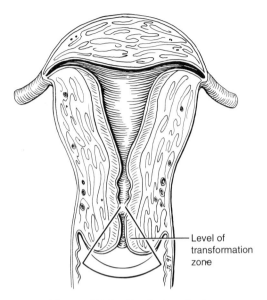

Level of transformation zone

Figure 42.3. Cervical conization.

Cervical conization, or cone biopsy of the cervix, is a minor surgical procedure performed under general or regional anesthesia. Usually performed with scalpel and scissors (cold knife conization), conization is now also performed with a laser or with a heated wire loop, the LEETZ loop (which stands for loop electrocervical excision of the transformation zone). As seen in Figure 42.3, a cone-shaped specimen is removed from the cervix, which encompasses the SCJ, all identified lesions on the exocervix, and a portion of the endocervical canal, whose extent depends on whether the ECC was positive or negative. This more extensive specimen allows the pathologist to fully ascertain the extent and severity of disease so that appropriate therapy may be selected. If the margins of disease cannot be established, the patient will then require either further conization therapy or close follow-up, depending on the severity of the lesions encountered and the wishes of the patient for further childbearing. The risks of the procedure include infection, blood loss, and anesthesia. For women who desire further childbearing there are the additional risks of cervical incompetence if the internal cer-

vical os is compromised and reduced cervical capacity to facilitate sperm transport due to loss of mucus-secreting glands.

Prior to the advent of colposcopic evaluation of abnormal Pap smears, most patients with abnormal screening Pap smears were destined to undergo cervical conization, necessitating an anesthetic and brief hospitalization. Colposcopy in the clinic setting has eliminated the need for conization in the majority of patients.

Treatment of Cervical Intraepithelial Neoplasia

The underlying concept in the treatment of CIN is that excision or ablation of the superficial precursor lesion will avoid progression to carcinoma. Because these lesions are superficial and usually confined to the visible and easily accessible SCJ, simple office techniques that require minimal or no anesthesia and that have little risk usually suffice. Controversy exists about the appropriateness of specific therapies for lesions of different severity and extent; ongoing research is designed to determine optimal therapies for each situation.

Cryocautery is a popular outpatient method used to treat low grade CIN. The procedure involves covering the SCJ and all identified lesions with a "mushroom-tipped" stainless steel probe, which is then supercooled with circulating liquid nitrogen or carbon dioxide. The size and shape of the probe depends on the size and shape of the cervix. The most commonly employed freezing technique involves a 3-minute freeze followed by a 5-minute thaw period with a repeat 3-minute freeze (Fig. 42.4). The thaw period between the two freezing episodes allows the damaged tissue from the first freeze to become edematous and swell with intracellular fluid. With the second freeze, the edematous cellular architecture is refrozen and extends the damaged area slightly deeper into the tissue. Healing after cryotherapy may take up to 4 or 5 weeks since the damaged tissue slowly sloughs and is replaced

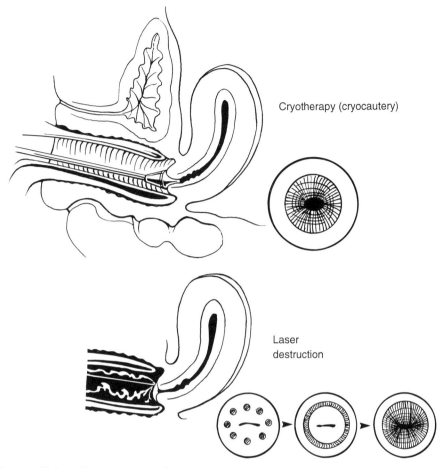

Cryotherapy (cryocautery)

Laser destruction

Figure 42.4. Ablation of cervical intraepithelial neoplasia: Cyrotherapy and laser ablation.

by new cervical epithelium. This process is associated with profuse watery discharge often mixed with necrotic cellular debris. It can be assumed that the entire healing process has been completed within 2 months and usually the next follow-up Pap smear is done 12 weeks following the freezing to ascertain the effectiveness of the procedure. The cure rates for this technique for low grade cervical intraepithelial neoplasia approach 90%.

More recently, colposcopically directed *laser therapy* has been employed to ablate lesions involving cervical intraepithelial neoplasia. Because of the precision imparted by the colposcopic direction of the fine laser beam as well as the precise control of depth of ablation available by varying the laser

beam's power and width, many physicians prefer laser ablation to "less precise" techniques. Each lesion may be addressed specifically and ablated. In addition, ablation of the entire SCJ is often performed (Fig. 42.4). Although the technology is more sophisticated than cryocautery, long-term cure rates with this technique are similar to that for cryocautery. An advantage of laser theapy is that it can be used for high grade intraepithelial lesions because the depth of ablation can be adjusted to accommodate the extent of the lesion.

On occasion, low grade epithelial lesions involving only focal areas of the squamocolumnar junction are treated by *excisional biopsy* performed at the time of colposcopy. There are no data comparing the outcomes of this therapy to limited lesion ablation by either laser or cryocautery.

The most commonly employed technique of surgical excision is *cervical conization*. Cervical conization can be done for diagnosis, as discussed. If an entire lesion is removed (i.e., the lesion margins are clear), the procedure may also be therapeutic. This may be especially valuable for women who wish future pregnancy. An alternative to conization is excision of the cone by hot wire loop, the LEETZ loop, a procedure done in the clinic setting. Long-term follow-up data of this treatment modality are as yet unavailable, although preliminary findings are promising.

Follow-Up of Treatment of Cervical Intraepithelial Neoplasia

Patients who have been treated for cervical intraepithelial neoplasia need to be followed more frequently than patients presenting for annual health examinations. The patient is usually advised to return for a follow-up examination and Pap smear in approximately 3 months. At this time, the healing process has been completed, and the generation of new cells from the squamocolumnar junction should be free of inflammation and reparative changes that were caused by the treatment. If a follow-up Pap smear is done too soon after ablative or excisional treatment, it may be misinterpreted because of the abnormal-appearing cellular architecture secondary to the healing process. The patient usually receives repeat Pap smear assessment at 3-month intervals to complete 1 year. Assuming the Pap smears remain normal, they may be done at 6-month intervals for the second year, and if these two are normal, patients may resume having annual Pap smear assessments beginning the third year. However, these patients should be counseled that they are at greater risk in the future for recurrent abnormalities of the Pap smear and should be encouraged to avail themselves of annual health care checkups to include the Pap smear.

CERVICAL CARCINOMA

Until approximately 10 years ago, cervical cancer was the most common gynecologic malignancy, with a ratio of 2:1 over endometrial carcinoma. Now the cervical carcinoma to endometrial carcinoma ratio has almost reversed; endometrial carcinoma rates are twice that for invasive cervical carcinoma. Approximately 16,000 new cases of invasive cervical carcinoma are diagnosed annually.

The average age at diagnosis for invasive cervical cancer is approximately 50, although the disease may occur in the very young as well as the very old patient. In studies following patients with advanced cervical intraepithelial neoplasia, this precursor is seen to precede the occurrence of invasive carcinoma on the average of 10 years. In some patients, however, this transformation time may be considerably less; for still other patients, cervical cancer may not be preceded by CIN.

The *etiology* of cervical cancer is unknown. There is ample evidence that advanced *cervical intraepithelial neoplasia* arising in the squamous epithelium of the cervical transformation zone will often progress to invasive squamous cell cervical carcinoma. Similar to such cervical intraepithelial neoplasia, the *human papilloma virus* has been implicated as an etiologic cofactor in the development of cervical carcinoma. Studies involving genetic probes have identified papilloma virus DNA fragments within areas of invasive cervical carcinoma. Other etiologic associations are also similar to those for CIN, including *factors related to the male ejaculation, the immature transformation zone, the number of different sexual partners, and cigarette smoking. Immunocompromised patients* are a special group who seem more susceptible to this disease.

About 90% of cervical cancer is of the squamous cell variety. Somewhat less than 10% of cervical cancers are adenocarcinomas arising from the endocervical glands. Three rare types of cervical cancer are also encountered: clear cell carcinoma associated with diethylstilbestrol exposure in utero, sarcoma, and lymphoma. In general, the evaluation

Table 42.2
Clinical Stages of Carcinoma of the Cervix Uteri (FIGO, Revised 1985)

Stage	Characteristics
I	Carcinoma is strictly confined to cervix (extension to corpus should be disregarded)
IA	Preclinical carcinoma
IA1	Minimal microscopically evident stromal invasion
IA2	Microscopic lesions no more than 5 mm depth measured from base of epithelium surface or glandular from which it originates, and horizontal spread not to exceed 7 mm
IB	All other cases of stage I: occult cancer should be marked "occ"
II	Carcinoma extends beyond cervix but has not extended to pelvic wall; it involves vagina, but not as far as lower third
IIA	No obvious parametrial involvement
IIB	Obvious parametrial involvement
III	Carcinoma has extended to pelvic wall; on rectal examination there is no cancer-free space between tumor and pelvic wall; tumor involves lower third of vagina; all cases with hydronephrosis or nonfunctioning kidney should be included, unless they are known to be due to another cause
IIIA	No extension to pelvic wall, but involvement of lower third of vagina
IIIB	Extension to pelvic wall, or hydronephrosis or nonfunctioning kidney due to tumor
IV	Carcinoma has extended beyond true pelvis or has clinically involved mucosa of bladder or rectum
IVA	Spread of growth to adjacent pelvic organs
IVB	Spread to distant organs

and treatment of squamous cell and adeno-carcinoma of the cervix are similar. The discussions that follow reflect this similarity and apply to these two most common cervical carcinomas.

Survival rates for cervical carcinoma reflect the extent of disease at the time of diagnosis. Stage I has over 91% 5-year survival, whereas stages II A, IIIA, and IV are 83, 45, and 14%, respectively.

Clinical Evaluation of Cervical Cancer

There is *no classic historical presentation* for cervical cancer. Two symptoms are classically described as associated with cervical carcinoma, although both have other more common causes: *postcoital bleeding and abnormal uterine bleeding. Other symptoms* are determined by the organs or organ systems encountered as the cancer spreads, and hence by the pattern of spread: direct invasion to contiguous structures and by lymphatics to distant sites of metastasis.

Visible lesions on the cervix should be biopsied. Lesions that should be considered for immediate biopsy include all new exophytic, friable, or bleeding lesions. These are readily differentiated from more common, normal variations of cervical anatomy such as nabothian cysts or condylomata. Pap smears are sometimes negative in this situation because exfoliative cells from frank cancer may be so distorted as to be uninterpretable. When a visible lesion is present, colposcopic assessment need not be done unless the results of the direct biopsy do not confirm cancer.

The *clinical staging of cervical carcinoma is the process by which the severity and extent of disease is assessed so that appropriate therapy may be undertaken.* Staging is based on the International Federation of Gynecology and Obstetrics (FIGO) Staging Classification (1985) presented in Table 42.2. This is a convention based both on the histologic assessment of sample tumor for cell type and estimated virulence and on physical examination and laboratory study to ascertain the physical extent of disease. It has been adopted because of the very predictable manner in which *cervical carcinoma spreads by direct invasion and by lymphatic metastasis*. Cervical carcinoma spreads through the cervical and paracervical lymphatics, through the parametria, and into the regional lymph nodes. Cervical carcinoma also spreads by direct extension proximal into the endocervical canal or distally into the vagina. In patients with primary lymphatic spread, the ascent of disease from the regional lymph glands proceeds to the deep pelvic nodes including the external and internal iliac node chain, the common iliac node chain, and periaortic node chain (Fig. 42.5). Accordingly, advanced stages include a description of tumor beyond the cervix, into the vagina or parametria (stage II); directly to the lateral pelvic wall, or the lower third of the vagina (stage III); or widespread disease, including but not limited to the bladder or rectum (stage IV). Adjunctive studies that may be useful include evaluation of the urinary tract by intravenous pyelography and cystoscopy or bowel tract by proctosigmoidoscopy or barium enema, blood chemistries with emphasis on liver and renal function, and computed tomography studies on a selective basis. Computed tomography has been of special value in evaluating the extent of lymphatic involvement, given the difficulty in performing and interpreting bipedal lymphangiography, the other procedure used in some institutions for this evaluation. Other studies are done on a selective basis using randomized treatment protocols in an effort to determine the most efficacious treatment.

Management of Cervical Carcinoma

Once there has been histologic confirmation of invasive cervical carcinoma, it is imperative to refer the patient to a gynecologic oncologist for appropriate surgical and/or radiation therapy.

The *mainstays of treatment* for invasive cervical carcinoma include *radical surgical therapy and/or pelvic irradiation*. In general, surgical therapy is indicated for most patients with stage I disease and selected patients with stage II disease because of the limited yet predictable extent of spread in these early stages. *Radical surgical therapy* includes radical hysterectomy aimed at removing all of the central disease, that is, disease not only in the cervix itself but in all the adjacent paracervical, parametrial, and vaginal tissue. In addition, surgical eradication of the local and regional lymph nodes is an important part of radical surgical therapy (pelvic lymphadenectomy). The presence or absence of tumor in the lymph nodes sampled defines, in part, the extent of disease and the need for further therapy, either radiation therapy or perhaps chemotherapy. It should be emphasized that simple hysterectomy with removal of the cervix is inadequate treatment for invasive cervical carcinoma. In young women who are treated surgically, ovarian preservation is usually advisable to provide the patient with the long-term benefits from endogenous estrogen secretion. Ovarian retention presents no additional risk to the patient since cervical carcinoma neither spreads through the adnexal structures nor is estrogen-dependent.

Radiation therapy is reserved for patients with stage 1B or 2A disease who are poor surgical candidates and for all patients with more advanced disease. The basis for radiation therapy in more advanced disease is the likelihood for more extensive regional nodal involvement. Even with stage III disease extending to the lateral pelvic wall, approximately one third of patients will be cured with primary radiation therapy. Both high dose external beam therapy and intracavitary irradiation are used for most patients. Fortunately, the adjacent nongynecologic structures, such as the bladder and distal colon, tolerate these treatments fairly well without significant untoward effects. Currently, these combined radiation methods are calculated specifically by individual patient needs to maximize therapeutic radiation to the tumor sites and potential spread areas, while minimizing the amount of radiation to adjacent uninvolved tissues. *Complications of radiation therapy* include radiation cys-

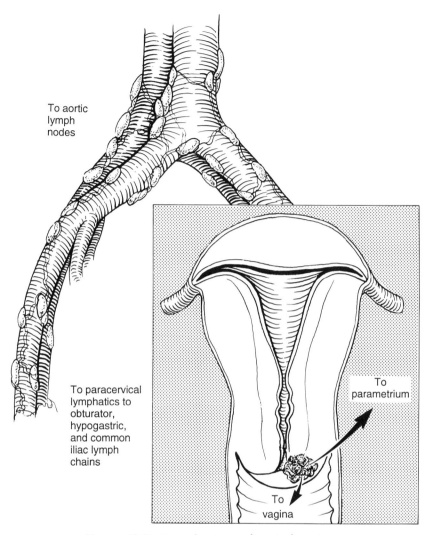

To aortic
lymph
nodes

To paracervical
lymphatics to
obturator,
hypogastric,
and common
iliac lymph
chains

To
parametrium

To
vagina

Figure 42.5. Spread patterns of cervical carcinoma.

titis and radiation proctitis, which are usually relatively easy to manage when appropriate radiation doses have been calculated. Other more unusual complications include intestinal fistula, small bowel obstruction, or difficult to manage hemorrhagic proctitis or cystitis. It should be remembered that the tissue damage and fibrosis incurred by radiation therapy progresses over many years and that these effects may complicate long-term management.

Most authorities believe that radical surgical excision and pelvic lymphadenectomy offer distinct advantages over radiation therapy for earlier stage disease. These include the potential for preservation of ovarian function in young women, preservation of sexual function, and avoidance of long-term radiation effects. On the other hand, certain operative complications such as hemorrhage, damage to local nerves supplying the bladder, and urinary vaginal fistula may develop from radical pelvic surgery. It is important for the risks and benefits of each form of therapy to be explained to the patient and treatment performed based on individual patient selection.

Table 42.3
5-Year Survival for Treated Cervical Carcinoma

FIGO stage[a]	5-year survival
	%
O	100
I-A	99
I-B	85–90
II-A	73–80
II-B	68
III-A	45
III-B	36
IV-A	15
IV-BH	2

[a]FIGO, International Federation of Gynecology and Obstetrics.

Follow-up of patients with cervical carcinoma is best done by gynecologic oncologists who will use specific long-term protocols. Most oncology centers will follow patients in a specialized clinic for at least 5 years. When there is recurrence, 90% will reoccur within this time period. The 5-year survival for various stages of cervical carcinoma are shown in Table 42.3.

Treatment for recurrent disease is associated with poor cure rates. Most chemotherapeutic protocols have only limited usefulness and are reserved for palliative efforts. Likewise, specific "spot" radiation to areas of recurrence also provides only limited benefit. Occasional patients with central recurrence— that is, recurrence of disease in the upper vagina or the residual cervix and uterus in radiation patients—may benefit from ultraradical surgery with partial or total pelvic exenteration. These candidates are few, but when properly selected, may benefit from this aggressive therapy.

FURTHER READINGS

Clarke-Pearson DL, Dawood MY. Green's gynecology: essentials of clinical practice. 8th ed. Boston: Little, Brown & Co., 1990.
_____. Chapter 25. Intraepithelial diseases of the lower genital tract. 493–508.
_____. Chapter 26. Cervical cancer. 509–520.
Herbst A, Mishell D, Stenchever M, Droegemueller W. Comprehensive gynecology. 2nd ed. St. Louis, MO: CV Mosby, 1992.
_____. Chapter 26. Herbst A. Intraepithelial neoplasia of the cervix. 821–860.
_____. Chapter 27. Herbst A. Malignant disease of the cervix. 861–894.

SELF-EVALUATION

Case 42-A

A 24-year-old college student, G1P0010, presents for her annual pelvic examination and Pap smear and renewal of her oral contraceptive. History and physical examination are unremarkable. Her Pap smear is subsequently reported as CIN-III.

Question 42-A-1

The most appropriate next step in this patient's management is:

A. repeat Pap smear in 1 year
B. repeat Pap smear now
C. colposcopy with ECC and directed biopsy
D. excisional biopsy
E. cervical conization

Answer 42-A-1

Answer: C

CIN-III atypia on screening examination requires histologic diagnosis so that appropriate treatment can be selected. Repeat Pap smear is another screening test and is thus inappropriate. Conization for diagnostic purposes is needed only if colposcopy and biopsy prove inadequate.

Question 42-A-2

The colposcopy was satisfactory. The ECC was negative. Two biopsies were taken. Both are reported as normal.

The most appropriate next step in this patient's management is:

A. repeat Pap smear in 1 year
B. repeat Pap smear now
C. colposcopy with ECC and directed biopsy
D. exisional biopsy
E. cervical conization

Answer 42-A-2

Answer: E

There is a "two-step" discrepancy between the screening Pap smear (CIN-III) and diagnostic biopsy results ("normal"), i.e., the source of the original abnormal Pap smear has yet to be found. This must be resolved before appropriate therapy can be suggested. Conization is appropriate, and may, in addition, be curative.

Case 42-B

A 46-year-old mother of four presents with a complaint of postcoital spotting. Her last Pap smear was 2 years ago and was normal. On physical examination, a 1 × 2 cm friable mass is found on the anterior lip of her cervix. The remainder of her physical examination is normal.

Question 42-B-1

The most appropriate next step in this patient's management is:

A. no further management indicated
B. Pap smear now
C. colposcopy with ECC and directed biopsy
D. exisional biopsy

E. cervical conization

Answer 42-B-1

Answer: B

Both a Pap smear and immediate biopsy are indicated. If cervical carcinoma is discovered, staging and appropriate therapy may be begun immediately. The Pap smear may be unreliable in frank carcinoma and should not be relied upon solely in the presence of a grossly visible lesion.

Question 42-B-2

For further consideration: Invasive squamous cell carcinoma of the cervix is discovered and appears to be confined to the cervix after full evaluation. What are the patient's treatment options? What are the risks and benefits of each? She is, understandably, very frightened and worried that she will not live to see her children (ages 13 and 15) graduate from college. What can, or should, you tell her? How reassuring should you be?

chapter 43

UTERINE LEIOMYOMA AND NEOPLASIA

Uterine enlargement due to leiomyoma (fibroids, myomas) is *common* in clinical practice. It is estimated that up to *30% of American women have these benign tumors*, although the majority do not present with significant symptoms and do not require hysterectomy. Histologically, these benign tumors represent localized proliferation of smooth muscle cells. When these tumors are symptomatic, the most *frequent clinical manifestations* include:

1. *Pain*, including secondary dysmenorrhea;
2. *Bleeding*, most common menorrhagia (increased amount and duration of flow);
3. *Pressure symptoms*, related to the size and number of these tumors filling the pelvic cavity.

Leiomyoma also represents an important clinical entity since, as *pelvic masses*, there may be a necessity to investigate them as if they were a malignancy. They are considered *hormonally responsive tumors* in that the growth potential of these tumors is related to *estrogen* production, often with rapid growth in the late reproductive or perimenopausal years. Menopause generally brings about cessation of tumor growth and even atrophy.

In less than 1% of cases, *malignancy* may arise in these tumors, usually *leiomyosarcoma*. Malignancy is more typical in older patients, especially postmenopausal patients who present with rapidly enlarging uterine masses and postmenopausal bleeding, unusual vaginal discharge, and pelvic pain. An enlarging uterine mass in a postmenopausal patient should be evaluated with considerably more concern for malignancy than in a younger woman. Other cell types may be involved in this form of malignancy. These *heterologous mixed tumors* contain other sarcomatous tissue elements not necessarily found only in the uterus.

LEIOMYOMAS

Symptoms

The clinical symptoms associated with uterine fibroids are a frequent reason for women to seek medical advice. Although smooth muscle tumors may occur anywhere in the body in women, they most commonly occur within the uterus or as an appendage to the uterus (Fig. 43.1). Gross and histologic changes may occur in uterine fibroids and historically these changes have been termed forms of "degeneration." The most common types of change include: *red degeneration*, hemorrhagic changes associated with rapid growth; *hyaline degeneration*, hyalinization of the smooth muscle elements, which occurs commonly after the menopause; *calcification*, calcific replacement of inactive smooth muscle elements, which occurs after menopause; and *sarcomatous change*, malignant degeneration, which is discussed later in this chapter.

Bleeding is the most common presenting symptom in uterine fibroids. Although the kind of abnormal bleeding may vary, the most common presentation includes the development of progressively heavier menstrual flow lasting longer than the normal duration (*menorrhagia*). This bleeding results from significant distortion of the endometrial cavity by the underlying tumor. This contributes to three generally accepted *mechanisms for increased bleeding*:

1. Alteration of normal myometrial contractile function in the small artery and arteriolar blood supply underlying the endometrium;

397

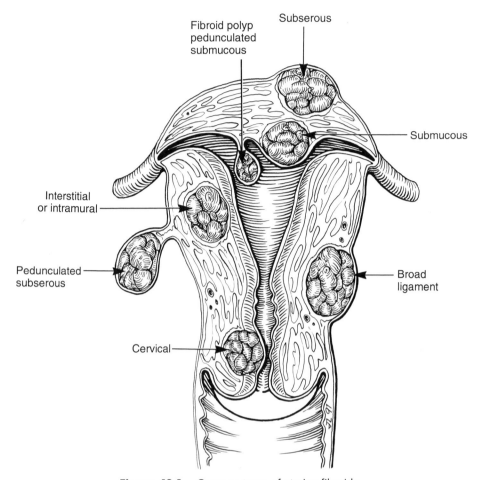

Figure 43.1. Common types of uterine fibroids.

2. Inability of the overlying endometrium to respond to the normal estrogen/progesterone menstrual phases, which contribute to efficient sloughing of the endometrium;
3. Pressure necrosis of the overlying endometrial bed, which exposes vascular surfaces that bleed in excess of that normally found with endometrial sloughing.

Characteristically, the best example of a type of leiomyoma contributing to this bleeding pattern is the so-called submucous leiomyoma. In this variant, the majority of the distortion created by the smooth muscle tumor projects toward the endometrial cavity rather than toward the serosal surface of the uterus. Enlarging intramural fibroids likewise may contribute to excessive bleeding if they become large enough to significantly distort the endometrial cavity.

Blood loss from this type of menstrual bleeding may occasionally be heavy enough to contribute to chronic iron deficiency anemia and, rarely, to profound acute blood loss. The occurrence of isolated submucous (subendometrial) leiomyomata is unusual. Commonly these are found in association with other types of leiomyomata, as seen in Figure 43.1.

Another common presenting complaint from uterine leiomyomata is that of *progressive increase in "pelvic pressure."* This may be a sense of progressive pelvic fullness and/or the sensation of a pelvic mass. Most commonly, this is caused by slowly enlarging intramural

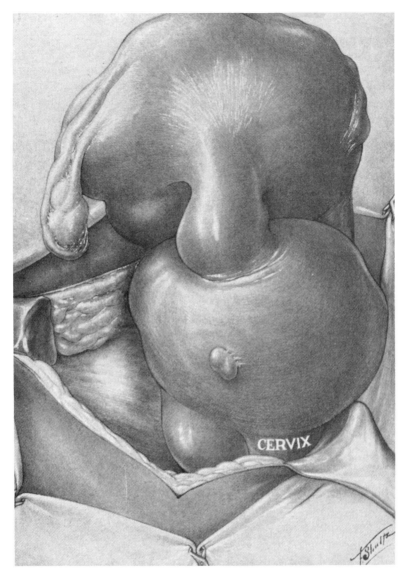

Figure 43.2. Large uterine fibroids at time of abdominal hysterectomy.

or subserous myomas, which on occasion, may attain a massive size (Fig. 43.2). This type of leiomyoma is the most easily palpated on bimanual or abdominal examination and contributes to a characteristic "lumpy-bumpy" or cobblestone sensation when multiple myomas are present. Occasionally, these large myomas present to the physician as a large asymptomatic pelvic mass.

Another spectrum of presentation includes patients who develop progressively worsen-ing *pelvic pain*. For many patients, this pain is manifest by the onset of secondary dysmenorrhea. Other pain symptoms may be due to rapid enlargement of a leiomyoma, resulting in areas of tissue necrosis or areas of sub-necrotic vascular ischemia, which contribute to alteration in myometrial response to prostaglandins similar to the mechanism described for primary dysmenorrhea. Occasionally, torsion of a peduculated myoma can occur, resulting in acute pain. Dull, intermittent low midline cramping pain is the clinical presentation when a submucous (subendometrial) myoma becomes pedunculated and progressively prolapses through the internal os of the cervix.

Diagnosis of Leiomyomata

The *diagnosis* of these tumors is usually made by clinical examination, including abdominal and bimanual palpation, or imaging studies. In addition, irregularities of the uterine cavity can be detected at the time of endometrial curettage. Often the diagnosis is made incidentally by pathologic assessment of a uterine specimen removed for other indications.

When appreciated clinically by *abdominopelvic examination*, uterine leiomyomata have characteristic qualities. These include the presence of a large midline mobile pelvic mass with an irregular contour; the mass usually has a characteristic "hard feel" or solid quality. This is often appreciated as separate from adnexal disease, although on occasion when a subserosal myoma becomes pedunculated it may be interpreted as a solid adnexal mass.

Of the available *imaging studies, pelvic ultrasound* is the most commonly used for confirmation of uterine myomas. The ultrasonographer can usually demonstrate areas of (acoustic shadow) hypoechogenicity amid otherwise normal myometrial patterns and can usually see a distorted endometrial stripe. Although solid leiomyomata share these characteristics, occasionally cystic components may also be seen as hypoechogenic areas and are consistent in appearance with myomas undergoing degeneration. Adnexal structures, including the ovaries, are usually identifiable separate from these masses. This is reassuring information, i.e., the pathology is uterine in nature and not adnexal, which has an associated higher risk of malignancy. Other studies that may be used include *computerized axial tomography* and *magnetic resonance imaging*. These studies are of relatively little cost-benefit value. They are expensive, time-consuming tests, which usually give no more information than found with clinical examination alone or clinical examination plus ultrasonography.

Endometrial cavity tissue sampling, through either outpatient office biopsy or outpatient dilation and curettage, may provide additional information necessary to make the diagnosis of leiomyomata uteri. Office sampling is unreliable to confirm this diagnosis since most of the sampling devices are not large enough to obtain the leiomyomatous elements and only "scratch the surface" of the endometrial cavity. However, an indirect appreciation for uterine enlargement may be gained by uterine sounding, which is part of this procedure.

Dilation and curettage may provide relevant information since larger tissue specimens including small submucous (subendometrial) myomas may be obtained. In addition, exploration by the sharp curette will often confirm the distortion of the uterine cavity suggestive of impingement by intramural myomas. For the patient with pedunculated intracavitary myomas, curettage may be not only diagnostic but also therapeutic, as removal of the pedunculated intracavity myomas results in relief from the patient's bleeding and pain symptoms.

Hysteroscopy may also be used to evaluate the enlarged uterus by directly visualizing the endometrial cavity. The increased size of the cavity can be documented and submucous fibroids can be visualized.

Treatment of Uterine Fibroids

The majority of patients with uterine myomas do not require surgical treatment. For example, if patients present with menstrual aberrations in the late reproductive or perimenopausal years, the endometrial cavity should be assessed by outpatient sampling to exclude significant endometrial hyperplasia or cancer. If the patient's bleeding is not heavy enough to cause significant alteration in hygiene or life-style and is not contributing to iron deficiency anemia, reassurance and observation may be all that are necessary. Assessment of further uterine growth, especially in the case of rapidly enlarging myomas, may be done by repeat pelvic examinations and assisted by serial pelvic ultrasound measurements. Rarely, uterine fibroids impinge upon the ureter, causing hydroureter and hydronephrosis. This is more likely the case when the fibroid grows laterally from the uterus between the leaves of the broad ligament. An attempt may be made to minimize uterine bleeding by using intermittent progestin supplementation, if patients are anovulatory, and/or prostaglandin synthetase inhibitors, which decrease the amount of secondary dysmenorrhea and in some cases the amount of menstrual flow. If there is significant endometrial cavitary distortion by large intramural or submucous myomas, hormonal supplementation will be of minimal benefit since the excessive bleeding is usually related to profound anatomic and vascular distortion. This conservative approach can potentially be utilized until the time of the menopause.

Surgical treatment by *myomectomy* is occasionally warranted in younger patients whose fertility is comprised by the presence of myomas, creating significant intracavitary distortion.

Although *hysterectomy* is commonly performed for uterine myomas, *indications* should be specific and well documented, including the presence of one or more of the following:

1. Excessively heavy *bleeding* that causes anemia or significant life-style and hygiene problems;
2. Intractable pelvic *pain* and progressive secondary dysmenorrhea;
3. Rapidly enlarging *size* and associated worsening of pelvic pressure;
4. Presence of *enlargement in the postmenopausal* years (Enlargement of uterine myoma despite the absence of significant endogenous estrogen production suggests an increased possibility for the presence of sarcoma.);
5. *Pressure symptoms* associated with the uterine myomas.

Because uterine leiomyomata are "estrogen-dependent" benign neoplasms, newer treatments to include *pharmacologic inhibition of estrogen secretion have been used as temporizing measures*. This is particularly applicable in the perimenopausal years when women are more likely anovulatory with relatively more endogenous estrogen production. Pharmacologic removal of the ovarian estrogen source can be achieved by suppression of the hypothalamic-pituitary—ovarian axis through the use of gonadotropin-releasing hormone agonists. This treatment is usually reserved as temporary treatment (3–6 months) of very large uterine myomas in preparation for treatment by hysterectomy, but can also be used as a temporizing medical therapy until the natural menopause occurs. GnRH agonists not only can result in a reduction in uterine size, but also technically easier surgery with markedly diminished blood loss. In patients with an adequate endogenous estrogen source this treatment will not permanently reduce the size of uterine myomas as withdrawal of the medication commonly results in growth of the myomas. Although less successful, other pharmocologic agents such as danazol have also been used as medical treatment for myomas by reducing endogenous production of ovarian estrogen.

The ultimate decision as to definitive surgical treatment by hysterectomy should include an assessment of the patient's future reproductive plans as well as careful assessment of clinical factors, including the amount and timing of bleeding, the degree of enlargement of the leiomyomata, and the associated disability rendered to the individual patient. The presence of uterine myomas alone does not necessarily warrant hysterectomy.

LEIOMYOSARCOMA

Uterine sarcomas represent an *unusual gynecologic malignancy* accounting for approximately *3% of cancers involving the body of the uterus*. Progressive uterine enlargement occurring in the postmenopausal years should not be assumed to be due to simple uterine leiomyomata, as appreciable endogenous ovarian estrogen secretion is absent, thereby minimizing this as a potential cause for progressive uterine enlargement. In addition, postmenopausal women on low dose hormone replacement therapy are not at risk for stimulation of uterine enlargement since the doses of estrogen given are low and unlikely to stimulate regrowth of preexisting uterine fibroids. In this situation, uterine sarcoma (leiomyosarcoma) should be considered. Other symptoms of uterine sarcoma include postmenopausal bleeding, unusual pelvic pain coupled with uterine enlargement, and an increase in unusual vaginal discharge. As with endometrial sampling in patients with myomas, this procedure in the postmenopausal patient may not provide the sufficient histologic information to diagnose sarcoma. This leaves surgical removal as the method of most reliable diagnosis. Accordingly, hysterectomy is usually indicated in patients with documented, and especially progressive, uterine enlargement.

The virulence of uterine sarcoma is directly related to the number of mitotic figures and cellular proliferation as defined histologically. In addition, these tumors are more likely to spread hematogenously than endometrial adenocarcinoma. When uterine sarcoma is suspected, patients should undergo typical tumor survey to include assessment for distant metastatic disease. At the time of hysterectomy, it is necessary to thoroughly explore the abdomen and sample commonly affected node chains including the iliac and periaortic areas. The staging for uterine sarcoma is surgical and identical to that for endometrial adenocarcinoma.

The overall rate of survival for patients with uterine sarcoma is considerably worse than that for those with endometrial adenocarcinoma. Only 50% of patients survive 5 years. Adjunctive radiation therapy and chemotherapy provide little additional benefit as primary adjuvant therapy or as therapy for recurrent disease. Unlike the adenocarcinoma endometrial counterparts, these tumors are not responsive to hormonal treatment with high dose progestins.

FURTHER READINGS

Droegemueller W. Benign gynecologic lesions. In: Herbst AL, Mishell DR, Stenchever MA, Droegemueller W, eds. Comprehensive gynecology. 2nd ed. St. Louis, MO: CV Mosby, 1992.

Herbst AL. Neoplasic diseases of the uterus. In: Herbst AL, Mishell DR, Stenchever MA, Droegemueller W, eds. Comprehensive gynecology. 2nd ed. St. Louis, MO: CV Mosby, 1992.

SELF-ASSESSMENT

Case 43-A

A 43-year-old G3P3 woman presents with an 8 month history of progressively longer and heavier menstruation. Her last two cycles have included clotted blood flow for the first 5 days of each menstrual period with another 5 days of relatively normal menstrual flow. Prior to 8 months ago, her menstruation included 6 days of "average flow." She has no other problems except that in the last few months she has felt tired.

Physical examination reveals a woman of normal height and weight with a resting pulse of 90. Her blood pressure is normal. General physical examination is unremarkable with the exception of a suprapubic "fullness." On pelvic examination, there is old menstrual blood in the vault. The cervix is smooth and on bimanual examination the uterus is consistent with approximately 14 week gestational size with multiple surface irregularities. Finger stick hematocrit done by your office nurse is 27%.

Question 43-A-1

The most likely diagnosis is:

A. endometrial hyperplasia
B. uterine fibroids
C. endometrial carcinoma
D. gestational trophoblastic disease
E. leiomyosarcoma of the uterus

Answer 43-A-1

Answer: B

This patient typifies the history and physical findings of a perimenopausal woman with probable fibroid tumors of the uterus. Significant aspects of her history include progressive menorrhagia with associated anemia as detected in your office. Physical examination is consistent with uterine fibroids as the most likely diagnosis. To confirm this diagnosis, ultrasonography can be performed. This ultrasound can also serve as baseline comparison for future studies. This patient should also have screening endometrial biopsy to rule out endometrial lesions and iron replacement therapy. The possibility of hormonal suppression should be discussed. Finally, a risk/benefit discussion regarding the possibility of hysterectomy should be undertaken, particularly in light of her age and severity of symptoms.

Case 43-B

A 64-year-old woman is referred to you by another physician requesting a second opinion. This patient had an uneventful menopause at the age of 54 and has not been on hormone replacement therapy. In the last 3 months she has had intermittent vaginal bleeding, and on physical examination the referring physician detected a uterus that he thought was consistent with approximately 12-week gestational size and somewhat irregular. Previous examination done by him 1½ years ago was entirely normal. Endometrial sampling done by him last week revealed atrophic endometrium. The uterine cavity sounded to 11 cm at that time. Your physical examination confirms his findings.

Question 43-B-1

Definitive treatment for this patient should include:

A. long-term progestin hormonal suppression
B. gonadotropin-releasing hormone agonists
C. dilation and curettage
D. total abdominal hysterectomy and bilateral salpingo-oophorectomy
E. vaginal hysterectomy

Answer 43-B-1

Answer: D

This patient illustrates features highly suggestive of uterine sarcoma. She is postmenopausal and has little potential for endogenous stimulation of preexisting fibroids. Knowledge of a normal examination 1½ years prior with current findings of a markedly enlarged uterus in this age group should alert the clinician to the possibility of uterine leiomyosarcoma. Although imaging studies might be useful and endometrial sampling is mandatory, definitive treatment for this patient is an abdominal hysterectomy with bilateral salpingo-oophorectomy.

chapter 44

ENDOMETRIAL HYPERPLASIA AND CANCER

Endometrial carcinoma is the most common genital tract malignancy, accounting for approximately 38,000–40,000 new cases annually. It is considered the best example of an "estrogen-dependent" neoplasm. Fortunately, patients with this disease usually present early in the disease course with some form of abnormal uterine bleeding, particularly postmenopausal bleeding. Accordingly, the screening for this disease by endometrial sampling is highly accurate and should be used liberally in patients at risk. Risk factors for the development of endometrial carcinoma include clinical factors associated with an estrogen-rich environment. With early diagnosis and surgical treatment, survival rates can be excellent.

Endometrial carcinoma may represent the endpoint of precursor lesions including atypical hyperplasias and/or intraepithelial neoplasia of the endometrial lining. Included in this chapter is a discussion of the spectrum of abnormal changes found in the endometrium ranging from simple hyperplasia to invasive adenocarcinoma of the endometrium.

The *underlying pathophysiologic process* in development of endometrial hyperplasia and endometrial cancer is overgrowth of the endometrium in response to an estrogen-dominant hormonal milieu. Sources of estrogen may be glandular (ovarian) or extraglandular (peripheral conversion or exogenous source) (Table 44.1). As explained later, endometrial hyperplasia may range from a simple hyperplastic response through an atypical hyperplastic response to an overt carcinomatous change. Endometrial hyperplasia is more common in perimenopausal women who do not ovulate regularly and postmenopausal women. Postmenopausal women are subject not only to residual estrogen stimulation from the ovary, but also estrogen is produced by conversion of androgenic precursors in peripheral fat stores. Obese women are at higher risk for endometrial hyperplasia and carcinoma. Approximately three quarters of patients with invasive endometrial carcinoma are diagnosed in their postmenopausal years. Of the remaining cases of endometrial cancer, most occur at the time of anovulation during the perimenopausal years (from their mid-forties through their early fifties), whereas a small number occur in younger patients who have been chronically anovulatory.

ENDOMETRIAL HYPERPLASIA

The relationship between estrogen production and endometrial growth (proliferation) is clear. Endometrial proliferation represents a normal part of the menstrual cycle and occurs during the follicular or estrogen-dominant phase of the cycle. With continued estrogen stimulation through either endogenous mechanisms or by exogenous administration, simple endometrial proliferation will become endometrial hyperplasia (Fig. 44.1). *Endometrial hyperplasia* is the "abnormal proliferation of both glandular and stromal elements showing altered histologic architecture." True endometrial proliferation is a simple overabundance of normal endometrium, whereas endometrial hyperplasia involves histologic features with cellular architectural abnormalities. When proliferation

Table 44.1
Estrogen Sources

Endogenous
  Glandular
    Estradiol (ovary)
    Estrone (ovary)
  Peripheral
    Estrone (fat)
  Tumor
    Granulosa cell of ovary (an uncommon tumor
      and source)
Exogenous
  Medications
    Conjugated estrogen (mostly estrone)
    Lyophilized estradiol
    Cutaneous patches
    Vaginal creams

becomes "hyperplasia" is not clear, although studies showing sequential change suggest it requires 6 months or longer of "unopposed estrogen" stimulation.

Histologic *variations of endometrial hyperplasia* include cystic glandular hyperplasia, adenomatous hyperplasia, and atypical adenomatous hyperplasia. Unlike cervical carcinoma precursors, there is no uniform agreement that each of these lesions will progress to endometrial cancer if left untreated. In addition, these histologic variants can occur in only small foci of an otherwise normal endometrium, revealing that these changes may not necessarily involve the entire endometrial cavity at the same time. It should be remembered that the microscopic picture as judged by a pathologist may not represent the complete anatomic picture.

Risk factors for endometrial hyperplasia are the same as for endometrial carcinoma, i.e., any features contributing to an increased estrogen environment. The sources of estrogen are listed in Table 44.1. Table 44.2 identifies those patients at increased risk for unopposed estrogen stimulation.

Cystic Endometrial Hyperplasia

Cystic endometrial hyperplasia is *the least significant form* of endometrial hyperplasia. It is not commonly associated with progression to or the occurrence of endometrial carcinoma, although it is considered a modest risk factor as a precursor lesion. In this variety of hyperplasia, both glandular elements and stromal cell elements proliferate excessively. Cystic glandular hyperplasia should not be confused with a normal postmenopausal variant—cystic involution of the endometrium—which is histologically not a hyperplastic condition.

Adenomatous Hyperplasia

Endometrial adenomatous hyperplasia represents an *abnormal proliferation of primarily glandular elements without concomitant proliferation of stromal elements*. This gives the endometrium a "crowded" picture, frequently with glands appearing almost "back to back." It is thought that adenomatous hyperplasia represents a true intraepithelial neoplastic process and is occasionally found coexisting with areas of endometrial adenocarcinoma; however, it may also be found microscopically in small areas within normal proliferative endometrium.

Atypical Adenomatous Hyperplasia

Adenomatous hyperplasia, which *contains significant numbers of glandular elements exhibiting cytologic atypia and disordered maturation*, is considered particularly important as a *precursor lesion to endometrial carcinoma*. This so-called "carcinoma in situ of the endometrium" has at least a 20–30% risk for malignant transformation.

DIAGNOSIS AND MANAGEMENT OF THE ENDOMETRIAL HYPERPLASIAS

The diagnosis of endometrial hyperplasia can be made by taking a sample of the endometrium for histologic evaluation. This is most easily accomplished by any of a number of different atraumatic aspiration devices available for office use (e.g., Pipelle, Vabra). The routine *Pap smear* is *not reliable* in diagnosing endometrial hyperplasia or cancer; however, this diagnosis must be considered when atypical endometrial cells are found on the Pap smear and an appropriate evaluation undertaken.

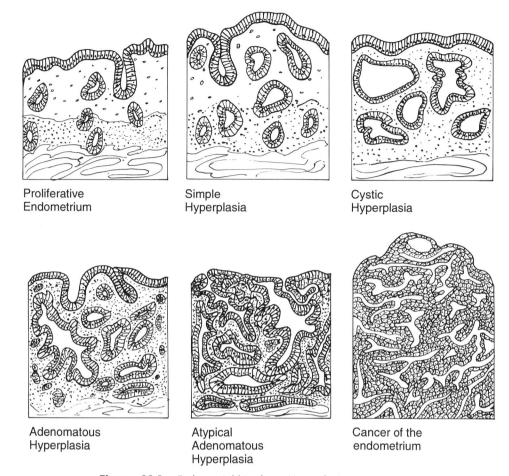

Proliferative Endometrium

Simple Hyperplasia

Cystic Hyperplasia

Adenomatous Hyperplasia

Atypical Adenomatous Hyperplasia

Cancer of the endometrium

Figure 44.1. Endometrial histology: Hyperplasia to carcinoma.

Table 44.2
Patients at Risk for Unopposed Estrogen Exposure

Patients using exogenous estrogen alone
Patients with history of chronic anovulation
Obese postmenopausal women
Patients with "late" menopause (patients >55 years old)

The most common *indication for endometrial sampling* is *abnormal bleeding* with liberal consideration given to endometrial aspiration *in patients over the age of 35 who present with abnormal uterine bleeding*. After ruling out pregnancy by simple urine pregnancy testing, patients can be adequately sampled with relatively little discomfort. Further management is usually dictated by the results of the biopsy specimen. Dilation and curettage can also be used for diagnostic sampling of the endometrium, although it is usually reserved for patients in whom outpatient sampling is technically difficult or in cases where outpatient sampling has been nondiagnostic.

Sometimes the office endometrial biopsy will be reported as "insufficient tissue for diagnosis." In, for example, a postmenopausal woman not on estrogen replacement, this data may be sufficient, as it is compatible with the suspected atrophic condition of the endometrium. In other cases, the clinical suspicion of a possible hyperplastic endometrial process may be high enough to warrant D&C to more fully sample the endometrial cavity. Although office endometrial biopsy is considered a sufficient technique for endometrial sampling, clinical judgment as to its interpretation must be applied in each clinical situation.

If *simple hyperplasia, cystic hyperplasia, or adenomatous hyperplasia* of the simple variety has been diagnosed by tissue sample, medical treatment is usually offered. In most cases, *medical treatment* involves the administration of a form of synthetic progesterone (progestin) in doses that will inhibit and eventually reverse the hyperplastic response evoked by estrogen stimulation. Progestin therapy works to alter the enzymatic pathways, which eventually convert endogenous estradiol to weaker estrogens, as well as to decrease the number of estrogen receptors in the endometrial glandular cells. Progestins have a net effect of decreasing endometrial glandular proliferation and, when administered for sufficient period of time or in high enough doses, will actually render the endometrium atrophic. In addition, with progestin withdrawal, the endometrium is sloughed, analogous to corpus luteum progesterone withdrawal in a normal menstrual cycle (the so-called "chemical D&C").

Atypical adenomatous hyperplasia is usually treated surgically by *hysterectomy* since it is this variant that is much more likely to become endometrial carcinoma. This treatment decision is usually fairly clear since the majority of patients with this disorder will be in their late reproductive or perimenopausal years. In the younger patient with chronic anovulation and associated atypical adenomatous hyperplasia, longer term *progestin management* after thorough endometrial curettage may be employed to allow the patient to try to become pregnant. Patients who are treated medically for atypical adenomatous hyperplasia should be treated with regular progestin-induced endometrial sloughing and/or ovulation induction as well as followed with periodic endometrial sampling (once to twice per year) so that treatment response can be gauged.

ENDOMETRIAL POLYPS

Most endometrial polyps represent *focal accentuated benign hyperplastic processes.* Their histologic architecture is characteristic and may commonly be found in association with other types of endometrial hyperplasia. Polyps occur most frequently in perimenopausal or immediately postmenopausal age women, when the ovary is characterized by unopposed estrogen production due to chronic anovulation. The most common presenting symptom is abnormal bleeding. Often small polyps may be incidentally found as part of endometrial aspiration or curettage done for evaluation of the bleeding problem. Rarely, a large polyp may begin to protrude through the cervical canal, and the patient will present not only with bleeding irregularities, but also with low dull midline pain as the cervix is slowly dilated and effaced. The appearance of these on speculum examination is quite striking. In these cases, surgical removal is necessary to reduce the amount of bleeding as well as prevent infection from the exposed endometrial surface. *Less than 5% of polyps show malignant change*, and when they do, they may represent any endometrial histologic variant.

ENDOMETRIAL CARCINOMA

Although the *relationship between endometrial hyperplasias and estrogen* dominance is clear, the mechanism behind the ultimate change from hyperplastic variations to endometrial carcinoma is less clear. Certainly, estrogen is implicated because of its association with the antecedent hyperplasia, but the actual stimulus to malignant degeneration is unknown. It remains standard teaching to consider endometrial carcinoma as an "estrogen-dependent neoplasm."

The diagnosis of endometrial cancer is most frequently made by *endometrial sampling* after a patient presents with abnormal uterine bleeding. Special consideration should be given to the patient who presents *with postmenopausal bleeding*, i.e., bleeding that occurs after 6 months of amenorrhea in a patient

Table 44.3
FIGO Surgical Staging of Endometrial Carcinoma (1988)

Stage IA G123:	Tumor limited to endometrium
IB G123:	Invasion to less than one half of the myometrium
IC G123:	Invasion to more than one half of the myometrium
Stage IIA G123:	Endocervical glandular involvement only
IIB G123:	Cervical stromal invasion
Stage IIIA G123:	Tumor invading serosa, adnexa, or both; and/or positive peritoneal cytology
IIIB G123:	Vaginal metastases
IIIC G123:	Metastases to pelvic and/or paraaortic lymph nodes
Stage IVA G123:	Tumor invades bladder, bowel mucosa, or both
IVB:	Distant metastases including intraabdominal and/or inguinal lymph node

Rules related to staging
1. Because corpus cancer is now surgically staged, procedures previously used for differentiation of stages are no longer applicable, e.g., the findings of D&C to differentiate between stage I and stage II.
   It is appreciated that there may be a small number of patients with corpus cancer who are treated primarily with radiation therapy. If that is the case, the clinical staging adopted by FIGO in 1971 would still apply but use of that staging system would be noted.
2. Ideally, the width of the myometrium is measured along with the width of tumor invasion.

who has been diagnosed as menopausal. In this group of patients, it is mandatory to assess the endometrium histologically since the chance of having an endometrial carcinoma is approximately 15%. Other gynecologic assessments should also be made including careful physical and pelvic examination as well as a screening Pap smear.

Because of the current International Federation of Gynecology and Obstetrics (*FIGO*) *staging of endometrial carcinoma* (1988) (Table 44.3), differential sampling of the endocervical canal and endometrial cavity prior to therapy is less important now than with previous staging criteria. Fractional curettage should, however, be kept in mind for patients who are not surgical candidates because of other risk factors, i.e., patients whose primary treatment is radiotherapy.

ROUTE OF SPREAD OF ENDOMETRIAL CARCINOMA

Knowledge of the route of spread of endometrial cancer guides the surgeon toward thorough surgical assessment of potentially involved tissues and serves as the basis for the recently accepted FIGO staging system. Endometrial carcinoma usually spreads throughout the endometrial cavity first and then begins to invade the myometrium, endocervical canal, and eventually, lymphatics. Hematogenous spread occurs with endometrial carcinoma more readily than in cervical cancer or ovarian cancer. Invasion of adnexal structures may occur via lymphatics or direct implantation through the fallopian tubes. Once there is extrauterine spread to the peritoneal cavity, cancer cells have access to the entire abdominal pelvic cavity and may spread in a fashion similar to ovarian cancer. Unusual histologic subtypes, including *papillary serous adenocarcinoma* and *clear cell adenocarcinoma* of the endometrium, tend to be more agressive in abdominopelvic spread than the more common adenocarcinoma of the endometrium. Microscopic spread may also be present despite the absence of gross abdominal pelvic lesions. Accordingly, cytologic assessment of peritoneal washings is important at the outset of surgical treatment for endometrial carcinoma. The current FIGO guidelines for the surgical staging of endometrial carcinoma emphasizes the need for thorough surgical assessment of the abdominopelvic cavity to include sampling of both periaortic and pelvic lymph nodes when depths of invasion are more than one third of the myometrial thickness or in cases where there are obvious peritoneal foci of tumor.

PROGNOSTIC FACTORS FOR ENDOMETRIAL CARCINOMA

The single most important prognostic factor for endometrial carcinoma is histologic grade. Histologically poorly differentiated tumors are associated with a considerably poorer prognosis because of the likelihood of extrauterine spread through adjacent lymphatics and peritoneal fluid. This is true even of relatively limited lesions. Therefore, this finding is important in both the initial surgical management of the patient and, more importantly, is of significance in deciding on adjunctive therapy via radiation or chemotherapy. *Depth of myometrial invasion is the second most important prognostic factor.* When the tumor has invaded greater than one third of the thickness of the myometrium, the prognosis is markedly worsened. Other factors that have prognostic value include the original tumor volume both within the uterus and defined by extrauterine spread, lymphatic involvement, and hematogenous spread.

Survival rates vary widely, depending on the grade of tumor and depth of penetration into the myometrium. A patient with a grade I tumor that does not invade the myometrium has a 95% 5-year survival rate, whereas a patient with a poorly differentiated (grade III) tumor with deep myometrial invasion may have a 5-year survival rate of only 20%.

TREATMENT OF ENDOMETRIAL CARCINOMA

As a surgically staged disease, *primary surgical treatment* is *the cornerstone of management.* After opening the abdomen, peritoneal washings are obtained. The abdominopelvic cavity is manually and visually explored, and then a total abdominal hysterectomy with bilateral salpingo-oophorectomy is performed. The decision to include pelvic and/or periaortic nodes is determined by the depth of myometrial invasion as judged by the attending pathologist.

Adjunctive therapy after hysterectomy, which may include *external beam radiation*, has been shown to significantly reduce the risk of pelvic and vaginal recurrence. Preoperative radiation may be given to those patients with obvious endocervical involvement and/or to reduce a bulky endometrial tumor.

The first line of *treatment for recurrent disease* is hormonal and includes various *progestin preparations* given in high doses. Approximately one third of these patients will have a short-term (less than 5 years) response, and approximately 15% will have a long-term response (greater than 5 years). A major advantage of high dose progestin therapy is its minimal complication rate. *Chemotherapy* with drugs including Adriamycin (doxorubicin) and cisplatin produce occasional favorable short-term results but long-term remissions with these therapies are rare.

The use of *estrogen replacement therapy* in patients previously treated for endometrial carcinoma is controversial. Recent data suggest that for well-differentiated, minimally invasive endometrial carcinoma that has not recurred within 5 years estrogen and progestin replacement therapy may be safe. However, cautious assessment of long-term risk versus benefits of hormone replacement therapy should be accorded each patient.

FURTHER READINGS

Clarke-Pearson DL, Dawood MY. Benign disease of the uterus: leiomyomas, adenomyosis, hyperplasia, and polyps. In: Green's gynecology: essentials of clinical practice. 8th ed. Boston: Little, Brown & Co, 1990: 357–372.

Clarke-Pearson DL, Dawood MY. Endometrial cancer and uterine sarcoma. In: Green's gynecology: essentials of clinical practice. 8th ed. Boston: Little, Brown & Co, 1990:521–530.

Droegemueller W. Benign gynecologic lesions. In: Herbst AL, Mishell DR, Stenchever MA, Droegemueller W, eds. Comprehensive gynecology. St. Louis, MO: CV Mosby, 1992:491.

Herbst A. Neoplastic diseases of the uterus. In: Herbst AL, Mishell DR, Stenchever MA, Droegemueller W, eds. Comprehensive gynecology. St. Louis, MO: CV Mosby, 1992:895.

SELF-EVALUATION

Case 44-A

A 62-year-old woman whose last normal menstrual period was 7 years ago presents with a 2-month history of intermittent vaginal bleeding. She has had two children (ages 39 and 40) and is in generally good health and currently taking no medications. Physical examination reveals a patient of average height and weight and normal blood pressure. Pelvic examination shows some atrophy of the vaginal mucosa with a small and smooth cervix without evidence of blood. Bimanual examination demonstrates a small, firm, anteflexed uterus of normal size with an unremarkable adnexal examination. Rectovaginal examination is negative and the stool is guaiac negative.

Question 44-A-1

Having performed Pap smears of both the exocervix and cervical canal, your next diagnostic assessment should be to:

A. Await results of Pap smear before further assessment.
B. Obtain vaginal maturation index for estrogen production.
C. Obtain pelvic ultrasound.
D. Perform endometrial biopsy.
E. Schedule for dilation and curettage.

Answer 44-A-1

Answer: D

This case illustrates a high risk history for endometrial carcinoma: new onset postmenopausal bleeding. Despite having normal physical and pelvic examinations, this patient has approximately a 15% risk of endometrial carcinoma. The Pap smear is unreliable in detecting this neoplasm and it is mandatory to obtain endometrial sampling. The preferable technique for this is by office biopsy. Dilation and curettage is reserved for patients in whom the clinician encounters technical difficulty or there is an inadequate office sample.

Case 44-B

A 27-year-old patient comes in with a 3-year history of progressively infrequent menstrual periods. Her menarche was age 17, she has never had "monthly periods" but has always had six or seven periods per year. In the last 3 years she has had only two or three menstrual periods per year. She has also been unable to become pregnant. Her last bleeding episode was 2 months ago. Physical examination reveals a woman 5 feet 4 inches tall weighing 180 pounds with a normal pelvic examination. After a negative pregnancy test, an endometrial biopsy performed as part of her infertility assessment reveals adenomatous hyperplasia.

Question 44-B-1

The most efficacious treatment for this patient would be:

A. pharmacologic ovulation induction
B. intermittent short-term progestin therapy
C. oral contraceptives
D. dilation and curettage
E. artificial insemination

Answer 44-B-1

Answer: A

This patient has chronic anovulation with resultant hyperplasia of the endometrium. Because she is also infertile, the optimal treatment of ovulation induction may help enable her to become pregnant, also reversing the hyperplasia by the production of progesterone. Other therapy such as intermittent progestin use and/or oral contraceptive use may treat the endometrial hyperplasia problem but would not address the infertility concern. Adenomatous hyperplasia without atypia carries a low risk for malignancy. Therefore, aggressive surgical treatment such as D&C is not warranted. Likewise, dilation and curettage is no better a diagnostic tool than office sampling. Artificial insemination is of no value in a chronically anovulatory patient. For completeness, other etiology for oligomenorrhea in the patient should also be assessed, e.g., pituitary or thyroid dysfunction.

For further consideration: What if the patient were not trying to conceive? What then would be the best therapy? What if the patient were 47 years old rather than 27 years old, with atypical adenomatous hyperplasia?

chapter 45

OVARIAN AND ADNEXAL DISEASE

The area between the lateral pelvic wall and the cornu of the uterus medially is referred to as the *adnexal space* or *adnexae*. This area includes the ovaries, fallopian tubes, the upper portion of the broad ligament and mesosalpinx, and remnants of the embryonic müllerian duct. Within the adnexal space, the organs most commonly affected by disease processes are the ovaries and fallopian tubes.

This chapter describes the physiologic variations of the ovary and fallopian tubes that can mimic disease as well as the benign and malignant ovarian and fallopian tube neoplasms. It also illustrates how nongynecologic structures in the region, such as the bowel and bladder, may produce symptoms that can be confused with "gynecologic" adnexal disease. Pelvic infection, ectopic pregnancy, and endometriosis are discussed in separate chapters.

THE "ADNEXAL SPACE" AND ASSOCIATED NONGYNECOLOGIC DISEASE

In addition to the reproductive organs, parts of the urinary and gastrointestinal tracts are located in the adnexal space. The most common urologic disorders are upper and lower *urinary tract infection*, and less commonly, *renal and ureteral calculi*. Even rarer are anatomic abnormalities such as a *ptotic kidney*, which may present as a solid pelvic mass. An isolated *pelvic kidney* may likewise present as an asymptomatic solid cul-de-sac mass. Right adnexal signs and symptoms are associated with acute *appendicitis*, which should be considered in the differential diagnosis of acute right lower quadrant pain. Less commonly, symptoms in the right adnexa may be related to intrinsic *inflammatory bowel disease* involving the ileocecal junction. Left-sided bowel disease involving the rectosigmoid is seen more often in older patients, as in acute or chronic diverticular disease. Because of the age of these patients and the proximity of the left ovary to the sigmoid, *sigmoid diverticular disease* is included in the differential diagnosis of a left-sided adnexal mass. Finally, left-sided pelvic pain or a mass may be related to *rectosigmoid carcinoma*.

THE OVARIES

Pelvic examination is central in evaluation of the ovary. Symptoms that may arise from physiologic and pathologic processes of the ovary must be correlated with physical examination findings. Also, since some ovarian conditions are asymptomatic, incidental physical examination findings may be the only information available when an evaluation begins. Interpretation of examination findings requires knowledge of the physical characteristics of the ovary during the stages of the life cycle.

In the *premenarchal age group*, the *ovary should not be palpable*. If it is, a pathologic condition is presumed and further evaluation is necessary.

In the *reproductive age group*, the normal *ovary is palpable about one-half of the time*. Important considerations include ovarian size, shape, consistency (firm or cystic), and mobility. In reproductive age women taking oral contraceptives, the ovaries are palpable less frequently and are smaller and more symmetrical than in women who are not using contraceptives.

In the *postmenopausal* patient, the ovaries are functionally quiescent except for some androgen production. These ovaries are no longer responsive to gonadotropin secretion, and therefore, their surface follicular activity diminishes over time, disappearing in most women within 3 years of the onset of natural menopause. Women who are close to the natural menopause are more likely to have residual functional cysts. In general, palpable ovarian enlargement in a postmenopausal patient should be assessed more critically than in a younger woman because the incidence of ovarian malignant neoplasm is increased in this group.

One quarter of all ovarian tumors in postmenopausal women are malignant, while in reproductive age women only about 10% of ovarian tumors are malignant. Indeed, this risk was considered so great in the past that the presence of any ovarian enlargement in a postmenopausal woman was an indication for surgical investigation, the so-called palpable postmenopausal ovary (PPO) syndrome. With the advent of more sensitive pelvic imaging techniques to assist in diagnosis, routine removal of minimally enlarged postmenopausal ovaries is less common. If the patient is within 3 years of natural menopause, and transvaginal ultrasonography confirms the presence of a simple, unilocular cyst of less than 5 cm in diameter, the management may be serial pelvic and transvaginal ultrasound examinations. Masses that are larger or appear complex on ultrasonography are best managed surgically.

Functional Ovarian Cysts

Functional ovarian cysts are not neoplasms but rather anatomic variations arising as a result of normal ovarian function. They may present as an asymptomatic adnexal mass or become symptomatic, requiring evaluation and possibly treatment.

When an ovarian follicle fails to rupture during follicular maturation, ovulation does not occur and a *follicular cyst* may develop. This, by definition, will involve a lengthen-ing of the follicular phase of the cycle with resultant secondary amenorrhea. Follicular cysts are lined by normal granulosa cells and the fluid contained within them is rich in estrogen.

A follicular cyst becomes clinically significant if it is large enough to cause pain or if it persists beyond one menstrual interval. For poorly understood reasons, the granulosa cells lining the follicular cyst persist through the time when ovulation should have occurred and continue to enlarge through the second half of the cycle. A cyst may enlarge beyond 5 cm and continue to fill with estrogen-rich follicular fluid from the thickened granulosa cell layer. Symptoms associated with a follicular cyst may include mild to moderate unilateral lower abdominal pain and alteration of the menstrual interval. The latter may be due to both failed subsequent ovulation and bleeding stimulated by the large amount of estradiol produced within the follicle. This estrogen-rich environment along with the lack of ovulation overstimulates the endometrium and causes irregular bleeding. Pelvic examination findings may include unilateral tenderness with a palpable mobile, cystic adnexal mass.

Given a patient with these findings, the physician must decide whether further diagnostic assessment and treatment are necessary. Pelvic ultrasonography is occasionally warranted in reproductive age patients who have cysts larger than 5 cm in diameter. Ultrasound characteristics include a unilocular simple cyst without evidence of blood or soft tissue elements and without evidence of external excrescences. For most patients, however, ultrasound confirmation is not required. Instead, the patient may be reassured and followed with a repeat pelvic examination in about 6–8 weeks. Most follicular cysts will spontaneously resolve during this time. Alternatively, an estrogen/progesterone-containing oral contraceptive may be given to suppress gonadotropin stimulation of the cyst. If the cyst persists, despite expectant management and/or oral contraceptive suppression, the presence of another type of cyst or neoplasm should be suspected.

On occasion, *rupture of a follicular cyst* may cause acute pelvic pain. Because release of follicular fluid into the peritoneum produces only transient symptoms, surgical intervention is rarely necessary.

A *corpus luteum cyst* is the other common type of functional ovarian cyst. It is related to the postovulatory, i.e., luteal dominant phase of the menstrual cycle. Two variations of corpus luteum cysts are encountered. The first is a slightly enlarged corpus luteum, which may continue to produce progesterone for longer than the usual 14 days. Menstruation is delayed from a few days to several weeks, although it usually occurs within 2 weeks of the missed period. Persistent corpus luteum cysts are often associated with dull lower quadrant pain. This pain and a missed menstrual period are the most common complaints associated with persistent corpus luteum cysts. Pelvic examination usually discloses an enlarged, tender, cystic or solid adnexal mass. Because of the triad of missed menstrual period, unilateral lower quadrant pain and adnexal enlargement, ectopic pregnancy is often considered in the differential diagnosis. A negative pregnancy test eliminates this possibility, whereas a positive pregnancy test mandates further evaluation as to the location of the pregnancy. Patients with recurrent persistent corpus luteum cysts may benefit from cyclic oral contraceptive therapy.

The second common type of corpus luteum cyst is the rapidly enlarging luteal phase cyst into which there is spontaneous hemorrhage. Sometimes called the *corpus hemorrhagicum*, this hemorrhagic cyst may rupture late in the luteal phase, resulting in the following clinical picture: a patient not using oral contraceptives, with regular periods, who presents with acute pain late in the luteal phase. Some patients present with evidence of hemoperitoneum as well as hypovolemia and require surgical resection of the bleeding cyst. In others, the acute pain and blood loss are self-limited. These pa-

tients may be managed with mild analgesics and reassurance.

Benign Ovarian Neoplasms

Although most ovarian enlargements in the reproductive age group are functional cysts, about 25% will prove to be nonfunctional ovarian neoplasms. In the reproductive age group, 90% of these neoplasms are benign, whereas the risk of malignancy rises to approximately 25% when postmenopausal patients are also included. Thus, ovarian masses in older patients and in reproductive patients where there is no response to oral contraceptives are of special concern. Unfortunately, unless the mass is particularly large or becomes symptomatic, these masses may remain undetected for some time. Many ovarian neoplasms are first discovered at the time of routine pelvic examination.

Ovarian neoplasms are usually categorized by the cell type of origin: (*a*) *epithelial cell tumors*, the largest class of ovarian neoplasm; (*b*) *germ cell tumors*, which includes the most common ovarian neoplasm in reproductive age women, the benign cystic teratoma or dermoid; and (*c*) *stromal cell tumors*. The classification of ovarian tumors by cell line of origin is presented in Table 45.1.

Benign Epithelial Cell Neoplasms

The exact *cell source for the development of epithelial cell tumors* of the ovary is unclear. However, the cells are characteristic of typical glandular epithelial cells: they contain microscopic glandular and secretory apparatus, they secrete into a luminal surface, and they are separated from underlying stroma by a basement membrane. Evidence exists to suggest that these cells are derived from mesothelial cells lining the peritoneal cavity. Since the müllerian duct-derived tissue becomes the female genital tract by differentiation of the mesothelium from the gonadal ridge, it is hypothesized that these tissues are also capable of differentiating into glandular tissue. Accordingly, the more common epithelial tumors of the ovary are grouped into serous,

Table 45.1
Histogenic Classification of All Ovarian Neoplasms

From celomic epithelium (epithelial)
  Serous
  Mucinous
  Endometrioid
  Brenner
From gonadal stroma
  Granulosa-theca
  Sertoli-Leydig (arrhenoblastoma)
  Lipid cell fibroma
From germ cell
  Dysgerminoma
  Teratoma
  Endodermal sinus (yolk sac)
  Choriocarcinoma
Miscellaneous cell line sources
  Lymphoma
  Sarcoma
  Metastatic
    Colorectal
    Breast
    Endometrial

Table 45.2
Histologic Classification of the Common Epithelial Tumors of the Ovary

Serous tumors
  Serous cystadenomas
  Serous cystadenomas with proliferating activity of the epithelial cells and nuclear abnormalities but with no infiltrative destructive growth (low potential malignancy)
  Serous cystadenocarcinoma
Mucinous tumors
  Mucinous cystadenomas
  Mucinous cystadenomas with proliferating activity of the epithelial cells and nuclear abnormalities but with no infiltrative destructive growth (low potential malignancy)
  Mucinous cystadenocarcinoma
Endometrioid tumors (similar to adenocarcinomas in the endometrium)
  Endometrioid benign cysts
  Endometrioid tumors with proliferating activity of the epithelial cells and nuclear abnormalities but with no infiltrative destructive growth (low potential malignancy)
  Adenocarcinoma
Brenner tumor
Unclassified carcinoma

mucinous, and endometrial neoplasms as shown in Table 45.2.

The most common epithelial cell neoplasm is the *serous cystadenoma*. Seventy percent of serous tumors are benign, approximately 10% will have intraepithelial cellular characteristics, which suggest that they are of low malignant potential, and the remaining 20% are frankly malignant by both histologic criteria and by clinical behavior. Benign tumors usually present clinically as cystic adnexal masses, which may be bilateral about 15% of the time. Typically, they are larger than functional ovarian cysts and may cause perceptive increasing abdominal girth. These tumors may occur in any age group, although they are more common in the peri- and postmenopausal patient. On ultrasonography, these cysts tend to appear multilocular, especially if they are large. The *treatment of serous tumors is surgical* because of the relatively high rate of malignancy. In the younger patient with smaller tumors, an attempt can be made to perform an ovarian cystectomy to try to minimize the amount of ovarian tissue removed. For large unilateral serous tumors

in young patients, unilateral oophorectomy with preservation of the contralateral ovary is indicated to maintain fertility. In patients past the reproductive age, bilateral oophorectomy along with hysterectomy may be indicated, not only because of the chance of future malignancy, but also because of the increased risk of a similar occurrence in the contralateral ovary.

Mucinous tumors are also of epithelial (mesothelial) cell origin. The *mucinous cystadenoma* is the second most common epithelial cell tumor of the ovary. The malignancy rate of 15% is lower than that for serous tumor, as is the 5% rate of bilaterality. These cystic tumors can become very large, sometimes filling the entire pelvis and extending into the abdominal cavity. In fact, when enormous cystic adnexal masses are found, mucinous cystadenomas should be suggested. Ultrasound assessment shows multilocular septation. Surgery is the treatment of choice.

A third type of benign epithelial neoplasm is the *endometrioid tumor*. The majority of benign endometrioid tumors take the form of endometriomas, which are cysts lined by well-differentiated endometrial-like glandular tissue. There is further discussion of this neoplasm under the heading Malignant Ovarian Neoplasms.

The *Brenner cell tumor* is an uncommon benign epithelial cell tumor of the ovary. This tumor is usually described as a solid ovarian tumor because of the large amount of stroma and fibrotic tissue that surrounds the epithelial cells. It is more common in older women and occasionally occurs in association with mucinous tumors of the ovary. When discovered as an isolated tumor of the ovary, it is relatively small compared to the large size attained often by the serous and especially by the mucinous cystadenomas. It is rarely malignant.

Benign Germ Cell Neoplasms

Germ cell tumors are derived from the primary germ cells. The tumors arise in the ovary and may contain relatively differentiated structures such as hair or bone. The most common tumor found in women of all ages is the *benign cystic teratoma*, also called a *dermoid cyst* or *dermoid*. Dermoids may contain differentiated tissue from all three embryonic germ layers (ectoderm, mesoderm, and endoderm). The most common elements found are of ectodermal origin, primarily squamous cell tissue such as skin appendages (sweat sebaceous glands) with associated hair follicles and sebum. It is because of this predominance of dermoid derivatives that the term "dermoid" is used. Other constituents of dermoids include central nervous system tissue, cartilage, bone, teeth, and intestinal glandular elements, most of which are found in well-differentiated form. One unusual variant is the *stroma ovarii*, in which functioning thyroid tissue is found. A dermoid cyst is frequently encountered as an asymptomatic unilateral cystic adnexal mass, which is mobile, nontender, and often felt anterior to the broad ligament, i.e., just under the abdominal examining fingers rather than deep in the pelvis. The diagnosis can be confirmed by ultrasound because of the peculiar pattern of echogenicity from inside the cyst due to its contents.

Treatment of benign cystic teratomas is necessarily surgical even though the rate of malignancy is less than 1%. Surgical removal is also required because of the possibility of ovarian torsion and rupture, resulting in intense chemical peritonitis and a potential surgical emergency. Approximately 10–20% of these cysts are bilateral, underscoring the need for examination of the contralateral ovary at the time of surgery.

Benign Stromal Cell Neoplasms

Stromal cell tumors of the ovary are usually considered solid tumors and are derived from specialized sex cord stroma of the developing gonad. These tumors may develop along primarily female cell type into *granulosa theca cell tumors* or into primarily male gonadal type of tissue, which are described as *Sertoli-Leydig cell tumor*. Both of these tumors are referred to as *functioning tumors* because of their hormone production. *Granulosa theca cell tumors primarily produce estrogenic components* and may be manifest in patients through feminizing characteristics, and *Sertoli-Leydig cell tumors produce androgenic components*, which may contribute to hirsutism or virilizing symptoms. These neoplasms occur with approximately equal frequency in all age groups including pediatric patients. When the granulosa cell tumor occurs in the pediatric age group, it may contribute to signs and symptoms of precocious puberty, including precocious thelarche and vaginal bleeding. Vaginal bleeding may also occur when this tumor develops in the postmenopausal years. Both the granulosa cell tumor and the Sertoli-Leydig cell tumor have malignant potential as discussed in the section on malignant tumors.

The *ovarian fibroma* occurs in approximately 10% of patients with ovarian neoplasms, but is unlike the other stromal cell tumors in that it does not secrete sex steroids. It is usually a small solid tumor with a smooth surface and occasionally will be clinically misleading because of the presence of ascites. The combination of benign ovarian fibroma coupled with ascites and right unilateral hydrothorax has historically been referred to as *Meigs syndrome*.

In summary, the following points regarding benign ovarian neoplasms can be made: (*a*) they are more common than malignant tumors of the ovary in all age groups; (*b*) the chance for malignant transformation increases with increasing age; (*c*) they warrant surgical treatment because of their potential for malignancy; (*d*) preoperative assessment may be assisted by the use of pelvic imaging techniques such as ultrasound; and (*e*) surgical treatment may be conservative for benign tumors, especially if future reproduction is desired.

Malignant Ovarian Neoplasms

Ovarian cancer is the *fifth most common of all cancers in women* in the United States and the *third most common gynecologic malignancy* with a frequency of approximately one fourth that of endometrial carcinoma. Yet, the *mortality rate of this disease is the highest of all the gynecologic malignancies*, primarily because early detection of the disease prior to widespread dissemination is difficult. Ovarian neoplasms are rarely symptomatic in early stages of disease, becoming symptomatic only after extensive metastasis. As yet, there is no effective screening test for ovarian cancer similar to the Pap smear for cervical cancer, so that approximately two thirds of the patients with ovarian cancer have advanced disease at the time of diagnosis. It is estimated that there will be approximately 21,000 new cases of ovarian cancer in 1992, and that 60% of these patients will die within 5 years. The most important demographic observation regarding ovarian cancer is that it *presents most commonly in the fifth and sixth decade of life*. There is a higher incidence of ovarian cancer in western European countries and in the United States, with 5–7 times greater than age-matched populations in the Far East. Caucasians are 50% more likely to develop ovarian cancer than blacks living in this country.

A woman's risk of developing ovarian cancer during her lifetime is approximately 1%. The risk increases with age until approximately 70 years of age, at which time it declines modestly. The certain epidemiologic factors associated with developing ovarian cancer include low parity, decreased fertility, and delayed childbearing. In small groups of patients, there appears to be a familial predisposition to the development of ovarian cancer (*cancer family syndrome*) with an autosomal dominant genetic transmission pattern. Some investigators have suggested a possible carcinogenic source introduced into the lower genital tract by way of the vagina that eventually reaches the ovary. Inert agents such as asbestos and talc can be found in the peritoneal mesothelial cells, although the role of these and other potentially carcinogenic agents is unclear. An association with viral exposure, in particular with prior infection with mumps virus, has been suggested.

Long-term suppression of ovulation may protect against the development of ovarian cancer, at least for epithelial cell tumors. It has been suggested that so-called incessant ovulation may predispose to neoplastic transformation of the epithelial cell surfaces of the ovary. Oral contraceptives that cause anovulation appear to be modestly protective against the occurrence of ovarian cancer. No evidence exists to implicate the use of postmenopausal hormone replacement therapy in the development of ovarian cancer.

Pathogenesis and Diagnosis

Malignant ovarian epithelial cell tumors spread primarily by direct extension within the peritoneal cavity because of direct cell sloughing from the ovarian surface. This process explains the observation that there is often widespread peritoneal dissemination of these cancers at the time of diagnosis, even with relatively small primary ovarian lesions. Although epithelial cell ovarian cancers also spread by lymphatic and blood-borne routes, it is the direct extension into the virtually unlimited space of the peritoneal cavity that contributes to their late clinical presentation.

The early diagnosis of ovarian cancer is also made difficult because of the *lack of effective screening tests*. Approximately 60% of patients have advanced disease at the time of diagnosis. Refined imaging techniques (especially transvaginal ultrasonography) and serum tumor markers such as Ca 125 offer promise for the future. Much work remains, however, before these or similar tests are considered accurate or cost-effective. Currently, serum tumor markers have been shown to be useful in the *follow-up* of previously treated epithelial cell neoplasms of the ovary but not for detection. Until these techniques are shown to be efficacious, detection is limited by the physician's skill in the gynecologic physical examination.

Histologic Classification

Malignant ovarian neoplasms are usually categorized by the cell type of origin similar to their benign counterparts: (*a*) *malignant epithelial cell tumors*, which are the most common type; (*b*) *malignant germ cell tumors*; and (*c*) *malignant stromal cell tumors* (Table 45.1). Most malignant ovarian tumors have histologically similar but benign counterparts. The relationship between a benign ovarian neoplasm and its malignant counterpart is clinically important. If the benign counterpart is found in a patient, removal of both ovaries is strongly considered because of the possibility of future malignant transformation in the remaining ovary. The decision as to removal of one or both ovaries, however, must be individualized based on age, type of tumor, and future risks. For example, it has been shown that approximately 10% of seemingly benign epithelial cell tumors may contain histologic evidence of intraepithelial neoplasia, commonly referred to as borderline malignancies, or "tumors of low malignant potential."

Staging

The staging of ovarian carcinoma is based on extent of spread of tumor and histologic evaluation of the tumor. The International Federation of Gynecology and Obstetrics (FIGO) classification of ovarian cancer is presented in Table 45.3.

Epithelial Cell Ovarian Carcinoma

About 90% of all ovarian malignancies are of the epithelial cell type. These are thought to represent abnormalities in the differentiation of the pleuripotential mesothelial cells (which were derived embryologically from the gonadal ridge) that occupy parts of the visceral peritoneum. The ovary contains these cells as part of an ovarian capsule just overlying the actual stroma of the ovary. When these mesothelial cell elements are situated over developing follicles, they go through metaplastic transformation whenever ovulation occurs. Repeated ovulation is, therefore, associated with the histologic change in these cells derived from celomic epithelium.

The *malignant epithelial serous tumors (serous cystadenocarcinoma)* are the most common malignant epithelial cell tumors. About 50% of these cancers are thought to be derived from their benign precursors (serous cystadenoma), and as many as 30% of these tumors are bilateral at the time of clinical presentation. They are typically multiloculated and often have external excrescences on an otherwise smooth capsular surface.

Another epithelial cell variant, which contains cells reminiscent of endocervical glandular mucous secreting cells, is the *malignant mucinous epithelial tumor* (the *mucinous cystadenocarcinoma*). These tumors have a lower rate of bilaterality (10–15%) and can be among the largest of ovarian tumors, often measuring greater than 20 cm. They may be associated with widespread peritoneal extension with thick mucinous ascites, termed *pseudomyxomatous peritonei*.

Endometrioid Tumors. Endometrioid epithelial cell tumors are the second most com-

Table 45.3
FIGO Staging for Primary Carcinoma of the Ovary[a]

Stage I	*Growth limited to the ovaries*	
	Stage Ia	Growth limited to one ovary; no ascites containing malignant cells. No tumor on the external surface; capsule intact.
	Stage Ib	Growth limited to both ovaries; no ascites containing malignant cells. No tumor on the external surface; capsule intact.
	Stage Ic	Tumor either stage Ia or Ib but with tumor on the surface of one or both ovaries; or with capsule ruptured; or with ascites present containing malignant cells or with positive peritoneal washings.
Stage II	*Growth involving one or both ovaries with pelvic extension*	
	Stage IIa	Extension and/or metastases to the uterus and/or tubes
	Stage IIb	Extension to other pelvic tissues
	Stage IIc	Tumor either stage IIa or IIb but with tumor on the surface of one or both ovaries; or with capsule(s) ruptured; or with ascites present containing malignant cells or with positive peritoneal washings.
Stage III	*Tumor involving one or both ovaries with peritoneal implants outside the pelvic and/or positive retroperitoneal or inguinal nodes. Superficial liver metastasis equals Stage III. Tumor is limited to the true pelvis, but the histologically proven malignant extension to small bowel or omentum.*	
	Stage IIIa	Tumor grossly limited to the true pelvis with negative nodes but with histologically confirmed microscopic seeding of abdominal peritoneal surfaces.
	Stage IIIb	Tumor of one or both ovaries with histologically confirmed implants of abdominal peritoneal surfaces; none exceeding 2 cm in diameter. Nodes negative.
	Stage IIIc	Abdominal implants >2 cm in diameter and/or positive retroperitoneal or inguinal nodes.
Stage IV	*Growth involving one or both ovaries with distant metastasis. If pleural effusion is present, there must be positive cytologic test results to allot a case to stage IV. Parenchymal liver metastasis equals stage IV.*	

[a]FIGO, International Federation of Gynecology and Obstetrics.

mon type of epithelial cell malignancy of the ovary, constituting about 20% of all ovarian cancers. These tumors contain histologic features similar to endometrial carcinoma. Endometrioid tumors may arise in association with a primary endometrial carcinoma, making it difficult to determine whether they are primary to the ovary or metastatic from the endometrium. Only about 10% of these tumors are found in association with endometriosis, and even fewer are known to have progressed from benign endometriotic precursors.

Of the remaining epithelial cell carcinomas of the ovary, *clear cell carcinomas* are thought to arise from mesonephric elements and *Brenner tumors* are thought to arise uncommonly (less than 5%) from their benign counterpart. Interestingly, Brenner tumors occur approximately 10% of the time in the same ovary that contains mucinous cystadenoma; the reason for this is unclear.

Germ Cell Tumors

Germ cell tumors constitute less than 5% *of all ovarian malignancies.* However, they are *the most common ovarian cancers in women under the age of 20,* making up 60% of the malignant tumors discovered in this age group. Germ cell tumors may be functional, producing human chorionic gonadotropin (hCG) or α-fetoprotein (AFP), both of which can be used as tumor markers. The most common germ cell malignancies are *dysgerminoma and immature teratoma.* Other tumors are recognized as *mixed germ cell tumors, endodermal sinus tumors, and embryonal tumors.* There has been remarkable progress in treatment of this group of tumors in the last 10 years. Improved chemotherapeutic and radiation protocols have resulted in greatly improved 5-year survival rates.

Dysgerminomas are unilateral in about 90% of patients. They are the *most common type of germ cell tumor seen in patients with gonadal dysgenesis.* These tumors often arise in benign counterparts called the gonadoblastoma. The tumors are particularly *radiosensitive*, rendering adjunctive therapy efficacious.

Because of the young age of patients with dysgerminomas, removal of only the involved ovary with preservation of the uterus and contralateral tube and ovary may be considered if the tumor is less than approximately 10 cm and if there is no evidence of extraovarian spread. Unlike the epithelial cell tumors, these malignancies are more likely to spread via lymphatic channels, and therefore the pelvic and periaortic lymph nodes must be assessed carefully at the time of surgery. If disease has spread outside the ovaries, conventional hysterectomy and bilateral salpingo-oophorectomy are necessary, usually followed by postoperative radiation to the abdomen and pelvis. Chemotherapy is usually reserved for primary treatment failures. The prognosis of these tumors is generally excellent. The overall 5-year survival rate for patients with dysgerminoma is approximately 90–95% when the disease is limited to one ovary of less than 10 cm in size.

Immature teratomas are the malignant counterpart of benign cystic teratomas (dermoids). These are the *second most common germ cell cancer* and are *most often found in women under the age of 25.* They are usually unilateral, although on occasion a benign counterpart may be found in the contralateral ovary. Because these tumors are rapidly growing, they may produce painful symptomatology relatively early due to hemorrhage and necrosis during the rapid growth process. As a result, the diagnosis is made when the disease is limited to one ovary in two thirds of these young women. As with dysgerminoma, if an immature teratoma is limited to one ovary, unilateral oophorectomy is sufficient. The 5-year survival is over 80% for patients with well-differentiated tumors.

Rare Germ Cell Tumors. *Endodermal sinus tumor* and *embryonal cell carcinoma* are uncommon malignant ovarian tumors for which there has been a remarkable improvement in cure rate. Prior to 10 years ago, these tumors were almost uniformly fatal. New chemotherapeutic protocols have resulted in an overall 5-year survival of over 60%. These tumors typically occur in childhood and adolescence with the primary treatment being surgical resection of the involved ovary followed by combination chemotherapy. The endodermal sinus tumor produces α-fetoprotein, whereas the embryonal cell carcinoma produces both α-fetoprotein and β-hCG.

Gonadal Stromal Cell Tumors

This unusual group of tumors is characterized by hormone production, hence their designation as *functioning tumors.* The hormonal output from these tumors is usually in the form of female or male sex steroids or, on occasion, adrenal steroid hormones.

The *granulosa cell tumor is the most common in this group.* These tumors occur in all ages, although in older patients they are more likely to be benign. Granulosa call tumors *may secrete large amounts of estrogen*, which *in 15–20% of older women may cause endometrial hyperplasia or endometrial carcinoma.* Thus, endometrial sampling is especially important when ovarian tumors such as the granulosa tumor are estrogen producing. Measurement of estrogen levels as a reflection of tumor dissemination has not been found useful nor has follow-up of estrogen production been suggested as a useful tumor marker. The survival of patients with this neoplasm is contingent on factors similar to those for other tumors, in particular, whether or not the tumor has ruptured at the time of surgical exploration. Surgical treatment should include extirpation of the uterus and both ovaries in postmenopausal women as well as in women of reproductive age who no longer wish to remain fertile. In a young woman with the lesions limited to one ovary with an intact capsule, unilateral oophorectomy with careful surgical staging may be adequate. This tumor may demonstrate recurrences up to 10 years later. This is especially true with large tumors that have a 20–30% chance of late recurrence.

Sertoli-Leydig cell tumors (arrhenoblastoma) are the rare *testosterone-secreting counterparts to the granulosa cell tumor*. They usually occur in older patients and should be suspected in the differential diagnosis of peri- or postmenopausal patients with hirsutism or virilization and an adnexal mass. Treatment of these tumors is similar to that for other ovarian malignancies in this age group and is based on extirpation of uterus and ovaries.

Other stromal cell tumors include *fibromas* and *thecomas*, which very rarely demonstrate malignant counterparts, the *fibrosarcoma* and *malignant thecoma*.

Other Ovarian Malignancies

Very rarely, the ovary may be the site of initial manifestation of *lymphoma*. These are usually found in association with lymphoma elsewhere, although there have been case reports of primary ovarian lymphoma. Once the diagnosis has been made, management is similar to that for lymphoma of other origin.

Malignant mesodermal sarcomas are another rare type of ovarian tumor, which usually show aggressive behavior and are diagnosed at late stages. The survival rate is poor and clinical experience with these tumors is limited.

Cancer Metastatic to the Ovary

Classically, the term *Krukenberg tumor* describes an ovarian tumor that is metastatic from other sites such as the gastrointestinal tract, breast, and endometrium. Most of these tumors are bilateral and associated with widespread metastatic disease. Cancers metastatic to the ovary account for about 5–10% of ovarian malignancies. In 10% of patients with cancer metastatic to the ovary, an extraovarian primary site cannot be demonstrated. In this regard, it is important to consider ovarian preservation versus "prophylactic" oophorectomy at the time of hysterectomy in patients who have a strong family history (first-degree relatives) of epithelial ovarian cancer, primary gastrointestinal tract cancer, or breast cancer. In patients previously treated for cancer or gastrointestinal cancer, consideration should be given to the incidental removal of the ovaries at the time of hysterectomy because these patients have a high predilection for development of ovarian cancer.

FALLOPIAN TUBES

Normal fallopian tubes cannot be palpated and are generally not considered in the differential diagnosis of adnexal disease *in the asymptomatic patient*. There are common problems involving the fallopian tubes, including ectopic pregnancy, salpingitis/hydrosalpinx/tubo-ovarian abscess, and endometriosis, but these are generally symptomatic.

Primary fallopian tube carcinoma is rare, accounting for less than 1% of all gynecologic cancers. It is *usually diagnosed at laparotomy* when surgery is performed for other indications since a tubal neoplasm cannot be differentiated from other adnexal masses by history or physical examination. As in ovarian cancer, patients may have a history of vague, chronic, lower abdominal pain or they may be asymptomatic. Progression is also *similar to ovarian carcinoma*, with intraperitoneal metastases and ascites. Histologically, these tumors are most usually similar to serous cystadenocarcinoma of the ovary. Surgical and/or adjunctive treatment is similar to that for ovarian cancer also. The 70% 5-year survival for stage I disease is not as good as that for stage I ovarian serous tumors.

GENERAL PRINCIPLES IN THE SURGICAL MANAGEMENT OF OVARIAN AND FALLOPIAN TUBE MALIGNANCY

Primary surgical therapy is indicated in the majority of ovarian malignancies regardless of stage. This surgery is based on the principle of *cytoreductive surgery, or "tumor debulking"*. The rationale for cytoreductive surgery is that adjunctive radiotherapy and chemotherapy are more effective when all tumor masses are reduced to less than 1 cm in size (see Chapter 40, "Cell Biology and Principles of Cancer Therapy"). Because direct peritoneal seeding is the primary method of intraperitoneal spread, multiple adjacent structures commonly contain tumor, resulting in cytoreductive procedures that are often quite extensive. Each procedure includes:

1. Peritoneal cytology is obtained; this is used to assess microscopic spread of tumor. Samples are taken immediately after entering the abdomen before extensive surgery has been undertaken. Gross ascites is aspirated and submitted for cytologic analysis. If there is no gross ascites, saline irrigation is used to "wash" the peritoneal cavity in an attempt to find microscopic disease. The "wash" is then submitted for cytologic assessment.
2. To visually and by palpation determine the extent of disease, thorough inspection and palpation is done, including the uterus, fallopian tubes and ovaries, surfaces of the pelvis, the right and left pericolic gutters, the omentum, the upper abdominal viscera including the surface of the liver and spleen, and the undersurface of the diaphragm.
3. Partial omentectomy is usually performed, with or without gross evidence of tumor involvement.
4. Sampling of the pelvic and periaortic lymph nodes is done, especially in earlier stage disease of stromal cell and germ cell tumors, which have a higher likelihood of lymphatic spread. In the absence of gross disease, biopsies are obtained from the pelvic peritoneum and peritoneum of the right and left upper and lower pericolic gutters.

Based on the histologic evaluation of all samples, a rational program of adjunctive radio- or chemotherapy may be undertaken.

Follow-up currently consists of clinical history and examination, various imaging studies such as ultrasound and/or CT, and in epithelial cell tumors, the use of serum tumor markers such as Ca 125. One other area of special consideration for ovarian cancer patients is the *second look laparotomy*. This procedure is reserved for patients who have no clinically evident disease after the completion of primary surgical therapy and a standard course of adjunctive chemotherapy. If the patient has been rendered clear of gross disease at the time of surgery, and if she has undergone a course of standard chemotherapy for presumed microscopic residual disease, it is often difficult to know whether residual disease remains. Therefore, many ovarian cancer treatment protocols include second look laparotomy to ascertain if residual disease remains.

FURTHER READINGS

Clarke-Pearson D, Dawood MY. Green's gynecology: essentials of clinical practice. 8th ed. Boston: Little, Brown & Co, 1990.

DiSaia PJ, Creasman WT. Clinical gynecologic oncology. 3rd ed. St. Louis, MO: CV Mosby, 1989.

Herbst AL, Mishell DR, Stenchever MA, Droegemueller W. Comprehensive gynecology. 2nd ed. St. Louis, MO: CV Mosby, 1992.

SELF-EVALUATION

Case 45-A

A 23-year-old G1P1001 describes a new, crampy pain in her right pelvis over the last 3 days. Her LMP was 3 weeks ago and was normal. She uses a diaphragm for contraception and her urine pregnancy test is negative. On pelvic examination a 3 × 4 cm tender cystic mass is found in the right adnexa. The remainder of her examination is normal.

Question 45-A-1

The best management at this time would be to schedule:

A. a return visit in 1 week
B. a return visit to the office in 2 months
C. a return visit to the office in 1 year
D. a diagnostic laparoscopy
E. an exploratory laparotomy

Answer 45-A-1

Answer: B

Although the differential diagnosis includes various tumors and benign gynecologic pathology, the most likely diagnosis is a "functional" ovarian cyst, i.e., a follicular or corpus luteum cyst. A return visit is necessary, as a functional cyst will resolve, whereas other pathology will not; 2 months is a reasonable time, whereas 1 year is too long. Surgical intervention is far too aggressive a measure at this time. Transvaginal or transabdominal ultrasound will provide additional information as to size and consistency of the mass and should be ordered on a case-by-case basis.

Question 45-A-2

Which medications are appropriate for this patient at this time?

A. oral contraceptives
B. oral progesterone
C. oral estrogen
D. GnRH agonist
E. oral doxycycline

Answer 45-A-2

Answer: A

Gonadotropin suppression with oral contraceptives can be used in a patient with a functional ovarian cyst, although this is not a "required" management. It would be particularly appropriate if the patient were to express a desire to switch to oral contraceptive pills for contraception purposes also. Indeed, no medication, i.e., watchful expectation, would also be an acceptable management. Progesterone and estrogen would not aid in cyst resolution. No evidence of infection was given, hence antibiotic therapy is not indicated. GnRH agonist would eliminate gonadotropin stimulation of the ovary, but would be overtreating this clinical situation.

Question 45-A-3

The mass persists after 2 months of oral contraceptive therapy; in fact, it is now 2 cm larger. Ultrasound examination confirms a cystic mass. Ca 125 is within normal ranges, as are all other laboratory evaluations.

At exploratory laparotomy, a cystic mass is found without any other pelvic abnormalities.

An ovarian cystectomy is performed. The final pathology report is: serous epithelial tumor of low malignant potential.

For further consideration: What are the implications of this finding? What is the risk of actual cancer for this patient? What is the best course of action? Observation? CAT scan? Second look laparotomy? Hysterectomy and bilateral salpingo-oophorectomy; and if so, when?

Case 45-B

A 53-year-old woman notices increased facial and body hair and a deepening tone of voice. On physical examination, the patient has considerable coarse facial hair and a 3 × 4 cm, firm left adnexal mass.

Question 45-B-1

The serum concentration of which of the following hormones would most likely be elevated?

A. hCG
B. progesterone
C. estradiol
D. testosterone

Answer 45-B-1

Answer: D

The history and physical examination are most consistent with a Sertoli-Leydig cell tumor, the rare testosterone-secreting counterpart to the granulosa cell tumor.

Question 45-B-2

The best management at this time would be to schedule:

A. a transvaginal pelvic ultrasound examination
B. a return visit to the office in 2 months
C. a return visit to the office in 1 year
D. a diagnostic laparoscopy
E. an exploratory laparotomy

Answer 45-B-2

Answer: E

Exploratory laparotomy and total abdominal hysterectomy with bilateral salpingo-oophorectomy are indicated. Temporizing with a probable ovarian malignancy in a post-menopausal patient is not appropriate. Ultrasound evaluation might offer more information about the characteristics of the adnexal mass, but would not alter the surgical management.

Question 45-B-3

For further consideration: Assuming a Sertoli-Leydig cell tumor is found and removed, what advice should be offered this patient about her hirsutism? About her deepened voice? About the risk of other malignancy?

chapter 46

GESTATIONAL TROPHOBLASTIC DISEASE

Gestational trophoblastic neoplasia (GTN), which represents *a rare variation of pregnancy*, is limited in most instances to a benign disease called *molar pregnancy*. This disorder includes neoplasms that are derived almost entirely from abnormal placental (trophoblastic) proliferation. Molar pregnancy may in turn be divided into *complete mole* (no fetus) and *incomplete mole* (fetus plus molar degeneration). Fewer than 10% of patients with GTN will develop persistent or malignant disease. Fortunately, persistent or malignant GTN is very responsive to effective chemotherapy.

Key features of gestational trophoblastic neoplasia include: its consistent clinical presentation; reliable means of diagnosis with pathognomonic ultrasound findings; presence of specific tumor marker (quantitative serum hCG); availability of effective surgical treatment; sensitivity to chemotherapy when GTN is persistent or malignant; and reliable long-term follow-up through assessment of quantitative hCG levels.

The disease has a number of *characteristic features* including: (*a*) the potential for malignant transformation, (*b*) clinical presentation as a pregnancy, (*c*) profound hormonal changes found in association with the abnormal proliferation of trophoblastic tissue, (*d*) genetic makeup, and (*e*) and high sensitivity to chemotherapeutic agents.

The *etiology* of this disorder is unknown. It has been observed that the incidence varies among different national and ethnic groups with the highest occurring among oriental women living in Asia (up to 1 in 200 pregnancies) and the lowest incidence occurring in Caucasian women of Western European and United States origins (approximately 1 in 2000 pregnancies). The recurrence rate is approximately 2%. It is more common in very young women and in women at the end of their reproductive years. It is associated with dietary deficiencies, such as folic acid. The classification of gestational trophoblastic disease is described in Table 46.1. Since persistent gestational trophoblastic neoplasia may follow simple molar pregnancy, an appreciation of the latter's clinical presentation, histology, clinical risk factors, and long-term follow-up are necessary to thoroughly treat the patient with this unusual tumor.

HYDATIDIFORM MOLE (MOLAR PREGNANCY)

A complete hydatidiform mole includes abnormal proliferation of the syncytiotrophoblast and replacement of normal placental trophoblastic tissue by *hydropic placental villi*. Complete moles do not include the formation of a fetus, and fetal membranes are characteristically absent. *Partial moles* are characterized by focal trophoblastic proliferation and degeneration of the placenta and are associated with a chromosomally abnormal fe-

Table 46.1
Classification of Gestational Trophoblastic Disease

Molar pregnancy
  Complete mole
  Partial mole
Persistent gestational trophoblastic neoplasia
  Histologically benign
  Persistent-histologically benign
  Persistent-histologically malignant

427

tus. In this form of molar pregnancy, trophoblastic proliferation is largely from the cytotrophoblast.

The *genetic constitution* of these two types of molar pregnancy is different. Complete moles are entirely of paternal origin as a result of the fertilization of a blighted ovum by a haploid sperm, which then reduplicates. Accordingly, the karyotype of a complete mole is 46,XX. The fetus of a partial mole is usually a triploidy, the most common being 69,XXY. The triploidy is comprised of one haploid set of maternal chromosomes and two haploid sets of paternal chromosomes, which arise from dispermic fertilization. Of the two varieties, the complete mole is more common (approximately 90% of molar pregnancies). Although the potential for malignant transformation is greater in complete moles, partial moles may also undergo this change and, therefore, both varieties should be followed in a similar fashion to minimize the chance for malignant sequelae.

Clinical Presentation

Clinically, patients with molar pregnancy of either variety may present with findings consistent with pregnancy but also with uterine size/dates discrepancy, exaggerated subjective symptoms of pregnancy, and bleeding suggestive of spontaneous abortion. Of these symptoms, *bleeding* is the most characteristic and occurs in most patients early in the second trimester of pregnancy. The bleeding is usually painless. The patient also may experience the passage of tissue as fragments of the edematous trophoblast are passed through the dilated cervical os. Most patients have already been *diagnosed as pregnant*, having had a positive pregnancy test. There is a *uterine dates/size discrepancy* in two thirds of patients. The uterus may be either too large or too small for gestational age, usually larger than expected. This discrepancy, coupled with late first or early second trimester bleeding, usually leads the clinician to perform ultrasound imaging of the uterus, which confirms the di-

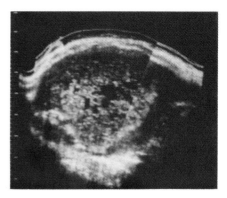

Figure 46.1. "Snowstorm" appearance of complete mole on ultrasound examination.

agnosis of molar pregnancy by its characteristic "snowstorm" appearance (Fig. 46.1).

Molar pregnancies may present with *other signs and symptoms* including visual disturbances, severe nausea and vomiting, marked pregnancy-induced hypertension (preeclampsia), proteinuria, and rarely, clinical hyperthyroidism. Some patients experience tachycardia and shortness of breath arising from intense hemodynamic changes to associated acute hypertensive changes. In these patients hyperflexia may also be found. Physical examination reveals not only the dates/size discrepancy of the uterine fundus and absent fetal heart tones, but also changes associated with developing preeclampsia. Occasionally, bimanual pelvic examination may reveal large *adnexal masses* (theca lutein cysts), which represent marked enlargement of the ovaries as a result of high levels of hCG stimulation.

The clinical presentation of partial molar pregnancy is similar to those for complete mole, although typically the patient presents at a more advanced gestational age (after the 20th week of pregnancy). Vaginal bleeding is less common than with complete moles. Uterine growth that is less than that expected for the gestational age, especially if coupled with rapidly developing hypertension, may be the first clinical indication. Because of the growth/dates discrepancy, ultrasonography is obtained, which reveals molar degeneration of the placenta and frequently a grossly abnormal fetus.

Laboratory Assessment

The laboratory assessment of molar pregnancy is critical for both treatment and follow-up. After the molar pregnancy has been confirmed by imaging studies, laboratory documentation is necessary to ascertain *the level of hCG*. These levels are extremely high in molar pregnancy and not only *help classify risk category but also serve as a sensitive tumor marker in the long-term follow-up* of these patients. In addition, other valuable studies include a baseline chest x-ray to check for metastatic disease, assessment of hemoglobin and hematocrit, and selected other tests, depending on whether or not the patient has signs of preeclampsia and/or hyperthyroidism. Prior to treatment, blood should be obtained for blood type and Rh and screened for antibodies in case blood replacement is necessary. This is particularly important for patients who undergo uterine evacuation, as there is the significant potential for extensive blood loss during the procedures. Similar laboratory studies should be obtained whether the patient has partial or complete mole.

Treatment

In most cases of *molar pregnancy*, the definitive treatment is prompt *removal of the intrauterine contents*. Uterine evacuation is done most expeditiously by dilation of the cervix followed by *suction curettage*. After suction curettage with an atraumatic plastic cannula, *gentle sharp curettage* may be performed to provide small amounts of myometrial tissue for separate pathologic assessment. This is used to ascertain whether there has been myometrial invasion.

In cases of *partial mole*, a similar procedure may be carried out, with the additional need for larger grasping instruments to remove the abnormal fetus. With cases involving enlargement of the uterus beyond 24 weeks gestational size, an alternative to suction evacuation is induction of labor with

Table 46.2
Conditions That Define High Risk Gestational Trophoblastic Disease

Uterus >16 week size
Theca-lutein cysts
Marked trophoblastic proliferation and/or anaplasia
Hyperthyroidism

prostaglandin vaginal suppositories. In general, *the larger the uterus, the greater the risk of pulmonary complications* associated with trophoblastic emboli, fluid overload, and anemia. This is particularly true in patients with extreme degrees of associated pregnancy-induced hypertension (preeclampsia) since patients may experience concomitant hemoconcentration and alteration in vascular hemodynamics. In these patients, uterine evacuation by prostaglandin stimulation may be safer.

Occasional patients in the older reproductive age group may be best served by hysterectomy, which assures removal of the entire primary neoplasm. This is especially true in patients with "high risk" disease as described in Table 46.2. This treatment should be reserved for patients who have no interest in further childbearing and/or have other indications for hysterectomy.

The *bilaterally enlarged multicystic ovaries (theca-lutein cysts)*, arising from massive follicular stimulation by large amounts of systemic hCG, do not represent malignant changes. This enlargement invariably regresses after the molar pregnancy has been evacuated, and, therefore, *does not* require surgical removal. This is especially important in the patient undergoing abdominal hysterectomy as the primary treatment.

Postevacuation Management

Because of the predisposition for recurrent nonmalignant or malignant disease, patients should be followed closely for at least 1 year. *The removed molar tissue* should be examined carefully to identify hyperplastic and/or anaplastic proliferation. The small tissue sample

Table 46.3
Posttreatment Follow-up for Molar Pregnancy

General physical and pelvic examination and
    baseline chest x-ray at 2 weeks
Serum quantitative hCG level every 2 weeks until
    normal (0–5 mIU)
Serum quantitative hCG monthly for 1 year after
    obtaining first normal level
Assurance of contraception for 1 year (oral
    contraceptives preferred unless contraindicated)
Early ultrasound examination and quantitative hCG
    level for future pregnancy

Table 46.4
Clinical Classification of Malignant GTN

Nonmetastatic GTD (not defined in terms of good
    versus poor prognosis)
Metastatic GTD
    Good prognosis: absence of high risk factors
      Pretreatment hCG level <40,000 mIU/ml
        serum β-hCG
      <4-months' duration of disease
      No evidence of brain or liver metastasis
      No significant prior chemotherapy
      No antecedent term pregnancy
    Poor prognosis: any single high risk factor
      Pretreatment hCG level >40,000 mIU/ml
        serum β-hCG
      >4-months' duration of disease
      Brain and/or liver metastases
      Failed prior chemotherapy
      Antecedent term pregnancy

provided by the sharp curettage specimen obtained after removal of the bulk of the mole is especially useful for the pathologic examination. RhoGAM should be given as indicated in a normal pregnancy.

Follow-up consists primarily of *periodic physical examination* including pelvic examination and the *assessment of quantitative hCG levels* according to the schedule outlined in Table 46.3. Following these guidelines assures the physician: that recurrent disease is not developing; that an intercurrent pregnancy (within 1 year) is not causing an increase in hCG levels; and that with future pregnancy, another molar pregnancy is ruled out early since the recurrence rate for these patients is approximately 5 times the initial

rate (1 in 400 in the United States). Effective contraception is recommended in the first year of follow-up.

METASTATIC/MALIGNANT GESTATIONAL TROPHOBLASTIC NEOPLASIA

Recurrent benign gestational trophoblastic neoplasia and/or malignant transformation of this disease *(choriocarcinoma)* occurs in less than 10% of patients with antecedent molar pregnancy. Early identification and treatment of recurrence is critically important. Failure of quantitative hCG levels to regress suggests that further therapy is needed. Common sites of persistent or metastatic disease include the uterus, adjacent pelvic structures, the lungs, and the brain. Treatment of persistent gestational trophoblastic disease may involve the use of a number of potentially effective chemotherapeutic agents. What should be remembered is that gestational trophoblastic neoplasia, even in its malignant form, is highly sensitive to chemotherapy and is considered a "prototype" for tumors that are sensitive to these agents.

Generally, nonmetastatic persistent gestational trophoblastic neoplasia is completely treated by single agent chemotherapy. The prognosis for malignant GTN is more complex, divided into good and poor prognosis categories as seen in Table 46.4. The World Health Organization (WHO) has developed a prognostic scoring system for gestational trophoblastic neoplasia, which takes into account a number of epidemiologic and laboratory findings (Table 46.5). Chemotherapeutic agents used include both single agent treatment with methotrexate and dactinomycin or a combination chemotherapy, which includes methotrexate/dactinomycin/chlorambucil (MAC). Other chemotherapeutic agents are being tested and may be effective as well. Where chemotherapy is indicated, the treatment protocol depends on whether patients fall into the "good prognosis" metastatic group or the "poor prognosis" metastatic group.

Table 46.5
WHO Prognostic Scoring System for Gestational Trophoblastic Disease[a]

Prognostic factor	Score[b]			
	0	1	2	4
Age	≤39	>39		
Antecedent pregnancy	HM	Abortion; ectopic	Term	
Interval (months)[c]	<4	4–6	7–12	>12
hCG level (IU/liter)	<10^3	10^3–10^4	10^4–10^5	>10^5
ABO blood groups (female × male)		O × A	B	
		A × O	AB	
Largest tumor (cm)	<3	3–5	>5	
Site of metastasis		Spleen, kidney	GI tract, liver	Brain
Number of metastases		1–3	4–8	>8
Prior chemotherapy			Single drug	Multiple drugs

[a]WHO, World Health Organization; HM, hydatidiform mole; GI, gastrointestinal.
[b]Low risk, ≤4; intermediate risk, 5–7; high risk, ≥8.
[c]Interval: time between antecedent pregnancy and start of chemotherapy.

FURTHER READINGS

Herbst AL. Gestational trophoblastic disease. In: Herbst AL, Mishell DR, Stenchever MA, Droegemueller W, eds. Comprehensive gynecology. St. Louis, MO: CV Mosby, 1992:1043.

Soper JT. Gestational trophoblastic disease. In: Clarke-Pearson DL, Dawood MY, eds. Green's gynecology: essentials of clinical practice, 8th ed. Boston: Little, Brown & Co, 1990:565–574.

SELF-EVALUATION

Case 46-A

A 38-year-old woman presents for prenatal care. Her last normal menstrual period was approximately 3 months ago. For the past 5 or 6 days, she has experienced light vaginal spotting, and she has been bothered by rather intense "morning sickness" for the past 4 weeks. She has been able to tolerate fluids and a few small meals, but generally does not have a normal appetite.

Physical examination reveals a blood pressure of 150/100, urine shows 3+ protein, the uterine fundus measures approximately 16 week size, and there is an absence of fetal heart tones as assessed by ultrasound. Pelvic examination shows the cervix to be fingertip dilated with a small amount of blood at the os. Bimanual examination confirms an enlarged uterus consistent with approximately 16 week size, and there is a suggestion of bilateral adnexal masses.

Question 46-A-1

Which of the following should be done immediately?

A. Obtain quantitative serum hCG.
B. Obtain pelvic ultrasound.
C. Begin 24-hour urine collection for total protein.
D. Obtain fetal heart rate reading with fetal monitor.
E. Initiate hypertension workup.

Answer 46-A-1

Answer: A, B

This problem typifies a number of features of molar pregnancy including uterine dates/size discrepancy, acute pregnancy-induced hypertension (preeclampsia), absence of fetal development, and bilateral theca-lutein cysts. The diagnosis can be most readily made by obtaining an ultrasound. This should be done first to confirm the diagnosis, after which treatment will include treatment of the preeclampsia to prevent seizures and plans for expeditious uterine evacuation. A quantitative serum β-hCG is drawn as a baseline value, to which postevacuation β-hCG evacuations may be compared.

Case 46-B

A 22-year-old woman returns for her fourth postoperative follow-up examination since undergoing a suction curettage for an incomplete mole (trophoblastic degeneration of the triploidy fetus) 5 weeks ago. The initial quantitative hCG titer drawn at the time of her diagnosis was 40,000 mIU. The serum titer drawn 2 weeks ago was 1,500 mIU. The serum titer obtained yesterday shows a quantitative hCG level of 4,500 mIU.

Question 46-B-1

The most appropriate therapy at this point should be:

A. a simple hysterectomy
B. hysterectomy and bilateral salpingo-oophorectomy
C. radiation therapy
D. dilation and curettage
E. chemotherapy

Answer 46-B-1

Answer: D, then E

This case is typical of a patient with persistent trophoblastic disease, as illustrated by rapidly falling serum β-hCG titers followed by resurgence a few weeks later. Given her young age and low risk category, single agent chemotherapy is most appropriate to treat this problem. Prior to beginning chemotherapy, she should have another dilation and curettage to obtain enough tissue to characterize the type of persistent trophoblast. It should be remembered, however, that dilation and curettage may not always reveal the presence of persistent trophoblast since it can be present outside the uterine cavity and/or in metastatic sites.

chapter 47

ETHICS IN OBSTETRICS AND GYNECOLOGY

Ethics in obstetrics and gynecology has some unique characteristics that are illustrated by the following cases.

First Case: A Jehovah's Witness, hemorraging from a placenta previa, who needs a cesarean section. Do we give blood against the patient's expressed wishes (a form of battery), even to save her life? Do we allow her to die while we deliver her child safely—motherless?

Second Case: A pregnant woman who uses cocaine. Should the mother-to-be who uses cocaine be held accountable for the condition (including death) of her unborn child?

Third Case: A markedly neurotic child-abusing mother with several children who refuses contraception. Should we require contraceptive Norplant implants for this woman?

Fourth Case: A 33-year-old woman dying of cervical cancer who has been given a high dose of morphine to try to abate her increasing and prolonged pain, but whose respirations have dropped to 3/minute. Should we give her a narcotic antagonist or let her die, a side effect of the medication for her intractable pain?

The ethical quandaries demonstrated in these four cases present a challenge to clarify the way we think about ethical problems in medicine that is relevant to whatever area of medicine is eventually chosen as a specialty.

There is a substantial literature that presents methods of thinking about ethical issues, which is quite helpful. By utilizing this literature, you will not be solely dependent upon your personal reaction to a problem or upon your intuition. Indeed, the use of ethical principles allows us to make better medical choices by standing back and reflecting on these problems rather than either by not dealing with them or by reacting randomly based on emotions, personal bias, or social pressures.

How can you identify the basic ethical dilemmas of a case? What sort of systematic approach is helpful? The answers to these questions are illustrated by detailed analysis of the first case.

A 24-year-old G2P1001 Jehovah's Witness with a complete placenta previa is transferred from the antepartum care unit to labor and delivery with the onset of bleeding (two cups of bright red blood over 10 minutes). Her husband, also a Jehovah's Witness, and her mother who is not a member of that group accompany her. She rapidly loses one liter of blood, and evidence of fetal distress is found on the electronic fetal monitor. She reaffirms her absolute refusal of blood or blood products even though an emergency cesarean section is proposed for her own and her fetus's survival. Her blood pressure is dropping despite rapid hydration. She becomes unconscious. The anesthesiologist says she will probably die with the insults of anesthesia and surgery without blood transfusion. The patient's mother demands that you give her daughter blood. The husband refuses. The fetal heart tracing demonstrates severe fetal distress consistent with profound fetal damage or death, and you begin the cesarean section and deliver a healthy 7 pound girl with Apgar scores of 2 and then 8 with resuscitation. The mother survives the surgery, but in recovery her blood pressure drops to 50/0 postoper-

Table 47.1
Areas of Concern and Associated Ethical Principles in Clinical Medical Ethics: A Functional Scheme for Clinical Ethical Decision Making

Ethical concern:	MEDICAL INDICATION What is the best treatment? What are the alternatives?		Ethical concern:	PATIENT PREFERENCES What does the patient want?
Ethical principle:	BENEFICENCE The duty to promote the good of the patient		Ethical principle:	AUTONOMY Respect for the patient's right to self-determination
Ethical concern:	QUALITY OF LIFE What impact will the proposed treatment or lack of it have on the patient's life?		Ethical principle:	SOCIOECONOMIC ISSUES What does the patient want? What are the needs of society?
Ethical principle:	NONMALEFICENCE The duty not to inflict harm or injury		Ethical principle:	JUSTICE The patient should be given what is "due."

atively, and she remains unconscious and on a ventilator with a central venous pressure of 0. The patient's mother screams, "You are killing her! She is my only child!" Her husband firmly reminds you of the religious beliefs he and his wife share and warns you that his attorney is available if needed. What is the right thing to do?

The first step is to try to separate this emotional case into ethically separate concerns. An analytical scheme (Table 47.1) from the book *Clinical Ethics* is useful for this purpose. Separating a case into four areas of concern allows us to fit each particular problem in a "family" of ethical issues that are associated with particular principles central to medical ethics. This process of systematic analysis and reflection is medical ethics.

Considering the first case, we could ask, "What was the *medical indication* for the cesarean section?" Clearly, both child and mother would die without surgery. Continuing acute hemorrhage from placenta previa has no potential therapy other than surgical delivery and removal of the placenta. Support of the cardiovascular system with blood products is medically indicated. Yet, this patient has clearly stated her *preference*: she will not accept blood products, both while no acute problem is present or after. She believes that blood is directly opposed to God's will and that receiving blood, even against

her wishes, will permanently and negatively affect her spiritual self. She does not feel life under such circumstances (i.e., after receiving blood) to be acceptable. Blood transfusion is more likely to produce a better quality of life, that is, survival without neurologic or major organ sequelae. Without blood products her survival is questionable, and even with survival her risk for prolonged ICU stay, cardiac failure, renal failure, and hematologic sequelae are much greater. Considering *socioeconomic issues*, we wonder how this newborn child will do without her mother. In addition, what is the validity of the cost of care in an ICU for the sequelae resulting from the patient's choice when other patients need the ICU bed? What about the grandmother's concerns? Is the husband coercing the patient to not accept blood? Is he coercing the physician with comments about his attorney, or is that his right to protect his wife? What would the law say if we gave the patient blood without permission?

The first case is complex, but it is clear that the patient's choice to refuse blood products is an underlying issue. Does this patient's autonomous refusal constitute a real choice, and if so, should we accept it? While the law has much to say about the rights of individuals to choose or refuse care, the choice here to not give blood is based on the great respect for the right of patients to determine their care that medical ethics has supported. There is much literature regarding autonomy and refusal of blood products that can be accessed to illuminate these choices.

In more general terms, the medical indications for a proposed management always need to be as clear and as "scientific" as possible. Is the benefit of what is proposed clearly greater than the harm that might be caused or is the benefit at a level that makes the harm acceptable? Consider the fourth case—the 33 year old dying slowly of cervical cancer. She is at risk from the pain medication needed to alleviate her suffering. Is the relief of pain so great a benefit that the decreased respiratory rate and potential respiratory arrest are acceptable? Consider the third case—the mother who refuses contraception yet abuses her children. Is Norplant medically indicated for the child-abusing patient? Does she have a medical contraindication to its use? Remember that before proceeding with a proposed treatment, the benefit to the patient must be clear. If the benefit is unclear but the treatment ongoing, the issues are still more complex. Consider a variation in the case of the patient with cervical cancer. She is also not able to eat because of the pain and the family requests TPN. It will make them "feel better about things." Many would consider that TPN was medically futile and question the ethics of its continued use. The group of cases related to *medical indications* involve such concerns as benefit (or *beneficence*) and the related concept of futility.

The cases that can be categorized under *patient preferences* revolve around the principle of *autonomy*, the respect we hold for the patient's right to choose care. It is important to note that the physician-patient relationship emphasizes a relationship between *the* physician and *the* patient. Even in obstetrics, where the consequences of patient choices on another potential life can be significant, the primacy of the physician-patient (versus physician-fetus relationship) is paramount. What the patient wants and her capacity to make those choices are in question here. Consider the second case: Does the drug-using mother have the capacity to make decisions about her unborn child? By reason of the effect of the drugs, has she lost the capacity for acceptable decision making? Is society bound by her decision making? What about the rights of the unborn child? Consider the fourth case: Is the dying patient whose mentation is potentially clouded by impending death and the medications used for pain relief capable of decisions about her care?

Quality of life issues are always important. The absence of pain in a terminal cancer patient may significantly improve the quality of her living, even if the length of time is shortened. Some patients may consider the diminution of quality of life with potential permanent neurologic damage or loss of time with children arising as a result of blood loss (as in the first case) so significant that they will accept blood despite their religious beliefs. So the harms of treatment or no treatment framed in the context of a particular patient's life are what must be considered. In a sense, this deals with *nonmaleficence*: the duty to not harm patients while treating them. Harm clearly must be framed in the patient's circumstances. In the fourth case, prolonged life may not be valued if significant pain or a elongated hospital stay are the quality of life that must be accepted. That becomes unacceptable "harm" to that patient. Yet, as in the first case, the quality of life after blood transfusion may be acceptable for the added time to be spent with her children and the diminished risk of major organ damage. The benefits of proposed therapy must be framed in the outcome of that therapy for good or ill.

Finally, all the *socioeconomic issues* that surround a particular case should be considered. It is here that the concerns of the children and mother and father and other relatives, and concerns about legal issues and issues of cost, are addressed. Threats to sue, angry families, and "dumping" of patients without health insurance or money to pay for health care, as examples, can so overwhelm the health care team that the real ethical issues of a case (for example, the capacity to choose or futility) are not considered. Socioeconomic issues, while important in making final choices about care, generally should not override clear medical indications or clear patient preferences. When socioeconomic considerations are deeply divided from what is medically indicated or what a patient prefers, they cause problems. For example, in the fourth case, the 33-year-old mother cannot die at home near her children because of medical cost regulations, and in the first case, the sequelae of refused blood products and prolonged ICU stay deny a bed to a patient with complications of leukemia therapy so that this care has to be delivered in another institution away from trusted physicians. These outcomes appear unfair or unjust and illustrate cases dealing with the ethical principle of *justice*, and how to determine allocation of resources.

What are the unique ethical problems of obstetrics and gynecology? Clearly, maternal and fetal conflicts and how we define procreation and family are uniquely poignant in obstetrics and gynecology.

The primary concern of physicians is the best care of their patients. This has been true since Hippocrates admonished us "to do away with the suffering of the sick." Special interest groups have variously defined the "rights" of the fetus so that, at times, the primacy of duty to the patient (mother) seems in question. Yet there never has been a time in the development of medical ethics or in the opinions expressed by the American College of Obstetricians and Gynecologists that the fetus is considered to take precedence over the mother in considerations of medical care or the therapeutic alliance of physician and patient. This is valuable to keep in mind when considering these problems.

Abortion would be the first example of these considerations, where the controversy can be so emotional and damaging that an ethical discussion cannot occur. Consistent with our primary duty to the patient, those circumstances where survival of the mother would be seriously compromised by the maintenance of pregnancy are the least controversial. Clearly, preservation of the patient-mother's life and loss of the fetus would

be supported by many viewers. As the "case" gets further away from this clearer situation, the discussion becomes more complex. It is valuable to explore what we define as "human" before we define loss of a fetus as loss of a human life. What are elements of humanness and when are they achieved in pregnancy? Is ability to survive independent of the mother significant? Is the potential to achieve those elements defining "human" pertinent? These are important issues to explore before considering, for example, a case such as elective abortion at 12 weeks or selective pregnancy reduction.

Defining these issues also helps in consideration of the "rights" of pregnant women to engage in behavior or activities that put the fetus at some risk, such as use of cocaine, alcohol, smoking, or refusal of cesarean section for fetal indication. At what level of "human" development or potential, if at all, does concern for fetal outcomes override the patient-mother's autonomous choices? In what sort of case might we reasonably override expressed patient wishes in order to preserve fetal life? For example, how does drug use interact with capacity to choose? Consider the second case: Is the drug-using mother's decision to continue to use drugs during pregnancy acceptable? Is an acutely intoxicated mother's decision to refuse cesarean section for fetal indications acceptable?

Looking at the many changes in reproductive endocrinology, the idea of a clearest case may help sort out the ethical discussions. What, for example, is the clearest set of relationships between parents and children? Biologically, the relationship between mother donating the egg and a father donating the sperm in vivo without augmentation is the paradigm case. The relationship of this family unit, with the parental responsibilities for financial support, history, culture, and education has been the traditional paradigm for family in our culture. How these elements change with a group of cases will vary. Adoption by mother/father pair; adoption by single parent; adoption by two mothers or two fathers; in vitro combination of egg from mother and father; in vitro combination of unrelated sperm with the maternal egg; or the varieties of gestational pattern with surrogacy and egg and sperm donation are all variations on the original theme. How far from our paradigm family is acceptable? Why? What do we do with the "extra" fertilized or harvested eggs from IVF? How is this different or the same as the issue of humanness or potential for humanness that we raised when discussing abortion?

SUMMARY

In obstetrics-gynecology, as in all medicine, there is potential to utilize the skills and concepts of medical ethics. To do so requires methods of systematic reflection to delineate the ethical problems and to analyze these problems further. The analytical framework described in Table 47.1 helps identify ethical issues, placing them in specific areas, associating them with some principles and families of cases. Further analysis comparing a case to a "paradigm" case, may be helpful. Finally, obtaining recent papers on the issues from MED-ETHX in Medline or the medical library will bring together varying authors' views on the ethical issues surrounding a given clinical situation.

FURTHER READINGS

Association of Professors of Gynecology and Obstetrics. Exploring issues in obstetrics and gynecology: medical ethics, 1990.

Jonsen A, Siegler M, Winslade W. Clinical ethics. New York: Macmillan, 1982.

Levine C, ed. Cases in bioethics: selections from the Hasting Center report New York: St. Martin's Press, 1989.

Veatch RM. Medical ethics. New York: Jones and Bartless, 1989.

SELF-EVALUATION

There are no clear answers in medical ethics, only questions to which we should apply a logical scheme for analysis in order to make best decisions possible.

Consider the following situations. Apply the decision matrix presented in this chapter to decide how YOU would analyze each.

Case 47-A

Your patient is a 28-year-old G3P3003 whose ethnic background and religious views place high value on a male offspring. She has had three girls. She is now 12 weeks pregnant and requests you test for gender and abort a female pregnancy. She notes she must have a son for her husband and can barely afford a fourth child in any event.

Do you do the test? Do you abort the pregnancy if it is female? If you do and she returns with another pregnancy, do you continue the process to its logical conclusion: a male fetus or a complication so that further pregnancy is not possible? What if the husband insists? What if the mother is unsure? What if her attorney reminds you that it is her body, not yours, and her decision? What if your attorney reminds you that the public relations outcome of this case stinks either way you choose?

Case 47-B

A 26-year-old G7P6006 arrives at an estimated 37–41 weeks gestation in labor. She has had no prenatal case. She is an abuser of drugs and alcohol and is high on cocaine she ingested just before entering the hospital. When placed on an electronic fetal monitor with external probes, decelerations are noted but the patient will not permit adjustment of the tocodynamometer to allow characterization of the decelerations, nor will she permit rupture of membranes for placement of a scalp clip. What do you do? A cesarean section because you cannot evaluate the fetus effectively and it may be in distress? Wait and see if the patient will calm down and allow appropriate fetal assessment? Is the patient competent to make decisions having just taken cocaine? Does the fetus have a right to a "good birth?" If you let the patient labor and deliver vaginally and the baby is brain damaged, are you liable? If you do a cesarean section and the baby is O.K. but the mother has a serious complication, are you liable?

FIGURE CREDITS

2.2   Redrawn from Dennon EH. Forceps deliveries. 2nd ed. Philadelphia: FA Davis, 1964:35.

2.7   Bassett LW, Gold RH. Introduction to mammography. In: Mitchell GW Jr, Bassett LW, eds. The female breast and its disorders: essentials of diagnosis and management. Baltimore: Williams & Wilkins, 1990:121–122.

2.8   Wentz AC. Infertility. In: Jones HW III, Wentz AC, Burnett LS, eds. Novak's textbook of gynecology. 11th ed. Baltimore: Williams & Wilkins, 1988:292.

2.9   Nichols DH, Randall CL. Vaginal surgery. 3rd ed. Baltimore: Williams & Wilkins, 1989:164.

2.11 Nichols DH, Randall CL. Vaginal surgery. 3rd ed. Baltimore: Williams & Wilkins, 1989:179.

2.12 Jones HW III. Cervical intraepithelial neoplasia. In: Jones HW III, Wentz AC, Burnett LS, eds. Novak's textbook of gynecology. 11th ed. Baltimore: Williams & Wilkins, 1988: 667.

3.1   Adapted from Moore KL. The developing human: clinically oriented embryology. 4th ed. Philadelphia: WB Saunders, 1988.

3.2   Adapted from Moore KL. The developing human: clinically oriented embryology. 4th ed. Philadelphia: WB Saunders, 1988.

3.3   Adapted from Moore KL. The developing human: clinically oriented embryology. 4th ed. Philadelphia: WB Saunders, 1988.

3.4   Burnett LS. Anatomy. In: Jones HW III, Wentz AC, Burnett LS, eds. Novak's textbook of gynecology. 11th ed. Baltimore: Williams & Wilkins, 1988:41.

3.6   Burnett LS. Anatomy. In: Jones HW III, Wentz AC, Burnett LS, eds. Novak's textbook of gynecology. 11th ed. Baltimore: Williams & Wilkins, 1988:57.

3.7   Garrey MM, Govan ADT, Hodge CH, Callander R. Gynae-
      cology illustrated. Baltimore: Williams & Wilkins, 1972:26.

3.8   Garrey MM, Govan ADT, Hodge CH, Callander R. Gynae-
      cology illustrated. Baltimore: Williams & Wilkins, 1972:29.

3.9   Garrey MM, Govan ADT, Hodge CH, Callander R. Gynae-
      cology illustrated. Baltimore: Williams & Wilkins, 1972:38.

5.1   Courtesy of American College of Obstetricians and Gynecol-
      ogists, Washington, D.C.

5.2   Courtesy of American College of Obstetricians and Gynecol-
      ogists, Washington, D.C.

7.1   Scott JR, DiSaia PJ, Hammond CB, Spellacy WN, eds. Dan-
      forth's obstetrics and gynecology. 6th ed. Philadelphia: JB
      Lippincott, 1990.

16.1 Adapted from Friedman E. Labor: clinical evaluation and
      management. 2nd ed. East Norwalk, CT: Appleton & Lange,
      1978.

18.3 Courtesy of the Division of Maternal-Fetal Medicine, De-
      partment of Obstetrics and Gynecology, University of Ten-
      nessee at Memphis.

18.4 Courtesy of the Division of Maternal-Fetal Medicine, De-
      partment of Obstetrics and Gynecology, University of Ten-
      nessee at Memphis.

21.3 Bassett LW. Mammographic features of malignancy. In:
      Mitchell GW Jr, Bassett LW, eds. The female breast and its
      disorders: essentials of diagnosis and management. Baltimore:
      Williams & Wilkins, 1990:143.

21.4 Bassett LW. Mammographic features of malignancy. In:
      Mitchell GW Jr, Bassett LW, eds. The female breast and its
      disorders: essentials of diagnosis and management. Baltimore:
      Williams & Wilkins, 1990:139.

30.1 Cartwright PS. Ectopic pregnancy. In: Jones HW III, Wentz
      AC, Burnett LS, eds. Novak's textbook of gynecology. 11th
      ed. Baltimore: Williams & Wilkins, 1988:479.

30.2 Wentz AC, Cartwright PS. Recurrent and spontaneous abor-
      tion. In: Jones HW III, Wentz AC, Burnett LS, eds. Novak's
      textbook of gynecology. 11th ed. Baltimore: Williams & Wil-
      kins, 1988:345.

30.3 Wentz AC, Cartwright PS. Recurrent and spontaneous abortion. In: Jones HW III, Wentz AC, Burnett LS, eds. Novak's textbook of gynecology. 11th ed. Baltimore: Williams & Wilkins, 1988:345.

30.4 Cartwright PS. Ectopic pregnancy. In: Jones HW III, Wentz AC, Burnett LS, eds. Novak's textbook of gynecology. 11th ed. Baltimore: Williams & Wilkins, 1988:489.

31.1 Nichols DH, Randall CL. Vaginal surgery. 3rd ed. Baltimore: Williams & Wilkins, 1989:85.

32.2 Wentz AC. Endometriosis. In: Jones HW III, Wentz AC, Burnett LS, eds. Novak's textbook of gynecology. 11th ed. Baltimore: Williams & Wilkins, 1990:309.

34.2 Speroff L, Glass RH, Kase NG. Clinical gynecologic endocrinology and infertility. 4th ed. Baltimore: Williams & Wilkins, 1989:93.

34.3 Speroff L, Glass RH, Kase NG. Clinical gynecologic endocrinology and infertility. 4th ed. Baltimore: Williams & Wilkins, 1989:94.

34.4 Marshall JC, Odell WD. The menstrual cycle—hormonal regulation, mechanisms of anovulation, and responses of the reproductive tract to steroid hormones. In: DeGroot LJ, ed. Endocrinology. 2nd ed. Philadelphia: WB Saunders, 1989: 1946.

46.1 Hobbins JC, Winsberg F, Berkowitz RL. Ultrasonography in obstetrics and gynecology. 2nd ed. Baltimore: Williams & Wilkins, 1983.

42.3 Jones HW III. Cervical intraepithelial neoplasia. In: Jones HW III, Wentz AC, Burnett LS, eds. Novak's textbook of gynecology. 11th ed. Baltimore: Williams & Wilkins, 1988: 667.

43.2 Entman SS. Uterine leiomyoma and adenomyosis. In: Jones HW III, Wentz AC, Burnett LS, eds. Novak's textbook of gynecology. 11th ed. Baltimore: Williams & Wilkins, 1988: 444.

TABLE CREDITS

15.1 Modified from Friedman EA. Labor: clinical evaluation and management. 2nd ed. East Norwalk, CT: Appleton & Lange, 1978.

19.1 Herbert WNP, Cefalo RC. Management of postpartum hemorrhage. Clin Obstet Gynecol 1984;27:139–147.

19.2 Herbert WNP, Cefalo RC. Management of postpartum hemorrhage. Clin Obstet Gynecol 1984;27:139–147.

19.3 Herbert WNP, Cefalo RC. Management of postpartum hemorrhage. Clin Obstet Gynecol 1984;27:139–147.

28.1 Courtesy of American College of Obstetricians and Gynecologists and Centers for Disease Control.

32.1 American Fertility Society. Revised American Fertility Society Classification of Endometriosis 1985. Fertil Steril 1985;43: 351.

41.3 International Federation of Gynecology and Obstetrics. Annual report on the results of treatment in gynecologic cancer. Int J Gynecol Obstet 1989;28:189–190.

APGO OBJECTIVES INDEX

This index is different from the usual Subject Index. It is designed to help the reader study a topic designated in one of the APGO objectives.

The objectives are listed on the left. On the right are the pages in the book where there are major discussions of the topic.

INDEX

Page numbers in italics denote figures; those followed by "t" denote tables.

447